# The Biology of Cancer

# The Biology of Cancer

Editor: Kimberly Craig

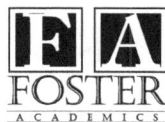

**FOSTER ACADEMICS**

www.fosteracademics.com

www.fosteracademics.com

**FA**
FOSTER
ACADEMICS

**Cataloging-in-Publication Data**

The biology of cancer / edited by Kimberly Craig.
    p. cm.
Includes bibliographical references and index.
ISBN 978-1-63242-881-3
1. Cancer. 2. Cancer--Molecular aspects. 3. Cancer--Genetic aspects. 4. Cancer cells.
5. Tumors--Genetics. I. Craig, Kimberly.
RC261 .B56 2020
616.994--dc23

Foster Academics,
118-35 Queens Blvd., Suite 400,
Forest Hills, NY 11375, USA

ISBN 978-1-63242-881-3 (Hardback)

# Contents

# Preface

This book aims to highlight the current researches and provides a platform to further the scope of innovations in this area. This book is a product of the combined efforts of many researchers and scientists, after going through thorough studies and analysis from different parts of the world. The objective of this book is to provide the readers with the latest information of the field.

Cancer can be thought as a complex adaptive system with emerging properties at different biological scales. The study of the disease using this approach requires an integration of systems biology to cancer research. Tumors are characterized by the presence of genomic and epigenetic anomalies, which alter the functions and interactions of different molecules and networks relative to the local environment. Cancer systems biology thus offers a holistic study of cancer by taking into account its genetics, clinical or preclinical manifestation, signaling networks, cellular behavior, histology and epidemiology. Such a study can be aided using high-throughput technologies that enable genomic analyses of mutations, methylation, copy number variations and rearrangements both at cellular and tissue levels. These also facilitate robust analyses of RNA and microRNA expression data, and protein and metabolite levels. Cancer systems biology is an upcoming field of science that has undergone rapid development over the past few decades. It presents researches and studies performed by experts across the globe on the biology of cancer. As this field is emerging at a rapid pace, the contents of this book will help the readers understand the modern concepts and applications of the subject.

I would like to express my sincere thanks to the authors for their dedicated efforts in the completion of this book. I acknowledge the efforts of the publisher for providing constant support. Lastly, I would like to thank my family for their support in all academic endeavors.

**Editor**

# Key elements involved in Epstein–Barr virus-associated gastric cancer and their network regulation

Jing-jing Jing, Ze-yang Wang, Hao Li, Li-ping Sun and Yuan Yuan*

## Abstract

**Background:** The molecular mechanism of Epstein–Barr virus (EBV)-associated gastric cancer (EBVaGC) remains elusive. A collection of molecular regulators including transcription factor and noncoding RNA (ncRNAs) may affect the carcinogenesis of EBVaGC by regulating the expression and function of key genes. In this study, integration of multi-level expression data and bioinformatics approach was used to identify key elements and their interactions involved in mechanism of EBVaGC and their network regulation.

**Methods:** Data of the gene expression profiling data sets (GSE51575) was downloaded from GEO database. Differentially expressed genes between EBVaGC and normal samples were identified by GEO2R. Gene ontology and pathway enrichment analyses were performed using R packages Cluster profiler. STRING database was used to find interacting proteins between different genes. Transcription factors in differentially expressed genes were obtained from TF Checkpoint database. Using Cytoscape, we built transcription factor regulation network. miRNAs involved in the gene-interacting proteins and the miRNA-targeted lncRNA were predicted through miRWalk. Using ViRBase, EBV related miRNA regulation network was built. Overlapping genes and regulators of the above three networks were further identified, and the cross network was constructed using Cytoscape software. Moreover, the differential expressions of the target genes and transcription factors in the cross network were explored in different molecular subtypes of GC using cBioPortal. By histological verification, the expression of two main target genes in the cross network were further analyzed.

**Results:** A total of 104 genes showed differential expressions between EBVaGC and normal tissues, which were associated with digestion, G-protein coupled receptor binding, gastric acid secretion, etc. Pathway analysis showed that the differentially expressed genes were mainly enriched in gastric acid secretion and protein digestion and absorption. Using STRING dataset, a total of 54 proteins interacted with each other. Based on the transcription factor network, the hub transcription factors IRX3, NKX6-2, PTGER3 and SMAD5 were identified to regulate their target genes SST and GDF5, etc. After screening and matching in miRwalk datasets, a ceRNA network was established, in which the top five miRNAs were hsa-miR-4446-3p, hsa-miR-5787, hsa-miR-1915-3p, hsa-miR-335-3p and hsa-miR-6877-3p, and the top two lncRNAs were RP5-1039K5.19 and TP73-AS1. According to the EBV related miRNA regulation network, CXCL10 and SMAD5 were found to be regulated by EBV-miR-BART1-3p and EBV-mir-BART22, respectively. By overlapping the three networks, CXCL10, GDF5, PTGER3, SMAD5, miR-6877-3p, RP5-1039K5.19, TP73-AS1, EBV-miR-BART1-3p and EBV-mir-BART22 were found to be key elements of regulation mechanism of EBVaGC. CXCL10, GDF5, PTGER3 and SMAD5 were also differentially expressed among the four molecular subtypes of GC. The histological verification

*Correspondence: yuanyuan@cmu.edu.cn
Tumor Etiology and Screening Department of Cancer Institute
and General Surgery, The First Hospital of China Medical University, Key
Laboratory of Cancer Etiology and Prevention (China Medical University),
Liaoning Provincial Education Department, Shenyang, Liaoning, China

experiment showed differential expressions of the two main target genes GDF5 and CXCL10 between EBVaGC and non-tumor tissues as well as EBVnGC.

**Conclusion:** In the current study, our results revealed key elements and their interactions involved in EBVaGC. Some hub transcription factors, miRNAs, lncRNAs and EBV related miRNAs were observed to regulate their target genes. Overlapping genes and regulators were observed in diverse regulation networks, such as CXCL10, GDF5, PTGER3, SMAD5, miR-6877-3p, RP5-1039K5.19, TP73-AS1, EBV-miR-BART1-3p and EBV-mir-BART22. Moreover, CXCL10, GDF5, PTGER3 and SMAD5 were also differentially expressed among the four molecular subtypes of GC. The histological verification experiment showed differential expressions of the two main target genes GDF5 and CXCL10 between EBVaGC and non-tumor tissues as well as EBVnGC. Therefore, the identified key elements and their network regulation may be specifically involved in EBVaGC mechanisms.

**Keywords:** Transcription factor, Noncoding RNA, Gene regulatory network, Bioinformatics, EBV-associated gastric cancer

## Background

Gastric cancer (GC) is the fourth most common cancer in the world, ranking second in the causes of cancer death [1]. It is a complex disease with great heterogeneity that can be divided into four molecular groups based on genomic characteristics and clinical features, including chromosomal instability (CIN), genomically stable (GS), microsatellite instability (MSI) and EBV-associated GC (EBVaGC) [2]. EBV is detected in GC cells rather than in noncancerous gastric mucosa, and shows a clonal nature in neoplastic cells. It is therefore considered to have a causal role in GC [3, 4]. Molecular characterization of EBVaGC has been described recently [2]. However, the pathogenic mechanism of EBVaGC remains elusive.

Gene misregulation plays a critical role in tumorigenesis and progression [5]. Regulation of gene expression includes a great variety of mechanisms that increase or decrease the specific gene products. Gene regulatory network is a collection of molecular regulators that interact with each other to govern the gene expression and function, which has been getting increasing attention for facilitation of gaining insight into the transcriptional and epigenetic regulation patterns in cancers [6, 7]. At the transcriptional level, transcription factors (TFs) are the main regulators. They can bind to the DNA regions of enhancer or promoter adjacent to the target genes that they regulate [8, 9]. Noncoding RNAs (ncRNAs) have been shown to regulate gene expression serving as an important type of epigenetic regulation mechanism [10, 11]. Two of the main types of ncRNAs, which are microRNAs (miRNAs) and long ncRNAs (lncRNAs), can suppress each other as competing endogenous RNAs (ceRNAs) and form a regulatory ceRNA network (lncRNAs–miRNAs–mRNAs) to regulate target mRNAs [12]. In addition, not only mammals but also viruses encode miRNAs. EBV was the first virus in which viral miRNAs were found. Recently, it has been commonly accepted

that EBV also encodes for plenty of miRNAs, such as BART cluster and BHRF cluster [13, 14]. These miRNAs were observed to promote viral latency or cancer development by targeting both viral and cellular genes [15–17].

Given the importance of TFs and ncRNAs, it is of great interest to construct gene regulatory networks based on TFs and ncRNAs for exploring the biological processes of EBVaGC. With the increasing availability of multi-level expression data from cancer and normal tissues, new opportunities for the extraction and integration of large data sets such as gene expression omnibus (GEO) may help to provide a more comprehensive understanding of cancer [18, 19]. In this study, we integrated expression data to identify differentially expressed mRNAs and the corresponding TFs, miRNAs, and lncRNAs involved in EBVaGC. Regulatory networks including TF–mRNA, lncRNA–miRNA–mRNA, EBV encoded miRNA–mRNA and their overlap were analyzed, which possibly provide a new avenue for investigating the regulation mechanisms of EBVaGC.

## Materials and methods

### Microarray data

GSE51575 is an mRNA profiling for EBVaGC. By downloading the GSE51575 microarray data, the adjacent normal tissues from 26 gastric cancer patients were used as control to be compared with 12 EBVaGC tissues.

### Data processing

As an interactive online tool, GEO2R (http://www.ncbi.nlm.nih.gov/geo/geo2r/) can be used to compare two or more sets of samples to determine differentially expressed genes in the GEO series [20]. In order to ensure the accuracy of the results, we used GEO2R to filter differentially expressed genes between EBVaGC and normal samples separately in each of the data sets. $FDR < 0.05$ and $|logFC| > 4$ were considered statistically significant. Duplicate gene probes and unspecific probes will be removed.

### Gene ontology and Kyoto encyclopedia of genes and genomes (KEGG) pathway enrichment analyses
Gene ontology analysis (GO) is a major bioinformatics tool to unify the representation of genes and gene products [21]. It contains three categories of terms including cellular component, molecular function, and biological process. KEGG is a set of databases containing information about genomes, biological pathways, diseases and chemicals [22]. GO and KEGG pathway enrichment analyses were performed using R packages Cluster profiler. $P < 0.05$ was considered statistically significant.

### Construction of transcription factor regulation network
STRING database was used to find interacting proteins between different genes [23]. Cytoscape software was used to screen for the hub protein. TF Checkpoint database was used to find the TFs in differentially expressed genes. The TFs in the PPI network were considered as the hub TFs. Using Cytoscape [24], we built transcription factor regulation network.

### Construction of ceRNA regulatory network
miRWalk is a database that can predict miRNA target genes [25]. We conducted a systematic analysis on the interaction between significantly modulated miRNAs and mRNAs considering an inverse expression correlation using MiRwalk. We ordered miRNAs on the basis of the connection numbers of target genes to select the top five miRNAs as hub miRNA. We then predicted the miRNA–targeted lncRNA in similar ways through miRWalk. The top 2 lncRNAs were selected as the hub lncRNA. Cytoscape software was used to construct ceRNA interaction network. These selected hub miRNAs and lncRNAs indicated that they can regulate more differentially expressed genes.

### Construction of EBV related miRNA regulation network
ViRBase (http://www.rna-society.org/virbase) is an online tool that can predict virus-host ncRNA-associated interactions [26]. Using ViRBase, we predicted the EBV related miRNA. Then we built the EBV related miRNA regulation network by Cytoscape.

### Construction of cross network
Overlapping genes and regulators of the above three networks were further identified, and the cross network was constructed using Cytoscape software.

### Exploring differential expressions of the target genes and transcription factors in the cross network in different molecular subtypes of GC using cBioPortal
Using cBioPortal (http://cbioportal.org), a web resource for exploring, visualizing, and analyzing multidimensional cancer genomics data [27], we analyzed the mRNA expressions of the target genes and TFs in the cross network in four different subtypes of GC (EBVaGC, GS–GC, MSI–GC, CIN–GC). $P < 0.05$ was considered to be statistical significant.

### Verification experiment of the target genes in the cross network using human tissues
Further, using 10 pairs of tumor tissues (5 EBVaGC and 5 EBVnGC) and adjacent non-tumor tissues, we detected the mRNA expression of two main target genes GDF5 and CXCL10 (approved by the Human Ethics Review Committee of the First Hospital of China Medical University). EBV was identified by the expression of EBV-encoded small RNA (EBER). In situ hybridization (ISH) with a complementary digoxigenin-labeled oligomer was used to detect the EBER according to the manufacturer's instructions (EBER Detection Kit, ZSGB-BIO). The hybridization signal was detected by diaminobenzidine (DAB) and positive nuclear signal was recognized as dark brown nuclear staining under light microscopy (Fig. 1). Sections from a patient with known EBER-positive GC were used for a positive control. Quantitative real-time PCR was used to detect the mRNA expression. The primers were listed in Additional file 1: Table S1. $P < 0.05$ was considered to indicate significant differences.

## Results
### Identification of differentially expressed genes in EBVaGC
According to differential expression analysis, a total of 216 gene probes showed differences, among which 199 genes were low expressed in EBVaGC and 17 genes were highly expressed in EBVaGC (Fig. 2). After removing the duplicate gene probes and unspecific probes, 100 low expressed genes and 4 highly expressed genes were remained. The identified differentially expressed genes were listed in Additional file 1: Table S2.

### GO and KEGG pathway functional enrichment analyses
As shown in Fig. 3, differentially expressed genes were mainly associated with digestion, G-protein coupled receptor binding, gastric acid secretion and so on. Differential genes were mainly located in cytoplasmic vesicle lumen. By KEGG enrichment analysis, the differential genes were mainly associated with the gastric acid secretion and protein digestion and absorption (Table 1).

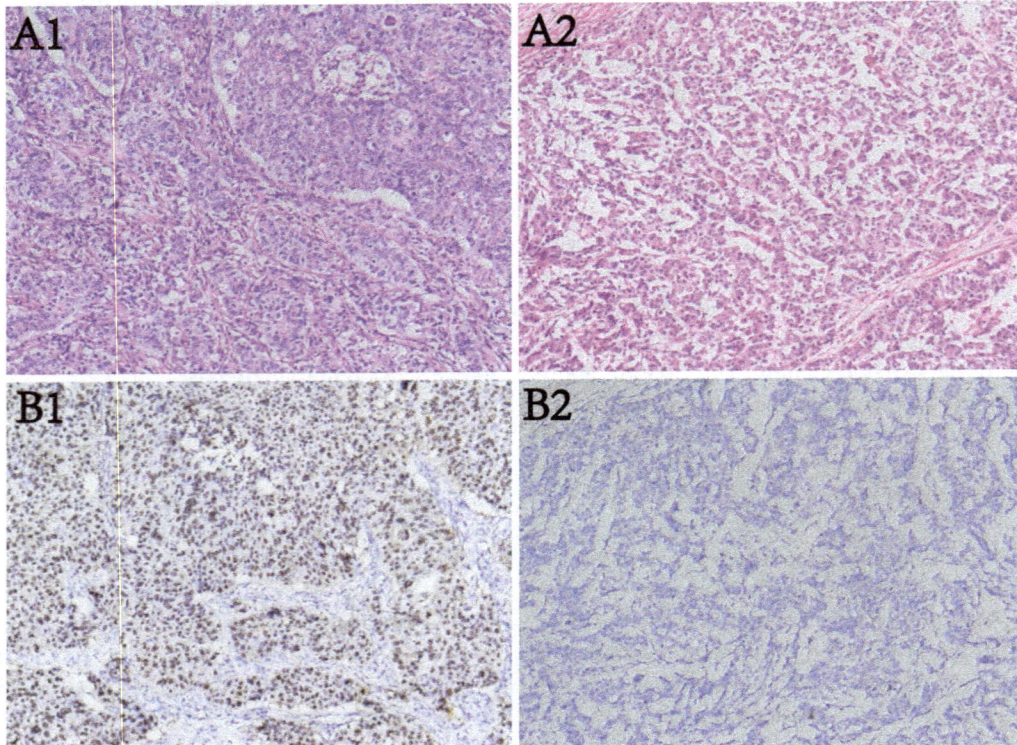

**Fig. 1** Detection of Epstein–Barr virus encoded small RNAs (EBERs) by in situ hybridization in gastric cancer tissues. A1&A2: H&E staining of EBVaGC and EBVnGC. B1&B2: EBER positive and negative staining in the nuclei of tumor cells (original magnification × 100)

### Transcription factor regulation network

We then built the transcription factor regulation network based on differential expressed 104 genes. Using STRING dataset, a total of 54 proteins interacted with each other. Using CytoScape, the hub transcription factors were IRX3, NKX6-2, PTGER3, and SMAD5, targeting SST and GDF5 separately. As shown in Fig. 4, orange circles indicate common genes, blue dots indicate transcription factors, and size increases with degree. Compared with normal tissues, the expression levels of the four hub transcription factors IRX3, NKX6-2, PTGER3, and SMAD5 were down-regulated, with the logFC value of $-4.39$, $-5.83$, $-4.18$ and $-4.64$, separately.

### ceRNA regulation network

After screening and matching in miRwalk datasets, an integrated lncRNA–miRNA–mRNA network was established. The top five miRNAs were hsa-miR-4446-3p, hsa-miR-5787, hsa-miR-1915-3p, hsa-miR-335-3p and hsa-miR-6877-3p. A total of 47 genes were regulated by hub miRNAs. The top two lncRNAs were RP5-1039K5.19 and TP73-AS1 (Fig. 5).

### EBV related miRNA regulation network

Using ViRBase, we predicted the EBV related miRNA regulation network. After screening and matching, we found CXCL10 and SMAD5 were regulated by EBV related miRNA in the difference expression genes. CXCL10 was regulated by ebv-miR-BART1-3p, while SMAD5 was regulated by ebv-mir-BART22 (Fig. 6).

### Cross network

Overlapping genes and regulators were observed in the cross network, including CXCL10, GDF5, PTGER3, SMAD5, miR-6877-3p, RP5-1039K5.19, TP73-AS1, EBV-miR-BART1-3p and EBV-mir-BART22 (Fig. 7). As for the two main target genes, compared with normal tissues, the expression of GDF5 was down-regulated while the CXCL10 was up-regulated significantly, with the logFC value of $-4.77$ and $4.97$, separately.

### Differential expressions of the target genes and transcription factors in the cross network in different molecular subtypes of GC

According to the mRNA expression data of different types of GC from cBioPortal, significant differences

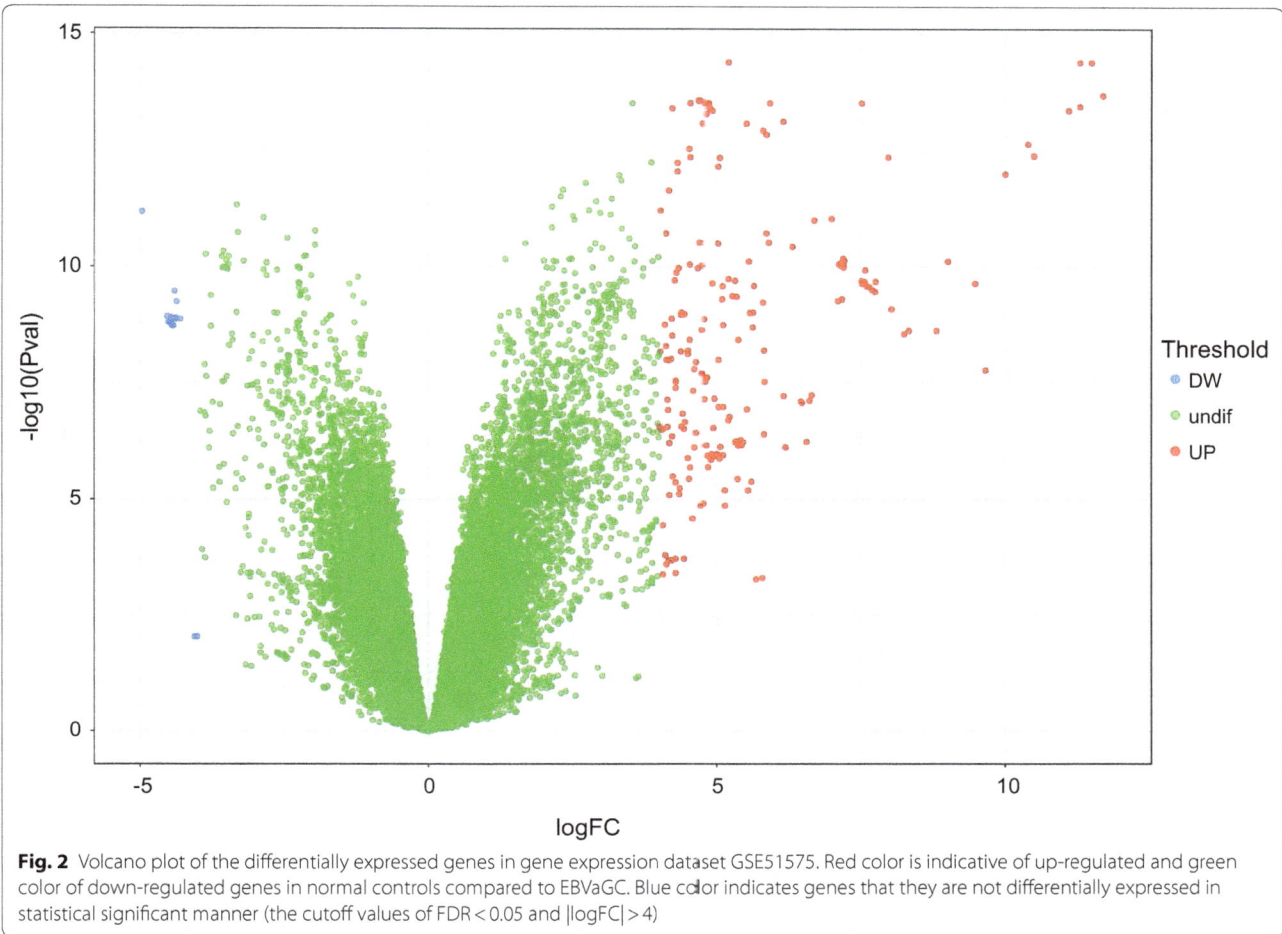

**Fig. 2** Volcano plot of the differentially expressed genes in gene expression dataset GSE51575. Red color is indicative of up-regulated and green color of down-regulated genes in normal controls compared to EBVaGC. Blue color indicates genes that they are not differentially expressed in statistical significant manner (the cutoff values of FDR < 0.05 and |logFC| > 4)

were observed between EBVaGC and EBVnGC for GDF5, CXCL10, SMAD5 and PTGER3 (P < 0.001, P < 0.001, P = 0.002 and P < 0.001). As for the four sub-types of GC, CXCL10 expression was significantly up-regulated in EBVaGC than in GS-GC, MSI-GC and CIN-GC (all P < 0.001). The expression levels of GDF5, SMAD5 and PTGER3 in EBVaGC were the lowest in the four subtypes (all P < 0.001). The significant differences were observed between EBVaGC and GS-GC for GDF5 (P < 0.001), and between EBVaGC and GS-GC/CIN-GC for SMAD5 (P < 0.001/P = 0.003) and PTGER3 (P < 0.001/P = 0.021) (Table 2).

### Verification of the target genes expression in the cross network

The results from human tissue verification of the two target genes showed that the gene expression level was lower in EBVaGC compared with that in non-tumor tissues for GDF5 (P = 0.043), and marginal difference was also observed between EBVaGC and EBVnGC (P = 0.076). As for CXCL10, its expression was higher

in EBVaGC than that in control group with a borderline significance (P = 0.080). There is significant difference between EBVaGC and EBVnGC for CXCL10 (P = 0.047) (Table 3).

### Discussion

The genetic and epigenetic regulation mechanisms can be clarified by examining mRNAs, TFs, miRNAs, lncRNAs and their networks. Our study conducted integrated analysis of gene regulatory networks based on TFs, miRNAs and lncRNAs targeting differentially expressed genes, and revealed key elements and their interactions associated with molecular mechanisms of EBVaGC.

Firstly, a total of 104 differentially expressed genes between EBvaGC and normal controls were identified from GEO databases using the GEO2R program in the present research. The functional analysis showed that these genes were mainly associated with digestion, G-protein coupled receptor binding, gastric acid secretion, etc. KEGG enrichment analysis also illustrated that

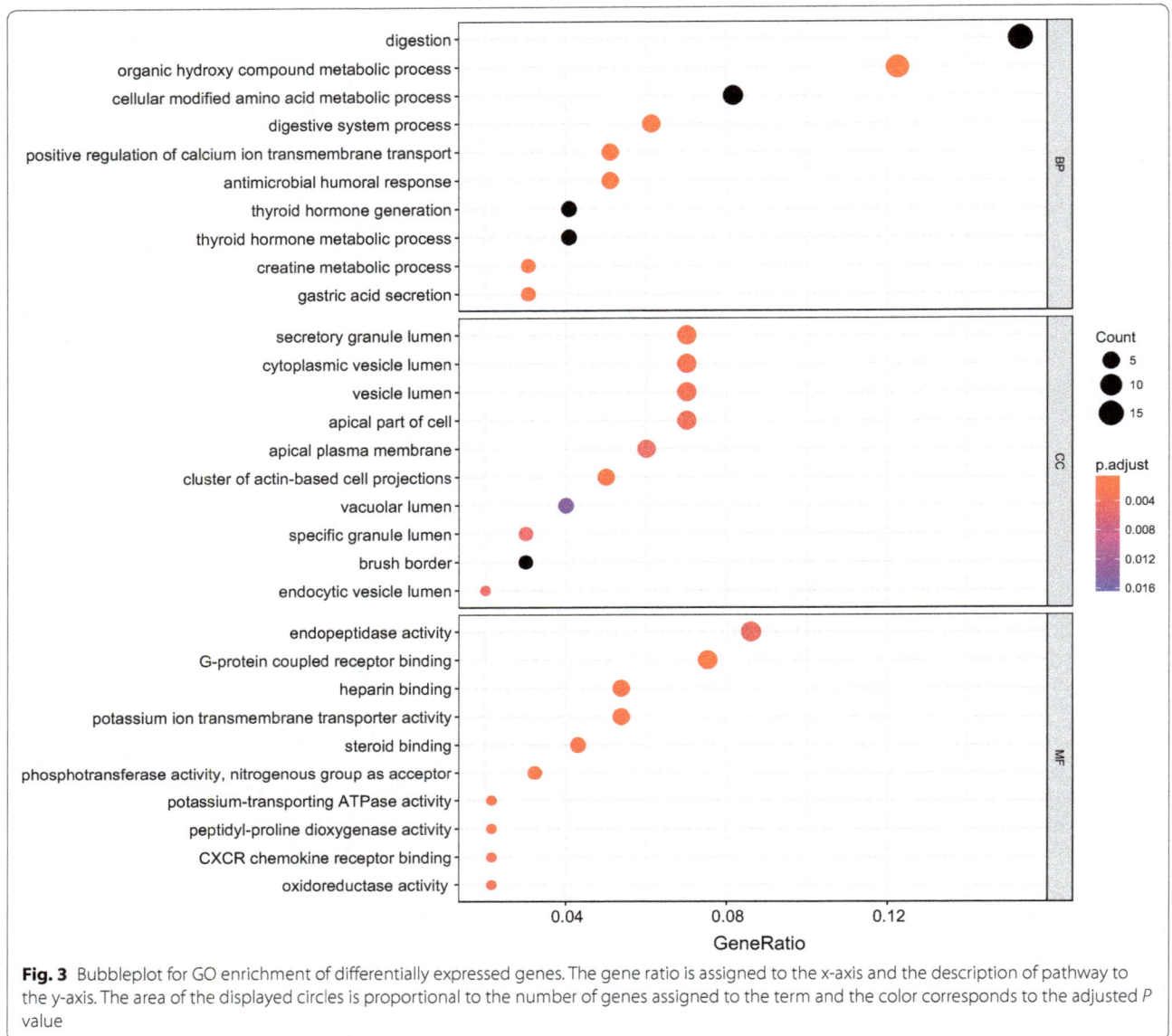

**Fig. 3** Bubbleplot for GO enrichment of differentially expressed genes. The gene ratio is assigned to the x-axis and the description of pathway to the y-axis. The area of the displayed circles is proportional to the number of genes assigned to the term and the color corresponds to the adjusted *P* value

**Table 1  KEGG enrichment analysis for the differential expressed genes**

| ID | Description | Gene ratio | Bg ratio | P value | P adjust | q value | Gene ID | Count |
|----|-------------|------------|----------|---------|----------|---------|---------|-------|
| hsa04971 | Gastric acid secretion | 6/54 | 75/7383 | 1.58E−05 | 0.0012128 | 0.0010942 | 495/496/6750/3773/9992/887 | 6 |
| hsa04974 | Protein digestion and absorption | 6/54 | 90/7383 | 4.48E−05 | 0.0017241 | 0.0015556 | 643834/1280/1358/6564/10136/23436 | 6 |

the differential genes were mainly involved in the gastric acid secretion and protein digestion and absorption. Acid secretion exerts the greatest impact of all gastric functions on the occurrence of stomach disorders [28]. Our findings highlighted the probable importance of the

regulation of these key genes and vital biological behaviors in EBVaGC, which warranted further investigations.

Furthermore, a set of gene regulatory networks were constructed by targeting these differentially expressed genes. At transcriptional level, studies have revealed that gene misregulation is often due to the aberrant expression

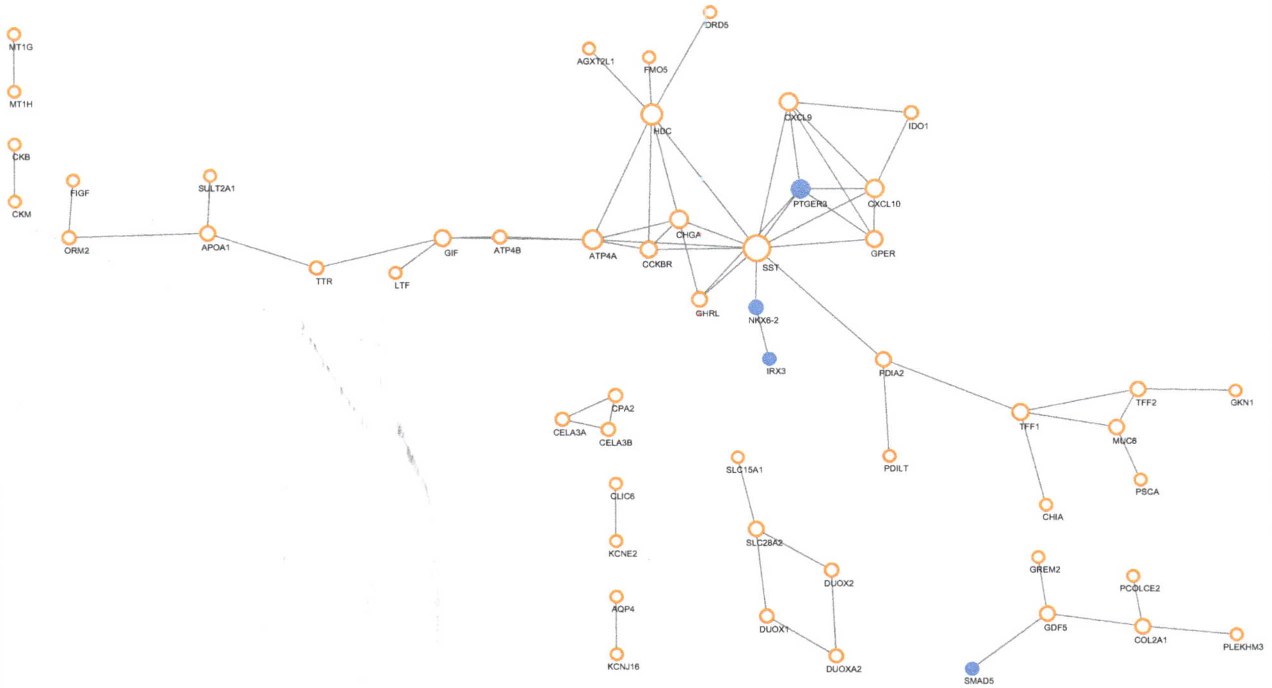

**Fig. 4** Transcription factor regulatory network (orange circles indicate common genes, blue dots indicate transcription factors, and size increases with degree)

of TFs. Based on the TF network, we identified some hub TFs associated with EBVaGC, including IRX3, NKX6-2, PTGER3 and SMAD5. Iroquois homeobox 3 (IRX3) plays vital roles in embryonic development, it has recently been reported to participate in tumor progression. Choi et al. [29] found that NKX6 participated in differentiation of gastrin-producing G cells in the stomach antrum. Prostaglandin E-receptor was observed to induce growth inhibition in gastric cancer cells [30]. Nagasako et al. [31] reported that up-regulated SMAD5 mediated apoptosis of gastric epithelial cells induced by Helicobacter pylori infection. These TFs may individually or comprehensively participate in EBVaGC pathogenesis by regulating their target genes, such as SST (Somatostatin) and GDF5 (growth differentiation factor 5). SST is important for regulating motor activity and the secretion of gastrin-stimulated gastric acid in the gastrointestinal tract [32], and GDF5 serves as a regulator of cell growth and differentiation in both embryonic and adult tissues. Their aberrant expressions were reported to be associated with varieties of cancers [33–36].

Noncoding RNAs (ncRNAs) are also important part of the regulatory network involved in post-transcriptional regulation of genes. By building ceRNA network, our results also revealed several novel miRNAs and lncRNAs that were possibly involved in gene regulation

associated with EBVaGC. The top five miRNAs were hsa-miR-4446-3p, hsa-miR-5787, hsa-miR-1915-3p, hsa-miR-335-3p and hsa-miR-6877-3p. Kim et al. [37] observed that miR-4446-3p was upregulated by compression in breast cancer cells. Aberrantly expression of miR-5787 was supposed significantly down-regulated in serum and might be involved in the process of glucose metabolism in colorectal cancer [38]. miR-1915 inhibits Bcl-2 to modulate multidrug resistance by increasing drug-sensitivity of human colorectal cancer cells [39]. Overexpression of miR-335 significantly inhibited cell proliferation, migration and invasion in GC cells [40]. Little is known about miR-6877-3p, the only research reported that its expression was associated with ovary development in cyprinus carpio [41]. In addition, two unreported lncRNAs, RP5-1039K5.19 and TP73-AS1 were identified in the ceRNA regulation network, which may become the candidate targets for in-depth study of EBVaGC.

Additionally, miRNAs are not solely produced by metazoans, but also by viruses, which opened a new window for the research. Up to date, 44 mature EBV coding miRNAs have been identified, many of which have been proven to promote carcinogenesis by targeting host genes [13]. In our study, we built an EBV related miRNA regulation network and found that CXCL10 and SMAD5 were regulated by EBV-miR-BART1-3p and

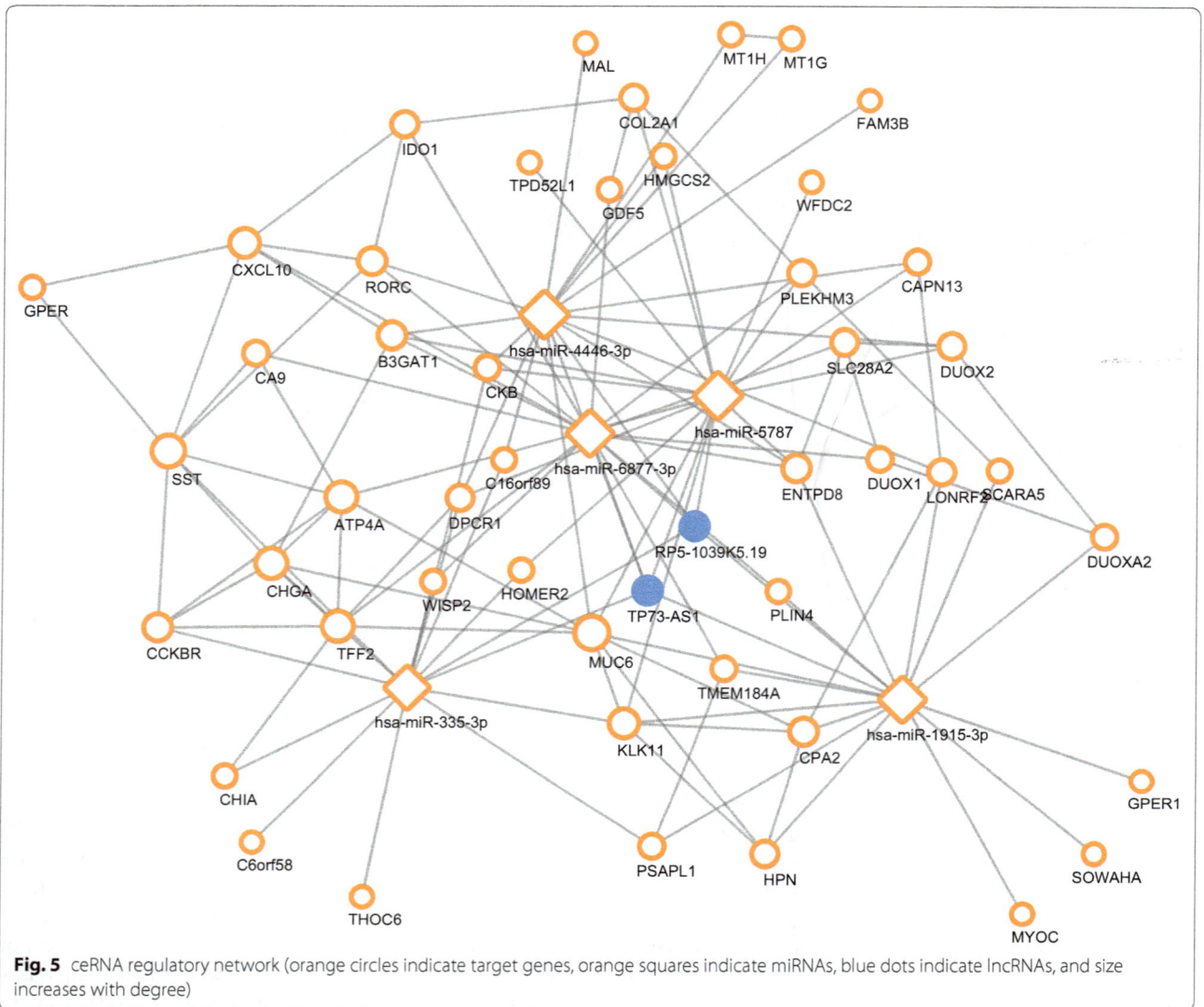

**Fig. 5** ceRNA regulatory network (orange circles indicate target genes, orange squares indicate miRNAs, blue dots indicate lncRNAs, and size increases with degree)

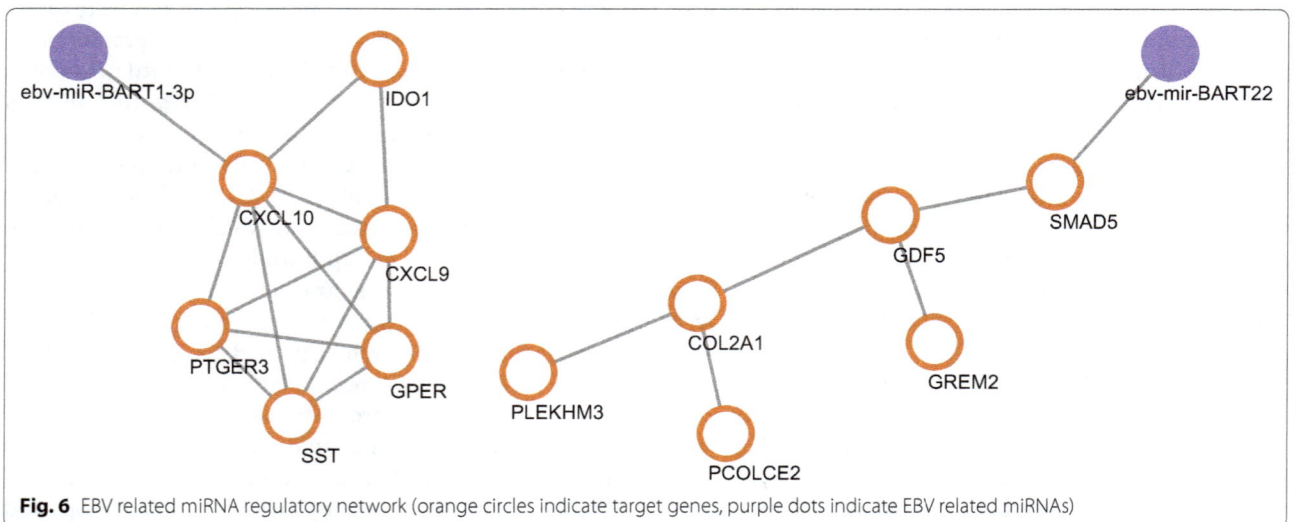

**Fig. 6** EBV related miRNA regulatory network (orange circles indicate target genes, purple dots indicate EBV related miRNAs)

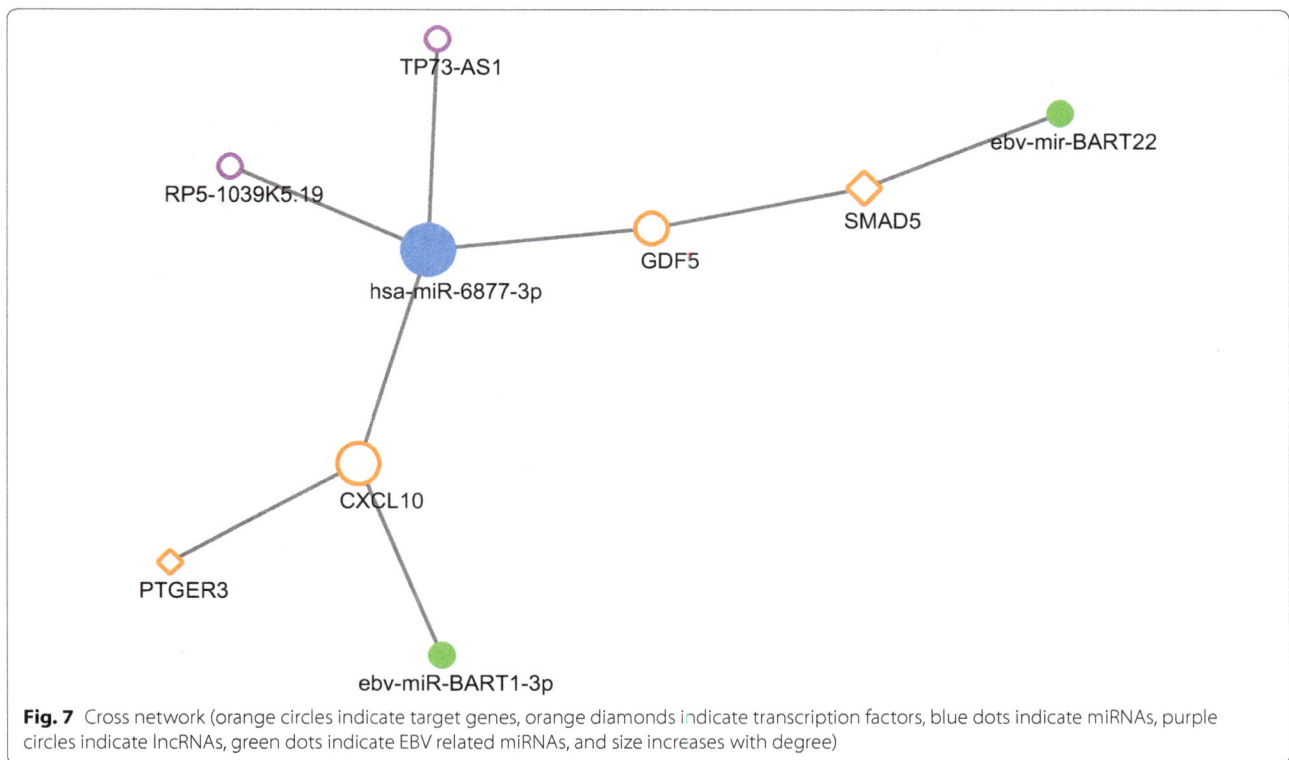

**Fig. 7** Cross network (orange circles indicate target genes, orange diamonds indicate transcription factors, blue dots indicate miRNAs, purple circles indicate lncRNAs, green dots indicate EBV related miRNAs, and size increases with degree)

EBV-mir-BART22. EBV-miR-BART1 was observed to be involved in regulating metabolism-associated genes [42] and induced tumor metastasis [43] in nasopharyngeal carcinoma. Zhou et al. [44] found that CXCL10/CXCR3 axis can promote the invasion of GC via PI3 K/AKT pathway-dependent MMPs production. As for EBV-mir-BART22, it is a brand new miRNA without prior study. Interestingly, its target gene SMAD5 was also identified as a hub TF associated with EBVaGC in our study.

Intriguingly, when taking an overview on the various regulation networks in the current study, some overlapping genes and regulators were observed in the cross network. Firstly, CXCL10 was the common target gene in the three diverse regulation networks. It could be regulated by the transcription factor PTGER3, miR-6877-3p and EBV-miR-BART1-3p at the same time. Secondly, GDF5 was the target gene of transcription factor SMAD5 and miR-6877-3p. Moreover, SMAD5 was simultaneously regulated by EBV-mir-BART22. In addition, both CXCL10 and GDF5 were in the same ceRNA network that they can be regulated by miR-6877-3p and the two unreported lncRNAs, RP5-1039K5.19 and TP73-AS1. Furthermore, the expression levels of GDF5, CXCL10, SMAD5 and PTGER3 were also different between EBVaGC and EBVnGC. There were also differences between EBVaGC and other molecular subtypes of GC

for these genes. In addition, in the histological verification experiment, differential expressions of the two main target genes GDF5 and CXCL10 were observed between EBVaGC and non-tumor tissues as well as EBVnGC. These results indicate that GDF5 and CXCL10 and their misregulation may play important roles specifically in EBVaGC related mechanisms. CXCL10 is a strong angiostatic factors, and it may be involved in the recruitment of tumour-infiltrating T cells [45]. It has been reported that TGF-β produced by breast cancer cells induces the GDF5 expression in the endothelial cells, which in its turn stimulates the angiogenesis both in vivo and in vitro [46]. Dysregulation of these two genes may lead to the activation of pathways related to cancer hallmarks like angiogenesis and tumour-promoting inflammation to promote EBVaGC, which needs further investigated. These identified key elements and their network regulation may offer new perspectives on mechanisms of EBVaGC.

## Conclusion

In summary, in current study, we provided a framework for revealing the key elements and their regulatory network involved in EBVaGC. Some hub TFs associated with EBVaGC, including IRX3, NKX6-2, PTGER3 and SMAD5 were found to regulate their target genes.

**Table 2 The mRNA expressions of target genes and TFs in the cross network in different molecular subtypes of GC by cBioPortal database**

| Gene | Tpye of GC | Sample number | mRNA expression | |
|------|-----------|---------------|------------------|---------|
| | | | Mean ± SD | P value |
| GDF5 | EBVaGC | 29 | 2.11 ± 2.52 | Ref |
| | EBVnGC | 311 | 5.16 ± 9.55 | <0.001 |
| | | | | <0.001* |
| | EBVaGC | 29 | 2.11 ± 2.52 | Ref |
| | GS-GC | 47 | 10.46 ± 12.75 | <0.001 |
| | MSI-GC | 62 | 2.12 ± 2.68 | 0.995 |
| | CIN-GC | 202 | 4.85 ± 9.57 | 0.120 |
| CXCL10 | EBVaGC | 30 | 6061.34 ± 6.56 | Ref |
| | EBVnGC | 346 | 759.53 ± 1.21 | <0.001 |
| | | | | <0.001* |
| | EBVaGC | 30 | 6061.34 ± 6.56 | Ref |
| | GS-GC | 50 | 352.97 ± 412.44 | <0.001 |
| | MSI-GC | 73 | 1523.12 ± 2.11 | <0.001 |
| | CIN-GC | 223 | 600.72 ± 743.04 | <0.001 |
| SMAD5 | EBVaGC | 30 | 1165.21 ± 557.37 | Ref |
| | EBVnGC | 346 | 1446.01 ± 459.22 | 0.002 |
| | | | | <0.001* |
| | EBVaGC | 30 | 1165.21 ± 557.37 | Ref |
| | GS-GC | 50 | 1638.22 ± 483.08 | <0.001 |
| | MSI-GC | 73 | 1355.35 ± 330.26 | 0.058 |
| | CIN-GC | 223 | 1432.59 ± 479.20 | 0.003 |
| PTGER3 | EBVaGC | 30 | 78.20 ± 91.63 | Ref |
| | EBVnGC | 346 | 191.35 ± 235.51 | <0.001 |
| | | | | <0.001* |
| | EBVaGC | 30 | 78.20 ± 91.63 | Ref |
| | GS-GC | 50 | 405.75 ± 309.97 | <0.001 |
| | MSI-GC | 73 | 101.47 ± 108.61 | 0.610 |
| | CIN-GC | 223 | 172.69 ± 218.64 | 0.021 |

* P value for overall comparison among four subgroups

**Table 3 Histological verification of the mRNA expressions of GDF5 and CXCL10**

| Gene | Group | mRNA expression | |
|------|-------|------------------|---------|
| | | Mean ± SD | P value |
| GDF5 | EBVaGC vs CON | 0.025 ± 0.038 vs 0.254 ± 0.418 | *0.043* |
| | EBVnGC vs CON | 0.096 ± 0.096 vs 0.118 ± 0.199 | 0.893 |
| | EBVaGC vs EBVnGC | 0.025 ± 0.038 vs 0.096 ± 0.096 | 0.076 |
| CXCL10 | EBVaGC vs CON | 0.867 ± 1.440 vs 0.205 ± 0.281 | 0.080 |
| | EBVnGC vs CON | 0.206 ± 0.138 vs 0.154 ± 0.164 | 0.686 |
| | EBVaGC vs EBVnGC | 0.867 ± 1.440 vs 0.206 ± 0.138 | *0.047* |

CON adjacent non-tumor tissue

We also identified five miRNAs hsa-miR-4446-3p, hsa-miR-5787, hsa-miR-1915-3p, hsa-miR-335-3p, hsa-miR-6877-3p and two unreported lncRNAs, RP5-1039K5.19 and TP73-AS1 in the ceRNA regulation network. EBV related miRNAs EBV-miR-BART1-3p and EBV-mir-BART22 were observed to regulate CXCL10 and SMAD5. Further, some overlapping genes and regulators were observed in the three diverse regulation networks, such as CXCL10, GDF5, PTGER3, SMAD5, miR-6877-3p, RP5-1039K5.19, TP73-AS1, EBV-miR-BART1-3p and EBV-mir-BART22. Moreover, CXCL10, GDF5, PTGER3 and SMAD5 were also differentially expressed among the four molecular subtypes of GC. The histological verification experiment showed differential expressions of the two main target genes GDF5 and CXCL10 between EBVaGC and non-tumor tissues as well as EBVnGC. Therefore, the misregulation of target genes GDF5 and CXCL10 may be specifically involved in EBVaGC mechanisms. This study provides a new insight into understanding the mechanism based on gene regulation of EBVaGC, and further molecular experiments are needed to confirm the findings.

**Authors' contributions**
JJ, ZW and HL collected the data; JJ and HL performed the statistical analysis; JJ and LS wrote the paper; JJ and ZW performed the verification experiments; YY conceived the study and revised the manuscript. All authors read and approved the final manuscript.

**Acknowledgements**
Not applicable.

**Competing interests**
The authors declare that they have no competing interests.

**Funding**
Not applicable.

**References**
1. Torre LA, Bray F, Siegel RL, Ferlay J, Lortet-Tieulent J, Jemal A. Global cancer statistics, 2012. CA Cancer J Clin. 2015;65(2):87–108.
2. Cancer Genome Atlas Research Network. Comprehensive molecular characterization of gastric adenocarcinoma. Nature. 2014;513(7517):202–9.
3. Marquitz AR, Mathur A, Shair KH, Raab-Traub N. Infection of Epstein-Barr virus in a gastric carcinoma cell line induces anchorage independence and global changes in gene expression. Proc Natl Acad Sci USA. 2012;109(24):9593–8.
4. Yau TO, Tang CM, Yu J. Epigenetic dysregulation in Epstein–Barr virus-associated gastric carcinoma: disease and treatments. World J Gastroenterol. 2014;20(21):6448–56.
5. Lee TI, Young RA. Transcriptional regulation and its misregulation in disease. Cell. 2013;152(6):1237–51.

5. Lee TI, Young RA. Transcriptional regulation and its misregulation in disease. Cell. 2013;152(6):1237–51.

6. Singh AJ, Ramsey SA, Filtz TM, Kioussi C. Differential gene regulatory networks in development and disease. Cell Mol Life Sci. 2018;75(6):1013–25.

7. Doane AS, Elemento O. Regulatory elements in molecular networks. Wiley Interdiscipl Rev. 2017;9(3):e1374.

8. Latchman DS. Transcription factors: an overview. Int J Biochem Cell Biol. 1997;29(12):1305–12.

9. Libermann TA, Zerbini LF. Targeting transcription factors for cancer gene therapy. Curr Gene Ther. 2006;6(1):17–33.

10. Macfarlane LA, Murphy PR. MicroRNA: biogenesis, function and role in cancer. Curr Genomics. 2010;11(7):537–61.

11. Kung JT, Colognori D, Lee JT. Long noncoding RNAs: past, present, and future. Genetics. 2013;193(3):651–69.

12. Salmena L, Poliseno L, Tay Y, Kats L, Pandolfi PP. A ceRNA hypothesis: the Rosetta Stone of a hidden RNA language? Cell. 2011;146(3):353–8.

13. Cai X, Schafer A, Lu S, Bilello JP, Desrosiers RC, Edwards R, Raab-Traub N, Cullen BR. Epstein-Barr virus microRNAs are evolutionarily conserved and differentially expressed. PLoS Pathog. 2006;2(3):e23.

14. Grundhoff A, Sullivan CS, Ganem D. A combined computational and microarray-based approach identifies novel microRNAs encoded by human gamma-herpesviruses. RNA. 2006;12(5):733–50.

15. Choy EY, Siu KL, Kok KH, Lung RW, Tsang CM, To KF, Kwong DL, Tsao SW, Jin DY. An Epstein–Barr virus-encoded microRNA targets PUMA to promote host cell survival. J Exp Med. 2008;205(11):2551–60.

16. Zheng XH, Lu LX, Cui C, Chen MY, Li XZ, Jia WH. Epstein-Barr virus mir-bart1-5p detection via nasopharyngeal brush sampling is effective for diagnosing nasopharyngeal carcinoma. Oncotarget. 2016;7(4):4972–80.

17. Iizasa H, Wulff BE, Alla NR, Maragkakis M, Megraw M, Hatzigeorgiou A, Iwakiri D, Takada K, Wiedmer A, Showe L, et al. Editing of Epstein–Barr virus-encoded BART6 microRNAs controls their dicer targeting and consequently affects viral latency. J Biol Chem. 2010;285(43):33358–70.

18. Kononen J, Bubendorf L, Kallioniemi A, Barlund M, Schraml P, Leighton S, Torhorst J, Mihatsch MJ, Sauter G, Kallioniemi OP. Tissue microarrays for high-throughput molecular profiling of tumor specimens. Nat Med. 1998;4(7):844–7.

19. Arsanious A, Bjarnason GA, Yousef GM. From bench to bedside: current and future applications of molecular profiling in renal cell carcinoma. Mol Cancer. 2009;8:20.

20. Barrett T, Wilhite SE, Ledoux P, Evangelista C, Kim IF, Tomashevsky M, Marshall KA, Phillippy KH, Sherman PM, Holko M, et al. NCBI GEO: archive for functional genomics data sets–update. Nucleic Acids Res. 2013;41(Database issue):991–5.

21. The Gene Ontology. (GO) project in 2006. Nucleic Acids Res. 2006;34(Database issue):322–6.

22. Kanehisa M, Furumichi M, Tanabe M, Sato Y, Morishima K. KEGG: new perspectives on genomes, pathways, diseases and drugs. Nucleic Acids Res. 2017;45(D1):D353–61.

23. von Mering C, Huynen M, Jaeggi D, Schmidt S, Bork P, Snel B. STRING: a database of predicted functional associations between proteins. Nucleic Acids Res. 2003;31(1):258–61.

24. Shannon P, Markiel A, Ozier O, Baliga NS, Wang JT, Ramage D, Amin N, Schwikowski B, Ideker T. Cytoscape: a software environment for integrated models of biomolecular interaction networks. Genome Res. 2003;13(11):2498–504.

25. Dweep H, Sticht C, Pandey P, Gretz N. miRWalk–database: prediction of possible miRNA binding sites by "walking" the genes of three genomes. J Biomed Inform. 2011;44(5):839–47.

26. Li Y, Wang C, Miao Z, Bi X, Wu D, Jin N, Wang L, Wu H, Qian K, Li C, et al. ViRBase: a resource for virus-host ncRNA-associated interactions. Nucleic Acids Res. 2015;43(Database issue):D578–82.

27. Gao J, Aksoy BA, Dogrusoz U, Dresdner G, Gross B, Sumer SO, Sun Y, Jacobsen A, Sinha R, Larsson E, et al. Integrative analysis of complex cancer genomics and clinical profiles using the cBioPortal. Sci Signal. 2013;6(269):l1.

28. Ramsay PT, Carr A. Gastric acid and digestive physiology. Surg Clin North Am. 2011;91(5):977–82.

29. Choi MY, Romer AI, Wang Y, Wu MP, Ito S, Leiter AB, Shivdasani RA. Requirement of the tissue-restricted homeodomain transcription factor Nkx6.3 in differentiation of gastrin-producing G cells in the stomach antrum. Mol Cell Biol. 2008;28(10):3208–18.

30. Okuyama T, Ishihara S, Sato H, Rumi MA, Kawashima K, Miyaoka Y, Suetsugu H, Kazumori H, Cava CF, Kadowaki Y, et al. Activation of prostaglandin E2-receptor EP2 and EP4 pathways induces growth inhibition in human gastric carcinoma cell lines. J Lab Clin Med. 2002;140(2):92–102.

31. Nagasako T, Sugiyama T, Mizushima T, Miura Y, Kato M, Asaka M. Up-regulated Smad5 mediates apoptosis of gastric epithelial cells induced by Helicobacter pylori infection. J Biol Chem. 2003;278(7):4821–5.

32. Harris AG. Somatostatin and somatostatin analogues: pharmacokinetics and pharmacodynamic effects. Gut. 1994;35(3 Suppl):S1–4.

33. Li H, Liu JW, Liu S, Yuan Y, Sun LP. Bioinformatics-based identification of methylated-differentially expressed genes and related pathways in gastric cancer. Dig Dis Sci. 2017;62(11):3029–39.

34. Pedraza-Arevalo S, Hormaechea-Agulla D, Gomez-Gomez E, Requena MJ, Selth LA, Gahete MD, Castano JP, Luque RM. Somatostatin receptor subtype 1 as a potential diagnostic marker and therapeutic target in prostate cancer. Prostate. 2017;77(15):1499–511.

35. Enescu AS, Margaritescu CL, Craitoiu MM, Enescu A, Craitoiu S. The involvement of growth differentiation factor 5 (GDF5) and aggrecan in the epithelial-mesenchymal transition of salivary gland pleomorphic adenoma. Roman J Morphol Embryol. 2013;54(4):969–76.

36. Margheri F, Schiavone N, Papucci L, Magnelli L, Serrati S, Chilla A, Laurenzana A, Bianchini F, Calorini L, Torre E, et al. GDF5 regulates TGFss-dependent angiogenesis in breast carcinoma MCF-7 cells: in vitro and in vivo control by anti-TGFss peptides. PLoS ONE. 2012;7(11):e50342.

37. Kim BG, Kang S, Han HH, Lee JH, Kim JE, Lee SH, Cho NH. Transcriptome-wide analysis of compression-induced microRNA expression alteration in breast cancer for mining therapeutic targets. Oncotarget. 2016;7(19):27468–78.

38. Yan S, Han B, Gao S, Wang X, Wang Z, Wang F, Zhang J, Xu D, Sun B. Exosome-encapsulated microRNAs as circulating biomarkers for colorectal cancer. Oncotarget. 2017;8(36):60149–58.

39. Xu K, Liang X, Cui D, Wu Y, Shi W, Liu J. miR-1915 inhibits Bcl-2 to modulate multidrug resistance by increasing drug-sensitivity in human colorectal carcinoma cells. Mol Carcinog. 2013;52(1):70–8.

40. Wang H, Zhang M, Sun G. Long non-coding RNA NEAT1 regulates the proliferation, migration and invasion of gastric cancer cells via targeting miR-335-5p/ROCK1 axis. Pharmazie. 2018;73(3):150–5.

41. Wang F, Jia Y, Wang P, Yang Q, Du Q, Chang Z. Identification and profiling of Cyprinus carpio microRNAs during ovary differentiation by deep sequencing. BMC Genomics. 2017;18(1):333.

42. Ye Y, Zhou Y, Zhang L, Chen Y, Lyu X, Cai L, Lu Y, Deng Y, Wang J, Yao K, et al. EBV-miR-BART1 is involved in regulating metabolism-associated genes in nasopharyngeal carcinoma. Biochem Biophys Res Commun. 2013;436(1):19–24.

43. Cai L, Ye Y, Jiang Q, Chen Y, Lyu X, Li J, Wang S, Liu T, Cai H, Yao K, et al. Epstein-Barr virus-encoded microRNA BART1 induces tumour metastasis by regulating PTEN-dependent pathways in nasopharyngeal carcinoma. Nat Commun. 2015;6:7353.

44. Zhou H, Wu J, Wang T, Zhang X, Liu D. CXCL10/CXCR3 axis promotes the invasion of gastric cancer via PI3K/AKT pathway-dependent MMPs production. Biomed Pharmacother. 2016;82:479–88.

45.  Eck M, Schmausser B, Scheller K, Brandlein S, Muller-Hermelink HK. Pleiotropic effects of CXC chemokines in gastric carcinoma: differences in CXCL8 and CXCL1 expression between diffuse and intestinal types of gastric carcinoma. Clin Exp Immunol. 2003;134(3):508–15.

46.  Afrem MC, CraiToiu S, Hincu MC, Manolea HO, Nicolae V, CraiToiu MM. Study of CK18 and GDF5 immunoexpression in oral squamous cell carcinoma and their prognostic value. Roman J Morphol Embryol. 2016;57(1):167–72.

# Research progresses in roles of LncRNA and its relationships with breast cancer

Xu Bin[1†], Yang Hongjian[2†], Zhang Xiping[2*] ⓘD, Chen Bo[3], Yang Shifeng[3] and Tang Binbin[4]

## Abstract

Some progresses have been made in research of long non-coding RNA (hereunder referred to as LncRNA) related to breast cancer. Lots of data about LncRNA transcription concerning breast cancer have been obtained from large-scale omics research (e.g. transcriptomes and chips). Some LncRNAs would become indices for detecting breast cancer and judging its development and prognosis. LncRNAs may affect genesis and development of breast cancer in multiple ways. Perhaps they could develop into potential targets for treating breast cancer if they are carcinogenic. Like those from other studies of breast cancer, many data gained from omics research remain to be validated by much experimental work. For instance, it is still necessary to demonstrate reliability of LncRNAs as indices for diagnosing breast cancer and judging its prognosis (particularly for various subtypes of breast cancer), effectiveness and feasibility of these genes for treating breast cancer as targets. In this paper, recent years' literatures about LncRNAs which are related to breast cancer are summarized and sorted out to review the research progresses in relationships between LncRNAs and breast cancer.

**Keywords:** LncRNA, Breast cancer, Promote, Inhibit, Target

## Introduction

As a type of non-coding RNAs with over 200 nucleotides, LncRNAs may regulate physiological functions of organisms from the perspectives of epigenetics, transcription and post-transcription. Some of them are discovered to be involved in some important processes of breast cancer, including genesis, development, drug resistance and metastasis of breast cancer (BC), while some others may inhibit these processes. No matter they promote or inhibit the processes of breast cancer, their common mechanism of action consists in that they impact proliferation, apoptosis, drug resistance or invasion of BC cells. Some attempts are being made to develop some LncRNAs into targets for treating BC, and biomarkers for diagnosing BC, judging its prognosis or predicting metastasis and survival. In this paper, these years' related literatures are collected, sorted out and summarized to review research progresses in relationships between LncRNAs and BC.

## A brief introduction to LncRNAs

Genomes of eukaryotes may transcript several types of RNAs, including protein-coding mRNAs, short and long non-coding RNAs (LncRNAs) [1]. From these RNAs, people have discovered that there are more non-coding RNAs than coding RNAs in human cells. According to encyclopedia of DNA elements (ENCODE), 76% human genomic DNA is transcribed into RNA [2]. The human genome project (HGP) indicates that only 2% genomic DNA is translated into protein [3], which reveals the existence of numerous non-coding RNAs. In these years' research, short non-coding RNAs such as microRNAs (miRNAs), small interfering RNAs (siRNAs) and snoRNAs have been extensively studied. Meanwhile, LncRNAs are receiving growing concerns. More and more evidences have shown that LncRNAs are not simply considered to emerge as by-products of genomes, but have plenty of definite cellular functions, many of which are connected with human diseases.

*Correspondence: zxp99688@sina.com
†Xu Bin and Yang Hongjian contributed equally to this work
2 Department of Breast Surgery, Zhejiang Cancer Hospital, Banshanqiao, No. 38 Guangji Road, Hangzhou 310022, Zhejiang, China
Full list of author information is available at the end of the article

LncRNAs are generally defined to be longer than 200 nucleotides and have no open reading frame that can be translated into protein. After analyzing genome tiling arrays and high-throughput sequencing of transcriptomes, numerous LncRNAs have been discovered. In these analyses, LncRNAs have been discovered to have complicated structures and origins, so researchers consider that they shall not be purely defined based on their length and non-coding. Research suggests that LncRNAs have some common characteristics as follows. (1) Coding LncRNAs are similar to genes of coding proteins in terms of chromatin states like H3K4me3 of promoters and H3K36me3 of transcribed regions [4]. (2) The expression of LncRNAs is regulated by multiple types of common transcription factors [5]. (3) Like coding genes, LncRNAs are transcribed with RNA polymerase II, generally spliced through spliceosomes and have poly A tails. According to the position of their DNA fragments in genomes, coding LncRNAs may be divided into five categories, including sense, antisense, bidirectional, intronic and intergenic LncRNAs. The position is more of less related to the functions of these genes.

In recent years, LncRNAs have drawn an increased attention because of their functions in the human diseases including cancers. They are involved in diverse biological processes such as cell proliferation, diferentiation, chromosome remodeling, epigenetic modulation, transcriptional and posttranscriptional modifcations [6, 7].

## Roles of LncRNAs

Some reports have claimed that more than 8000 types of LncRNAs have been discovered after a complete analysis of human genomes [8]. Some others have suggested that over 1000 types of LncRNAs are expressed in human beings and other mammals [4, 9]. In a word, there is a large amount of LncRNAs. However, the transcripts of several types of LncRNAs are not conservative among specimens with similar genetic relationships, and only over 200 types of LncRNAs have been investigated relatively clearly at present [10]. As a result, people question if all LncRNAs have biochemical functions, and to answer this question, further research shall be conducted.

The expression of most LncRNAs is tissue-specific. Among more than 200 types of LncRNAs which have been explored relatively clearly at present, many of them have been found to have functions in vitro, whereas only some of them have been demonstrated to function in vivo. It may be judged from current data that LncRNAs get involved in extensive biological and physiological processes, having distinct functions in different stages of these processes. Furthermore, LncRNAs, as crucial regulators for promoting or inhibiting tumor development, have been discovered to play their regulatory roles

from the perspectives of epigenetic, transcriptional and post-transcriptional levels. In view of their roles in development of BC, LncRNAs are classified into two types: (1) some LncRNAs that promote the development of BC and (2) some others that inhibit the development of BC. No matter they promote or inhibit the development of BC, their mechanism of action generally covers several aspects as follows: (1) affect proliferation and apoptosis of BC cells, (2) influence drug resistance of BC cells, (3) impact invasion of BC cells.

## LncRNAs that promote development of breast cancer

There is a range of LncRNAs that promote development of BC, and their functions have been preliminarily investigated. It is helpful for developing more effective means for diagnosing BC, judging its prognosis, predicting its genesis and intervening with the treatment. Hereunder, mechanisms related to these LncRNAs will be particularly introduced (see Fig. 1).

### Promoting proliferation of breast cancer cells or inhibiting apoptosis of breast cancer cells

#### H19

H19 is one of the first discovered LncRNAs, and located at the downstream of the sense of IGF2 in human genome. In multiple types of cancer, including BC, the expression of H19 is upregulated [11]. Compared with normal mammary tissues, the expression of H19 is higher in 72.5% of BC [12]. H19 may promote proliferation of BC cells when they are overexpressed in these cells. As a transcription factor, E2F1 may bind with promoters of H19 to enhance its expression and thereby lead to cell proliferation [13]. In addition, the overexpression of H19 in MDA-MB-231 contributes to the colony-forming efficiency and tumorigenic abilities in vivo [14]. In BC, the

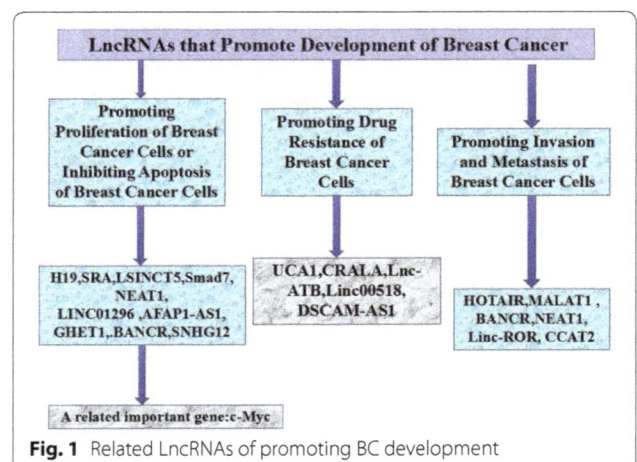

**Fig. 1** Related LncRNAs of promoting BC development

expression of H19 is higher in Estrogen receptor (ERα) positive cells, but in the ERα negative MDA-MB-231 cell line, ectopic overexpression of H19 is associated with increased proliferation [15]. It is clear that H19 is a category of LncRNAs that promote proliferation of BC cells.

### Steroid receptor RNA activator (SRA)

Steroid receptor RNA activator (SRA) sites may be transcribed into encoded mRNAs or non-coding LncRNAs. It is the first LncRNA that was discovered to be not impacted by epigenetic regulation or catalytic regulation of enzymes. Selectively impacted by steroid receptors, it is a gene that gets involved in transactivating dependence of steroid receptors [16]. SRR is found to have higher expression in BC tissues and serum [17]. However, it has been discovered in animal experiments that pure excess SRA is inadequate for causing BC. This indicates that SRA promotes BC, but can't lead to BC unless it acts together with other carcinogenic factors.

### LSINCT5

As a type of about 2.6 kb long stress LncRNA, LSINCT5 is generally located in nucleus, and its genes are transcribed by RNA polymerase III instead of RNA polymerase II [18, 19]. LSINCT5 is overexpressed in several types of BC cells, so is it in BC tissues. The proliferation of BC cells will be reduced if LSINCT5 is knocked out of them [19]. It is thus clear that LSINCT5 is effective for increasing proliferation of BC cells, so it is deemed to promote the genesis of BC. It will be helpful for developing related reagents and drugs for diagnosing and intervening with BC by intensively exploring LSINCT5.

### Smad7

As a type of genes located near Smad7 in mice, LncRNA-Smad7 has been reported to inhibit apoptosis of cancer cells with its expression in mammary epithelial cells and BC cell lines [20]. The anti-apoptotic functions of TGF-β may be mediated by suppressing the expression of LncRNA-Smad7. In contrast, ectopic expression of LncRNA-Smad7 may offset apoptosis induced by TGF-β receptor inhibitor. Nonetheless, LncRNA-Smad7 possibly only promotes the genesis of BC by affecting the apoptosis, because the knockout of its expression imposes no impacts upon TGF-β induced epithelial–mesenchymal transition, Smad2 phosphorylation or expression of Smad7. This indicates that LncRNA-Smad7 is a promoter of BC, but unlike other promoters, it merely inhibits apoptosis, so there would be new findings if it is further studied.

### NEAT1

The human nuclear enriched abundant transcript 1 (NEAT1) gene encodes two LncRNA isoforms that play a central role in nuclear paraspeckles, which function in regulating RNA splicing and transcription. NEAT1 has been reported to play a critical role in mouse mammary gland development. NEAT1 functions as an oncogenic factor in multiple types of cancer, including BC, and its expression is under the regulation of ERαsignaling, the miR-449b-5p/c-Met axis, and hypoxia responses [21]. Studies have demonstrated that LncRNA NEAT1 promotes cancer progression. NEAT1 promoted invasion through inducing epithelial–mesenchymal transition (EMT) and NEAT1 played a role in 5-fluorouracil (5-FU) resistance. LncRNA NEAT1 could be a new diagnostic biomarker and therapy target for BC [22].

The meta-analysis by Yang et al. [23] suggest that there was significant difference in the OS between high NEAT1 expression level group and low NEAT1 expression level group. A significantly shorter OS was shown in the patients with high NEAT1 expression level than that with low NEAT1 expression level. Thus, it is implied that the increased expression level of NEAT1 was associated with poor OS. The meta-analysis results suggest the prognostic role NEAT1 in prognosis in the patients with different types of cancer. However, due to several limitations of the included studies, larger-sample size, multi-center and higher-quality studies with consistent criteria for defining high NEAT1 expression level and low NEAT1 expression level may be required to further confirm the current findings in this study. Above all, all aforementioned types of LncRNAs promote proliferation and inhibit apoptosis. It is favorable for understanding other similar LncRNAs by acquiring certain knowledge about these types of LncRNAs. Meanwhile, it will be helpful for developing pertinent means for diagnosing and intervening with BC by intensively investigating these genes.

### LINC01296

LINC01296 exerts a tumor-promoting function in many cancers, in the regulation of proliferation and metastasis [24]. LINC01296 is up-regulated in both BC tissue samples and cells. Up-regulated LINC01296 is correlated with larger tumor size, positive lymph node metastasis, and advanced TNM stage of patients with BC. Additionally, Cox regression analysis confirmed LINC01296 as an independent prognostic indicator for patients with BC. LINC01296 may function as a potential prognostic predictor and therapeutic target for patients with BC [25].

### AFAP1-AS1

LncRNA actin filament-associated protein 1 antisense RNA 1 (AFAP1-AS1) is a newly recognized cancer-related lncRNA deriving from the antisense strand of DNA at the AFAP1 coding gene locus. A slew of new studies suggest that AFAP1-AS1 is involved in many kinds of malignant tumors. Evidence has increasingly shown that AFAP1-AS1 could probably serve as a novel potential molecular biomarker in tumor diagnosis and therapeutic target in tumor treatment. A series of studies provide detailed information to understand lncRNA AFAP1-AS1 role in various human cancers. LncRNA AFAP1-AS1 is an oncogene in tumors that have been studied so far, and it may act as a useful tumor biomarker and therapeutic target [26]. The expression of AFAP1-AS1 was up-regulated in human BC tissue and associated with malignancy status, high expression of AFAP1-AS1 had a poor prognosis in BC patients. Up-regulated lncRNA AFAP1-AS1 indicates a poor prognosis in BC patients [27].

### GHET1

Song et al.'s study for the first time revealed the biological functions of lncRNA gastric carcinoma highly expressed transcript 1 (GHET1) in BC. Their results demonstrated that GHET1 was up-regulated in BC tissues and cell lines, and promoted BC cell proliferation, invasion and migration by affecting EMT. Their research demonstrated that GHET1 was up-regulated in BC tissues and cell lines, and promoted BC cell proliferation, invasion and migration by affecting EMT [28].

### BANCR

The role of the LncRNA BRAF-regulated LncRNA 1 (BANCR) in BC has not yet been elucidated. The present study revealed that BANCR was overexpressed in BC cell lines and tissues, and could promote the clinical progression of disease, including increases in tumor size, lymph node metastasis and tumor-node-metastasis stage. BANCR overexpression could promote the clinical progression, metastasis and proliferation of BC and indicate poor prognosis of patients with BC. BANCR may therefore be a potential prognostic marker and therapeutic target of patients with BC [29]. BRAF-activated non-protein coding RNA (BANCR) is a novel and potential regulator of cancer cell proliferation and migration [30]. LncRNA BANCR is highly expressed in BC, which is significantly correlated with the prognosis of patients. The down-regulation of BANCR can inhibit the proliferation, invasion and metastasis capacities of MCF-7 cells [31].

### SNHG12

The long non-coding RNA (lncRNA) small nucleolar RNA host gene 12 (SNHG12) has a role in cell proliferation and migration. SNHG12 has been shown to play a role in a variety of human cancers [32]. The expression pattern of SNHG12 in BC and its clinical significance remains unclear. SNHG12 is upregulated in Triple-negative BC (TNBC), and its high expression is significantly correlated with tumor size and lymph node metastasis. Mechanistic investigations show that SNHG12 is a direct transcriptional target of c-MYC. SNHG12 contributes to the oncogenic potential of TNBC and may be a promising therapeutic target [33].

### A related important gene: c-Myc

Oncogenic c-Myc, which is located at chromosome 8q24, is one of the proto-oncogenic genes which is most frequently involved in human carcinogenesis [34]. Myc-induced transformation leads to the conversion from glucose to glutamine as the oxidizable substrate which is essential to maintain TCA cycle activity. c-Myc binds to the promoters and induces the expression of several crucial regulatory genes which are involved in glutaminolytic metabolism. It has been demonstrated that supra-physiological levels of Myc expression associated with oncogenic transformation are both necessary and sufficient for the induction of glutaminolysis to the excessive level that results in "glutamine addiction" specific to tumor cells.

The c-Myc mediates elevation of glutaminolysis in cancer cells. c-Myc promotes both glutamine uptake and glutamine catabolism. Because of c-Myc-mediated metabolic reprogramming, cancer cells tend to exhibit "glutamine addiction". This is a typical example of metabolic reprogramming in cancer cells with oncogene-addiction, suggesting a potential "Achilles' heel" of tumor cells that are addicted to glutamine metabolism in manner that is mediated by c-Myc [35]. The c-Myc/Max complex inhibits the ectopic differentiation of both types of artificial stem cells. Whereas c-Myc plays a fundamental role as a "double-edged sword" promoting both induced pluripotent stem cells generation and malignant transformation. Collectively, although the further research is warranted to develop the effective anti-tumor therapeutic strategy targeting Myc family, we should always catch up with the current advances in the complex functions of Myc family in highly-malignant and heterogeneous tumor cells to realize the precision medicine [36].

As a transcription factor, MYC's primary mode of transformation is through the pro-tumorigenic transcriptional dysregulation of a wide variety of processes including proliferation, cell size, apoptosis, and metabolism.

The alternative strategies of targeting MYC-driven cancers via selective inhibition of cellular pathways, like metabolism, that may selectively kill MYC-overexpressing cells have attractive therapeutic potential [37].

In a subset of neuroendocrine breast carcinoma tissues, the catalytic activity of EZH2 increases the number of the complex composed of N-Myc, AR, and EZH2-PRC2. Enhanced levels of EZH2 protein expression and EZH2 catalytic activity play a crucial role both in murine models overexpressing N-Myc and in human castration-resistant prostate cancer cells. N-Myc redirects EZH2 activity to N-Myc target gene promoters, resulting in the transcriptional suppression, whereas EZH2 inhibition reverses N-Myc-driven genetic regulation. Importantly, N-Myc sensitizes tumor cells to EZH2 inhibitors both in vitro and in vivo. In addition, N-Myc amplification rarely occurs in other lung cancer patho-histologic findings. N-Myc amplification also occurs in approximately 40% of neuroendocrine/small-cell prostate cancers, is commonly seen concurrently with amplification of the aurora kinase A gene (AURKA), and associated with poor prognosis.

Notably, downregulation of Myc interactor (NMI), a gatekeeper of epithelial phenotype, in breast tumors promotes mesenchymal, invasive and metastatic phenotype of the cancer cells. Aberrant miR-29 expression may account for reduced NMI expression in breast tumors and mesenchymal phenotype of cancer cells that promotes invasive growth. Reduction in NMI levels has a positive feedback machinery on miR-29 levels [36].

N-myc (MYCN), a member of the Myc family of basic-helix–loop–helix–zipper (bHLHZ) transcription factors, is a central regulator of many vital cellular processes. Overexpression of N-myc has been seen in a subset of BCs and correlates with poor prognostic features. Because phosphorylation of N-myc is directly regulated by Gsk3β, and indirectly by upstream signaling through the PI3K/Akt/mTOR pathway, targeting PI3K/Akt/mTOR may be an effective therapeutic approach [38]. NMI is an inducible protein whose expression is compromised in advanced stage breast cancer. Analysis of mRNA of NMI and miR-29 from patient derived breast cancer tumors showed a strong, inverse relationship between the expression of NMI and the miR-29. The related studies also revealed that in the absence of NMI, miR-29 expression is upregulated due to unrestricted Wnt/β-catenin signaling resulting from inactivation of GSK3β. Reduction in NMI levels has a feed-forward impact on miR-29 levels [39].

After neoadjuvant chemotherapy, 82.4% of patients showed pathologic partial response, with only 9.8% showing pathologic complete response. In multivariate analysis, MYC immunoreactivity and high MYC gain defined as MYC/nucleus $\geq 5$ were significant predictor factors for pathologic partial response. MYC may have a role in chemosensitivity to AC and/or docetaxel drugs. The analysis of MYC amplification may help in the identification of patients that may have a better response to AC + T treatment [40].

## Promoting drug resistance of breast cancer cells

The growth of ER-positive BC is mostly dependent upon estrogen, so anti-estrogen therapies are major means for treating this type of BC in clinical practices. Nevertheless, these therapies can't completely inhibit the growth of BC cells. BCAR4 (breast cancer antiestrogen resistance 4), as a type of LncRNA connected with resistance to tamoxifen which is an endocrine drug, may be detected in 10–27% BC samples. For patients with metastatic BC who are treated by tamoxifen, relatively high level of BCAR4 mRNA is associated with high degree of tumor malignancy and short survival. Certain report has suggested that in human BC cells ZR-75-1 and MCF7, cells can proliferate without estrogen and with various antiestrogen factors owing to artificial expression of BCAR4. Besides, BCAR4-induced resistance to endocrine drugs doesn't depend upon estrogen receptors. Therefore, BCAR4 promotes BC by strengthening drug resistance of BC cells. As a type of highly transformed genes, it makes the growth of cancer cells not depend upon estrogen and drug-resistant to antiestrogen therapies. As a result, it contributes to the genesis of tumors in vivo. Meanwhile, some researchers consider that BCAR4-based high tumor-specific expression would be used for treating anti-estrogen BC as target. The research of Godinho et al. has suggested that both ERBB2 and ERBB3 are upregulated in the BC cell ZR that expresses BCAR4. In their research, the activation of ERBB2/ERBB3 signaling pathway is considered to be the reason why BCAR4 promotes drug resistance of BC. BCAR4-positive patients with BC would benefit from BCAR4-targeted therapies. Shi et al. [41] have discovered that Lnc-ATB is upregulated in BC cells and tissues which are resistant to trastuzumab (i.e. a type of monoclonal antibody for immunotherapies and drug for targeted therapies). It can be induced and activated by TGF-β. By competitively binding with miR-200c, it may promote the resistance to trastuzumab and induce invasion-metastasis cascade to upregulate expressions of ZEB1 and ANF-217. As a result, EMT is caused. In addition, researchers have discovered that high-level Lnc-ATB is connected with the resistance of BC to trastuzumab. These research findings imply that perhaps Lnc-ATP would cause EMT and resistance to trastuzumab in patients with BC as a downstream factor of TGF-β. Furthermore, Jiang et al. [42] have reported that LncRNA HIF1A-AS2 and AK124454 may not only stimulate proliferation and invasion of BC cells, but also play certain roles in promoting resistance of triple-negative BC to paclitaxel. Possibly used as signals for recurrence of BC, HIF1A-AS2 and AK124454 can be also utilized for strengthening therapeutic effects of paclitaxel as a target.

It is thus clear that some LncRNAs may increase resistance of BC cells to endocrine drugs and those for targeted therapies, so as to promote the genesis of BC.

## UCA1

Recent studies reported that long non-coding RNAs (LncRNAs) might play critical roles in regulating endocrine resistance of BC. Urothelial carcinoma-associated 1 (UCA1) is an LncRNA with an oncogenic role in BC. Li et al.'s findings reveal that tamoxifen induces UCA1 upregulation in ER-positive BC cells in a HIF1α-dependent manner. UCA1 upregulation results in significantly enhanced tamoxifen resistance. miR-18a inhibitor reduced the sensitivity of MCF-7 cells to tamoxifen, while miR-18a mimics sensitized BT474 cells to tamoxifen. The upregulated UCA1 sponges miR-18a, which is a negative regulator of HIF1α. Therefore, UCA1 upregulation is further enhanced through a miR-18a-HIF1α feedback loop. In addition, our data also showed that miR-18a is a modulator of tamoxifen sensitivity due to its regulative effect on cell cycle proteins [43].

## CRALA

The expression levels of chemoresistance-associated long non-coding RNA (CRALA), a newly discovered long non-coding RNA, CRALA is upregulated in chemoresistant BC cell lines. Silencing of CRALA in chemoresistant BC cells resensitizes the cells to chemotherapy in vitro. The univariate and multivariate analysis showed that higher CRALA expression was significantly associated with poor prognosis in BC patients. The study findings indicate that CRALA expression may be an important biomarker for predicting the clinical response to chemotherapy and prognosis in BC patients. It is possible to target CRALA to reverse chemoresistance in BC patients [44].

## Lnc-ATB

Trastuzumab resistance (TR) is leading cause of mortality in Her-2-positive BCs, and the role of TGF-β-induced epithelial–mesenchymal transition (EMT) in trastuzumab resistance is well established, but the involvement of LncRNAs in trastuzumab resistance is still unknown. Shi et al. [41] identified long noncoding RNA activated by TGF-β (lnc-ATB) was the most remarkably upregulated LncRNA in TR SKBR-3 cells and the tissues of TR BC patients. They found that LncRNA-ATB, a mediator of TGF-β signaling, could predispose BC patients to EMT and trastuzumab resistance.

## Linc00518

Linc00518 expression increased nearly twofold and MRP1 level elevated about 2.5-fold in BC tissues as compared to that in adjacent normal tissues. Linc00518 could act as a molecular sponge of miR-199a to repress MRP1 expression. MRP1 depletion increased the sensitivity of MCF-7/ADR cells to ADR, VCR and PTX, and this effect was attenuated following miR-199a inhibition or linc00518 overexpression. Also, linc00518 silencing increased ADR-mediated anti-tumor effect in vivo. linc00518 downregulation reduced MDR by regulating miR-199a/MRP1 axis in BC [45].

## DSCAM-AS1

Ma et al. [46] investigate the influence of long noncoding RNA (LncRNA) DSCAM-AS1 on the propagation and apoptosis of tamoxifen-resistant (TR) BC cells via regulation of mircoRNA (miR)-137 and epidermal growth factor receptor pathway substrate 8 (EPS8). They think that LncRNA DSCAM-AS1 acts as a competing endogenous RNA of miR-137 and regulates EPS8 to promote cell reproduction and suppresses cell apoptosis in tamoxifen-resistant (TR) BC.

## Promoting invasion and metastasis of breast cancer cells
### HOTAIR

Gupta et al. [47] have discovered that the expression of HOTAIR (i.e. a type of LncRNA) increases to different extent in primary BC tissues compared with normal mammary tissues, while it is upregulated by several hundred times and even nearly 2000 times in metastatic BC tissues. However, its expression is not so consistently high in primary tumors. In primary BC tissues, the high expression of HOTAIR may be considered as an index of cancer metastasis and patients' survival [47, 48]. Additionally, highly expressed HOTAIR may enhance invasion of BC cells. Furthermore, high expression of HOTAIR has been discovered in in vivo experiments to more or less promote growth and spontaneous pulmonary metastasis of tumors. The knockout of HOTAIR may significantly decrease invasion of BC cells. In terms of its mechanism, it has been discovered that highly expressed HOTAIR induces site binding of PRC2 (i.e. polycomb repressive complex 2, a type of transcriptional inhibitor) and H3K27me3 (i.e. a kind of multiplex methylated histones) on 854 loci of genes, which are mostly downregulated by HOTAIR [47]. Chisholm et al. [49] have reported that in BC tissues, the expression of HOTAIR is positively correlated to EZH2, which is a subunit of PRC2. Compared with primary BC tissues, the expressions of both

HOTAIR and EZH2 are significantly upregulated in metastatic BC tissues. Meanwhile, the co-expression of these two genes has positive correlations with poor prognosis of patients. The long noncoding RNA HOTAIR (HOX transcript antisense intergenic RNA) has been reported to be a biomarker for various malignant tumors; however, its involvement in BC is not fully understood. Han et al.'s study suggests the higher expressions of HOTAIR and EZH2 among three BC cells. Furthermore, the downregulation of HOTAIR or silencing of EZH2 was noted to inhibit the proliferation, invasion, and migration of BC cells, while promoting their apoptosis [50].

### MALAT1

As a type of conservative LncRNAs, metastasis-associated lung adenocarcinoma transcript 1 (MALAT1) is highly expressed in multiple categories of cancer, including BC. The in vivo and in vitro experiments have demonstrated that MALAT1 may not only promote proliferation of triple negative BC cells, cancer development and metastasis, but also has negative correlations with the survival of patients with ER-negative HER-2 positive and triple negative BC in terms of its expression level [51]. In MCF7 (Luminal A) and MDA-MB-231 (triple negative), which belong to two kinds of cell lines, high-concentration 17b-Estradiol (E2) may not only inhibit cell proliferation, metastasis and invasion, but also reduce the level of MALAT1. The downregulation of MALAT1 may achieve similar effects, so E2 would impact cancer cells when the level of MALAT1 is decreased [52]. It has been discovered in research on MDA-MB-231 that KDM5B regulates MDA-MB-231 as a carcinogenic gene and the downregulation of KDM5B leads to lower expression of MALAT1 while decreasing invasion of cancer cells [53]. Above research indicates that MALAT1 has the potential to become an index for judging prognosis of BC and possibly turn into a target for treating BC.

The aforementioned studies suggest that both HOTAIR and MALAT1 may promote genesis and metastasis of BC by enhancing invasion of BC cells. Furthermore, MALAT1 may enhance proliferation of BC cells. Both LncRNAs are helpful for treating BC as targets for intervening with such cancer.

### BANCR

The present study revealed that LncRNA BRAF-regulated LncRNA 1 (BANCR) was overexpressed in BC cell lines and tissues, and could promote the clinical progression of disease, including increases in tumor size, lymph node metastasis and tumor-node-metastasis stage. BANCR overexpression could romote the clinical progression, metastasis and proliferation of BC and indicate poor prognosis of patients with BC. BANCR may therefore be a potential prognostic marker and therapeutic target of patients with BC [29].

### NEAT1

LncRNA NEAT1 was highly expressed in BC tissue, and the expression was also closely related to the tumor size and lymph node metastasis. Survival study also showed that the expression of lncRNA NEAT1 was closely related with prognosis of BC patients. LncRNA NEAT1 may act as an oncogene in BC, which can promote proliferation and metastasis of BC [54].

### Linc-ROR

Hou et al. [55] have discovered that linc-ROR was upregulated in breast tumor samples, and ectopic overexpression of linc-ROR in immortalized human mammary epithelial cells induced an epithelial-to-mesenchymal transition (EMT) program. Moreover, they showed that linc-ROR enhanced BC cell migration and invasion, which was accompanied by generation of stem cell properties. Their results indicate that linc-ROR functions as an important regulator of EMT and can promote BC progression and metastasis through regulation of miRNAs. Potentially, the findings of the related study implicate the relevance of linc-ROR as a possible therapeutic target for aggressive and metastatic breast cancers.

### CCAT2

The present study demonstrates that TAM-resistant cells show a higher level of long non-coding RNA CCAT2 expression compared with TAM-sensitive cells. Biologically, CCAT2 knockdown could inhibit proliferation and induce apoptosis in TAM-resistant cells exposed to TAM. Furthermore, knockdown of CCAT2 improves the sensitivity to TAM in TAM-resistant cells. Overall, the study results provide a novel therapeutic approach for TAM-resistant patients through depleting CCAT2 expression [56].

## LncRNAs that inhibit development of breast cancer

So far, some LncRNAs that inhibit BC from development have been explored relatively clearly. They have been discovered to mainly inhibit development of BC by inhibiting proliferation or stimulating apoptosis. See Fig. 2.

### Inhibiting proliferation of breast cancer cells or promoting their apoptosis
### ZFAS1

Research has suggested that Zfas1, located inside mammary ducts and acinus, is expressed differently during pregnancy and breastfeeding, which has been found to be

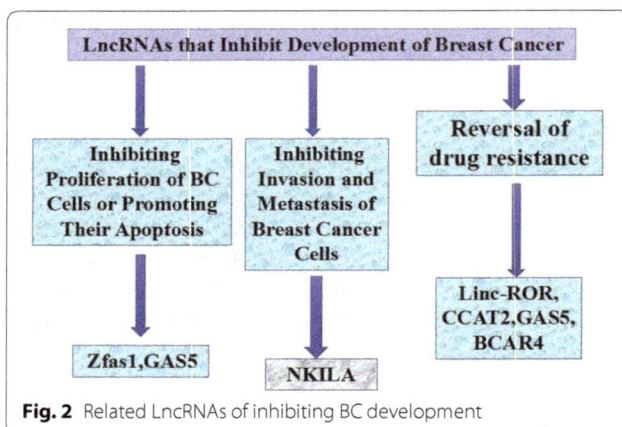

**Fig. 2** Related LncRNAs of inhibiting BC development

associated with breast development. After the knockout of Zfas1 from mammary epithelial cells, proliferation of cells is strengthened. Moreover, it has been found that the expression of Zfas1 is lower in BC tissues than that in normal breast tissues [57]. Hence, Zfas1 is a potential inhibitor of BC. Its functions and mechanism in the genesis of BC need to be further investigated, in hope of making certain contributions to developing means for intervening with and treating BC.

### GAS5

GAS5 is another LncRNA that may cause cell growth arrest and apoptosis. Compared with peripheral normal cells, LncRNA GAS5 is significantly downregulated in BC cells. Mourtada-Maarabouni et al. [58] have reported that in MCF10A and MCF7 (BC cell lines), overexpressed GAS5 may increase the apoptosis rate of these cells under UV radiation and intervention of cisplatin as an anticancer drug. In line with above research findings, Ozgur et al. [59] have reported that in apoptotic MCF7 cells under genotoxic stress, the expression of GAS5 is upregulated. In some cases, the growth arrest and apoptosis of BC cell lines can be just caused by ectopic expression of GAS5. Besides, the expression of GAS5 is high in cells under growth arrest induced by lack of nutrients or growth factors, as a result of which these cells become extremely sensitive to the stimuli promoting apoptosis [60]. It is thus clear that some LncRNAs may inhibit BC by suppressing cell proliferation and stimulating apoptosis. These LncRNAs are expected to be developed and employed for intervening with BC.

### Inhibiting invasion and metastasis of breast cancer cells

Recently, Liu et al. [61] have reported a new LncRNA known as NF-KappaB interacting LncRNA (NKILA). Upregulated by NF-κB, it binds with NF-κB/IκB to produce stable composites, so as to directly cover the

phosphorylated structural domains of IκB. As a consequence, IKK (IκB kinase) induced IκB phosphorylation and NF-κB are activated. Importantly, NKILA may prevent excessive activation of the NF-κB in mammary epithelial cells under inflammatory stimuli. In MDA-MB-231 (i.e. a BC cell line), NKILA may enhance apoptosis and reduce invasion. To sum up, NKILA may control invasion and metastasis of BC by inhibiting activation of NF-κB.

Thus, it may be inferred that some LncRNAs inhibit genesis and development of BC. In terms of its mechanism, it mainly plays its roles in inhibiting genesis and development of BC by suppressing proliferation of BC cells, or promoting apoptosis of these cells, or inhibiting invasion and metastasis of the cells. Nevertheless, no many LncRNAs have been discovered to be effective for inhibiting BC, and very few of them have been investigated from the perspective of their inhibition mechanism. It is hoped that researchers can discover more LncRNAs that can inhibit BC and examine them more clearly through their efforts.

### Reversal of drug resistance

Li et al.'s study explored the mechanism underlying long non-coding RNA ROR regulating autophagy on tamoxifen resistance in BC. These results indicate that inhibition of long non-coding RNA ROR reverses resistance to tamoxifen by inducing autophagy in BC [62]. The expression levels of chemoresistance-associated long non-coding RNA (CRALA), a newly discovered long non-coding RNA, were measured by quantitative real time-PCR in 79 pre-treatment biopsied primary BC samples. Small interfering RNAs were used to knockdown CRALA expression. The effect of CRALA on chemosensitivity was evaluated using cell growth assay. The study findings indicate that CRALA expression may be an important biomarker for predicting the clinical response to chemotherapy and prognosis in BC patients. It is possible to target CRALA to reverse chemoresistance in BC patients [44]. Gu et al. [63] investigates the role of LncRNA growth arrest-specific transcript 5 (GAS5) in tamoxifen resistance in BC. Their study demonstrates that GAS5 enhances the efficacy of tamoxifen in the treatment of BC and could be a novel prognostic biomarker.

BC antiestrogen resistance 4 (BCAR4) was identified in a functional screen for genes involved in tamoxifen resistance. BCAR4 is a strong transforming gene causing estrogen-independent growth and antiestrogen resistance, and induces tumor formation in vivo. Due to its restricted expression, BCAR4 may be a good target for treating antiestrogen-resistant BC [64]. BCAR4 may have clinical relevance for tumour aggressiveness and tamoxifen resistance. The research of Godinho et al. [65] suggests that BCAR4-positive breast tumours are driven by ERBB2/ERBB3 signalling. Patients with such tumours may benefit from ERBB-targeted therapy.

## Use of LncRNAs-related information

In spite of lack of complete and deep understanding about LncRNAs, people are not hindered from utilizing the conformed knowledge about these genes mainly for diagnosing BC, judging its prognosis and predicting its metastasis and survival.

### LncRNAs used as diagnostic markers

Ding et al. [66] have studied the possible applications of LncRNAs in diagnosing BC as a type of LncRNAs that exist among genes. They have found that lincRNA-BC2 and lincRNA-BC5 are generally upregulated by over twice in BC specimens compared with normal mammary tissues, whereas lincRNA-BC4 and lincRNA-BC5 are downregulated. For stage 3 BC, the expression of LincRNA-BC4 is significantly low, whereas the expression of lincRNA-BC5 is significantly high, and the expression of lincRNA-BC2 has significant positive correlations with LNM (lymph node metastasis). In particular, the expression of numerous LncRNAs is found to be highly associated with different molecular classification [67]. Furthermore, some research has suggested that LncRNAs in serum may be used for diagnosing genesis of BC. For instance, the expression of RP11-445H22.4 increases significantly in serum of patients with BC. The sensitivity and specificity for diagnosing BC with this are up to 92% and 74% respectively among Chinese people [68]. Liu et al. [69] aimed to develop a long noncoding RNA (LncRNA) expression signature that can predict response to tamoxifen. A set of LncRNAs (LINC01191, RP4-639F20.1 and CTC-429P9.3) associated with distant metastasis-free survival was established. Estrogen receptor-positive BC patients in the training series could be classified into high- and low-risk groups with significantly different distant metastasis-free survival values based on this signature. The LncRNA signature may have possible clinical implications in the selection of high-risk patients for tamoxifen therapy. It is thus clear that certain LncRNAs may be employed for diagnosing BC as biomarkers.

### LncRNAs used as prognostic biomarkers

Zhao et al. [70] have discovered a range of LncRNAs which may be used for differentiating patients with BC from low to high risks. The high expression of LINC00324 and low expressions of PTPRG-AS1 or SNHG17 are related to the relatively longer survival. Another study has suggested that SPRY4-IT1 promotes

proliferation of BC cells by upregulating the expression of ZNF703. In addition, increased expression of SPRY4-IT1 is connected with higher tumor volume and more severe pathological staging in patients with BC [71]. Hence, SPRY4-IT1 is a type of new prognostic biomarkers and potential candidates of therapeutic targets.

The overexpression of HOTAIR in BC tissues is discovered to be connected with higher invasiveness and metastasis, which implies that HOTAIR would become biomarkers for predicting overall survival. The expression of HOTAIR may independently forecast if ER-positive BC is metastatic. MALAT1 is discovered to have higher expression in primary BC and its expression further increases in the course of metastasis [72]. On the contrary, the expression of BC040587 [73], NBAT1 [74] and EGOT [75] is discovered to be downregulated in BC tissues, which is associated with poor prognosis. Additionally, the high expression of LINC00472 in BC tissues is connected with poor invasiveness of BC cells and relatively good therapeutic effects [76]. Related clinical and in vivo studies suggest that LINC00472 is a type of tumor inhibitors, so it is possibly valuable for judging prognosis and predicting therapeutic effects of BC in clinical practices. This suggests that some LncRNAs may be used for judging prognosis of BC as biomarkers and have a great prospect for application in clinical practices.

MALAT1 is a highly conserved LncRNA that is highly expressed in several types of cancer, including BC. It has been demonstrated by in vivo and in vitro studies that MALAT1 promotes proliferation, tumor development and metastasis of TNBC. In addition, the expression of MALAT1 has been reported to be negatively correlated to the survival of ER negative, lymph node negative patients of the Her-2 and TNBC molecular subtypes. It is particularly noteworthy that a recent study using genetic interventions with MALAT1 antisense nucleotides has achieved good effects for suppressing cancer development in mouse models with luminal B BC. These studies suggested that MALAT1 is expected to become a new biomarker for prognosis of BCs and a potential target for treating them [77].

### LncRNAs used for predicting drug resistance and survival as markers

LncRNAs have potential value for being used for predicting drug resistance and survival of BC as markers. The overexpression of BCAR4 (a type of LncRNAs) is discovered to be effective for forecasting the resistance to tamoxifen which is a type of estrogenic drugs. On the other hand, LINC00160 and LINC01016 (i.e. two kinds of LinRNAs) are discovered to be highly expressed in ER-positive BC compared with ER-negative BC and normal tissues, which is discovered to have significant negative correlations with the overall survival of luminal A BC [78]. Additionally, a special BC subtype may be identified by detecting whether CCAT2 is overexpressed, having poor responses to adjuvant chemotherapies based on cyclophosphamide, methotrexate and CMF [79]. At last, the research of Chen et al. [80] has shown that the overexpression of ROR (i.e. a kind of LncRNAs) is correlated to chemotherapy resistance, which suggests that ROR may be used for predicting such resistance as an indicator. It may be inferred from the above that some LncRNAs are likely to become markers for predicting drug resistance and survival of BC.

Therefore, researchers are exploring the applications of LncRNAs from multiple perspectives (mainly including diagnosis of BC, judgment of prognosis, prediction of drug resistance and survival) based on their existing knowledge about them. Although it still needs some time to put them into practices, it is believed that the explorations of their applications will be more elaborate with the promotion of pertinent studies in terms of their breadth and depth. Meanwhile, new applications will be constantly developed.

## Conclusion

LncRNAs belong to a type of common transcription products in genomes of human beings and mammals. Since their relationships with the genesis and development of tumors have received growing attention, the functions and mechanisms of actions of some LncRNAs have been investigated clearly in preliminary research. Nevertheless, a majority of LncRNAs remain to be further widely and deeply studied. With the improvement of research methods like the development of gene array technologies and high-throughput sequencing technologies, more categories of LncRNAs are expected to be discovered. As people acquire a deeper understanding of LncRNAs, some of these genes are likely to be developed into biomarkers for diagnosing BC, judging and predicting its prognosis. Nevertheless, LncRNAs have been rarely reported to be used for intervening with BC. Recent CRISPR/CAS9 gene editing technologies would play certain roles in developing LncRNAs as therapies. For example, they can be employed for targeted silencing of certain LncRNAs that promote the genesis of BC.

**Authors' contributions**
XB provided the idea of this paper, ZX wrote this paper, other authors participated in the translation and revision of this paper. All authors contributed to the intellectual context. All authors read and approved the final manuscript.

**Author details**
[1] Department of Surgery, Zhejiang Rehabilitation Medical Center, Hangzhou 310053, Zhejiang, China. [2] Department of Breast Surgery, Zhejiang Cancer Hospital, Banshanqiao, No. 38 Guangji Road, Hangzhou 310022, Zhejiang, China. [3] Department of Pathology, Zhejiang Cancer Hospital, Hangzhou 310022, Zhejiang, China. [4] Second Outpatient Department of Traditional Chinese Internal Medicine, Tongde Hospital of Zhejiang Province, Hangzhou 310012, Zhejiang, China.

**Acknowledgements**
Not applicable.

**Competing interests**
The authors declare that they have no competing interests. We claimed that this paper was original and would not have any financial interest in a company or its competitor, and that all authors meet criteria for authorship.

**Funding**
This study was supported by a foundation for the "1022 first level of innovative talents of Zhejiang Cancer Hospital, China (Grant Number: 2013102202) and Key platform technological project of Zhejiang medical science and hygiene (Grant Number: 2016ZDB003).

**References**
1. Kapranov P, Cheng J, Dike S, Nix DA, Duttagupta R, Willingham AT, Stadler PF, Hertel J, Hackermüller J, Hofacker IL, Bell I, Cheung E, Drenkow J, Dumais E, Patel S, Helt G, Ganesh M, Ghosh S, Piccolboni A, Sementchenko V, Tammana H, Gingeras TR. RNA maps reveal new RNA classes and a possible function for pervasive transcription. Science. 2007;316(5830):1484–8.
2. Pennisi E. Genomics. ENCODE project writes eulogy for junk DNA. Science. 2012;337(6099):1159–61.
3. Lander ES, Linton LM, Birren B, Nusbaum C, Zody MC, Baldwin J, et al. Initial sequencing and analysis of the human genome. Nature. 2001;409(6822):860–921.
4. Guttman M, Amit I, Garber M, French C, Lin MF, Feldser D, Huarte M, Zuk O, Carey BW, Cassady JP, Cabili MN, Jaenisch R, Mikkelsen TS, Jacks T, Hacohen N, Bernstein BE, Kellis M, Regev A, Rinn JL, Lander ES. Chromatin signature reveals over a thousand highly conserved large non-coding RNAs in mammals. Nature. 2009;458(7235):223–7.
5. Yang JH, Li JH, Jiang S, Zhou H, Qu LH. ChIPBase: a database for decoding the transcriptional regulation of long non-coding RNA and micro-RNA genes from ChIP-Seq data. Nucleic Acids Res. 2013;41(Database issue):D177–87.
6. Tian T, Gong Z, Wang M, Hao R, Lin S, Liu K, Guan F, Xu P, Deng Y, Song D, Li N, Wu Y, Dai Z. Identification of long non-coding RNA signatures in triple-negative breast cancer. Cancer Cell Int. 2018;17(18):103.
7. Quinn JJ, Chang HY. Unique features of long non-coding RNA biogenesis and function. Nat Rev Genet. 2016;17(1):47–62.
8. Cabili MN, Trapnell C, Goff L, Koziol M, Tazon-Vega B, Regev A, Rinn JL. Integrative annotation of human large intergenic noncoding RNAs reveals global properties and specific subclasses. Genes Dev. 2011;25(18):1915–27.
9. Khalil AM, Guttman M, Huarte M, Garber M, Raj A, Morales DR, Thomas K, Presser A, Bernstein BE, van Oudenaarden A, Regev A, Lander ES, Rinn JL. Many human large intergenic noncoding RNAs associate with chromatin-modifying complexes and affect gene expression. Proc Natl Acad Sci USA. 2009;106(28):11667–72.
10. Amaral PP, Clark MB, Gascoigne DK, Dinger ME, Mattick JS. lncRNAdb: a reference database for long noncoding RNAs. Nucleic Acids Res. 2011;39(Database issue):D146–51.
11. Doucrasy S, Coll J, Barrois M, Joubel A, Prost S, Dozier C, Stehelin D, Riou G. Expression of the human fetal bac h19 gene in invasive cancers. Int J Oncol. 1993;2(5):753–8.
12. Adriaenssens E, Dumont L, Lottin S, Bolle D, Leprêtre A, Delobelle A, Bouali F, Dugimont T, Coll J. Curgy JJ.H19 overexpression in breast adenocarcinoma stromal cells is associated with tumor values and steroid receptor status but independent of p53 and Ki-67 expression. Am J Pathol. 1998;153(5):1597–607.

13. Berteaux N, Lottin S, Monté D, Pinte S, Quatannens B, Coll J, Hondermarck H, Curgy JJ, Dugimont T, Adriaenssens E. H19 mRNA-like noncoding RNA promotes breast cancer cell proliferation through positive control by E2F1. J Biol Chem. 2005;280(33):29625–36.

14. Lottin S, Adriaenssens E, Dupressoir T, Berteaux N, Montpellier C, Coll J, Dugimont T, Curgy JJ. Overexpression of an ectopic H19 gene enhances the tumorigenic properties of breast cancer cells. Carcinogenesis. 2002;23(11):1885–95.

15. Collette J, Le Bourhis X, Adriaenssens E. regulation of human breast cancer by the long non-coding RNA H19. Int J Mol Sci. 2017;18(11):2319.

16. Vicent GP, Nacht AS, Zaurin R, Font-Mateu J, Soronellas D, Le Dily F, Reyes D, Beato M. Unliganded progesterone receptor-mediated targeting of an RNA-containing repressive complex silences a subset of hormone-inducible genes. Genes Dev. 2013;27(10):1179–97.

17. Lanz RB, Chua SS, Barron N, Söder BM, DeMayo F, O'Malley BW. Steroid receptor RNA activator stimulates proliferation as well as apoptosis in vivo. Mol Cell Biol. 2003;23(20):7163–76.

18. Dieci G, Fiorino G, Castelnuovo M, Teichmann M, Pagano A. The expanding RNA polymerase III transcriptome. Trends Genet. 2007;23(12):614–22.

19. Silva JM, Boczek NJ, Berres MW, Ma X, Smith DI. LSINCT5 is over expressed in breast and ovarian cancer and affects cellular proliferation. RNA Biol. 2011;8(3):496–505.

20. Arase M, Horiguchi K, Ehata S, Morikawa M, Tsutsumi S, Aburatani H, Miyazono K, Koinuma D. Transforming growth factor-β-induced lncRNA-Smad7 inhibits apoptosis of mouse breast cancer JygMC(A) cells. Cancer Sci. 2014;105(8):974–82.

21. Lo P-K, Zhang Y, Wolfson B, Gernapudi R, Yao Y, Duru N, Zhou Q. Dysregulation of the BRCA1/long non-coding RNA NEAT1 signaling axis contributes to breast tumorigenesis. Oncotarget. 2016;7(40):65067–89.

22. Li X, Wang S, Li Z, Long X, Guo Z, Zhang G, Zu J, Chen Y, Wen L. The lncRNA NEAT1 facilitates cell growth and invasion via the miR-211/HMGA2 axis in breast cancer. Int J Biol Macromol. 2017;105(Pt 1):346–53.

23. Yang C, Li Z, Li Y, Xu R, Wang Y, Tian Y, Chen W. Long non-coding RNA NEAT1 overexpression is associated with poor prognosis in cancer patients:a systematic review and meta-analysis. Oncotarget. 2017;8(2):2672–80.

24. Yu X, Pang L, Yang T, Liu P. lncRNA LINC01296 regulates the proliferation, metastasis and cell cycle of osteosarcoma through cyclin D1. Oncol Rep. 2018;40(5):2507–14.

25. Jiang M, Xiao Y, Liu D, Luo N, Gao Q, Guan Y. Overexpression of long noncoding RNA LINC01296 indicates an unfavorable prognosis and promotes tumorigenesis in breast cancer. Gene. 2018;30(675):217–24.

26. Ji D, Zhong X, Jiang X, Leng K, Xu Y, Li Z, Huang L, Li J, Cui Y. The role of long non-coding RNA AFAP1-AS1 in human malignant tumors. Pathol Res Pract. 2018. https://doi.org/10.1016/j.prp.2018.04.014.

27. Ma D, Chen C, Wu J, Wang H, Wu D. Up-regulated lncRNA AFAP1-AS1 indicates a poor prognosis and promotes carcinogenesis of breast cancer. Breast Cancer. 2018;Jul:5.

28. Song R, Zhang J, Huang J, Hai T. Long non-coding RNA GHET1 promotes human breast cancer cell proliferation, invasion and migration via affecting epithelial mesenchymal transition. Cancer Biomark. 2018;22(3):565–73.

29. Jiang J, Shi SH, Li XJ, Sun L, Ge QD, Li C, Zhang W. Long non-coding RNA BRAF-regulated lncRNA 1 promotes lymph node invasion, metastasis and proliferation, and predicts poor prognosis in breast cancer. Oncol Lett. 2018;15(6):9543–52.

30. Zhang J, Du Y, Zhang X, Li M, Li X. Downregulation of BANCR promotes aggressiveness in papillary thyroid cancer via the MAPK and PI3K pathways. J Cancer. 2018;9(7):1318–28.

31. Lou KX, Li ZH, Wang P, Liu Z, Chen Y, Wang XL, Cui HX. Long non-coding RNA BANCR indicates poor prognosis for breast cancer and promotes cell proliferation and invasion. Eur Rev Med Pharmacol Sci. 2018;22(5):1358–65.

32. Ruan W, Wang P, Feng S, Xue Y, Li Y. Long non-coding RNA small nucleolar RNA host gene 12 (SNHG12) promotes cell proliferation and migration by upregulating angiomotin gene expression in human osteosarcoma cells. Tumour Biol. 2016;37(3):4065–73.

33. Wang O, Yang F, Liu Y, Lv L, Ma R, Chen C, Wang J, Tan Q, Cheng Y, Xia E, Chen Y, Zhang X. C-MYC-induced upregulation of lncRNA SNHG12 regulates cell proliferation, apoptosis and migration in triple-negative breast cancer. Am J Transl Res. 2017;9(2):533–45.

34. Xu J, Chen Y, Olopade OI. MYC and breast cancer. Genes Cancer. 2010;1(6):629–40.

35. Yoshida GJ. Metabolic reprogramming:the emerging concept and associated therapeutic strategies. J Exp Clin Cancer Res. 2015;34:111.

36. Yoshida GJ. Emerging roles of Myc in stem cell biology and novel tumor therapies. J Exp Clin Cancer Res. 2018;37(1):173.

37. Camarda R, Williams J, Goga A. In vivo reprogramming of cancer metabolism by MYC. Front Cell Dev Biol. 2017;5:35.

38. Beltran H. The N-myc oncogene: maximizing its targets, regulation, and therapeutic potential. Mol Cancer Res. 2014;12(6):815–22.

39. Rostas JW, Pruitt HC, Metge BJ, Mitra A, Bailey SK, Bae S, Singh KP, Devine DJ, Dyess DL, Richards WO, Tucker JA, Shevde LA, Samant RS. microRNA-29 negatively regulates EMT regulator N-myc interactor in breast cancer. Mol Cancer. 2014;29(13):200. https://doi.org/10.1186/1476-4598-13-200.

40. Pereira CBL, Leal MF, Abdelhay ESFW, Demachki S, Assumpção PP, de Souza MC, Moreira-Nunes CA, Tanaka AMDS, Smith MC, Burbano RR. MYC amplification as a predictive factor of complete pathologic response to docetaxel-based neoadjuvant chemotherapy for breast cancer. Clin Breast Cancer. 2017;3:188–94.

41. Shi SJ, Wang LJ, Yu B, Li YH, Jin Y, Bai XZ. LncRNA-ATB promotes trastuzumab resistance and invasion-metastasis cascade in breast cancer. Oncotarget. 2015;6(13):11652–63.

42. Jiang YZ, Liu YR, Xu XE, et al. Transcriptome analysis of triple-negative breast cancer reveals an integrated mRNA-lncRNA signature with predictive and prognostic value. Cancer Res. 2016;76(8):2105–14.

43. Li X, Wu Y, Liu A, Tang X. Long non-coding RNA UCA1 enhances tamoxifen resistance in breast cancer cells through a miR-18a-HIF1α feedback regulatory loop. Tumour Biol. 2016;37(11):14733–43.

44. Li Y, Wang B, Lai H, Li S, You Q, Fang Y, Li Q, Liu Y. Long non-coding RNA CRALA is associated with poor response to chemotherapy in primary breast cancer. Thorac Cancer. 2017;8(6):582–91.

45. Chang L, Hu Z, Zhou Z, Zhang H. Linc00518 contributes to multidrug resistance through regulating the MiR-199a/MRP1 axis in breast cancer. Cell Physiol Biochem. 2018;48(1):16–28.

46. Ma Y, Bu D, Long J, Chai W, Dong J. LncRNA DSCAM-AS1 acts as a sponge of miR-137 to enhance tamoxifen resistance in breast cancer. J Cell Physiol. 2018. https://doi.org/10.1002/jcp.27105.

47. Gupta RA, Shah N, Wang KC, Kim J, Horlings HM, Wong DJ, Tsai MC, Hung T, Argani P, Rinn JL, Wang Y, Brzoska P, Kong B, Li R, West RB, van de Vijver MJ, Sukumar S, Chang HY. Long non-coding RNA HOTAIR reprograms chromatin state to promote cancer metastasis. Nature. 2010;464(7291):1071–6.

48. Sørensen KP, Thomassen M, Tan Q, Bak M, Cold S, Burton M, Larsen MJ, Kruse TA. Long non-coding RNA HOTAIR is an independent prognostic marker of metastasis in estrogen receptor-positive primary breast cancer. Breast Cancer Res Treat. 2013;142(3):529–36.

49. Chisholm KM, Wan Y, Li R, Montgomery KD, Chang HY, West RB. Detection of long non-coding RNA in archival tissue: correlation with polycomb protein expression in primary and metastatic breast carcinoma. PLoS ONE. 2012;7(10):e47998.

50. Han L, Zhang HC, Li L, Li CX, Di X, Qu X. Downregulation of long noncoding RNA HOTAIR and EZH2 induces apoptosis and inhibits proliferation, invasion, and migration of human breast cancer cells. Cancer Biother Radiopharm. 2018;33(6):241–51.

51. Jadaliha M, Zong X, Malakar P, Ray T, Singh DK, Freier SM, Jensen T, Prasanth SG, Karni R, Ray PS, Prasanth KV. Functional and prognostic significance of long non-coding RNA MALAT1 as a metastasis driver in ER negative lymph node negative breast cancer. Oncotarget. 2016;7(26):40418–36.

52. Zhao Z, Chen C, Liu Y, Wu C. 17β-Estradiol treatment inhibits breast cell proliferation, migration and invasion by decreasing MALAT-1 RNA level. Biochem Biophys Res Commun. 2014;445(2):388–93.

53. Bamodu OA, Huang WC, Lee WH, Wu A, Wang LS, Hsiao M, Yeh CT, Chao TY. Aberrant KDM5B expression promotes aggressive breast cancer through MALAT1 overexpression and downregulation of hsa-miR-448. BMC Cancer. 2016;16:160.

54. Zhang M, Wu WB, Wang ZW, Wang XH. lncRNA NEAT1 is closely related with progression of breast cancer via promoting proliferation and EMT. Eur Rev Med Pharmacol Sci. 2017;21(5):1020–6.

55. Hou P, Zhao Y, Li Z, Yao R, Ma M, Gao Y, Zhao L, Zhang Y, Huang B, Lu J. LincRNA-ROR induces epithelial-to-mesenchymal transition and contributes to breast cancer tumorigenesis and metastasis. Cell Death Dis. 2014;12(5):e1287.

56. Cai Y, He J, Zhang D. Suppression of long non-coding RNA CCAT2 improves tamoxifen-resistant breast cancer cells' response to tamoxifen. Mol Biol (Mosk). 2016;50(5):821–7.

57. Askarian-Amiri ME, Crawford J, French JD, Smart CE, Smith MA, Clark MB, Ru K, Mercer TR, Thompson ER, Lakhani SR, Vargas AC, Campbell IG, Brown MA, Dinger ME, Mattick JS. SNORD-host RNA Zfas1 is a regulator of mammary development and a potential marker for breast cancer. RNA. 2011;17(5):878–91.

58. Mourtada-Maarabouni M, Pickard MR, Hedge VL, Farzaneh F, Williams GT. GAS5, a non-protein-coding RNA, controls apoptosis and is downregulated in breast cancer. Oncogene. 2009;28(2):195–208.

59. Özgür E, Mert U, Isin M, Okutan M, Dalay N, Gezer U. Differential expression of long non-coding RNAs during genotoxic stress-induced apoptosis in HeLa and MCF-7 cells. Clin Exp Med. 2013;13(2):119–26.

60. Piao HL, Ma L. Non-coding RNAs as regulators of mammary development and breast cancer. J Mammary Gland Biol Neoplasia. 2012;17(1):33–42.

61. Liu B, Sun L, Liu Q, Gong C, Yao Y, Lv X, Lin L, Yao H, Su F, Li D, Zeng M, Song E. A cytoplasmic NF-kappaB interacting long noncoding RNA blocks IkappaB phosphorylation and suppresses breast cancer metastasis. Cancer Cell. 2015;27(3):370–81.

62. Li Y, Jiang B, Zhu H, Qu X, Zhao L, Tan Y, Jiang Y, Liao M, Wu X. Inhibition of long non-coding RNA ROR reverses resistance to tamoxifen by inducing autophagy in breast cancer. Tumour Biol. 2017;39(6):1010428317705790.

63. Gu J, Wang Y, Wang X, Zhou D, Shao C, Zhou M, He Z. Downregulation of lncRNA GAS5 confers tamoxifen resistance by activating miR-222 in breast cancer. Cancer Lett. 2018;10(434):1–10.

64. Godinho M, Meijer D, Setyono-Han B, Dorssers LC, van Agthoven T. Characterization of BCAR4, a novel oncogene causing endocrine resistance in human breast cancer cells. J Cell Physiol. 2011;226(7):1741–9.

65. Godinho MF, Sieuwerts AM, Look MP, Meijer D, Foekens JA, Dorssers LC, van Agthoven T. Relevance of BCAR4 in tamoxifen resistance and tumour aggressiveness of human breast cancer. Br J Cancer. 2010;12;103(8):1284–91.

66. Ding X, Zhu L, Ji T, Zhang X, Wang F, Gan S, Zhao M, Yang H. Long intergenic non-coding RNAs (LincRNAs) identified by RNA-seq in breast cancer. PLoS ONE. 2014;9(8):e103270.

67. Su X, Malouf GG, Chen Y, Zhang J, Yao H, Valero V, Weinstein JN, Spano JP, Meric-Bernstam F, Khayat D, Esteva FJ. Comprehensive analysis of long non-coding RNAs in human breast cancer clinical subtypes. Oncotarget. 2014;5(20):9864–76.

68. Xu N, Chen F, Wang F, Lu X, Wang X, Lv M, Lu C. Clinical significance of high expression of circulating serum lncRNA RP11-445H22.4 in breast

cancer patients: a Chinese population-based study. Tumour Biol. 2015;36(10):7659–65.

69. Liu R, Hu R, Zhang W, Zhou HH. Long noncoding RNA signature in predicting metastasis following tamoxifen treatment for ER-positive breast cancer. Pharmacogenomics. 2018. https://doi.org/10.2217/pgs-2018-0032.

70. Zhao W, Luo J, Jiao S. Comprehensive characterization of cancer subtype associated long non-coding RNAs and their clinical implications. Sci Rep. 2014;4:6591.

71. Shi Y, Li J, Liu Y, Ding J, Fan Y, Tian Y, Wang L, Lian Y, Wang K, Shu Y. The long noncoding RNA SPRY4-IT1 increases the proliferation of human breast cancer cells by upregulating ZNF703 expression. Mol Cancer. 2015;22(14):51.

72. Arun G, Diermeier S, Akerman M, Chang KC, Wilkinson JE, Hearn S, Kim Y, MacLeod AR, Krainer AR, Norton L, Brogi E, Egeblad M, Spector DL. Differentiation of mammary tumors and reduction in metastasis upon Malat1 lncRNA loss. Genes Dev. 2016;30(1):34–51.

73. Chi Y, Huang S, Yuan L, Liu M, Huang N, Zhou S, Zhou B, Wu J. Role of BC040587 as a predictor of poor outcome in breast cancer. Cancer Cell Int. 2014;14(1):123.

74. Hu P, Chu J, Wu Y, Sun L, Lv X, Zhu Y, Li J, Guo Q, Gong C, Liu B, Su S. NBAT1 suppresses breast cancer metastasis by regulating DKK1 via PRC2. Oncotarget. 2015;6(32):32410–25.

75. Xu SP, Zhang JF, Sui SY, Bai NX, Gao S, Zhang GW, Shi QY, You ZL, Zhan C, Pang D. Downregulation of the long noncoding RNA EGOT correlates with malignant status and poor prognosis in breast cancer. Tumour Biol. 2015;36(12):9807–12.

76. Shen Y, Katsaros D, Loo LW, Hernandez BY, Chong C, Canuto EM, Biglia N, Lu L, Risch H, Chu WM, Yu H. Prognostic and predictive values of long non-coding RNA LINC00472 in breast cancer. Oncotarget. 2015;6(11):8579–92.

77. Xiping Z, Bo C, Shifeng Y, Feijiang Y, Hongjian Y, Qihui C, Binbin T. Roles of MALAT1 in development and migration of triple negative and Her-2 positive breast cancer. Oncotarget. 2018;9(2):2255–67.

78. Jonsson P, Coarfa C, Mesmar F, Raz T, Rajapakshe K, Thompson JF, Gunaratne PH, Williams C. Single-molecule sequencing reveals estrogen-regulated clinically relevant lncRNAs in breast cancer. Mol Endocrinol. 2015;29(11):1634–45.

79. Redis RS, Sieuwerts AM, Look MP, Tudoran O, Ivan C, Spizzo R, Zhang X, de Weerd V, Shimizu M, Ling H, Buiga R, Pop V, Irimie A, Fodde R, Bedrosian I, Martens JW, Foekens JA, Berindan-Neagoe I, Calin GA. CCAT2, a novel long non-coding RNA in breast cancer: expression study and clinical correlations. Oncotarget. 2013;4(10):1748–62.

80. Chen YM, Liu Y, Wei HY, Lv KZ, Fu P. Linc-ROR induces epithelial–mesenchymal transition and contributes to drug resistance and invasion of breast cancer cells. Tumour Biol. 2016;37(8):10861–70.

# Paraoxonase 3 is involved in the multi-drug resistance of esophageal cancer

Dabing Huang[1,2,3,4,5‡], Yong Wang[1,2‡], Yifu He[1,2], Gang Wang[1,2], Wei Wang[1,2], Xinghua Han[1,2], Yubei Sun[1,2], Lin Lin[1,2], Benjie Shan[1,2], Guodong Shen[2,3,4,5], Min Cheng[2,3,4,5], Geng Bian[2,3,4,5], Xiang Fang[2,3,4,5], Shilian Hu[2,3,4,5†] and Yueyin Pan[1,2*†]

## Abstract

**Background:** Drug resistance prevents the effective treatment of cancers. DNA methylation has been found to participate in the development of cancer drug resistance.

**Methods:** We performed the wound-healing and invasion assays to test the effect of the paraoxonase gene PON3 on esophageal cancer (EC) cells. In addition, in vivo EC-derived tumor xenografts in nude mice were generated to test the effect of PON3 on the chemoresistance of EC cells.

**Results:** We found that PON3 is hypermethylated in drug-resistant EC cell line K150, which in-return down-regulates its expression. The following experiments by the forced changes of PON3 level in vitro and in vivo demonstrated that the PON3 expression negatively correlates with drug resistance in EC cells. Further wound-healing and invasion assays showed that PON3 suppresses the migration and invasion of EC cells.

**Conclusion:** Our data established that PON3 is associated with the EC drug resistance, which may serve as a biomarker for the potential therapeutic treatment of EC.

**Keywords:** Esophageal cancer, Multi-drug resistance, Methylation, PON3

## Background

Esophageal cancer (EC) is the eighth most common cancer worldwide, which arises from the inner lining of the esophagus [1, 2]. To date, the frequently used therapy for the treatment of EC is chemotherapy in combination with other therapeutic strategies. However, the prognosis of patients with EC remains poor and the 5-year survival rate is less than 20% [3]. This mainly results from the resistance to the commonly used drugs owing to the abuse of antibiotics [4]. There are limited salvage options for patients with refractory EC [5] and targeted therapies are not yet available. Therefore, there is an urgent need for understanding the mechanism of drug-resistance to guide the design of novel approaches for the treatment of EC.

The family of paraoxonase (PON) has three members, PON1, PON2 and PON3, that are located adjacent to each other on chromosome 7 in humans [6]. They share high levels of homology [7]. The expression level and specific activities of PON genes were found to be negatively correlated with several inflammatory disorders, such as cardiovascular diseases, type-2 diabetes, and inflammatory bowel disease [8, 9]. Moreover, PON3 expression is remarkably up-regulated in a variety of human cells, including cancer cells [10, 11]. Recent study suggested that PON3 promotes cell proliferation and metastasis by regulating PI3K/Akt in oral squamous cell carcinoma [12]. Despite the extensive studies of PON3 in cancer cells, the roles of PON3 in EC are rarely evaluated, especially the involvement in drug resistance. In this study, we investigated the roles of PON3 in EC cells and found that PON3 is related in various biological processes in EC cells, which will give us hints for a clinical therapy of EC.

*Correspondence: pyyahslyy@163.com
†Shilian Hu and Yueyin Pan are Co-corresponding authors
‡Dabing Huang and Yong Wang are Co-first authors
[1] Department of Oncology, the First Affiliated Hospital of USTC, Division of Life Sciences and Medicine, University of Science and Technology of China, Hefei 230001, Anhui, People's Republic of China
Full list of author information is available at the end of the article

## Methods

### Cell lines and culture

The eight K30, K450, K180, K150, TE-1, K510, K140 and K410 cell lines come from our laboratory. All cell lines were cultured in RPMI1640 (Biological Industries, Israel) +10% fetal bovine serum (Invitrogen, USA) and 1% glutamine at 37 °C in 5% $CO_2$.

### Bisulfite sequencing PCR (BSP) analysis

Genomic DNA was isolated by a standard phenol/chloroform purification method, verified by electrophoresis on an agarose gel, and treated by an ammonium bisulfite-based bisulfite conversion method. Then the PCR fragments from the converted DNA were sequenced and analyzed. Raw sequence data files were processed, and the area ratio (%) of C over C+T of the primary CpG dinucleotide was calculated as the % of methylation and plotted [13].

### Transient transfection assays and reagents

siRNA and scrambled (negative control, NC) sequences as well as a riboFECT CP transfection kit were supplied by Guangzhou RiboBio, China. A GFP-tagged PON3 overexpression construct (pReciever-M98) was purchased from Genecopia, Guangzhou, China (Catalog No.: EX-E0804-M98-5). Transfections of the above mentioned ribonucleic acid reagents and reporter plasmids were performed according to the manufacturer's instructions.

### Chemoresistance profiling ($IC_{50}$ determination)

All of the chemotherapeutic drugs used in this study were of clinical grade. To perform thiazolyl blue tetrazolium blue (MTT)-based cell proliferation assays, experimental groups of cells in the logarithmic phase of growth were seeded in triplicate in 96-well plates at a cell density of $0.5 \times 10^4$/well and treated with fourfold serially diluted drugs for 72 h. Then 10 µl (5 mg/ml) of MTT salt (Sigma) was added to the corresponding wells. The cells were incubated at 37 °C for another 4 h, and the reaction was stopped by lysing the cells with 150 µl of DMSO for 5 min. The optical density was measured at 570 nm. A group that received no drug treatment was used as a reference for calculating the relative cell survival rate.

### RNA analysis

Total RNA was isolated from cells during the logarithmic phase using TRIzol (Tiangen Biotech). For mRNA analysis, a cDNA primed by an oligo-dT was constructed using a PrimeScript RT reagent kit (Tiangen Biotech). The PON3 mRNA level was quantified using duplex-qRT-PCR analysis, wherein TaqMan probes with a different fluorescence profile were used to detect β-actin (provided by Shing Gene, Shanghai, China) in a FTC-3000P PCR instrument (Funglyn Biotech). Using the $2^{-\Delta\Delta Ct}$ method, target gene expression levels were normalized to the β-actin expression level before the relative levels of the target genes were compared.

### Western blot protein analysis

Cells were lysed with lysis buffer (60 mM Tris–HCl [pH 6.8], 2% SDS, 20% glycerol, 0.25% bromophenol blue, and 1.25% 2-mercaptoethanol) and heated at 95 °C for 10 min before electrophoresis/Western blot analysis. The primary anti-PON3 (17422-1-AP) antibodies and anti-GAPDH (60004-1-lg) antibodies were purchased from Proteintech (San Ying Biotechnology, China) and were recognized with anti-rabbit IgG peroxidase-conjugated antibody (30000-0-AP) (San Ying Biotechnology, China), followed by an enhanced chemiluminescence reaction (Thermo Fisher Scientific, Waltham, MA, USA). Relative levels of proteins were quantified using densitometry with a Gel-Pro Analyzer (Media Cybernetics, Rockville, MD, USA). The target bands over the GAPDH band were densitometrically quantified, as indicated under each band (Additional file 1).

### Wound-healing assays

For cell motility assays, cells stably expressing si-PON3, GFP-PON3 and the corresponding NC were seeded in 24-well plates and cultured to near confluence. After 6 h of culture in RPMI1640 without FBS, a linear wound was carefully made using a sterile 10 µl pipette tip across the confluent cell monolayer, and the cell debris was removed by washing with phosphate-buffered saline. The cells were incubated in RPMI1640 plus 10% FBS, and the wounded monolayers were then photographed at 0, 8, 12 and 20 h after wounding.

### In vitro invasion assays

Cell invasion assays were performed in a 24-well plate with 8 mm pore size chamber inserts (Corning, USA). For invasion assays, $1 \times 10^3$ cells stably expressing si-PON3, GFP-PON3 or NC were placed into the upper chamber in each well with the matrigel-coated membrane, which was diluted in serum-free culture medium. In the assay, cells were suspended in 100 µl of RPMI1640 without FBS when they were seeded into the upper chamber. In the lower chamber, 500 µl of RPMI1640 supplemented with 10% FBS was added. After incubation for 36 h at 37 °C and 5% $CO_2$, the membrane inserts were removed from the plate, and non-invading cells were removed with cotton swab from the upper surface of the membrane. Cells that moved to the bottom surface of the chamber were stained with 0.1% crystal violet for 30 min. The cells were then imaged and counted in at least 5 random fields using a CKX41 inverted microscope (Olympus, Japan). The assays were conducted in three independent times.

### Signaling pathway analysis

The reporter construct encodes the firefly luciferase reporter gene under the control of a basal promoter element (TATA box) joined to tandem repeats of a specific transcriptional response element. The cells were transfected in triplicate with each firefly luciferase reporter construct in combination with the Renilla luciferase-based control construct using the riboFECT CP transfection reagent, and both the luciferase activities were measured in the cell extracts 24 h after transfection. The luciferase activities (luciferase unit) of the pathway reporter relative to those of the negative control in the transfected cells were calculated as a measurement of the pathway activity.

### In vivo studies

Animal experiments were performed in accordance with the National Institutes of Health Guide for the Care and Use of Laboratory Animals. Male BALB/c nude mice between 3 and 4 weeks old were used for this study [14]. K510 cells were embedded in BD Matrigel Matrix (Becton, USA) and subcutaneously injected into two sites on the back of each mouse as follows: $1.0 \times 10^7$ cells/site for K510 into 2 sites/mouse, with 6 mice. Ten days after cell injection, all of the tumors were intratumorally injected with 2 nM NC/si-PON3 every 2 days. Ten days later, after four cell injections, three mice intraperitoneally received DDP (75 µg/mouse) once every other day. The remaining three mice in each group received PBS as a mock treatment control. The mice were euthanized on day 30 after four drug injections, and their tumors were weighed and imaged. Tumor weight was described as the mean ± S.D. The expression levels of PON3 and Ki67 proteins were measured using immunochemical analysis on 5 µm sections of formalin-fixed, paraffin-embedded tumor xenografts in nude mice. The antigens were retrieved by pre-treating the de-waxed sections in a microwave oven at 750 Watts for 5 min in citrate buffer (pH 6) processed with a Super Sensitive Link-Labeled Detection System (Biogenex, Menarini, Florence, Italy), and the slides were developed using 3-amino-9-ethylcarbazole (Dako, Milan, Italy) as a chromogenic substrate. After the slides were counterstained with Mayer's hematoxylin (Invitrogen), they were mounted in an aqueous mounting medium (Glycergel, Dako). Images were captured using a Leica DM 4000B microscope (Wetzlar, Germany), the relative level of each protein was calculated using Leica software (Wetzlar, Germany), and the percentage of the mock over the chemotherapeutically treated tumors was calculated and plotted.

### Statistical analysis

All of the results are represented as the mean ± standard deviation (SD) of three independent experiments. Two-tailed Student's $t$-test, one-way analysis of variance or Mann–Whitney U test was used to calculate statistical significance. All of the statistical analyses were performed with Microsoft Excel 2010 (Microsoft, Redmond, WA). A p-value of less than 0.05 was designated statistically significant.

## Results

### PON3 is hypermethylated in drug-resistant esophageal cancer cell line K150

To profile the drug resistance ability of the eight common EC cell lines (K30, K450, K180, K150, TE-1, K510, K140 and K410), we performed the $IC_{50}$ profiling against the four drugs CBCDA, 5-FU, VP-16 and DDP, which are frequently used for EC therapy. As shown in Fig. 1, the drug resistance index revealed that K510 is the most multi-drug sensitive cell lines, with the lowest $IC_{50}$ values against all the four drugs. In contrast, K150 is the most drug-resistant cell lines with relative drug resistance index of 12.48 (Fig. 1).

To find the insight that governs the drug-resistance of EC, we tested the expression pattern of the PON3 gene, which was previously reported to involve in drug-resistance [9]. First, we detected the methylation status of the PON3 promoter region in the eight EC cells by Bisulfite Sequencing PCR (BSP) assay. The results showed that 16 CpG sites among the total 20 CpG sites were methylated at varying ratios (Fig. 2). The average methylation ratio of the PON3 gene in K150 cells is approximately 6.4-folds higher than that in K510 cells (85.79:13.44, Fig. 2b). The results suggested that PON3 is hypermethylated in the drug-resistant EC cell line K150.

### The PON3 expression negatively correlates with drug resistance in EC cells

To determine whether the hypermethylation may affect the expression of PON3 in EC cells, we detected the expression levels of PON3 in the eight EC cell lines. The qRT-PCR assay revealed that the PON3 mRNA level is relatively lower in the drug-resistant cell lines K30 and K150, compared to the drug-sensitive cell lines K410 and K510 (Fig. 3a). In agreement with the mRNA level, the western blot assays also suggested that PON3 protein level is much lower in the drug-resistant cell lines K450, K140 and K150, but higher in the drug-sensitive cell lines K510 and K410 (Fig. 3b).

Next, we transfected si-PON3 to down-regulate the PON3 level in K510 cells and tested the drug-resistance ability against the four drugs. Indeed, transfection of si-PON3 decreased the level of PON3 at both protein and

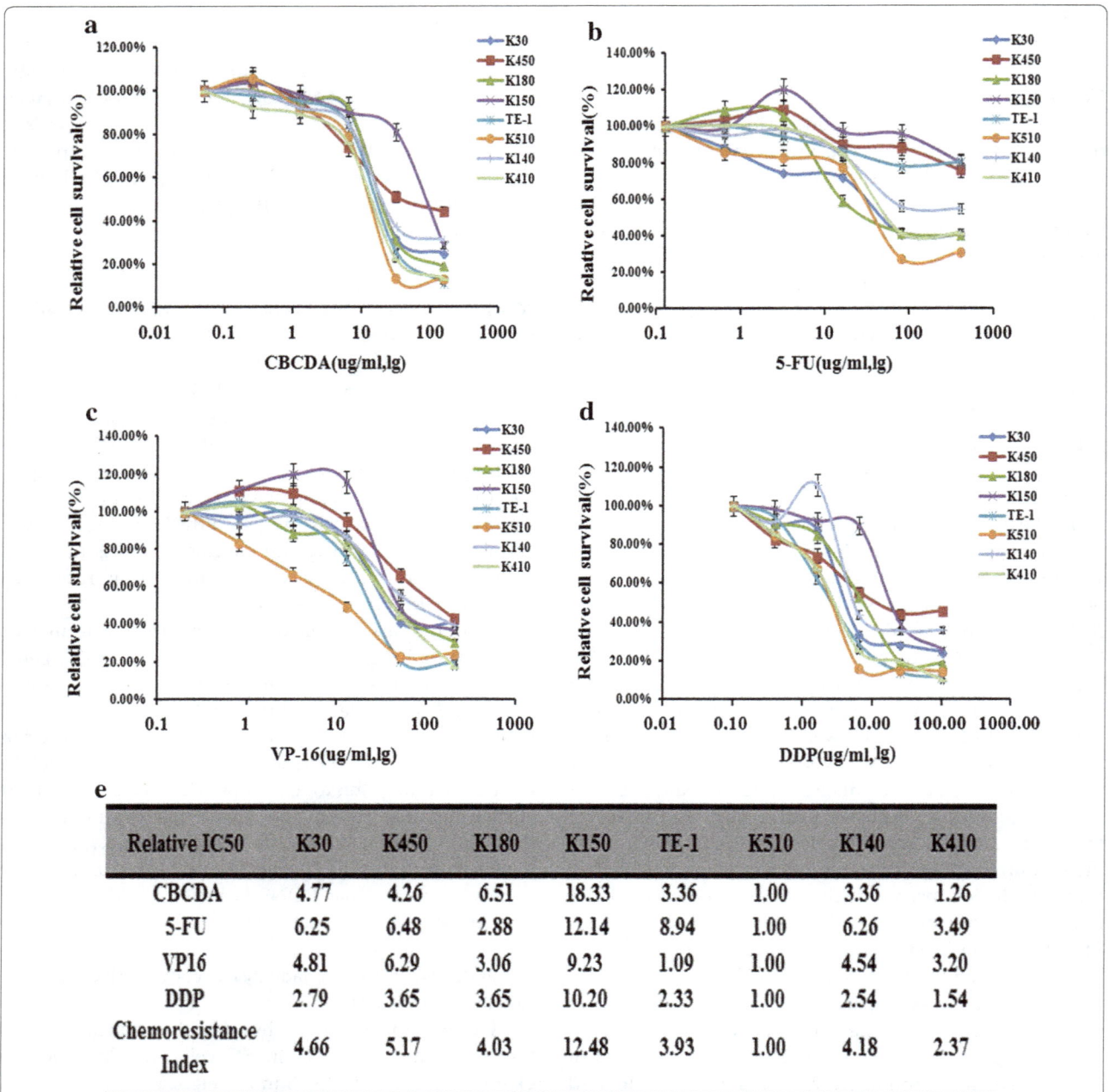

**a** Relative cell survival(%) vs CBCDA(ug/ml,lg)

**b** Relative cell survival(%) vs 5-FU(ug/ml,lg)

**c** Relative cell survival(%) vs VP-16(ug/ml,lg)

**d** Relative cell survival(%) vs DDP(ug/ml,lg)

**e**

| Relative IC50 | K30 | K450 | K180 | K150 | TE-1 | K510 | K140 | K410 |
|---|---|---|---|---|---|---|---|---|
| CBCDA | 4.77 | 4.26 | 6.51 | 18.33 | 3.36 | 1.00 | 3.36 | 1.26 |
| 5-FU | 6.25 | 6.48 | 2.88 | 12.14 | 8.94 | 1.00 | 6.26 | 3.49 |
| VP16 | 4.81 | 6.29 | 3.06 | 9.23 | 1.09 | 1.00 | 4.54 | 3.20 |
| DDP | 2.79 | 3.65 | 3.65 | 10.20 | 2.33 | 1.00 | 2.54 | 1.54 |
| Chemoresistance Index | 4.66 | 5.17 | 4.03 | 12.48 | 3.93 | 1.00 | 4.18 | 2.37 |

**Fig. 1** Drug resistance profiling of eight esophageal cancer cell lines. **a–d** $IC_{50}$ values of the four indicated chemotherapeutics for eight esophageal cancer cell lines. The cell survival rates were calculated as percentages relative to the mock treatment and plotted against lg μg/ml of drug. **e** The $IC_{50}$ (-fold) values relative to those of the most sensitive cell cine (K510) are presented in the table

mRNA levels, which are only 34% and 12%, respectively, of the control cells (Fig. 3c, d). Following the changes of the PON3 level in K510 cells, the cell death triggered by all four drugs was- reduced, except that against VP16 (Fig. 3e), indicating an increased drug-resistance capability. Conversely, we over-expressed GFP-tagged PON3 in K150 cells to further test the drug-resistance effect (Fig. 4a). The PON3 protein level was up-regulated by 1.77-folds following the over-expression of GFP-PON3 (Fig. 4b, c). As expected, the drug resistance ability was somewhat decreased, except that against VP16 (Fig. 4d). All these results suggest that PON3 is negatively correlated with the drug-resistance of EC cells.

**a**

PON3 bspf →

AGCTTCCCCATGGTCTCGGGGGTGCCCAGCGGCGACTGCGCG
　　　　　　　　　　　1　　　　　　　　2　3　　　4　5

GCGCCGAGAGCTCTCGGGGGCGCGGCGGGCGGTTCCTGCCT
6　7　　　　　　　8　　　　　9　10　11　　12

CGCGTACGGATTGGGGCCCGCTCGGCCCCGCCCGCACACGC
13　14　15　　　　　　16　　17　　　18　　19　　20

CTCCTACTTACCTGAG
← PON3 bspr

**b**

| CpGsites | K30 | K450 | K180 | K150 | TE1 | K510 | K140 | K410 |
|---|---|---|---|---|---|---|---|---|
| 4 | 78.23 | 36.29 | 36.22 | 88.26 | 49.37 | 12.36 | 71.18 | 62.59 |
| 5 | 82.26 | 41.12 | 30.41 | 97.59 | 65.06 | 24.99 | 62.28 | 59.52 |
| 6 | 65.29 | 70.25 | 17.15 | 70.26 | 50.96 | 16.34 | 63.36 | 77.81 |
| 7 | 46.55 | 69.33 | 20.15 | 71.20 | 78.22 | 20.29 | 60.02 | 69.49 |
| 8 | 76.36 | 68.05 | 22.21 | 72.25 | 91.02 | 26.33 | 88.81 | 80.06 |
| 9 | 90.26 | 19.63 | 9.66 | 91.33 | 86.26 | 10.51 | 81.88 | 77.88 |
| 10 | 81.20 | 21.44 | 41.02 | 80.63 | 55.28 | 29.48 | 70.14 | 50.20 |
| 11 | 39.26 | 77.12 | 9.26 | 81.79 | 65.22 | 8.99 | 80.89 | 86.35 |
| 12 | 59.00 | 62.12 | 6.39 | 85.69 | 60.06 | 9.34 | 92.26 | 81.41 |
| 13 | 88.69 | 64.55 | 3.20 | 90.03 | 47.24 | 6.39 | 98.28 | 80.62 |
| 14 | 92.36 | 63.23 | 4.55 | 91.05 | 86.22 | 8.25 | 65.20 | 41.11 |
| 15 | 41.26 | 74.25 | 61.25 | 93.26 | 19.69 | 10.28 | 91.06 | 33.61 |
| 16 | 52.36 | 50.25 | 8.55 | 93.34 | 80.66 | 7.49 | 83.31 | 77.89 |
| 17 | 95.26 | 49.22 | 5.59 | 90.23 | 46.28 | 2.51 | 17.22 | 26.59 |
| 18 | 77.22 | 67.05 | 14.09 | 85.38 | 70.11 | 9.33 | 62.33 | 77.88 |
| 19 | 82.02 | 66.06 | 30.32 | 90.36 | 71.88 | 12.11 | 69.64 | 90.48 |
| **Average** | **71.72** | **56.25** | **20.00** | **85.79** | **63.97** | **13.44** | **72.37** | **67.09** |

**c**

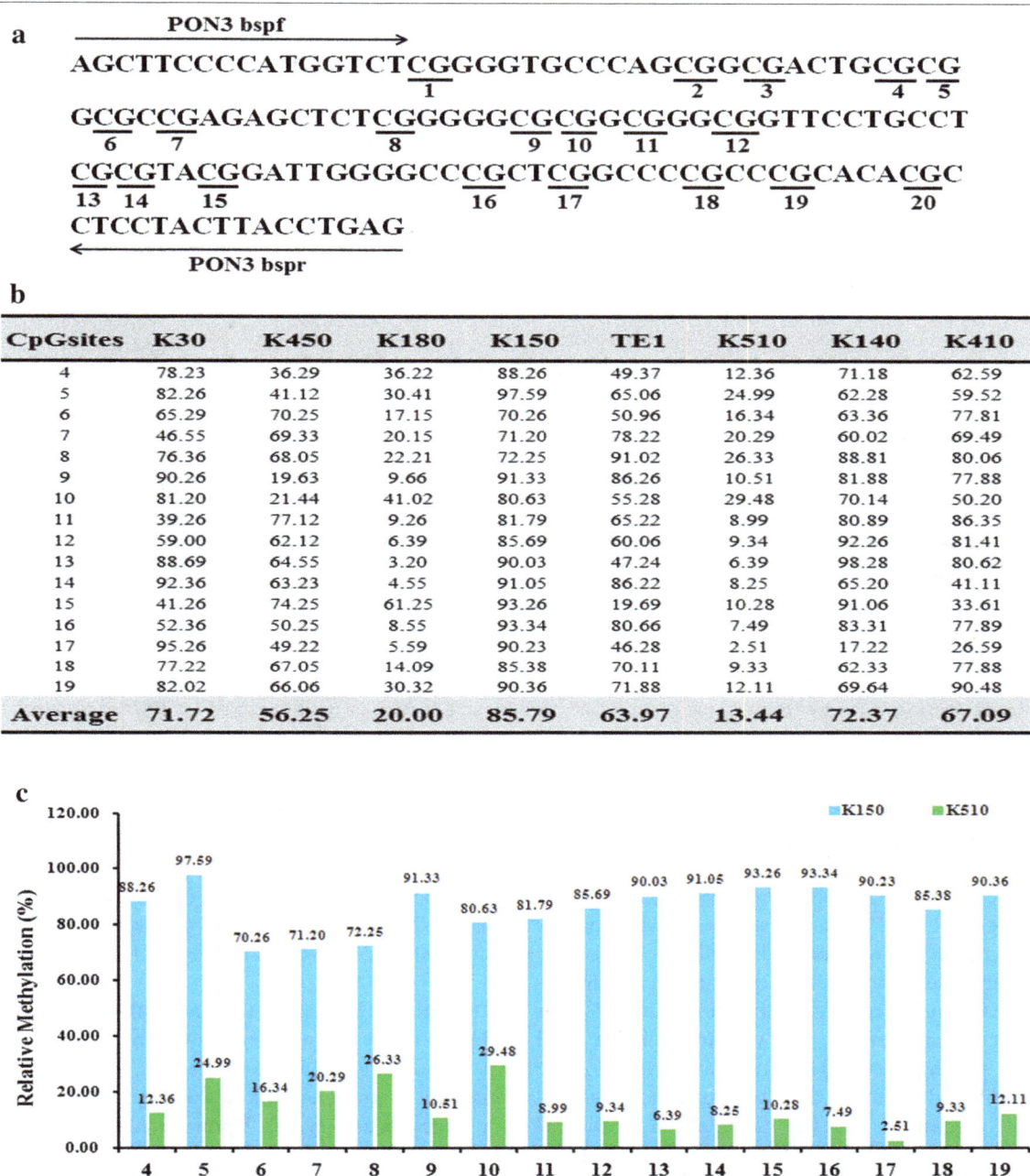

**Fig. 2** Differential methylation of the PON3 gene in eight esophageal cancer cell lines. **a** BSP primers and CpG dinucleotides of PON3 are shown. **b** Relative methylation levels (fold) of PON3 in eight esophageal cancer cell lines. **c** Methylation percentage at each CpG site in the K150 and K510 cells

## PON3 suppresses the migration and invasion of EC cells in vitro

The differential methylation state as well as the different expression level of PON3 in the EC cell lines indicate their potential roles in the metastasis of EC. We then compared the migration and invasion capability of K510 and K150 cells using the wound-healing and matrigel invasion assays, respectively. Compared to the control cells, transfection of si-PON3 into K510 cells significantly increased the migration capability, whereas transfection of GFP-PON3 into K150 cells largely decreased the migration capability (Fig. 5a). The results suggest that the

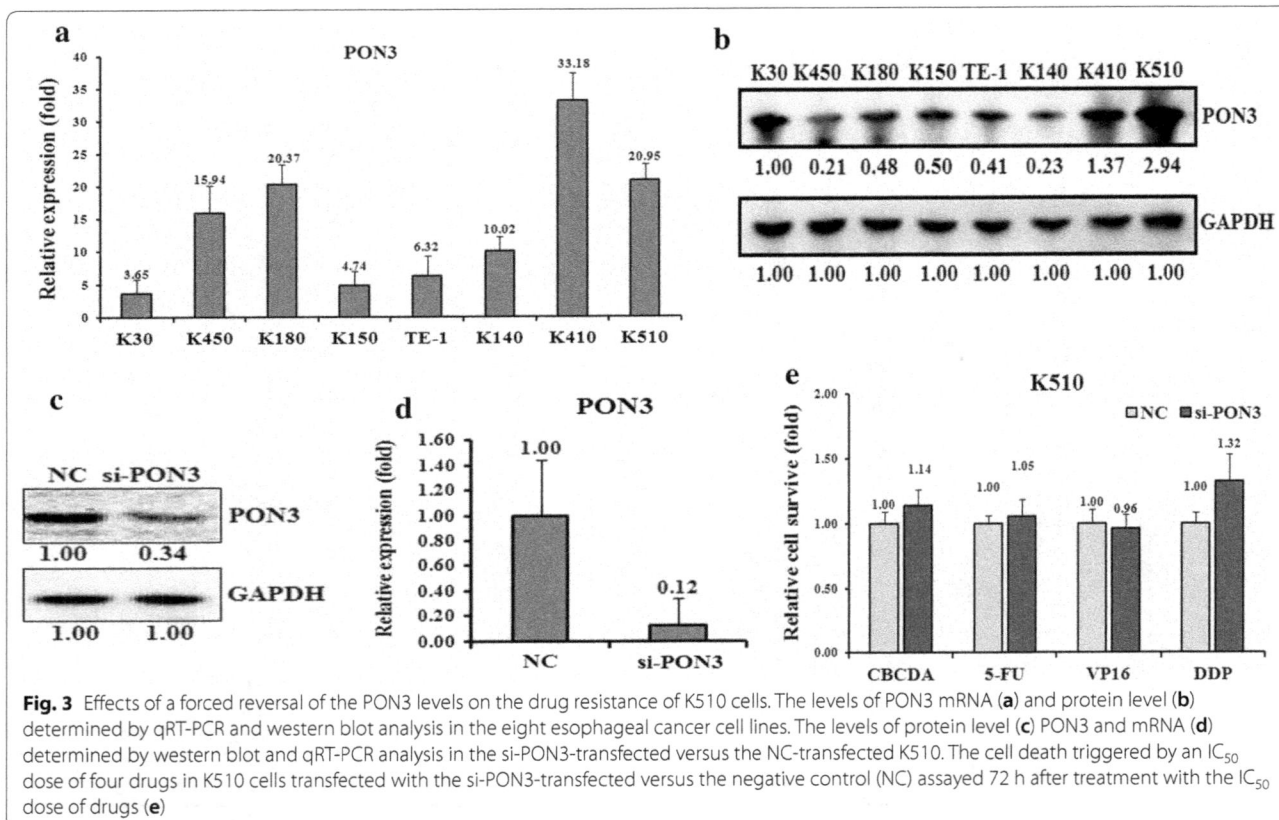

**Fig. 3** Effects of a forced reversal of the PON3 levels on the drug resistance of K510 cells. The levels of PON3 mRNA (**a**) and protein level (**b**) determined by qRT-PCR and western blot analysis in the eight esophageal cancer cell lines. The levels of protein level (**c**) PON3 and mRNA (**d**) determined by western blot and qRT-PCR analysis in the si-PON3-transfected versus the NC-transfected K510. The cell death triggered by an $IC_{50}$ dose of four drugs in K510 cells transfected with the si-PON3-transfected versus the negative control (NC) assayed 72 h after treatment with the $IC_{50}$ dose of drugs (**e**)

PON3 level negatively correlates with the migration of EC cells. Similar results are also found for the invasion assays, as revealed by the transfection of either si-PON3 into K510 cells, or GFP-PON3 into K150 cells (Fig. 5b). Taken together, PON3 might act as a negative regulator of both migration and invasion of EC cells.

To further understand the underlying molecular mechanisms of EC drug resistance, we measured the activities of the ten classical signaling pathways in both K510 and K150 cells. Among the ten pathways, the activities of five pathways differed by more than two-folds in K510 and K150 cells, suggesting that they might play a role in EC drug resistance. Among them, four pathways, p53/DNA damage, NF-κB, MAPK/ERK and PI3K/AKT showed higher activities in K510 cells, whereas cAMP/PKA showed higher activities in K150 cells (Fig. 6a). We then determined which of the five pathways were also affected by forced changes of the PON3 level in both K150 and K510 cells. As shown in Figure 6B and 6C, upon the repression of PON3 level by si-PON3 in K510 cells, the activities of p53/DNA damage, NF-κB, and PI3K/AKT were elevated, which correlate well with the negative regulation of these pathways by PON3 in K510 cells (Fig. 6c). We also transfected GFP-PON3 into K150 cells and measured the activities of these five pathways in K150 cells.

Following the increase of the PON3 level, the NF-κB and PI3K/AKT pathways were repressed (Fig. 6c), which is in agreement with the forced changes of PON3 level in K510 cells upon transfection of si-PON3. Overall, we propose that the NF-κB and PI3K/AKT pathways involve in the EC drug resistance mediated by the PON3 gene.

### PON3 inhibits both the growth and DDP drug resistance of K510-derived tumor xenografts in nude mice

To investigate the in vivo effect of PON3 on EC drug resistance, we generated a K510-derived tumor model in nude mice (Fig. 7a). Upon transfection of si-PON3, K510-derived tumors were approximately 2.4-folds heavier than the control cells, suggesting that PON3 inhibits tumor growth in vivo. In addition, after an intraperitoneal injection of DDP, the K510 tumors were much smaller than the control cells with the injection of PBS (Fig. 7b). Furthermore, the tumor weight for the si-PON3/DDP K510 mice was heavier than that in the DDP K510 mice (Fig. 7b). These results clearly indicated that PON3 inhibits both the growth and DDP drug resistance of K510-derived tumor xenografts in nude mice.

Further confirmation of the PON3 role in the DDP resistance of EC came from the immunohistological analysis of PON3 and Ki67 (an indicator of tumor cell

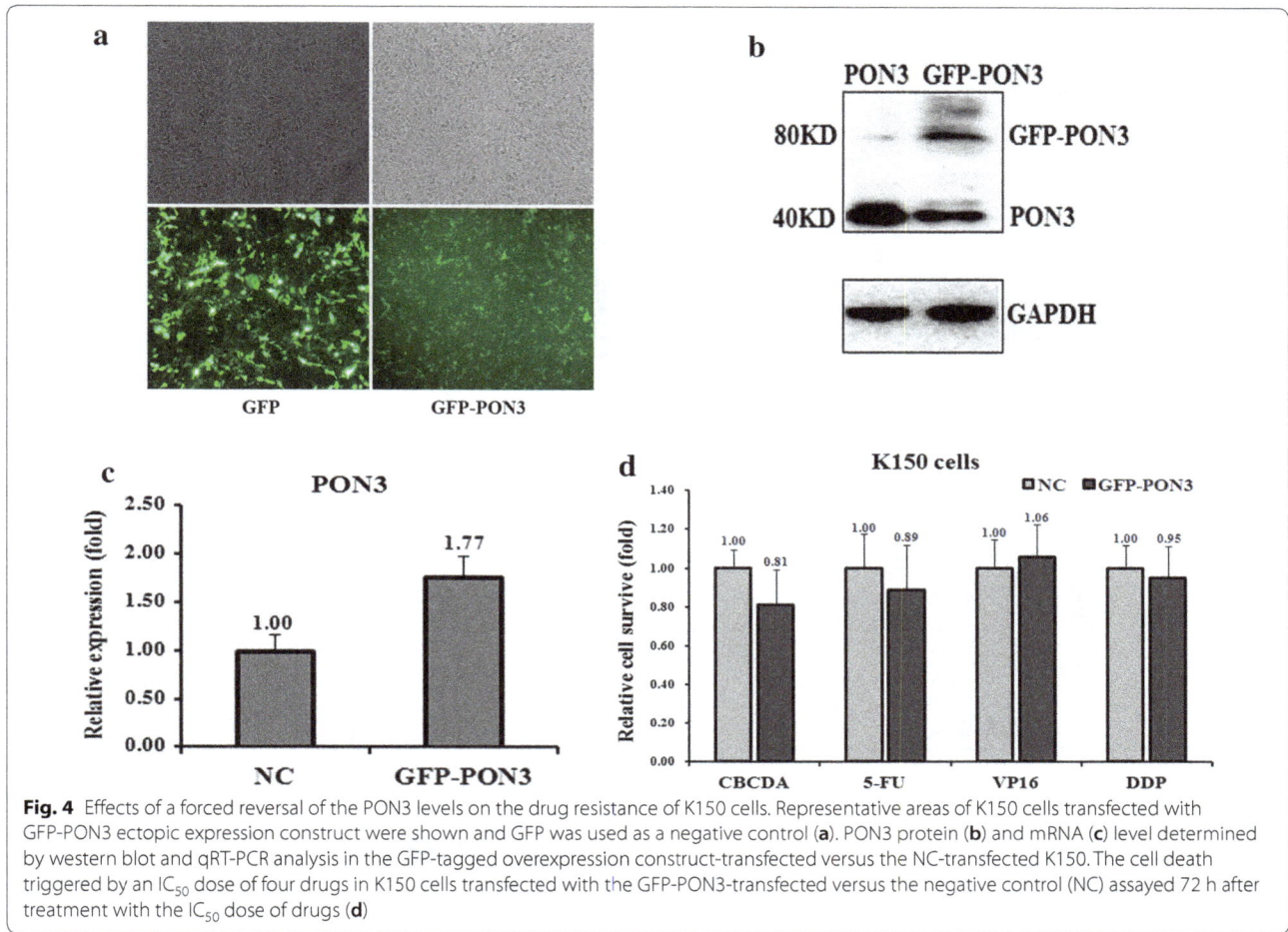

**Fig. 4** Effects of a forced reversal of the PON3 levels on the drug resistance of K150 cells. Representative areas of K150 cells transfected with GFP-PON3 ectopic expression construct were shown and GFP was used as a negative control (**a**). PON3 protein (**b**) and mRNA (**c**) level determined by western blot and qRT-PCR analysis in the GFP-tagged overexpression construct-transfected versus the NC-transfected K150. The cell death triggered by an $IC_{50}$ dose of four drugs in K150 cells transfected with the GFP-PON3-transfected versus the negative control (NC) assayed 72 h after treatment with the $IC_{50}$ dose of drugs (**d**)

proliferation) in the tumor sections of the DDP-treated versus PBS-treated mice (Fig. 7c). The intratumoral injection of si-PON3 into K510 indeed led to the decrease of the PON3 level in the tumor sections (Fig. 7c), which further confirmed that PON3 has a positive effect on both the growth and drug resistance of EC cell-derived tumor xenografts in nude mice

## Discussion

Accumulating evidences have been shown that DNA methylation play important roles in drug resistance of cancers, which prevents the effective treatment of cancers [15]. Altered DNA methylation patterns can influence the expression of genes [16]. Recent study on the profiling of gene-specific methylation levels in EC provides a useful approach for investigating the individual hypermethylated gene in EC [17]. Despite extensive studies revealed that methylation is a modulator of cancer, the understanding of DNA methylation on the effect of EC remains limited. In our study, we identified that the promoter region of PON3 is hypermethylated in drug resistant EC cell lines. The hypermethylation of PON3 in return down-regulates its expression in drug resistant EC cells. Furthermore, we showed that the PON3 level is negatively correlated with the drug-resistance of EC cells, and thus suppresses the EC drug resistance. In vivo experiments also found that PON3 inhibits tumor growth in nude mice. All these findings made us to propose that PON3 might be a tumor suppressor, considering its high methylation in the promoter region and low expression level in multiple cancers.

Paraoxonase 3 (PON3) belongs to the paraoxonase family that helps in preventing oxidative stress and anti-inflammatory [18]. This gene also involves in other diseases including cancer [19, 20]. PON3 gene has a high expression level in cancer tissues of the lung, liver and colon [11]. Previous studies also showed that PON3 is hypermethylated in colorectal cancer [9] and chordomas [21]. Notably, the genome-wide DNA methylation analysis identified that several genes, including PON3, are aberrantly methylated in the high-grade non-muscle invasive bladder cancer [22]. These findings suggest that

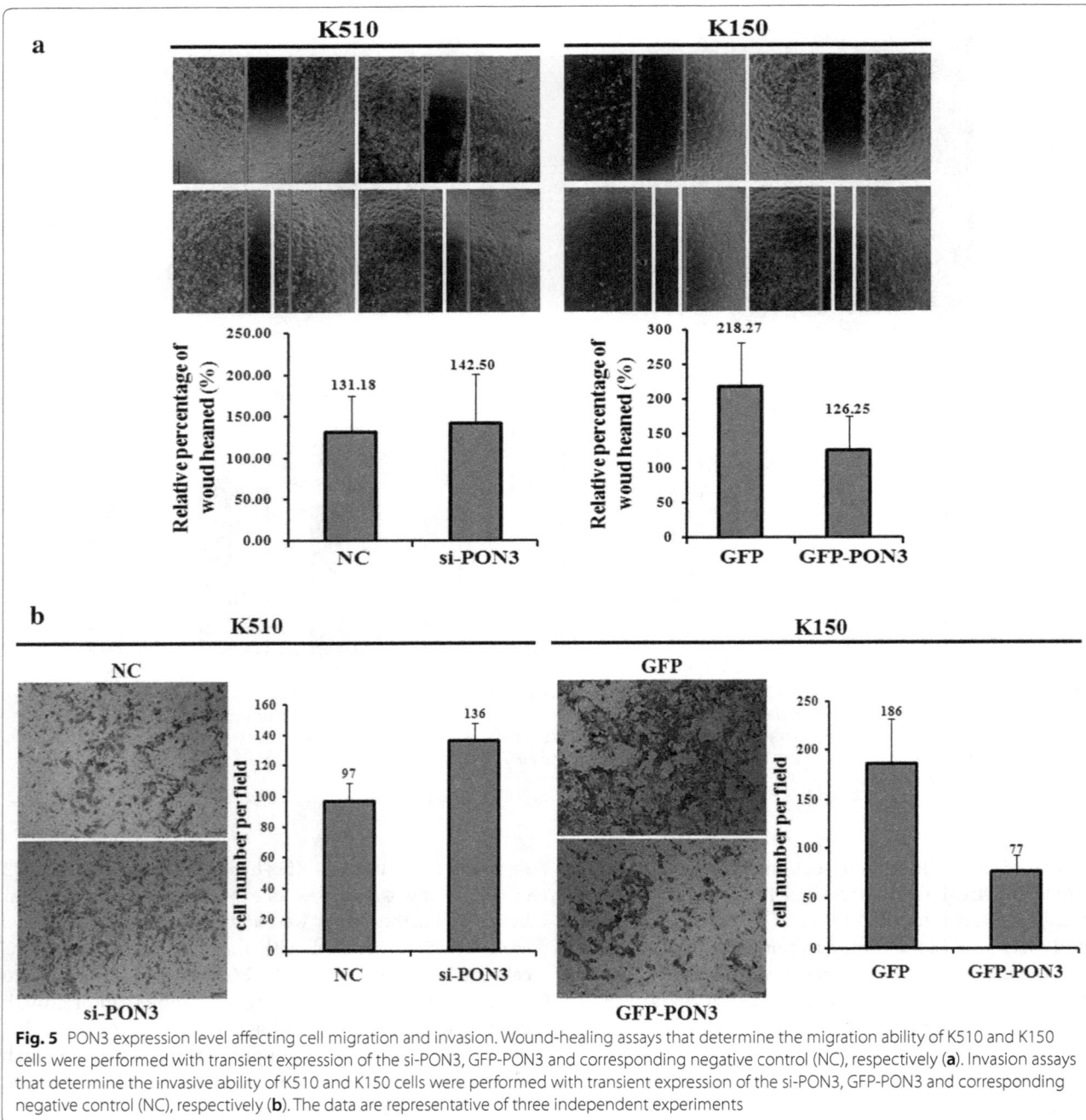

**Fig. 5** PON3 expression level affecting cell migration and invasion. Wound-healing assays that determine the migration ability of K510 and K150 cells were performed with transient expression of the si-PON3, GFP-PON3 and corresponding negative control (NC), respectively (**a**). Invasion assays that determine the invasive ability of K510 and K150 cells were performed with transient expression of the si-PON3, GFP-PON3 and corresponding negative control (NC), respectively (**b**). The data are representative of three independent experiments

epigenetic modifications are usually associated with the development and/or progression of different type of tumors [13, 23]. In accordance with previous studies, we identified that the promoter region of PON3 is hypermethylated in EC cancer. The hypermethylation of PON3 may serve as a marker of poor prognosis in human EC. Furthermore, the expression of PON3 negatively correlates with drug resistance in EC cells, and thus appears to act a biomarker for the drug resistance of EC cells. The study may provide a new potential therapeutic target in the treatment of EC. However, the detailed mechanism for the PON3-regulated drug resistance in EC cells remains to be clarified.

**a**

| Pathway | Transcription Factor | K150 | K510 | K510/K150 |
|---|---|---|---|---|
| Wnt | TCF/LEF | 125.36 | 150.25 | 0.834 |
| Notch | RBP-Jκ | 40.11 | 51.71 | 0.776 |
| p53/DNA Damage | p53 | 21.74 | 9.30 | 2.338 |
| TGFβ | SMAD2/3/4 | 10.51 | 15.44 | 0.681 |
| NFκB | NFκB | 950.25 | 77.54 | 12.255 |
| MAPK/ERK | Elk-1/SRF | 363.39 | 126.33 | 2.877 |
| cAMP/PKA | CREB | 8.69 | 107.52 | 0.081 |
| MAPK/JNK | FOS/JUN | 16.28 | 33.26 | 0.489 |
| PI3K/AKT | FOXO | 161.00 | 13.39 | 12.024 |
| PKC/Ca++ | NFAT | 152.11 | 110.62 | 1.375 |
| Negative Control | | 1.00 | 1.00 | 1.000 |

**b**

| Pathway | Transcription Factor | K150 | | K510 | |
|---|---|---|---|---|---|
| | | GFP | GFP-PON3 | NC | si-PON3 |
| p53/DNA Damage | p53 | 1.00±0.34 | 4.04±0.44 | 1.00±0.45 | 3.39±0.25 |
| NFκB | NFκB | 1.00±0.75 | 0.52±0.29 | 1.00±0.36 | 10.78±0.66 |
| MAPK/ERK | Elk-1/SRF | 1.00±0.42 | 3.09±0.40 | 1.00±0.40 | 0.77±0.57 |
| cAMP/PKA | CREB | 1.00±0.30 | 1.33±0.36 | 1.00±0.28 | 10.71±0.53 |
| PI3K/AKT | FOXO | 1.00±0.74 | 0.57±0.59 | 1.00±0.39 | 6.62±0.49 |

**c**

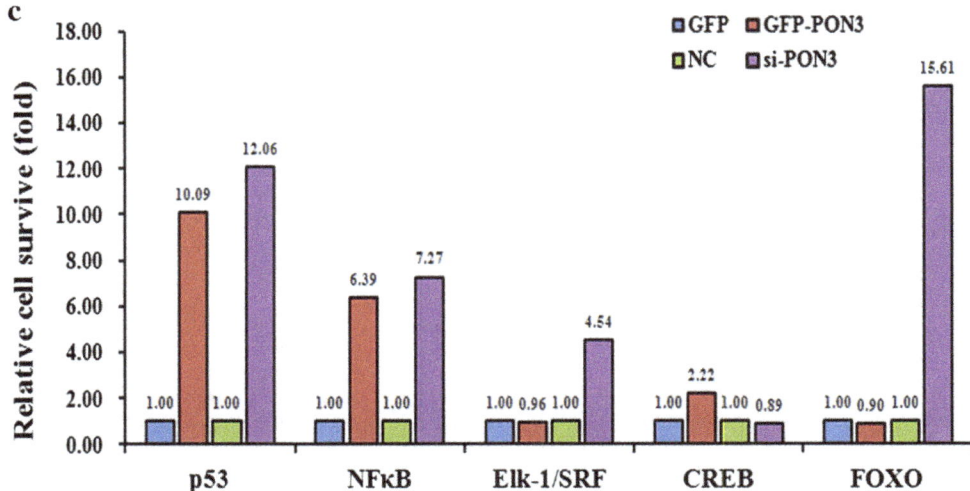

**Fig. 6** The effects of the forced reversal of PON3 levels on the activity of the signaling pathways in K150 versus K510 cells. The activities of the ten pathways in K150 versus K510 cells (**a**). The relative pathway activities in the PON3 siRNA- and GFP-PON3 versus the corresponding NC, which were transfected in K510 and K150 cells, respectively (**b**). The expression ratio of the five transcription Factors in the PON3 siRNA- and GFP-PON3 versus the corresponding NC- transfected in K510 and K150 cells, respectively (**c**)

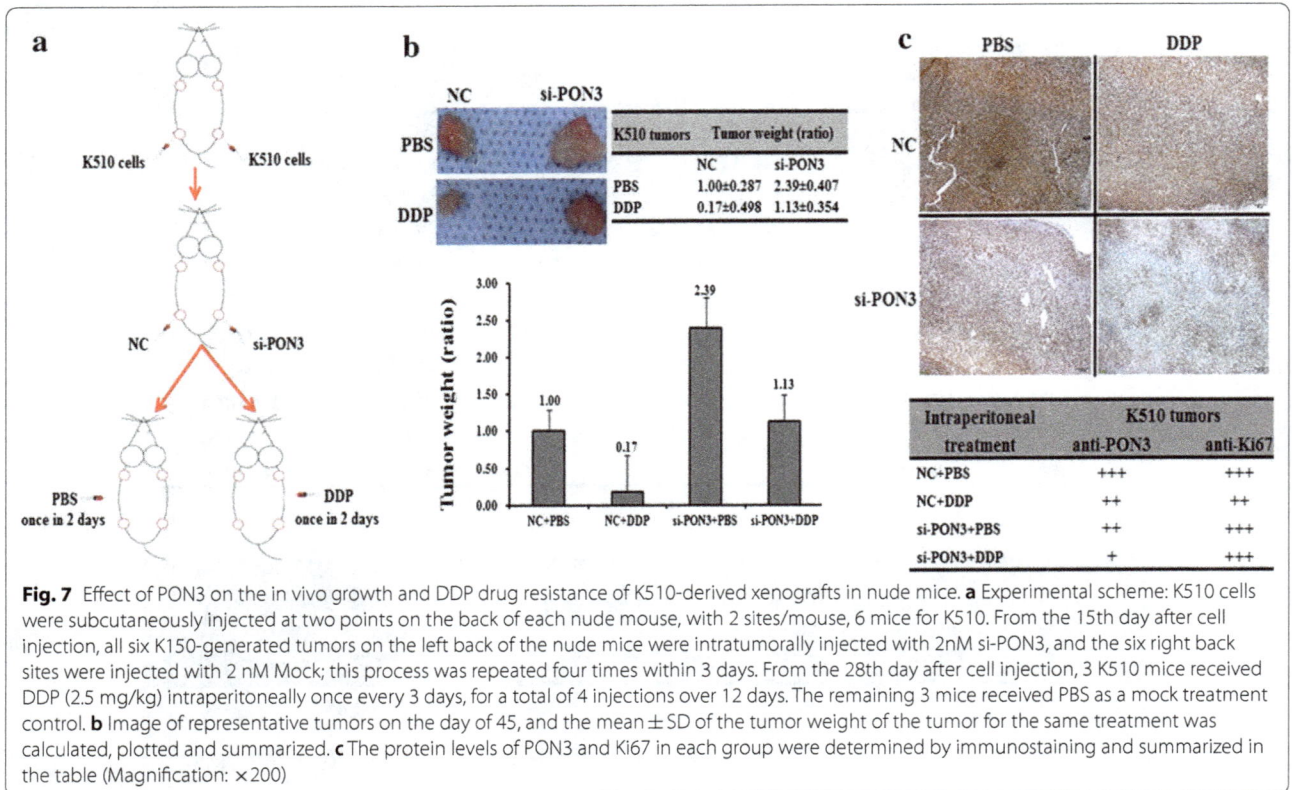

**Fig. 7** Effect of PON3 on the in vivo growth and DDP drug resistance of K510-derived xenografts in nude mice. **a** Experimental scheme: K510 cells were subcutaneously injected at two points on the back of each nude mouse, with 2 sites/mouse, 6 mice for K510. From the 15th day after cell injection, all six K150-generated tumors on the left back of the nude mice were intratumorally injected with 2nM si-PON3, and the six right back sites were injected with 2 nM Mock; this process was repeated four times within 3 days. From the 28th day after cell injection, 3 K510 mice received DDP (2.5 mg/kg) intraperitoneally once every 3 days, for a total of 4 injections over 12 days. The remaining 3 mice received PBS as a mock treatment control. **b** Image of representative tumors on the day of 45, and the mean ± SD of the tumor weight of the tumor for the same treatment was calculated, plotted and summarized. **c** The protein levels of PON3 and Ki67 in each group were determined by immunostaining and summarized in the table (Magnification: ×200)

## Conclusions

In this work, we identified that PON3 is associated with the multi-drug resistance of EC cancer. Our findings suggest that PON3 may serve as a biomarker for the potential therapeutic treatment of EC.

### Abbreviations
EC: esophageal cancer; BSP: bisulfite sequencing PCR; CBCDA: carboplatin; 5-FU: 5-fluorouracil; VP-16: etoposide phosphate; DDP: cisplatin; PON3: paraoxonase 3.

### Authors' contributions
DBH, YW, SLH and YYP made substantial contributions to conception and design, acquisition of data, and analysis and interpretation of data, and were involved in drafting and critically revising the manuscript for important intellectual content. DBH, YW and YYP was principally responsible for drafting the manuscript and for several cycles of revision of the manuscript. YFH, GW, WW, XHH, YBS, GDS, MC, GB and XF made substantial contributions to analysis and interpretation of data and were involved in critically revising the manuscript for important intellectual content. BJS, LL made substantial contributions to conception and design, and analysis and interpretation of data and was involved in drafting and critically revising the manuscript for important intellectual content. All authors read and approved the final manuscript.

### Author details
[1] Department of Oncology, the First Affiliated Hospital of USTC, Division of Life Sciences and Medicine, University of Science and Technology of China, Hefei 230001, Anhui, People's Republic of China. [2] Department of Oncology, The Affiliated Hospital of Anhui Medical University, Hefei 230001, Anhui, People's Republic of China. [3] Department of Geriatrics, the First Affiliated Hospital of USTC, Division of Life Sciences and Medicine, University of Science and Technology of China, Hefei 230001, Anhui, People's Republic of China. [4] Anhui Provincial Key Laboratory of Tumor Immunotherapy and Nutrition Therapy, Hefei 230001, Anhui, People's Republic of China. [5] Gerontology Institute of Anhui Province, Hefei 230001, Anhui, People's Republic of China.

### Acknowledgements
Not applicable.

### Competing interests
The authors declare that they have no competing interests.

### Funding
This work was supported by the Special Subsidy for Central Guidance of China (2017070503B041 granted to SLH), Anhui Provincial science and technology key projects (1501041142 granted to SLH), Anhui Provincial Key Laboratory of Tumor Immunotherapy and Nutrition Therapy (1606c08236 granted to SLH) and the Key research and development plan of Anhui Province (1704a0802148 granted to YYP).

### References
1. Torre LA, Bray F, Siegel RL, Ferlay J, Lortet-Tieulent J, Jemal A. Global cancer statistics, 2012. CA Can J Clin. 2015;65(2):87–108.
2. Chen W, Zheng R, Baade PD, Zhang S, Zeng H, Bray F, Jemal A, Yu XQ, He J. Cancer statistics in China, 2015. CA Cancer J Clin. 2016;66(2):115–32.

3.  Kim T, Grobmyer SR, Smith R, Ben-David K, Ang D, Vogel SB, Hoch-wald SN. Esophageal cancer—the five year survivors. J Surg Oncol. 2011;103(2):179–83.

4.  Katoh R, Takebayashi Y, Takenoshita S. Expression of copper-transporting P-type adenosine triphosphatase (ATP7B) as a chemoresistance marker in human solid carcinomas. Ann Thorac Cardiovasc Surg. 2005;11(3):143–5.

5.  Shim HJ, Cho SH, Hwang JE, Bae WK, Song SY, Cho SB, Lee WS, Joo YE, Na KJ, Chung IJ. Phase II study of docetaxel and cisplatin chemotherapy in 5-fluorouracil/cisplatin pretreated esophageal cancer. Am J Clin Oncol. 2010;33(6):624–8.

6.  Mochizuki H, Scherer SW, Xi T, Nickle DC, Majer M, Huizenga JJ, Tsui LC, Prochazka M. Human PON2 gene at 7q21.3: cloning, multiple mRNA forms, and missense polymorphisms in the coding sequence. Gene. 1998;213(1–2):149–57.

7.  Primo-Parmo SL, Sorenson RC, Teiber J, La Du BN. The human serum paraoxonase/arylesterase gene (PON1) is one member of a multigene family. Genomics. 1996;33(3):498–507.

8.  Camps J, Marsillach J, Joven J. The paraoxonases: role in human diseases and methodological difficulties in measurement. Crit Rev Clin Lab Sci. 2009;46(2):83–106.

9.  Baharudin R, Ab Mutalib NS, Othman SN, Sagap I, Rose IM, Mohd Mokhtar N, Jamal R. Identification of predictive DNA methylation biomarkers for chemotherapy response in colorectal cancer. Front Pharmacol. 2017;8:47.

10.  Witte I, Foerstermann U, Devarajan A, Reddy ST, Horke S. Protectors or traitors: the roles of PON2 and PON3 in atherosclerosis and cancer. J Lipids. 2012;2012:342806.

11.  Schweikert EM, Devarajan A, Witte I, Wilgenbus P, Amort J, Forstermann U, Shabazian A, Grijalva V, Shih DM, Farias-Eisner R, et al. PON3 is upregu-lated in cancer tissues and protects against mitochondrial superoxide-mediated cell death. Cell Death Differ. 2012;19(9):1549–60.

12.  Zhu L, Shen Y, Sun W. Paraoxonase 3 promotes cell proliferation and metastasis by PI3K/Akt in oral squamous cell carcinoma. Biomed Pharma-cother. 2017;85:712–7.

13.  Lv L, Deng H, Li Y, Zhang C, Liu X, Liu Q, Zhang D, Wang L, Pu Y, Zhang H, et al. The DNA methylation-regulated miR-193a-3p dictates the multi-chemoresistance of bladder cancer via repression of SRSF2/PLAU/HIC2 expression. Cell Death Dis. 2014;5:e1402.

14.  Lv L, Deng H, Li Y, Zhang C, Liu X, Liu Q, Zhang D, Wang L, Pu Y, Zhang H, He Y, Wang Y, Yu Y, Yu T, Zhu J. The DNA methylation-regulated miR-193a-3p dictates the multi-chemoresistance of bladder cancer via repres-sion of SRSF2/PLAU/HIC2 expression. Cell Death Dis. 2014;5:e1402.

15.  Edwards JR, Yarychkivska O, Boulard M, Bestor TH. DNA methylation and DNA methyltransferases. Epigenet Chromatin. 2017;10:23.

16.  Wajed SA, Laird PW, DeMeester TR. DNA methylation: an alternative pathway to cancer. Ann Surg. 2001;234(1):10–20.

17.  Haque MH, Gopalan V, Islam MN, Masud MK, Bhattacharjee R, Hossain MSA, Nguyen NT, Lam AK, Shiddiky MJA. Quantification of gene-specific DNA methylation in oesophageal cancer via electrochemistry. Anal Chim Acta. 2017;976:84–93.

18.  Rosenblat M, Draganov D, Watson CE, Bisgaier CL, La Du BN, Aviram M. Mouse macrophage paraoxonase 2 activity is increased whereas cellular paraoxonase 3 activity is decreased under oxidative stress. Arterioscler Thromb Vasc Biol. 2003;23(3):468–74.

19.  Devarajan A, Shih D, Reddy ST. Inflammation, infection, cancer and all that… the role of paraoxonases. Adv Exp Med Biol. 2014;824:33–41.

20.  Rull A, Garcia R, Fernandez-Sender L, Garcia-Heredia A, Aragones G, Beltran-Debon R, Marsillach J, Alegret JM, Martin-Paredero V, Mackness B, et al. Serum paraoxonase-3 concentration is associated with insulin sensitivity in peripheral artery disease and with inflammation in coronary artery disease. Atherosclerosis. 2012;220(2):545–51.

21.  Alholle A, Brini AT, Bauer J, Gharanei S, Niada S, Slater A, Gentle D, Maher ER, Jeys L, Grimer R, et al. Genome-wide DNA methylation profiling of recurrent and non-recurrent chordomas. Epigenetics. 2015;10(3):213–20.

22.  Kitchen MO, Bryan RT, Emes RD, Glossop JR, Luscombe C, Cheng KK, Zeegers MP, James ND, Devall AJ, Mein CA, et al. Quantitative genome-wide methylation analysis of high-grade non-muscle invasive bladder cancer. Epigenetics. 2016;11(3):237–46.

23.  Marofi F, Vahedi G, Solali S, Alivand M, Salarinasab S, Zadi Heydarabad M, Farshdousti Hagh M. Gene expression of TWIST1 and ZBTB16 is regulated by methylation modifications during the osteoblastic differentiation of mesenchymal stem cells. J Cell Physiol. 2018. https://doi.org/10.1002/jcp.27352.

# 4

# Genome editing of oncogenes with ZFNs and TALENs: caveats in nuclease design

Sumitra Shankar, Ahalya Sreekumar, Deepti Prasad, Ani V. Das and M. Radhakrishna Pillai[*] ⓘ

## Abstract

**Background:** Gene knockout technologies involving programmable nucleases have been used to create knockouts in several applications. Gene editing using Zinc-finger nucleases (ZFNs), Transcription activator like effectors (TALEs) and CRISPR/Cas systems has been used to create changes in the genome in order to make it non-functional. In the present study, we have looked into the possibility of using six fingered CompoZr ZFN pair to target the E6 gene of HPV 16 genome.

**Methods:** HPV 16[+ve] cell lines; SiHa and CaSki were used for experiments. CompoZr ZFNs targeting E6 gene were designed and constructed by Sigma-Aldrich. TALENs targeting E6 and E7 genes were made using TALEN assembly kit. Gene editing was monitored by T7E1 mismatch nuclease and Nuclease resistance assays. Levels of E6 and E7 were further analyzed by RT-PCR, western blot as well as immunoflourescence analyses. To check if there is any interference due to methylation, cell lines were treated with sodium butyrate, and Nocodazole.

**Results:** Although ZFN editing activity in yeast based MEL-I assay was high, it yielded very low activity in tumor cell lines; only 6% editing in CaSki and negligible activity in SiHa cell lines. Though editing efficiency was better in CaSki, no significant reduction in E6 protein levels was observed in immunocytochemical analysis. Further, in silico analysis of DNA binding prediction revealed that some of the ZFN modules bound to sequence that did not match the target sequence. Hence, alternate ZFN pairs for E6 and E7 were not synthesized since no further active sites could be identified by in silico analyses. Then we designed TALENs to target E6 and E7 gene. TALENs designed to target E7 gene led to reduction of E7 levels in CaSki and SiHa cervical cancer cell lines. However, TALEN designed to target E6 gene did not yield any editing activity.

**Conclusions:** Our study highlights that designed nucleases intended to obtain bulk effect should have a reasonable editing activity which reflects phenotypically as well. Nucleases with low editing efficiency, intended for generation of knockout cell lines nucleases could be obtained by single cell cloning. This could serve as a criterion for designing ZFNs and TALENs.

**Keywords:** Zinc-finger nucleases, TALEN, HPV, Cervical cancer, Gene editing

## Background

The field of gene therapy has advanced a lot with the advent of programming nucleases. Genome engineering involves the use of DNA-binding modules that can be combined with nucleases to impact genomic structure and function. This largely depends on the DNA-binding specificity and affinity of designed zinc-finger and TALE (Transcription activator like effectors) proteins. Recently

*Correspondence: mrpillai@rgcb.res.in
Rajiv Gandhi Centre for Biotechnology, Thiruvananthapuram, India

CRISPR/Cas system has also been used for genome editing experiments [1–4]. Such a knockout technology offers advantage over other approaches such that a specific area of the DNA could be modified with a single dose of administration of these molecules, thereby making permanent change in the genome at once and making it non-functional. Recent reports have shown that programmable nucleases could be used to correct mutations in diseases such as SCID (Severe Combined Immunodeficiency), Hemophilia, and sickle cell disease, etc. [5–7].

These tools have also been used to develop null pheno-types or make a gene non-functional by Non-Homologous End Joining (NHEJ)-mediated double strand break repair which leads to the introduction of small insertions or deletions at the targeted site, resulting in knockout of gene function via frame-shift mutations. In order to make them suitable for clinical applications, DNA binding specificity and affinity plays an important role. In addition to this, the nucleases have been designed as heterodimers to enhance cleavage specificity and reduced toxicity [8, 9].

The possibility of virtually targeting any region in the genome has attracted several researchers to use genome editing tools in their field of study. Genome editing is done using sequence-specific DNA-binding domains fused to a non-specific DNA cleavage module which allow efficient and precise modifications in the gene of interest causing DNA double-strand breaks (DSBs), thereby stimulating the cellular DNA repair mechanisms [10]. Zinc-finger (ZFNs) and transcription activator-like effector proteins (TALENs) are two such DNA binding proteins that could be engineered to target specific gene of interest. Efficiency of targeted gene editing depends on the affinity and specificity of DNA-binding of these nucleases. ZFNs have been successfully applied to excise HIV-I proviral DNA [11] and this has opened up new possibilities of ZFN/TALEN application to target other viral genomes as well. There are studies which have also shown that by combining zinc finger proteins with cell penetrating peptides, HPV-18 DNA replication was inhibited. This capability of these zinc finger fusion proteins to function as potent anti-viral drugs in transient replication assays has also been demonstrated [12]. ZFNs have also been used to target Hepatitis B Virus which prevent viral reactivation and replication [13, 14]. Similarly, TALEN was used to knockout *APOB* gene in order to investigate its role in Hepatitis C Virus infection [15]. These examples show that ZFNs or TALENs could be used to achieve a knockout since they share the same mode of action.

There are several publicly available open access selection approaches created to design zinc finger proteins as well as TALENs with customized specificity [16–19]. A number of software tools have been developed in which the binding specificity of hundreds of artificial and natural zinc fingers have been characterized by several research groups. In spite of advances in nuclease designs, there is still no assurance that the pair would work effectively for that particular target region in a particular system.

Here, ZFNs and TALENs were used to target Human Papillomavirus oncogenes. CompoZr ZFNs (from Sigma) were used to target *E6* gene of HPV 16. Although gene editing activity of the six-fingered CompoZr ZFNs in yeast based MEL-I assay showed activity greater than 50%, editing was found to be low in SiHa and CaSki cervical cancer cell lines was observed by endonuclease assays and immunofluorescence experiments. We looked at DNA binding prediction which revealed that sequences bound by ZFN modules did not match the exact target site hence, we screened for suitable ZFN pairs that could edit *E6* gene using publicly available computational tools. Since no useful target sites were obtained for ZFNs, we designed TALENs targeting *E6* which also did not yield any editing activity in these cell lines. We recently showed that TALENs successfully edited *E7* gene in SiHa cells [20]. We extended this editing study to another HPV$^{+ve}$ cell line CaSki and found similar editing efficiency. There was significant reduction in mRNA and protein levels of E7 after TALEN treatment. In the present study, we have compared the downstream effects of E7 and E6 oncogenes using these synthetic nucleases. From our study we observed that while E7 targeting by TALENs was very successful, E6 targeting by both ZFNs and TALENs turned out to be ineffective.

## Materials and methods
### Cell lines used
Two HPV 16$^{+ve}$ cell lines; SiHa and CaSki were used for experiments. These cell lines were grown in DMEM containing 10% FBS in $CO_2$ incubator at 37 °C. The presence of HPV 16 was confirmed by analyzing the presence of *E6* gene by PCR and also sequencing of *E6* gene in the genomic DNA was isolated from both the cell lines.

### Transfection
Transfection was done using Lipofectamine LTX plus reagent (Cat # 15338100, Invitrogen) as per manufacturer's instructions. The cells were seeded and cultured to reach 60–70% confluency and then transfected with ZFN plasmids (~ 5 μg) using lipofectamine LTX reagent and plus reagent. Briefly, the lipofectamine LTX-plus-DNA complex was prepared in opti-MEM I (Life technologies, USA) and incubated at room temperature for 25 min and then added to the culture plate in a dropwise manner. Plasmid carrying GFP (pGFPmax, Amaxa) was transfected as control to monitor transfection efficiency. Genomic DNA was isolated from both the cell lines and subjected to further analyses.

### Preparation of ssODN
The ssODNs donor template sequences which have a BAMH1 site (underlined) *ATGATATAATATTAGAAT GTGTGTACTGCAAGCAACAGTTACTGCGGATCC GAGGTATATGACTTTGCTTTTCGGGATTTATGCATA GTATATAGA* were synthesized as normal oligonucleotides and purified by PAGE (Sigma). ssODNs were diluted

with RNase free water to 100 μM, and stored at − 20 °C. For ssODN nucleofection, 10 μM of working solution of ssODN was mixed with 5 μg of *ZFN* plasmids before nucleofection. Cells were grown at 37 °C and 5% $CO_2$ after nucleofection. For nucleofection, solution R (82 μl) and supplement of 18 μl were mixed with cells and program A-028 was used (Amaxa) was used.

### TALEN assembly and sequencing

This was done using *Sidansai Biotechnology* TALEN assembly kit (Cat# GL201305-3), according to the vendor's protocol. Briefly, TALE modules and their backbone vector for right arm and left arm were mixed with solution 1, 2 and 3 and keep the tubes in the thermal cycler with a ligation program 37/25° for 20 cycles. Then the ligation mix was transformed into DH5α strain. Colony PCR was done to confirm the positive clones. Then plasmids were isolated from positive clones and sequenced using ABI 310 mix (Bigdye terminator v 3.1, Applied Biosystems). TALEN vector backbone contained the following elements CMV-SP6-3XFlag-NLS-N′-[TALE]-C′-FokI-IRES-puro-pA. TALEN targeting *E6* gene contained 18 modules on both arm and a spacer of 19 nucleotides while TALEN targeting *E7* contained 18 modules on both arm and a spacer of 21 nucleotides.

### CompoZr zinc finger nucleases

ZFNs targeting *E6* gene were designed and constructed by Sigma-Aldrich (St Louis, MO, USA, Lot Number: 08231013MN). The selection of modules, cloning and validation of the ZFNs by Yeast MEL-I assay [21] was performed by Sigma-Aldrich. ZFN design involved using an archive of pre-validated two-finger and one-finger modules. ZFNs used for this study are heterodimers containing Fok I variant EL, KK. The target region was scanned for several positions for which suitable modules existed in the archive. pZFN plasmid contains CMV promoter and BGH polyA tail.

### T7E1 mismatch endonuclease assay

In order to monitor the gene editing, T7E1 mismatch nuclease assay was carried out [22]. For this, genomic DNA was isolated from both the cell lines and PCR for *E6* gene was performed in control and ZFN treated samples. Similarly, PCR was done in TALEN treated cells targeting E6. 10 μl of the PCR products from control and treated samples were taken and subjected to the following program in a thermocycler.

95 °C 10 min
95–85 °C − 2 °C/s
85–25 °C − 0.1 °C/s
4 °C ∞

After the reaction was complete, 1 μl of T7E1 (Cat # M0302S) enzyme and 2 μl of 10× buffer 2 was added to the PCR samples and incubated at 37 °C for 20 min. The digestion product was run in a 2.0% agarose gel and the result was recorded in the gel documentation system (Bio-Rad).

### Nuclease resistance assay

Nuclease resistance assay was also done to confirm the gene editing in SiHa and CaSki cells. Briefly, *E6* gene was amplified from DNA extracted from control and treated samples. 5 μl of the PCR product was digested with HPyChIV4 (Cat # R0619S) enzyme. The interpretation of result is that the control DNA gets completely digested whereas the treated population of cells which have undergone gene editing will give an uncut product. The intensity of the uncut product was analyzed by image J software to measure ZFN editing activity.

### RT-PCR analysis

Isolation of total RNA and cDNA synthesis were carried out as per manufacturer's instructions. RNA was isolated from the SiHa cells using DNA/RNA kit (Qiagen Cat # 80204) and ∼ 1 μg of RNA was transcribed into cDNA using MMLV reverse transcriptase (Promega Cat# M1701), 0.5 μl of dNTPs, 0.5 μl of RNase inhibitor, 4 μl of reverse random primer in a total volume of 20 μl. Specific transcripts were amplified using gene-specific primers:

*HPV E6*
Forward: 5′-ATGCATGGAGATACACCTACATTG-3′,
Reverse: 5′-CATTACATCCCGTACCCTCTTC-3′;
*HPV E7*
Forward: 5′-ATGCACCAAAAGAGAACTGCAATGT-3′,
Reverse: 5′-TTACAGCTGGGTTTCTCTACGTG-3′;
*β-actin*
Forward: 5′-AGACTTCGAGCAGGAGATG-3′,
Reverse: 5′-CTTGATCTTCATGGTGCTAGG-3′

Amplifications were carried out for 25 cycles on a Veriti Thermal cycler (Applied Biosystems) and the products were visualized by ethidium bromide staining after electrophoresis on 2% agarose gel. The bands corresponding to specific transcripts were scanned using a densitometer and normalized against the values corresponding to *β-actin* transcript bands.

### Immunofluorescence

Further to confirm whether ZFN-mediated gene editing resulted in reduction of *E6* and *E7* expression levels in vitro, an immunocytochemical analysis was carried out using specific antibodies. For this, 72 h after treatment, SiHa cells were washed with 1× PBS and fixed in 4% PFA. Cells were then permeabilized with acetone:

methanol (1:1) for 20 min and blocked with 3% BSA for 1 h followed by overnight incubation anti-E6 (1:100, Santacruz, Cat # SC460) and anti-E7 (1:100, Santacruz, Cat # Sc 6981) antibody. After washing three times with 1× PBS, the cells were incubated with secondary bodies in appropriate dilutions (1:400, anti-mouse FITC; Life technologies, Cat# A21200). The cells were counterstained with DAPI (D1306, Thermofisher Scientific) and mounted in 80% glycerol and sealed. Images were taken in confocal laser scanning microscope (Nikon).

In order to further account for the editing, we assessed the expression of 53BP1, a marker for DNA damage by immunocytochemical analysis. Fourteen hours after treatment SiHa cells were washed with PBS and fixed in 4% PFA. Cells were permeabilized with acetone: methanol (1:1) for 20 min and blocked with 3% BSA for 1 h followed by overnight incubation of anti-53BP1 (1:100, Cell signaling Cat # 4937). Cells were then washed with PBS followed by 1 h incubation with anti-rabbit FITC (1:100, Sigma Cat # F9887) and were counterstained with DAPI. Cells were then washed and mounted in 80% glycerol. Images were taken in confocal laser scanning microscope (Nikon).

### Statistical analysis
Results are expressed as mean ± SEM of at least three separate experiments. Statistical analyses were done using Student's t test to determine the significance of the differences between the various conditions.

### Software and tools used for ZFN design

- ZIFIT: It combines OPEN, CODA and modular assembly to screen for zinc finger proteins [23].
- SAPTA: Scoring algorithm for predicting TALEN activity. This tool evaluates and assigns scores of several target sites that give an estimate of predicted TALEN activities [24].
- TALEN-T: TAL effector nucleotide targeter v 2.0 (Cornell University). It is a tool for designing pairs of TALENs to target a specific gene sequence and screens for off-target effects [25].
- B1H screens of C2H2-ZF domains: predicting DNA-binding specificities for C2H2-ZF proteins [26].

## Results
### CompoZr ZFN pair targeting E6 gene demonstrated high editing activity in Yeast Mel I assay but not in cervical cancer cell lines
E6 gene is 477 bp long and it is known to have three exons and two introns [27]. For a simple gene disruption, the first criterion is to target coding exons towards the

beginning of the gene which may create mutations leading to complete abolition of the gene and be less likely to generate truncated protein artifacts with residual biological activity. The second criterion is to screen for unique areas in the genome in order to minimize off-target effects [28]. Based on these design parameters, CompoZr ZFNs (Sigma Aldrich) were designed spanning a region of 117–159 nt in the E6 gene sequence (Fig. 1a, b). This target site was checked for sequence similarity within human genome and showed no match to any genomic sequence. The nuclease pair targeting this region contained six fingers (ZFN amino acid sequence shown in Additional file 1: Figure S1A) on either side of the target site with a spacer region of five nucleotides (Fig. 1c) ZFN editing activity (arbitrary units in y-axis) was analyzed using Yeast based Mel-I assay which showed greater than 50% activity than that of the positive control at 6 h post-induction (Fig. 1d). With a high activity for Mel-I assay, we further assessed the gene editing activity of CompoZr ZFNs in HPV positive cell lines.

Before commencing our experiments on editing with HPV 16 E6 gene, we checked for the presence of HPV-16 in SiHa and CaSki cell lines. PCR analysis revealed the presence of both E6 and E7 genes in SiHa and CaSki cells which was absent in C33A, an HPV$^{-ve}$ cell line (Additional file 1: Figure S1B). Presence of E6 gene in SiHa and CaSki cell lines was further confirmed by PCR and sequencing. Sequencing of the portion of genomic DNA confirmed that indeed these cells contain HPV-E6 and E7 genes (Additional file 1: Figure S1C, D).

Next, we transfected both SiHa and CaSki cells with ZFNs and obtained more than 70% efficiency in transfection in both the cells. Approximately 72 h post-transfection, cells were harvested and genomic DNA was extracted. Then a PCR was performed to amplify E6 gene followed by T7E1 assay to detect NHEJ events. PCR products were amplified followed by denaturation and then gradual re-annealing of the products. T7E1 assay suggested that ~ 6% indels were obtained for E6 in CaSki Cell line (Fig. 1e) whereas negligible activity (only ~ 0.1% indels) was obtained in SiHa cell line (Fig. 1f). These results were further corroborated by complementary nuclease resistance assay (NRA) which also showed a similar result for both CaSki (Fig. 1g) and SiHa cells (Fig. 1h). Further, immunocytochemical analysis for double strand breaks was done using 53bp1 antibody and very few cells containing ZFNs showed double stranded breaks in CaSki cell lines (Fig. 2A–H). We did not check in SiHa cells since these cells showed a negligible editing activity in T7E1 assay. With 6% editing in CaSki, we analyzed whether ZFN-mediated editing could actually reduce the E6 levels in these cells. In order to check this, PCR for E6 gene was carried out and

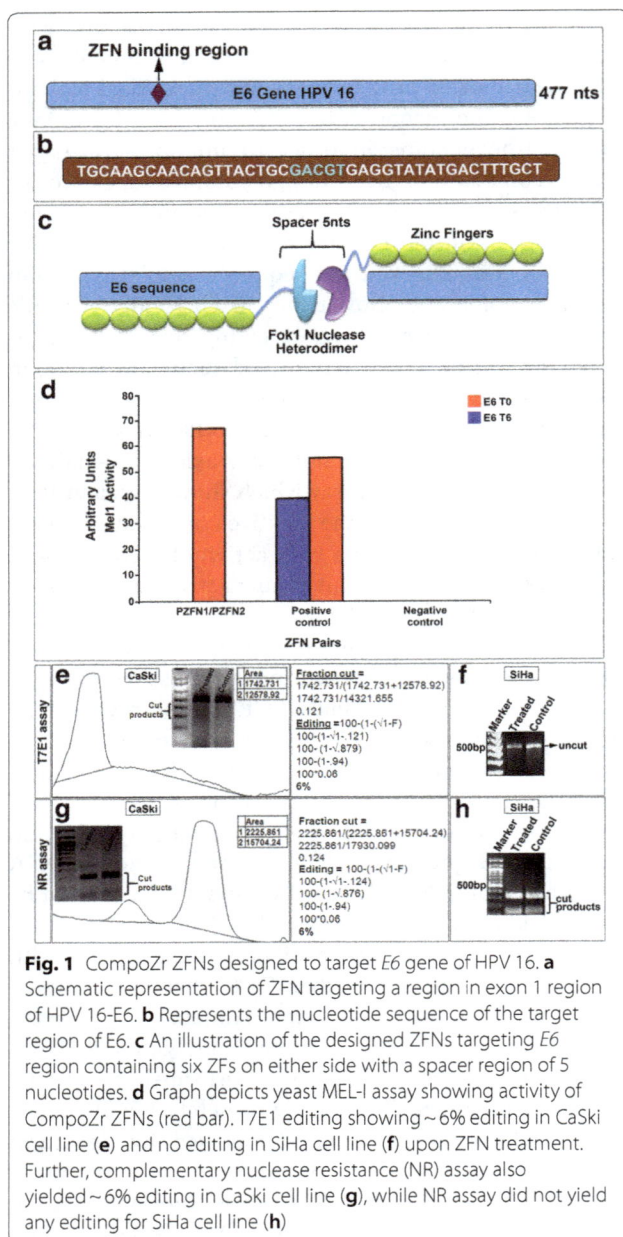

**Fig. 1** CompoZr ZFNs designed to target *E6* gene of HPV 16. **a** Schematic representation of ZFN targeting a region in exon 1 region of HPV 16-E6. **b** Represents the nucleotide sequence of the target region of E6. **c** An illustration of the designed ZFNs targeting *E6* region containing six ZFs on either side with a spacer region of 5 nucleotides. **d** Graph depicts yeast MEL-I assay showing activity of CompoZr ZFNs (red bar). T7E1 editing showing ~6% editing in CaSki cell line (**e**) and no editing in SiHa cell line (**f**) upon ZFN treatment. Further, complementary nuclease resistance (NR) assay also yielded ~6% editing in CaSki cell line (**g**), while NR assay did not yield any editing for SiHa cell line (**h**)

complementary nuclease assay could be done along with T7E1 assay to validate the efficacy of the treatments (Additional file 2: Figure S2C, D). Another group was treated with Nocodazole (Additional file 2: Figure S2E) synchronize all the cells to the same stage of cycle in order to enhance editing before sodium butyrate treatment. We observed that none these treatments improved the editing activity for E6 gene neither in SiHa nor in CaSki cells. Our data suggests that CompoZr ZFNs did not seem to be a successful strategy for E6 editing according to the RT-PCR results, but immunofluorescence assay indicated that some of the CaSki cells were observed to contain significant spots for 53BP1 which suggests that low editing efficiency masked the end point i.e. cells with no E6 phenotypic expression. Still, single cell cloning, and further analysis could probably yield a positive result.

Then we checked if CompoZr ZFN sequences bound to their target site. There have been many reports where ZFNs have failed to produce significant activity and there are many studies which study zinc finger protein binding to its target site. Recently, newer tools are emerging to assess and predict DNA binding to respective target sites. Hence, we performed an in silico analysis using B1-H screens which predicted that some of the modules in CompoZr ZFN 1 and 2 did not match exact binding to the target site (Fig. 4). This method takes into account additional DNA binding DNA–amino acid binding contacts, and higher order interactions that are responsible for specificity. Altogether, our data suggested that editing of HPV-E6 gene was not effective using CompoZr ZFNs.

### Screening for ZFNs targeting E6 of HPV 16 using ZIFIT and Zif Predict tools did not yield any active ZFN pairs

Since ZFNs designed to target E6 gene did not yield any activity, we then screened for other ZFNs to target *E6*. ZFNs targeting HPV-E6 were screened using various open access platforms such as CoDA, OPEN, Modular assembly, Sangamo, Toolgen, Barbas and Zif Predict (Fig. 5). CoDA and OPEN have been reported to give high success rates in editing. For E6 gene of HPV 16 CoDA (Context dependent assembly) that accounts for context dependency and utilizes well characterized N and C terminal finger pools, did not give any hits. OPEN, which has well characterized zinc finger arrays for GNN and TNN triplets [29] showed a few hits for E6 gene, but their prediction scores showed that they were inactive. Likewise, Modular assembly, Sangamo, Toolgen and Zif Predict also failed to yield any target sites for E6. For Modular assembly, it is well known that the likelihood for success depends on more number of GNN triplets as they have been very well validated. However, Barbas modules gave several ZFN target sites for E6 but only one of the half sites showed a high GNN score. All these analyses in

did not find any editing (Fig. 3a). Further, immunocytochemical analysis was carried out with antibody specific to E6. We did not observe any significant difference in E6 levels in CaSki cell line after treatment when we checked by immunocytochemical (Fig. 3b–g) as well as western blot (Fig. 3h) analyses. This suggested that though editing could be observed at gene level, it was not reflected phenotypically.

We further treated cell lines with sodium butyrate to check if there is any interference due to methylation (Additional file 2: Figure S2A, B). Single stranded oligonucleotide (ssODN) treatment was done so that

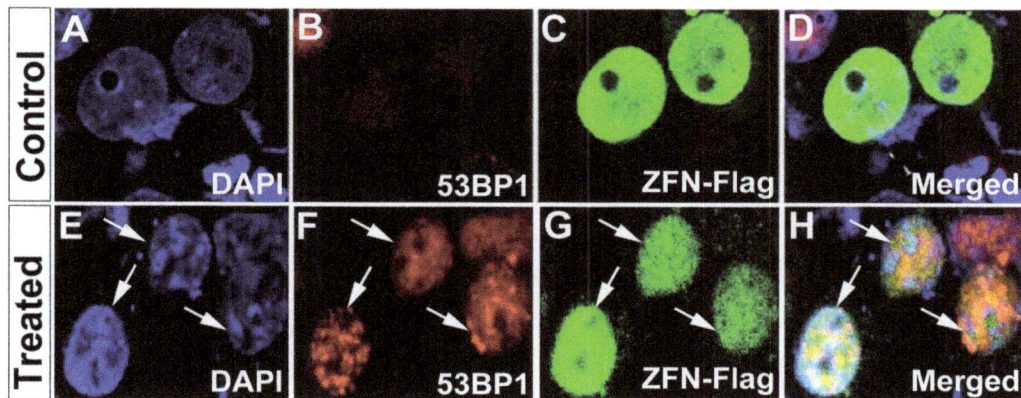

**Fig. 2** ZFN mediated editing indicated by 53bp1 (red spots) in CaSki cells. **A–D** Control cells with vector alone (green) showed no red spots (53bp1). **E–H** Treated cells with CompoZr ZFNs flag tagged (FITC-green) showed red spots indicating double strand breaks. Magnification ×600

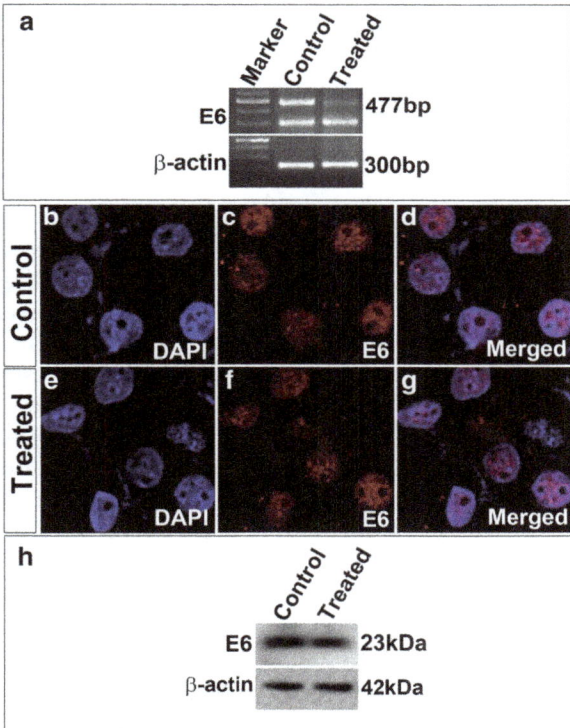

**Fig. 3** Expression analysis of E6 in CaSki cells showed no significant difference between control and treated groups. **a** RT-PCR data indicated that although full length E6 levels were decreased in treated, E6* spliced variant (300 bp) levels remained the same in both control and treated. This was further validated by immunocytochemical analysis for E6 proteins (**b–g**). ZFN treated CaSki cells showed no difference in E6 (red) levels after editing (**e–g**) when compared to control cells (**b–d**). Western blot analysis corroborated with the immunocytochemical analysis indicating no significant difference in E6 levels before and after treatment (**h**). Magnification ×600

our study indicated that identifying a proper ZFN pair to target HPV-E6 gene was difficult using publicly available tools. In silico analysis for ZFNs targeting E7 also did not yield any suitable hits (Additional file 3: Figure S3).

### TALEN pair designed to edit E7 gene showed editing in SiHa and CasKi cell lines

We designed TALENs to edit *E6* gene. Gene editing efficiency of TALENs designed using SAPTA TALEN software targeting *E6* was assessed. In silico, Off-target effects for were checked using TALEN-T software and were found to be zero. However, T7E1 assay for TALENs targeting at position 112 did not yield any editing activity in both the cell lines (Additional file 4: Figure S4). We also designed TALENs targeting position 57 and 284 which also did not yield editing activity in T7E1 assay in both cell lines (Additional file 4: Figure S4). Hence, we designed TALENs to target *E7* gene. TALENs designed targeting the position 44 of *E7* (Fig. 6a) were also found to yield T7E1 editing activity in CaSki cells in vitro (Fig. 6b). We recently reported that TALENs successfully edit *E7* gene in SiHa cells [20], leading to necrotic cell death. This was further corroborated by RT-PCR analysis for the transcripts corresponding to *E7* in both SiHa and CaSki cells. In both the cells the expression of *E7* was drastically reduced in TALEN-edited group (Fig. 6c, d). Immunocytochemical analysis for double strand breaks using 53bp1 antibody further confirmed the efficient editing by the designed TALENs in both SiHa and CaSki cells (Fig. 7a–h). All these results pointed towards an efficient editing of E7 mediated by TALENs in both SiHa as well as CaSki cells. Subsequent immunocytochemical analysis for E7 proteins in both SiHa (Fig. 8A–D) and CaSki (Fig. 8E, F) cells revealed that the TALEN-mediated editing also resulted in the reduction of target E7 proteins in both

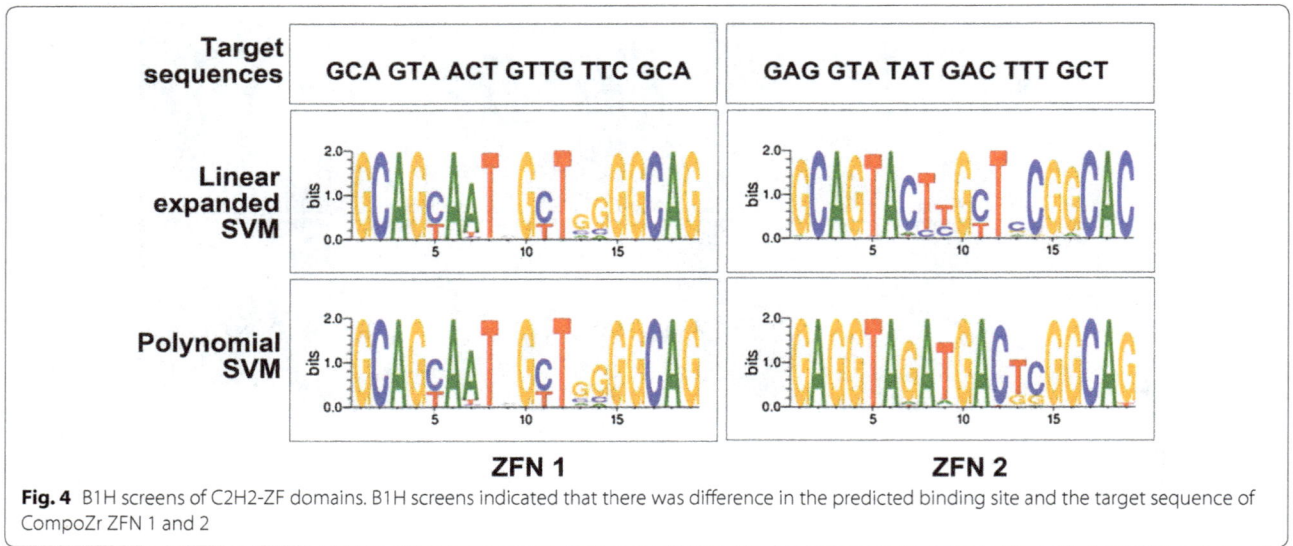

| Target sequences | GCA GTA ACT GTTG TTC GCA | GAG GTA TAT GAC TTT GCT |

**Fig. 4** B1H screens of C2H2-ZF domains. B1H screens indicated that there was difference in the predicted binding site and the target sequence of CompoZr ZFN 1 and 2

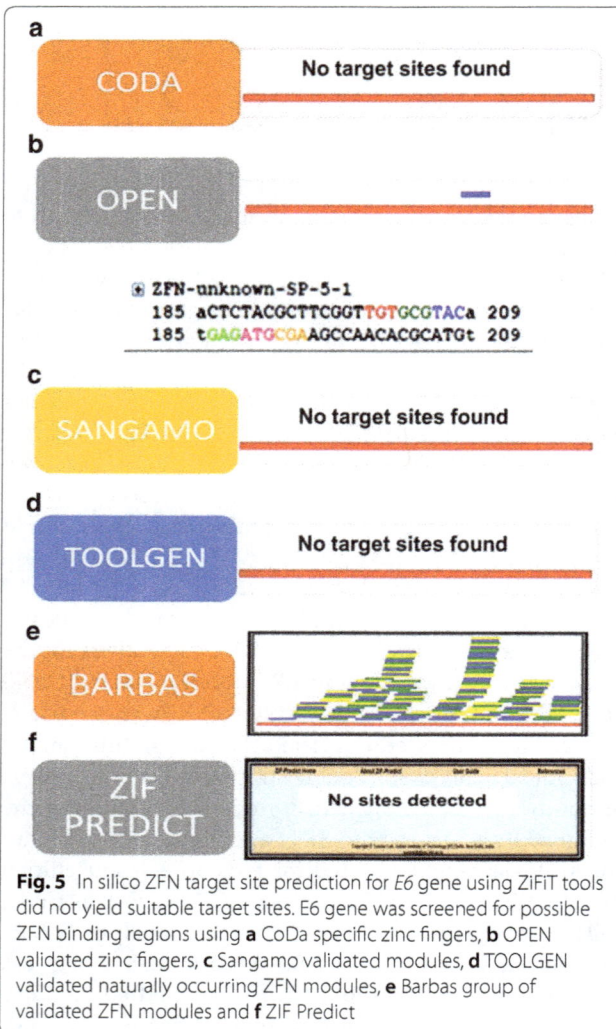

**Fig. 5** In silico ZFN target site prediction for *E6* gene using ZiFiT tools did not yield suitable target sites. E6 gene was screened for possible ZFN binding regions using **a** CoDa specific zinc fingers, **b** OPEN validated zinc fingers, **c** Sangamo validated modules, **d** TOOLGEN validated naturally occurring ZFN modules, **e** Barbas group of validated ZFN modules and **f** ZIF Predict

the cell lines. This was further corroborated by western blot analysis which also showed a marked decrease in E7 proteins in both SiHa and CaSki cells (Fig. 8I). Thus, our results suggested that although TALENs were effective in editing in *E7* gene it was unable to target *E6* gene.

**Discussion**

Gene editing using ZFNs and TALENs has been efficiently used in many systems. The ability to utilize a cell's endogenous repair system has made it possible to make alternations in the gene in a site-specific manner. The duration and magnitude of nuclease expression is an important parameter for both on target and off-target nuclease activity. Recently, CRISPR/Cas system has dominated the gene editing field because it does not require engineering of proteins that bind to DNA in a specific manner. In our study TALEN targeting *E7* gene generated cut products for T7E1 assay and E7 levels were also reduced in both cell lines as indicated in the immunofluorescence and RT- PCR analyses. Our data revealed that TALEN-mediated editing of HPV-*E7* gene showed a reduction in *E7* levels after treatment in both SiHa and CaSki cell lines. However, treating cell lines with TALEN targeting *E6* did not give any editing activity for *E6* gene. It has also been showed by Sander et al. [30] that ZFNs failed to induce any mutations in the gene of interest. The ZFN and TALEN targeting E6 were designed at an exon–intron boundary. TALEN pair designed at exon–intron boundary did not yield any mutations in the target gene [31].

Several ZFN design platforms were screened for E6 gene using publicly available platforms. Since E6 gene had few GNN triplets it indicated that ZiFiT could not

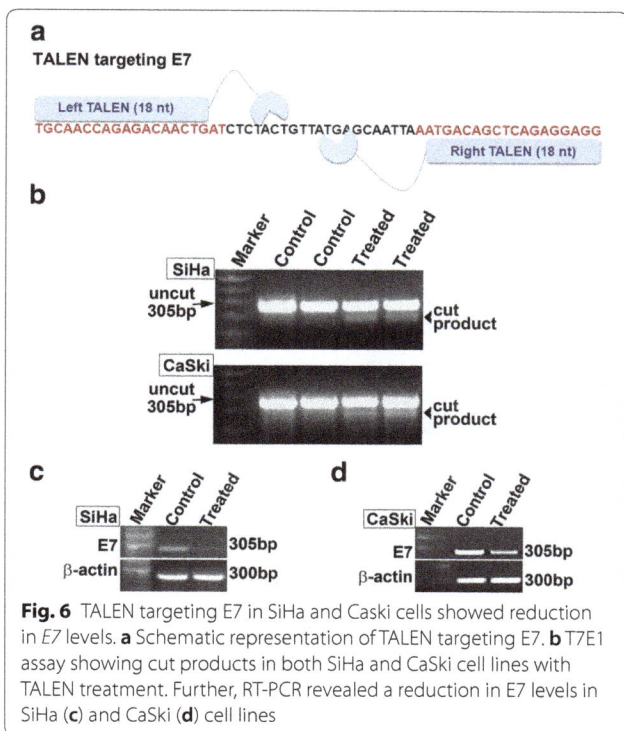

**Fig. 6** TALEN targeting E7 in SiHa and Caski cells showed reduction in *E7* levels. **a** Schematic representation of TALEN targeting E7. **b** T7E1 assay showing cut products in both SiHa and CaSki cell lines with TALEN treatment. Further, RT-PCR revealed a reduction in E7 levels in SiHa (**c**) and CaSki (**d**) cell lines

have been used to successfully design ZFNs to knock-out several genes. In silico analysis implied that limited GNN rich regions in *E6* and *E7* gene sequence of HPV 16 due to low GC content restricted the design options for ZFNs.

Since in silico tools did not yield suitable hits, we procured CompoZr ZFN for *E6* gene. Initial region of the *E6* gene was selected for gene knockout. CompoZr ZFN design for *E6* contained six fingers with more coverage of GNN triplets in the sequence. Genome editing includes many criteria such as number of fingers, spacer length and chromatin accessibility. Another critical factor to be considered is that the target exon should be present in all splice variants. Through this study, it was demonstrated by T7E1 and Nuclease resistance assay that CompoZr ZFNs showed some editing activity of *E6* gene in CaSki cells, but negligible activity in SiHa cell line. This could be attributed to the low editing levels of E6 gene exhibited by the ZFN pair. Further, there was no significant decrease in the levels of E6 in both the cell lines as shown by RT-PCR and immunofluorescence. Though the six-finger design had increased specificity, gene activity reduction due to additional fingers has been indicated in recent reports. It has been reported that the number of fingers and the number of nucleotides in the spacer region can affect the ZFN activity [33]. In their study, when they performed Cel I assay for 5 or 6 zinc fingers on either side showed no cleavage indicating that the ZFN pairs were not active. Similarly, when the spacer nucleotide size was 4, 5, 7 or 8, the activity of the 6 fingered ZFN pair was negligible. The ZFN pair used in our study had 6 fingers on each side with a spacer region of 5 nucleotides

provide suitable hits. On similar lines, in a study by Wayengara, where zinc finger arrays were used to target HPV 16 and HPV 18 genome using ZiFiT software, only a set of unpaired zinc finger arrays of length 9 bp were obtained for *E6* gene [32]. It is known that zinc fingers that recognize *GNN* triplets are well characterized and

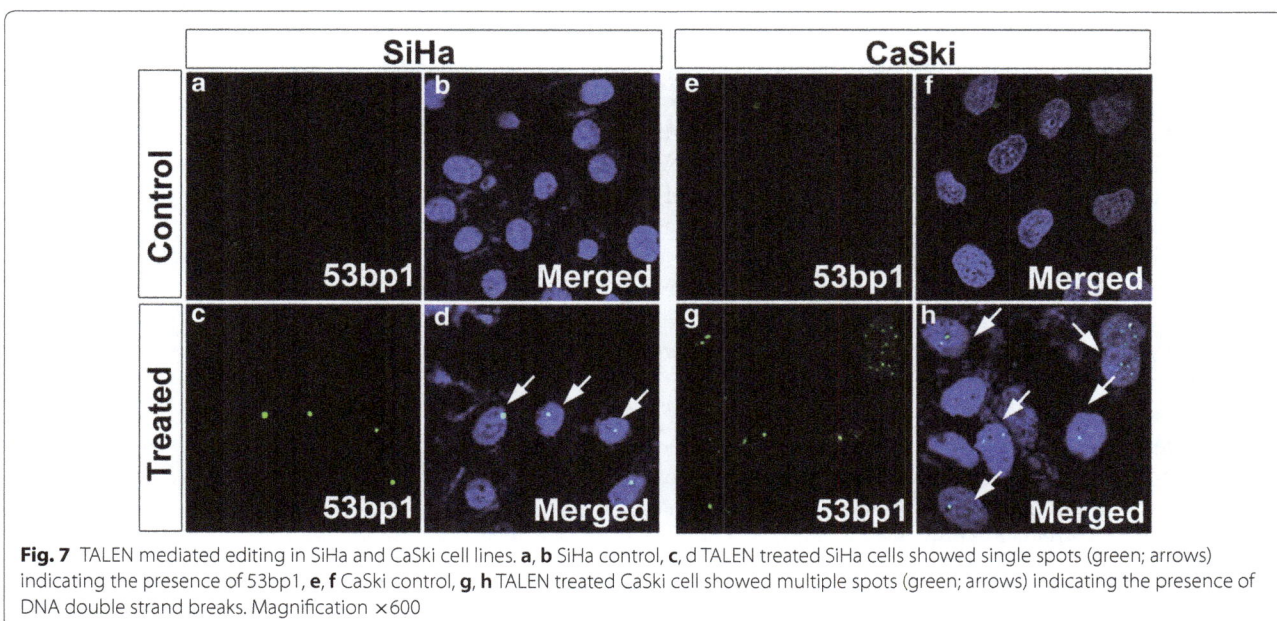

**Fig. 7** TALEN mediated editing in SiHa and CaSki cell lines. **a**, **b** SiHa control, **c**, d TALEN treated SiHa cells showed single spots (green; arrows) indicating the presence of 53bp1, **e**, **f** CaSki control, **g**, **h** TALEN treated CaSki cell showed multiple spots (green; arrows) indicating the presence of DNA double strand breaks. Magnification ×600

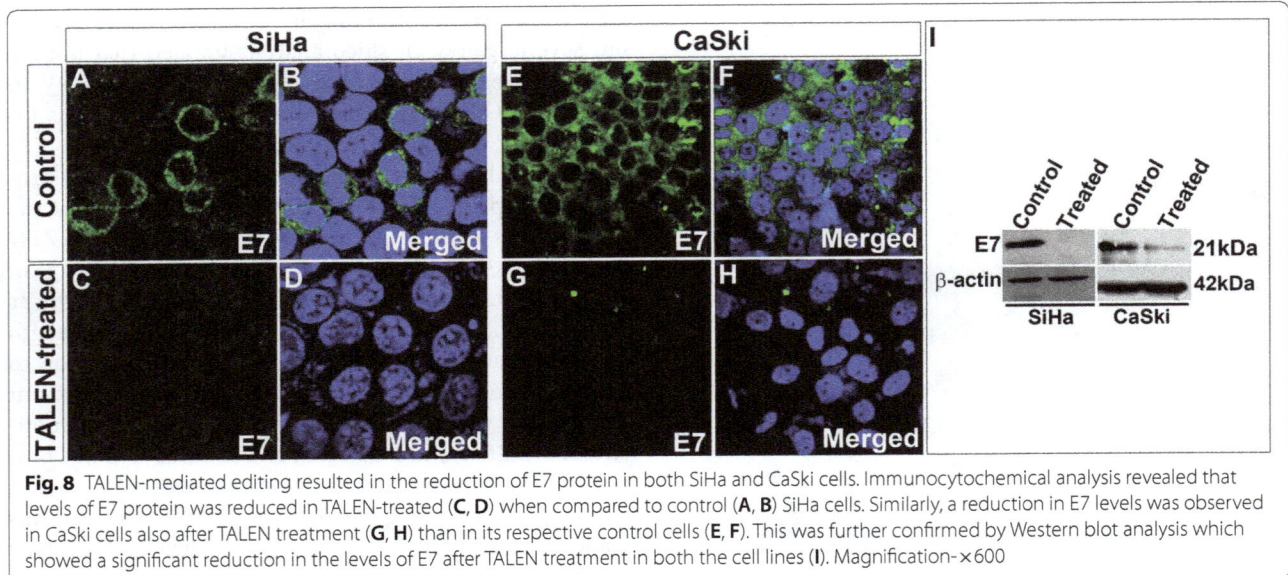

**Fig. 8** TALEN-mediated editing resulted in the reduction of E7 protein in both SiHa and CaSki cells. Immunocytochemical analysis revealed that levels of E7 protein was reduced in TALEN-treated (**C, D**) when compared to control (**A, B**) SiHa cells. Similarly, a reduction in E7 levels was observed in CaSki cells also after TALEN treatment (**G, H**) than in its respective control cells (**E, F**). This was further confirmed by Western blot analysis which showed a significant reduction in the levels of E7 after TALEN treatment in both the cell lines (**I**). Magnification-×600

which could possibly be a reason for the low activity that we observed.

Although activity levels of ZFN in SiHa and CaSki were low, yeast Mel-I assay showed greater than 50% activity after 6 h of induction. A recent report by Yang et al. [34], showed that among the three pairs of ZFNs only one exhibited very significant high activity in yeast MEL-I assay, but apparently this pair failed to show any activity in their cell system. This suggests that ZFNs validated in yeast based assay may not necessarily be active in tumor-derived cell lines or in vivo. Even commercial designs do not often work as expected which can be observed from yeast Mel-I assay which showed reasonable editing activity, but showed low level of editing activity in cell lines.

Usually in two finger modules, binding of each module enhances cooperative and specific base recognition of subsequent modules. Considering this factor and further extrapolating our analysis on CompoZr ZFN modules indicate that binding affinity and specificity of modules for both ZFNs could affect improper binding to their target triplets. This in turn would affect Fok-I dimerization which in turn would lead to poor cleavage of target site (Additional file 5: Figure S5).

This study points to the fact that nucleases with low editing activity may be useful in making knockout cell lines that are derived using single cell cloning. However, studies which require mass reduction of a particular gene, editing activity should be good enough and also reflect phenotypically. Therefore, nucleases intended for therapeutic applications should necessarily have good editing activity so that downstream phenotypic effects are prominent. In addition to this,

nuclease should also be optimized to reduce toxicity in such systems.

## Conclusions

Our study points to the fact that nucleases with low editing activity may be useful in making knockout cell lines that are derived using single cell cloning. However, studies which require mass reduction of a particular gene, editing activity should be good enough and also reflect phenotypically. Therefore, nucleases intended for therapeutic applications should necessarily have good editing activity so that downstream phenotypic effects are prominent. In addition to this, nuclease should also be optimized to reduce toxicity in such systems.

## Additional files

**Additional file 1: Figure S1.** Sequence analysis of HPV 16 *E6* and *E7* gene. (A) CompoZr ZFN sequences, (B) PCR showing the presence of *E6* and E7 in SiHa and CaSki cell lines. C33A, an HPV−ve cell line was used as a negative control. Sequencing PCR for *E6* gene in SiHa (C) and CaSki (D) cell lines, respectively.

**Additional file 2: Figure S2.** Methylation status did not affect the editing efficiency of TALENs and ZFNs. SiHa and CaSki cells treated with 10 mM sodium butyrate showed some editing by both TALEN and ZFN in CaSki (A), but not in SiHa cell line (B). Treatment with ssODN and Sodium butyrate did not yield any editing in either of the cell lines (C, D). Nocodazole was used to bring cells to the same phase of cell cycle and then treated with ZFNs and TALENs along with ssODN. No significant editing was observed in editing after Nocodazole treatment in both the cells (E).

**Additional file 3: Figure S3.** In silico ZFN target site prediction for E7 using following tools did not yield suitable target sites. *E6* gene was screened for possible ZFN pairs using (A) CoDa specific zinc fingers, (B) OPEN validated zinc fingers, (C) Sangamo validated modules, (D) TOOLGEN validated naturally occurring ZFN modules, (E) Barbas group of validated ZFN modules and F) ZFN predict.

**Additional file 4: Figure S4.** TALEN designed against E6 could not yield editing in both SiHa and Caski cells. (A) Schematic of three TALEN binding sites on E6 gene. (B, C) TALEN targeting sequence at position 284 and its T7E1 assay in SiHa and CaSki cells showed no significant editing. (D, E) TALEN targeting sequence at position 57 and its T7E1 assay in SiHa and CaSki cells showed no significant editing. (F, G) TALEN targeting sequence at position 112 and its T7E1 assay in SiHa and CaSki cells showed no significant editing.

**Additional file 5: Figure S5.** Improper binding of the designed CompoZr ZFNs led to poor editing of E6 in SiHa and CaSki cell lines. Binding of ZF modules is co-operative binding and since both the CompoZr ZFNs have some of the modules not binding to its predicted target site. This could have probably led to poor cleavage as was observed in the low cleavage efficiency obtained in SiHa and CaSki cell lines.

## Authors' contributions
SS conceived the idea, did the experiments and prepared the manuscript. AS carried out ssODN, NaBu and Nocodazole experiments, DP helped in carrying out FACS and Western blot experiments. AVD prepared the figures and critically evaluated the manuscript. MRP conceived the idea, supervised the study and prepared the manuscript. All authors read and approved the final manuscript.

## Acknowledgements
We would like to thank Prof. P. N. Rangarajan, Indian Institute of Science, Bangalore, India for his critical suggestions.

## Competing interests
The authors declare that they have no competing interests.

## Funding
This work was supported by funding from the Council of Scientific and Industrial Research, Government of India, Department of Biotechnology, Government of India and intramural funding from Rajiv Gandhi Centre for Biotechnology, Kerala, India. SS has been funded by Council for Scientific and Industrial Research: 10-2(5)/2007(ii)-E.U. II, AS has been funded by DBT, Govt. of India and DP has been funded by Junior Research Fellowship from the University Grants Commission [Order no. F.2-12/2003(SA-I)].

## References
1. Mali P, Yang L, Esvelt KM, Aach J, Guell M, DiCarlo JE, Norville JE, Church GM. RNA-guided human genome engineering via Cas9. Science. 2013;339:823–6.
2. Biagioni A, Chillà A, Andreucci E, Laurenzana A, Aargheri F, Peppicelli S, Del Rosso M, Fibbi G. Type II CRISPR/Cas9 approach in the oncological therapy. J Exp Clin Cancer Res. 2017;36(1):80.
3. Ye R, Pi M, Cox JV, Nishimoto SK, Quarles LD. CRISPR/Cas9 targeting of GPRC6A suppresses prostate cancer tumorigenesis in a human xenograft model. J Exp Clin Cancer Res. 2017;36:90.
4. Sekiba K, Yamaqami M, Otsuka M, Suzuki T, Kishikawa T, Ishibashi R, Ohno M, Sato M, Koike K. Transcriptional activation of the MICA gene with an engineered CRISPR-Cas9 system. Biochem Biophys Res Commun. 2017;486(2):521–5.
5. Hoban MD, Cost GJ, Mendel MC, Romero Z, Kaufman ML, Joglekar AV, Ho M, Lumaquin D, Gray D, Lill GR, et al. Correction of the sickle cell disease mutation in human hematopoietic stem/progenitor cells. Blood. 2015;125(17):2597–604.
6. Mashimo T, Kaneko T, Sakuma T, Kobayashi J, Kunihiro Y, Voigt B, Yamamoto T, Serikawa T. Efficient gene targeting by TAL effector nucleases coinjected with exonucleases in zygotes. Sci Rep. 2013;13:3–1253.
7. Deleidi M, Yu C. Genome editing in pluripotent stem cells: research and therapeutic applications. Biochem Biophys Res Commun. 2016;473(3):665–74.
8. Carroll D. Genome engineering with zinc-finger nucleases. Genetics. 2011;188(4):773–82.
9. Gaj T, Gersbach CA, Barbas CF 3rd. ZFN, TALEN, and CRISPR/Cas-based methods for genome engineering. Trends Biotechnol. 2013;31(7):397–405.
10. Wyman C, Kanaar R. DNA double-strand break repair: all's well that ends well. Annu Rev Genet. 2006;40:363–83.
11. Qu X, Wang P, Ding D, Li L, Wang H, Ma L, Zhou X, Liu S, Lin S, Wang X, et al. Zinc-finger-nucleases mediate specific and efficient excision of HIV-1 proviral DNA from infected and latently infected human T cells. Nucleic Acids Res. 2013;41(16):7771–82.
12. Mino T, Mori T, Aoyama Y, Sera T. Inhibition of human papillomavirus replication by using artificial zinc-finger nucleases. Nucleic Acids Symp Ser. 2008;52:185–6.
13. Weber ND, Stone D, Sedlak RH, De Silva Feelixge HS, Roychoudhury P, Schiffer JT, Aubert M, Jerome KR. AAV-mediated delivery of zinc finger nucleases targeting hepatitis B virus inhibits active replication. PLoS ONE. 2014;9(5):e97579.
14. Dreyer T, Nicholson S, Ely A, Arbuthnot P, Bloom K. Improved antiviral efficacy using TALEN-mediated homology directed recombination to introduce artificial primary miRNAs into DNA of hepatitis B virus. Biochem Biophys Res Commun. 2016;478(4):1563–8.
15. Schaefer EAK, Meixiong J, Mark C, Deik A, Motola DL, Fusco D, Yang A, Brisac C, Salloum S, Lin W, et al. Apolipoprotein B100 is required for hepatitis C infectivity and Mipomersen inhibits hepatitis C. World J Gastroenterol. 2016;22(45):9954–65.
16. Maeder ML, Thibodeau-Beganny S, Sander JD, Voytas DF, Joung JK. Oligomerized pool engineering (OPEN): an 'open-source' protocol for making customized zinc-finger arrays. Nat Protoc. 2009;4(10):1471–501.
17. Herrmann F, Garriga-Canut M, Baumstark R, Fajardo-Sanchez E, Cotterell J, Minoche A, Himmelbauer H, Isalan M. p53 gene repair with zinc finger nucleases optimised by yeast 1-hybrid and validated by Solexa sequencing. PLoS ONE. 2011;6(6):e20913.
18. Joung JK, Ramm EI, Pabo CO. A bacterial two-hybrid selection system for studying protein–DNA and protein–protein interactions. Proc Natl Acad Sci USA. 2000;97(13):7382–7.
19. Bae KH, Kwon YD, Shin HC, Hwang MS, Ryu EH, Park KS, Yang HY, Lee DK, Lee Y, Park J, et al. Human zinc fingers as building blocks in the construction of artificial transcription factors. Nat Biotechnol. 2003;21(3):275–80.
20. Shankar S, Prasad D, Sanawar R, Das AV, Pillai MR. TALEN based HPV-E7 editing triggers necrotic cell death in cervical cancer cells. Sci Rep. 2017;7:5500.
21. Doyon Y, McCammon JM, Miller JC, Faraji F, Ngo C, Katibah GE, Amora R, Hocking TD, Zhang L, Rebar EJ, et al. Heritable targeted gene disruption in zebrafish using designed zinc finger nucleases. Nat Biotechnol. 2008;26(6):702–8.
22. Kim HJ, Lee HJ, Kim H, Cho SW, Kim JS. Targeted genome editing in human cells with zinc finger nucleases constructed via modular assembly. Genome Res. 2009;19(7):1279–88.
23. Sander JD, Maeder ML, Reyon D, Voytas DF, Joung JK, Dobbs D. ZiFiT (Zinc Finger Targeter): an updated zinc finger engineering tool. Nucleic Acids Res. 2010;38(Web Server issue):W462–8.
24. Lin Y, Fine EJ, Zheng Z, Antico CJ, Voit RA, Porteus MH, Cradick TJ, Bao G. SAPTA: a new design tool for improving TALE nuclease activity. Nucleic Acids Res. 2014;42(6):e47.

25. Doyle EL, Booher NJ, Standage DS, Voytas DF, Brendel VP, VanDyk JK, Bogdanove AJ. TAL Effector-Nucleotide Targeter (TALE-NT) 2.0: tools for TAL effector design and target prediction. Nucleic Acids Res. 2012;40(1):W117–22.

26. Persikov AV, Singh M. De novo prediction of DNA-binding specificities for Cys2His2 zinc finger proteins. Nucleic Acids Res. 2014;42(1):97–108.

27. Tang S, Tao M, McCoy JP Jr, Zheng ZM. The E7 oncoprotein is translated from spliced E6*I transcripts in high-risk human papillomavirus type 16- or type 18-positive cervical cancer cell lines via translation reinitiation. J Virol. 2006;80(9):4249–63.

28. Byrne SM, Mali P, Church GM. Genome editing in human stem cells. Methods Enzymol. 2014;546:119–38.

29. Maeder ML, Thibodeau-Beganny S, Osiak A, Wright DA, Anthony RM, Eichtinger M, Jiang T, Foley JE, Winfrey RJ, Townsend JA, et al. Rapid "open-source" engineering of customized zinc-finger nucleases for highly efficient gene modification. Mol Cell. 2008;31(2):294–301.

30. Sander JD, Cade L, Khayter C, Reyon D, Peterson RT, Joung JK, Yeh JR. Targeted gene disruption in somatic zebrafish cells using engineered TALENs. Nat Biotechnol. 2011;29(8):697–8.

31. Ma L, Zhu F, Li Z, Zhang J, Li X, Dong J, Wang T. TALEN-based mutagenesis of lipoxygenase LOX3 enhances the storage tolerance of rice (*Oryza sativa*) seeds. PLoS ONE. 2015;10(12):e0143877.

32. Wayengera M. Zinc finger arrays binding human papillomavirus types 16 and 18 genomic DNA: precursors of gene-therapeutics for in situ reversal of associated cervical neoplasia. Theor Biol Med Model. 2012;9:30.

33. Shimizu Y, Sollu C, Meckler JF, Adriaenssens A, Zykovich A, Cathomen T, Segal DJ. Adding fingers to an engineered zinc finger nuclease can reduce activity. Biochemistry. 2011;50(22):5033–41.

34. Yang D, Yang H, Li W, Zhao B, Ouyang Z, Liu Z, Zhao Y, Fan N, Song J, Tian J, et al. Generation of PPARgamma mono-allelic knockout pigs via zinc-finger nucleases and nuclear transfer cloning. Cell Res. 2011;21(6):979–82.

# 5

# SKA3 promotes cell proliferation and migration in cervical cancer by activating the PI3K/Akt signaling pathway

Rong Hu[1,2†], Ming-qing Wang[1,2†], Wen-bo Niu[5†], Yan-jing Wang[3], Yang-yang Liu[6], Ling-yu Liu[1,2], Ming Wang[3], Juan Zhong[1,2], Hai-yan You[1,2], Xiao-hui Wu[1,2], Ning Deng[2], Lu Lu[4*] and Lian-bo Wei[1,2*]

## Abstract

**Background:** Cervical cancer (CC) is one of the most common cancers among females worldwide. Spindle and kine-tochore-associated complex subunit 3 (SKA3), located on chromosome 13q, was identified as a novel gene involved in promoting malignant transformation in cancers. However, the function and underlying mechanisms of SKA3 in CC remain unknown. Using the Oncomine database, we found that expression of SKA3 mRNA is higher in CC tissues than in normal tissues and is linked with poor prognosis.

**Methods:** In our study, immunohistochemistry showed increased expression of SKA3 in CC tissues. The effect of SKA3 on cell proliferation and migration was evaluated by CCK8, clone formation, Transwell and wound-healing assays in HeLa and SiHa cells with stable SKA3 overexpression and knockdown. In addition, we established a xenograft tumor model in vivo.

**Results:** SKA3 overexpression promoted cell proliferation and migration and accelerated tumor growth. We further identified that SKA3 is involved in regulating cell cycle progression and the PI3K/Akt signaling pathway via RNA-sequencing (RNA-Seq) and gene set enrichment analyses. Western blotting results revealed that SKA3 overexpression increased levels of p-Akt, cyclin E2, CDK2, cyclin D1, CDK4, E2F1 and p-Rb in HeLa cells. Additionally, the use of an Akt inhibitor (GSK690693) significantly reversed the cell proliferation capacity induced by SKA3 overexpression in HeLa cells.

**Conclusions:** We suggest that SKA3 overexpression contributes to CC cell growth and migration by promoting cell cycle progression and activating the PI3K–Akt signaling pathway, which may provide potential novel therapeutic targets for CC treatment.

**Keywords:** SKA3, Cervical cancer, Cell proliferation, Cell cycle, PI3K/Akt

## Background

Cervical cancer (CC) is the second most common type of gynecologic cancer worldwide [1], with approximately 500,000 newly diagnosed cases and 275,000 deaths every year [2]. Depending on the stage of the disease, 5-year survival rate ranges from approximately 5–50%, depending on the stage [3]. Furthermore, due to poor economic situations and delays in treatment, morbidity and mortality rates of CC remain very high in some developing countries due to poor economic situations and delays in treatment [4, 5]. It is well known that persistent infection with HPV is a major risk factor for CC due to the oncoproteins E6 and E7. These factors inactivate and degrade tumor suppressor p53 and retinoblastoma (Rb), causing cell cycle deregulation, genomic instability, and increased chromosomal aberrations and mutations in cellular genes [6]. Gene

*Correspondence: coinland@gzucm.edu.cn; wlb@smu.edu.cn
†Rong Hu, Ming-qing Wang and Wen-bo Niu contributed equally to this work
[1] Shenzhen Hospital, Southern Medical University, No. 1333, Xinhu Road, Bao'an District, Shenzhen 518101, Guangdong, China [4] The First Affiliated Hospital, Guangzhou University of Chinese Medicine, No.16 Baiyun Airport Road, Baiyun District, Guangzhou 510405, Guangdong, China
Full list of author information is available at the end of the article

network reconstruction has revealed cell cycle and anti-viral genes as major drivers of CC [7]. Current standard treatments for CC, including surgery and definitive chemoradiation, result in the loss of childbearing ability [8], and targeted therapeutic strategies have mainly focused on the HPV E6 and E7 oncogenic proteins [9]. Nevertheless, the outcome of current therapy strategies is still poor. Therefore, investigating the exact molecular mechanisms of CC may promote the identification of novel biomarkers and treatment targets, which is critical for improving the prognosis of these patients [10].

SKA3, a subunit located in the kinetochore outer layer of the SKA complex, is not only required for controlling and promoting proper mitotic exit during mitosis by cooperating with the NDC80 complex [11, 12] but also plays an important role in meiotic spindle migration and anaphase spindle stability [13]. Previous studies have reported that SKA3 participates in cancer pathogenesis and progression. SKA3 is frequently somatically mutated in breast cancer and has a role in cell growth [14]. A recent study showed that SKA3 is associated with patient outcome and aggressive disease development in several cancers [15]. By analyzing an Oncomine dataset, we found that SKA3 mRNA expression is higher in CC tissue than in normal tissue and may be associated with survival rate in CC patients. However, the detailed functions and underlying mechanisms of SKA3 in CC remain largely unknown.

Cell cycle progression critically depends on numerous regulatory processes that are often dysregulated in cancer [16]. Cyclin D in complexes with CDK4 or CDK6 and cyclin E in a complex with CDK2 regulate progression through the G1-S boundary of the cell cycle. These complexes phosphorylate and thereby prevent Rb from binding to E2F, which once released, drives cells from G1 into S phase [17, 18].

Some signaling pathways have been found to have important functions in the occurrence and progression of CC, such as the Notch1 ligand, Wnt/beta-catenin, p53, p38 MAPK, and PI3K/Akt/mTOR signaling pathways [19–22]. Overall, a deeper knowledge of signal transduction may provide new targets for tumor therapy. The phosphoinositide 3-kinase (PI3K)/Akt pathway is a classical and important signaling pathway involved in numerous cellular functions, including cell proliferation, survival, adhesion, migration and metabolism [23, 24]. Furthermore, PI3K/Akt signaling pathway controls proliferation, transformation, growth, apoptosis, drug resistance, and other processes in various types of cancers [25, 26]. Previous studies have shown that PI3K/Akt signaling pathway is closely associated with the occurrence and development of CC [27], and the pathway has become a potential target for the prevention and treatment of CC [28, 29].

This study was designed to investigate the role and mechanisms of SKA3 in CC both in vitro and in vivo. We hypothesized that SKA3 may play a very important role in the development and progression of CC. Importantly, SKA3 expression may indicate a poor prognosis and could serve as a potential therapeutic target in CC.

## Materials and methods

### Cell culture

HEK 293FT cells and human CC cell lines (HeLa, C4-I, CaSki, C-33A, HT-3, SiHa, SW756, MS751, ME-180) were purchased from the Chinese Academy of Science cell bank (Shanghai, China). The cell lines were authenticated by a Cell Line Authentication Service with an STR Profile Report (Genetic Testing Bio-technology, Suzhou, China). All CC cell lines were cultivated in RPMI-1640 medium supplemented with 10% fetal bovine serum (FBS) (Gibco, BRL), 100 units/mL penicillin and 100 μg/mL streptomycin (Gibco, New York, USA). HEK 293FT cells were maintained in DMEM (Gibco, BRL) supplemented with 10% FBS in a humidified atmosphere containing 5% $CO_2$ at 37 °C.

### Real-time quantitative PCR (RT-qPCR)

Total RNA was extracted using TRIzol reagent (TaKaRa, Dalian, China) and reverse transcribed into cDNA using a Prime Script RT Reagent Kit (TaKaRa), according to the manufacturer's instructions. RT-qPCR was performed with a CFX96™ Real-Time System (Bio-Rad Hercules, California, USA) using SYBR Green (SYBR Premix Ex Taq™ II; TaKaRa) for fluorescent quantification. The following cycling conditions were used: pre-denaturation at 95 °C for 30 s, 35 cycles of denaturation at 95 °C for 5 s, 35 cycles), annealing at 55–60 °C for 30 s, extension at 72 °C for 1 min) and a final extension at 72 °C for 10 min. Relative mRNA expression was calculated using the $2^{-\Delta\Delta Ct}$ method. The primers of SKA3 and β-actin were list in Table 1.

### Clinical specimens

A tissue microarray containing 100 samples of formalin-fixed, paraffin-embedded (FFPE) CC and para-carcinoma tissues with detailed clinical characteristics was purchased from Alenabio.com (CR1003, Xi an, China). Forty CC tissues and 10 normal tissues (each tissue was represented twice) were included on the tissue chip, which was evaluated by IHC staining to examine SKA3 expression. The 7th edition of the American Joint Committee on Cancer (AJCC) Cancer Staging Manual was used to reclassify the tumor-node-metastasis (TNM) staging. The clinical features of all patients are listed in Table 2. All procedures involving human subjects were performed in accordance with institutional and national research committee ethical standards.

## Overexpression plasmid construction and lentivirus infection

The coding sequence of the SKA3 gene was obtained from PUBGENE. The primers were obtained from The Beijing Genomics Institute (BGI) and were listed in Table 1. The SKA3 gene was first cloned into the PCDH lentiviral vector. After enzyme digestion and DNA sequencing, a recombinant plasmid containing a GFP reporter gene and FLAG tag was successfully constructed. The packaging plasmids pMD2.G and pSPAX2 were mixed with PCDH-SKA3 or PCDH-NC (control). All plasmids were transfected into HEK 293FT cells using Lipofectamine 2000 reagent (Invitrogen) to form lentiviral particles and generate stably transfected cell lines. Lentiviral particles were harvested and used to infect HeLa cells 48 h later. After selection with puromycin (1 mg/mL) (Sigma-Aldrich) for 2 weeks, western blotting was performed to validate SKA3 overexpression or knockdown in the stably transfected cells. SKA3 knockdown lentiviral particles were purchased from Genechem, and the sequence was listed in Table 1.

## CCK8 assay and clone formation assay

For the Cell Counting Kit-8 assay (CK04, Dojindo Kumamoto, Japan), stable HeLa cell lines were seeded at 5000 cells per well in 96-well plates. Cell viability was measured at 450 nm using a spectrophotometric plate reader from 0 to 7 days, and each experiment was performed in triplicate. For the clone formation assay, cells were plated at 500 cells per well in 6-well plates and cultured for 14 days. Clones were counted under an inverted microscope after the cells were fixed in methyl alcohol and stained with 0.5% crystal violet (Saiguo, Guangzhou, China). Clones containing > 50 cells were counted

for statistical analysis. Cells in each group were plated in three duplicate wells, and all experiments were repeated independently three times.

## Wound healing assay

Stable HeLa cells were plated in 6-well cell culture plates ($3 \times 10^6$ cells per well) and grown to near 100% confluence. The monolayers were scratched with a sterile 200-μL tip and washed with phosphate-buffered saline (PBS) to remove the detached cells. Then, the cells were then cultured in serum-free medium for 48 h. Images of cells migrating at the corresponding wound sites were captured at 0, 24, and 48 h using an inverted microscope (200×), and the wound size was measured by Image-pro plus 6.0. Data were collected from three independent experiments.

## Transwell migration assays

The transwell migration assay was carried out using 24-well MILLI cell Hanging Cell Culture Inserts (8 μm) (Corning, Bedford, MA, USA). The upper surface of Transwell chambers (8-mm pores; Corning) was used to assess the cell migration ability. Dishes were placed in a cell culture incubator for 1 h at 37 °C. Stable HeLa cells were harvested in 200 μL serum-free medium and plated in the upper chamber at a density of $1 \times 10^5$ cells per insert. The lower chambers were filled with 600 μL of medium supplemented with 20% FBS. After 24 h of incubation, the migrated cells on the membrane surface were fixed with methanol, stained with 0.5% crystal violet, and counted under an inverted microscope (200×). Data were collected from three independent experiments.

## Flow cytometry to detect the cell cycle and apoptosis

Stable HeLa cells ($3 \times 10^5$ cells per well) were plated in 6-well cell culture plates. For cell cycle analysis, cells were collected by trypsinization after 2 days, washed once with PBS, fixed in 70% alcohol at 4 °C overnight, and again washed with PBS. RNA helicase was added to the cells for 30 min at 37 °C. The cells were then stained with 400 μL of propidium iodide (PI) buffer (Chemo Metec, Allerod, Denmark), kept in a darkroom at 4 °C for

**Table 1  Sequences of primers and short RNA oligos**

| Gene | Forward primers | Reverse primers |
|------|-----------------|-----------------|
| SKA3 | 5′-CAGATCCCTCTTCACCTACGA-3′ | 5′-TCAACGTTTAAAGGGGGACA-3′ |
| β-Actin | 5′-GGCATCCTCACCCTGAAGTA-3′ | 5′-GGGGTGTTGAAGGTCTCAAA-3′ |
| Over-SKA3 | 5′-GCTCTAGAGCCACCATGGACCCTATCCGGAGCTTCTGC-3′ | 5′-CGGAATTCTCACTTGTCATCGTCATCCTTG TAGTCGTTTTCTTTGTTGCTGACATCTCGG ATG-3′ |
| Sh-SKA3 | CCGGCATGGACAGAACATCCGAGATCTCGAGATCTCGGATGTTCTGTCCATGTTTTTG | |

**Table 2 Clinical and pathological variables and the expression of SKA3 in 40 cases of cervical cancer**

| Parameters | Expression of SKA3 | | p-value |
|---|---|---|---|
| | Low | High | |
| Age (years) | | | 0.3598 |
| ≥ 50 | 2 (5%) | 15 (37.5%) | |
| < 50 | 4 (10%) | 19 (47.5%) | |
| TNM stage | | | 0.999 |
| I + II | 6 (15%) | 32 (80%) | |
| III + IV | 0 (0%) | 2 (5%) | |
| Clinical stage | | | 0.999 |
| I + II | 5 (12.5%) | 29 (72.5%) | |
| III + IV | 1 (2.5%) | 5 (12.5%) | |

30 min, and evaluated using a FACS flow cytometer (BD, Franklin Lakes, NJ, USA). For cell apoptosis analysis, cells were collected after transfection by trypsinization (without EDTA), washed once with PBS, added to 500 μL of 1× binding buffer, and stained with 5 μL of Annexin V-PE and 5 μL of 7-AAD. The mixture was incubated in the dark for 15 min and detected by flow cytometry. All experiments were repeated independently three times.

### In vivo xenograft tumor model

BALB/c nude mice (4–6 weeks old, male) were purchased from the Experimental Animal Centre of Southern Medical University and maintained under standard pathogen-free conditions, with 6 mice in each group. A sample of $1 \times 10^7$ HeLa cells with stable SKA3 overexpression or SKA3 knockdown or control plasmid resuspended in 200 μL of PBS was injected into the left, middle or right dorsal flank of the mice, respectively. To analyze tumor growth, tumor size was measured using calipers for 6 weeks according to the following formula: L*W*W*π/6, where L is the length and W is the width of the tumor. The tumor tissues were harvested, fixed, and paraffin-embedded before 4-mm tissue sections were obtained. All sections were subjected to immunohistochemistry (IHC) staining. All animal studies (including the mouse euthanasia procedure) were performed in compliance with the regulations and guidelines of Southern Medical University Institutional Animal Care and according to AAALAC and IACUC guidelines.

### Immunohistochemistry (IHC) staining

IHC staining was performed on formalin-fixed paraffin-embedded tumor tissue sections and a clinical tissue microarray chip. The sections were deparaffinized and rehydrated, and endogenous peroxidase activity was blocked by incubating the samples with 3% $H_2O_2$ for 15 min in the dark. Antigen retrieval was performed by heating in a pressure cooker in citrate buffer (Saiguo, Guangzhou, China) for 10 min. The samples were then incubated at room temperature for 40 min and washed three times with PBS. Next, 5% BSA was used to block nonspecific binding at room temperature for 30 min. The processed sections were incubated with a primary antibody overnight at 4 °C at the following dilutions: SKA3, 1:800 for the clinical tissue microarray chip and 1:200 for tumor sections (Abcam, Cambridge, MA, USA); Ki67, 1:100 (Abcam, Cambridge, MA, USA); Cyclin D1, 1:50 (Abcam, Cambridge, MA, USA); and CDK4, 1:50 (Abcam, Cambridge, MA, USA). The sections were washed 3 times with PBS and incubated with a biotinylated secondary antibody for 40 min at room temperature. Immunostaining signals were enhanced and visualized using the ABC staining system and DAB substrate kit (Vector Laboratories, CA, USA) according to the manufacturer's instructions. Signal intensity was scored as follows: 0 (no staining), 1 (weak staining), 2 (moderate staining), and 3 (strong staining). The percentage of positively stained cells was divided into four categories: < 25% (1), 25–50% (2), 51–75% (3), and > 76% (4). The final staining scores were calculated as the intensity × the staining percentage to achieve a score between 0 and 12. A final score > 6 was defined as high expression, and ≤ 6 was defined as low SKA3 expression.

### RNA-sequencing and gene set enrichment analysis (GSEA)

Total mRNA was extracted from HeLa cells stably overexpressing SKA3 or PCDH using an RNA extraction kit (Qiagen). RNA-Seq was performed using an Ion Proton system for next-generation sequencing according to the manufacturer's instructions. Sequenced reads were mapped to the hg19 genome using the Ion Torrent TMAP aligner with the 'map4' option. HTSeq-Count was used to quantify the aligned RNA-Seq reads against exon regions of genes in the RefSeq hg19 annotation.

GSEA was performed on mRNA expression datasets of HeLa cells with stable SKA3 overexpression and cells expressing the control plasmid using the C2 curated gene sets and C6 oncogenic signature gene sets (GSEA, Broad Institute) with the addition of a cell cycle signature. Gene signatures were considered enriched at FDR q-values < 0.05 and Family Wise Error Rate (FWER) p-values < 0.05.

### Western blotting

Cells were lysed in RIPA buffer, and the lysates were sonicated and pelleted by centrifugation. Protein concentrations were measured using a BCA protein assay kit (Thermo Fisher Scientific, Waltham, MA, USA). The lysates were mixed with 5× loading buffer, boiled for 15 min, and equally loaded on 10% SDS polyacrylamide gels. After electrophoresis, the proteins were transferred to PVDF membranes (Millipore, Billerica, MA, USA) at a constant current of 350 mA for 100 min. The PVDF membranes were blocked with 5% BSA in 1× TBST for 1 h and probed overnight at 4 °C with respective primary antibodies at dilutions suggested by the manufacturers. The following antibodies were used: anti-GAPDH (1:2000; Epitomics); anti-SKA3 (1:2000; Abcam); anti-FLAG tag (1:2000; Sigma); anti-Cdk4 (1:3000; Proteintech); anti-cyclin D1 (1:3000; Proteintech); anti-Cdk2 (1:2000; Proteintech); anti-cyclin E2 (1:2000; Proteintech) anti-p-Rb (1:2000; Proteintech); anti-E2F1 (1:3000; Abcam); anti-Akt (1:3000; Abcam); anti-p-Akt (1:3000; Abcam); anti-GSK-3β (1:2000; Sigma); anti-p21 (1:2000; Abcam); anti-p15 (1:2000; Epitomics); anti-foxo1 (1:2000; Epitomics); and anti-p-foxo1 (1:2000; Epitomics). The membranes were then incubated with a species-matched HRP-conjugated secondary antibody (1:10,000, Proteintech) for 1 h. Finally, the membranes were washed 3 times with 1× TBST (10 min each), and the blots were visualized with enhanced chemiluminescence (ECL) reagent using FUJI SUPER RX film or a CCD system (Imagestation 2000 MM, Kodak, NY, USA).

## Immunofluorescence

Cells were passaged until reaching 80% confluence and fixed with 4% paraformaldehyde for 15 min, washed 3 times with PBS (10 min each), permeabilized with 0.25% Triton X-100 for 10 min at room temperature, washed with 3 times PBS, and blocked with 5% BSA for 30 min. After washing with PBS, the cells were incubated at 4 °C overnight with an anti-E2F1 antibody (1:100, Abcam) and foxo1 antibody (1:50, Abcam). The cells were washed with PBS and incubated with a fluorescent-labeled secondary antibody (DyLight red 594, Abbkine, Amyjet) for 40 min in the dark and then later treated with DAPI for 10 min. Fluorescence was observed using a Leica inverted fluorescence microscope (Leica, Germany).

## Statistical analysis

Expression differences between normal tissues and CC tissues were calculated using a Chi squared test. Kaplan–Meier analysis was applied to determine the overall survival data. Cell proliferation and migration were analyzed using Student's t test or one-way ANOVA. All statistical analyses were performed with SPSS 20.0 software (SPSS Inc.), and differences were considered statistically

significant at $p < 0.05$. Data are representative of 3 independent experiments and presented as the mean ± SD.

## Results

### SKA3 expression was increased in CC patients and appeared to be a prognostic indicator of CC

The SKA3 gene, which is located on chromosome 13q, is associated with mitosis and cancer development. To determine the role of SKA3 in CC, we first analyzed data from the Oncomine database. We found the expression of SKA3 mRNA was higher in CC tissue than in normal tissue in both the Biewenga Cervix database ($p < 0.001$, Fig. 1a) and the Pyeon Multi-cancer database ($p < 0.001$, Fig. 1b). Next, we evaluated SKA3 expression in clinical CC patients by IHC staining of a human tissue microarray. The adjusted clinical characteristics included age, sex, pathological grade, American Joint Committee on Cancer (AJCC) stage, and TNM stage. SKA3 immunoreactivity was observed in the nucleolus and cytoplasm of both non-neoplastic epithelium and cancer cells, and SKA3 staining was obviously stronger in CC tissue than in normal tissue (score > 6, **$p < 0.01$, Fig. 1c), indicating that SKA3 may play an important role in CC development.

In addition, we downloaded raw survival data and SKA3 expression in CC from the TCGA Bio Portal (http://www.cbioportal.org/). The cut-off value was determined based on the median expression of individual genes. The raw survival rate of the 292 patients did not show significant differences ($p = 0.08$, Fig. 1d), mainly because of the small sample size and high rate of death among CC patients. According to the data, SKA3 expression may be associated with poor prognosis in CC. In addition, we examined the level of SKA3 mRNA expression in different CC cell lines and normal cervical cells, and the results suggested that SKA3 mRNA expression is higher in CC cells than in normal cells (**$p < 0.01$, Fig. 1e).

### SKA3 overexpression promoted cell proliferation, clone formation and migration in CC cells

To investigate the biological function of SKA3 on CC in vitro, stable CC cell lines (HeLa and SiHa) transfected with SKA3 overexpression, knockdown and control plasmids were established and confirmed by fluorescence microscopy and western blotting. Fluorescence microscopy showed that exogenous green fluorescent protein (GFP) was well expressed in HeLa and SiHa cells. Western blotting indicated that the level of SKA3 was significantly increased in HeLa and SiHa cells with SKA3 overexpression, however the opposite result was observed in cells with SKA3 knockdown, in which the FLAG tag was measured (vs. control vector, Fig. 2a). Next, we performed a CCK-8 assay to determine the

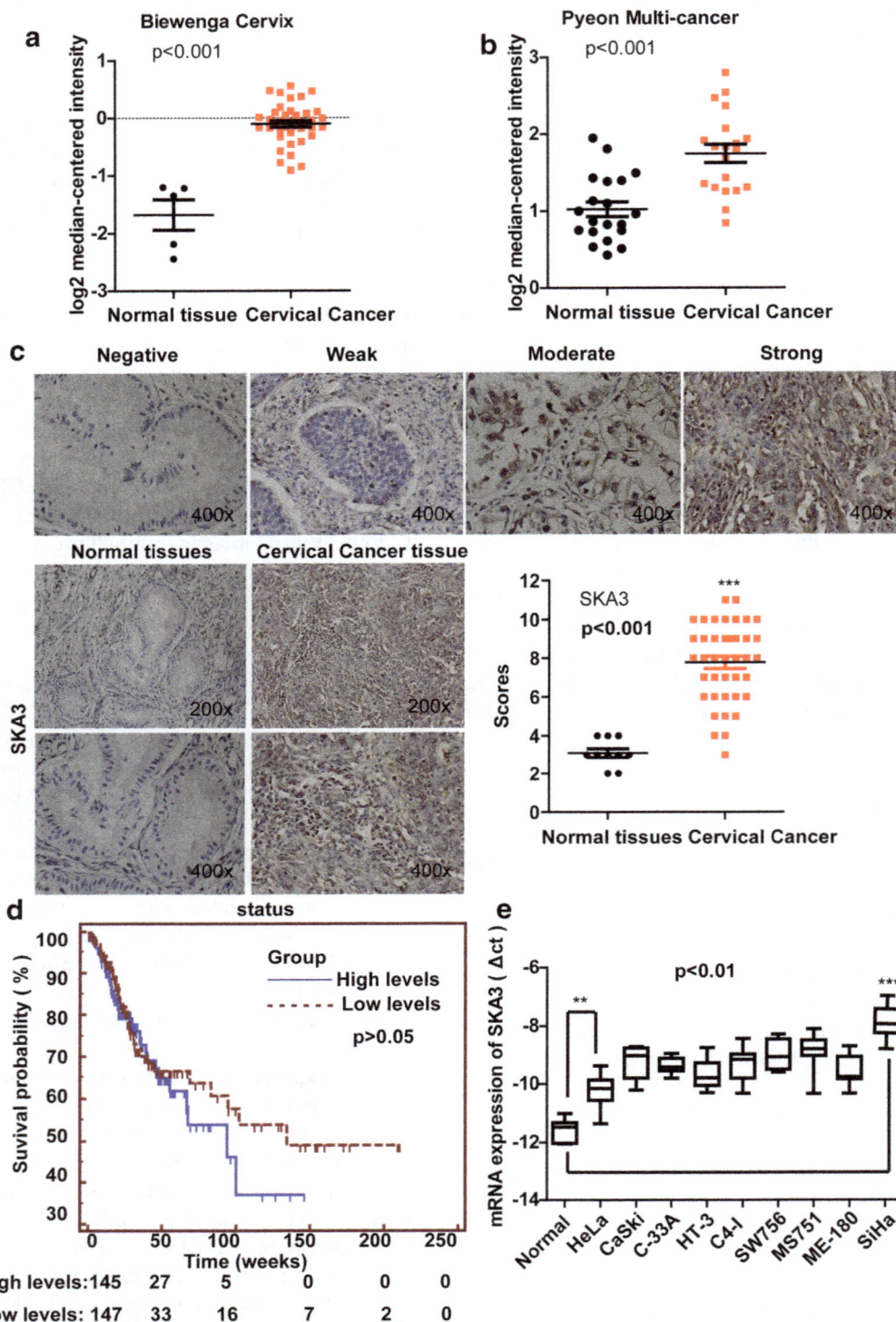

**Fig. 1** Expression of SKA3 is higher in CC tissue and appears to be correlated with overall patient survival. Data from the Oncomine database (https ://www.oncomine.org/) showed that mRNA expression of SKA3 is higher in CC tissue than in normal tissue. **a** Biewenga Cervix database; **b** Pyeon Multi-cancer database. The p-value was calculated using Student's t test (*p < 0.05, **p < 0.01). **c** Respective immunochemistry staining in a clinical tissue microarray of samples from CC patients and normal controls. **d** In a TCGA dataset, the overall survival of 292 CC patients was analyzed by Kaplan–Meier analysis. There was no significant difference between the two groups (p > 0.05, p = 0.08, patients with a high level of SKA3 vs. patients with a low level of SKA3). **e** The mRNA expression of SKA3 in different CC cell lines and normal cells; the levels of SKA3 in CC cells were higher than those in normal cervical cells (*p < 0.05, **p < 0.01)

effect of SKA3 on cell proliferation ability, and the results showed that SKA3 overexpression significantly promoted HeLa and SiHa cell proliferation from day 3 to day 7, but that SKA3 knockdown significantly suppressed HeLa and SiHa cell proliferation (vs. control vector, **p < 0.01, ##p < 0.01, Fig. 2b). Furthermore, a clone formation assay indicated that SKA3 overexpression significantly increased the number of HeLa and SiHa cell clones (**p < 0.01, ##p < 0.01, Fig. 2c).

In addition, we determined whether SKA3 can influence the migration of CC cells. A Transwell assay indicated that SKA3 overexpression promoted migration in HeLa and SiHa cells, whereas SKA3 knockdown suppressed the migration in both cell types (**p < 0.01, ##p < 0.01, Fig. 2d). Similar results were obtained in a wound-healing assay. Whereby the wound distance was narrower in HeLa and SiHa cells with stable SKA3 overexpression than in control cells after 48 h (**p < 0.01, ##p < 0.01, Fig. 2e). To further understand how SKA3 affects cell growth in CC, we performed a cell cycle analysis by flow cytometry. With stable SKA3 overexpression in HeLa and SiHa cells, the percentage of cells in G1 phase and G2 phase decreased, whereas that of cells in S phase increased (vs. control vector, *p < 0.05, **p < 0.01, Fig. 2f), indicating that SKA3 overexpression promoted cell proliferation in HeLa and SiHa cells by enhancing cell cycle progression. However, the effect of SKA3 overexpression and knockdown on cell apoptosis in HeLa and SiHa cells was not significant (vs. control vector, Additional file 1: Fig. S1). In general, our results demonstrate that SKA3 overexpression promotes cell proliferation, clone formation and migration in CC cells in vitro.

### SKA3 overexpression accelerated CC tumor growth in vivo

To determine the effect of SKA3 on CC tumor growth in vivo, xenograft mouse models were established by injecting HeLa cells with stable SKA3 overexpression into the left dorsal flank, cells with stable SKA3 knockdown into the right dorsal flank, and cells stably expressing the control plasmid into the middle dorsal flank of different animals. Tumor size was measured continually from 1 to 6 weeks. Our results showed that SKA3 overexpression significantly increased xenograft tumor growth (Fig. 3a). The tumor volume was significantly increased in

mice injected with HeLa cells stably overexpressing SKA3 from week 2 to week 6, whereas SKA3 knockdown inhibited tumor growth (vs. control vector, *p < 0.05, **p < 0.01, Fig. 3b). Furthermore, IHC staining was performed to evaluate the expression of Ki67, which is the most common indicator of cell proliferation. Ki67 and SKA3 levels were significantly increased in tumors with SKA3 overexpression (vs. control vector, *p < 0.05, **p < 0.01, Fig. 3c). Thus, we demonstrated SKA3 accelerates CC tumor growth in vivo.

### SKA3 overexpression promoted cell cycle progression by activating the PI3K–Akt pathway in CC

Because our results indicate that SKA3 might promote cell proliferation and cell cycle progression by favoring the G1-S transition, we next explored the molecular mechanisms of SKA3 in cell cycle progression. We evaluated gene expression using RNA-Seq analysis of mRNA isolated from HeLa cells with stable SKA3 overexpression and control vector expression. In GO enrichment, the term "cell cycle checkpoint" passed the filtering criteria (p = 0.0096, Fig. 4a). According to pathway enrichment based on the KEGG database, 19 pathways passed the filtering criteria, including the "PI3K/Akt signaling pathway" (p = 0.00027) and "cell cycle" (p = 0.0096, **p < 0.01, a representative pathway is shown in Fig. 4b). In addition, we performed GSEA for KEGG enrichment from MsigDB, and "PI3K/Akt signaling pathway" and "cell cycle" also passed the filtering criteria (**p < 0.01, Fig. 4c, d). The heat map shown in Fig. 4e indicates that the expression profiles of cell cycle-associated genes were substantially altered in HeLa cells overexpressing SKA3 (**p < 0.01). In an effort to determine the key downstream target of SKA3, we found two genes (Akt and CDK) involved in the PI3K/Akt pathway to be increased in HeLa cells overexpressing SKA3 (**p < 0.01, Fig. 4f).

Furthermore, we detected the expression of G1-S checkpoint proteins by western blotting. Levels of cyclin D1, cyclin E2, CDK4, p-Rb, E2F1 and p-Akt were higher in HeLa cells overexpressing SKA3, but levels of p15 and p27 were lower (vs. control vector, Fig. 5a). Immunofluorescence results further showed that SKA3 overexpression increased luciferase activity driven by the E2F motif (Fig. 5b). Because expression of cell cycle-related genes

(See figure on next page.)

**Fig. 2** Overexpression of SKA3 promotes HeLa and SiHa cell proliferation, clone formation and migration. **a** HeLa and SiHa cells with stable SKA3 overexpression, SKA3 knockdown and control plasmid expression were generated and confirmed by western blotting. **b** Proliferation of HeLa and SiHa cells with stable SKA3 overexpression, SKA3 knockdown and control plasmid expression was assessed using a CCK-8 assay. **c** Clone formation assay in HeLa and SiHa cells with stable SKA3 overexpression, SKA3 knockdown and control plasmid expression. The migration of HeLa and SiHa cells was examined by **d** a Transwell assay and **e** a wound-healing assay. **f** Representative cell cycle data were measured by flow cytometry in HeLa and SiHa cells with stable SKA3 overexpression, SKA3 knockdown and control plasmid. All data (mean ± SD; n = 3) were analyzed by Student's t test (*p < 0.05, **p < 0.01, over-SKA3 vs. control vector. #p < 0.05, ##p < 0.01, SKA3 knockdown vs. control vector)

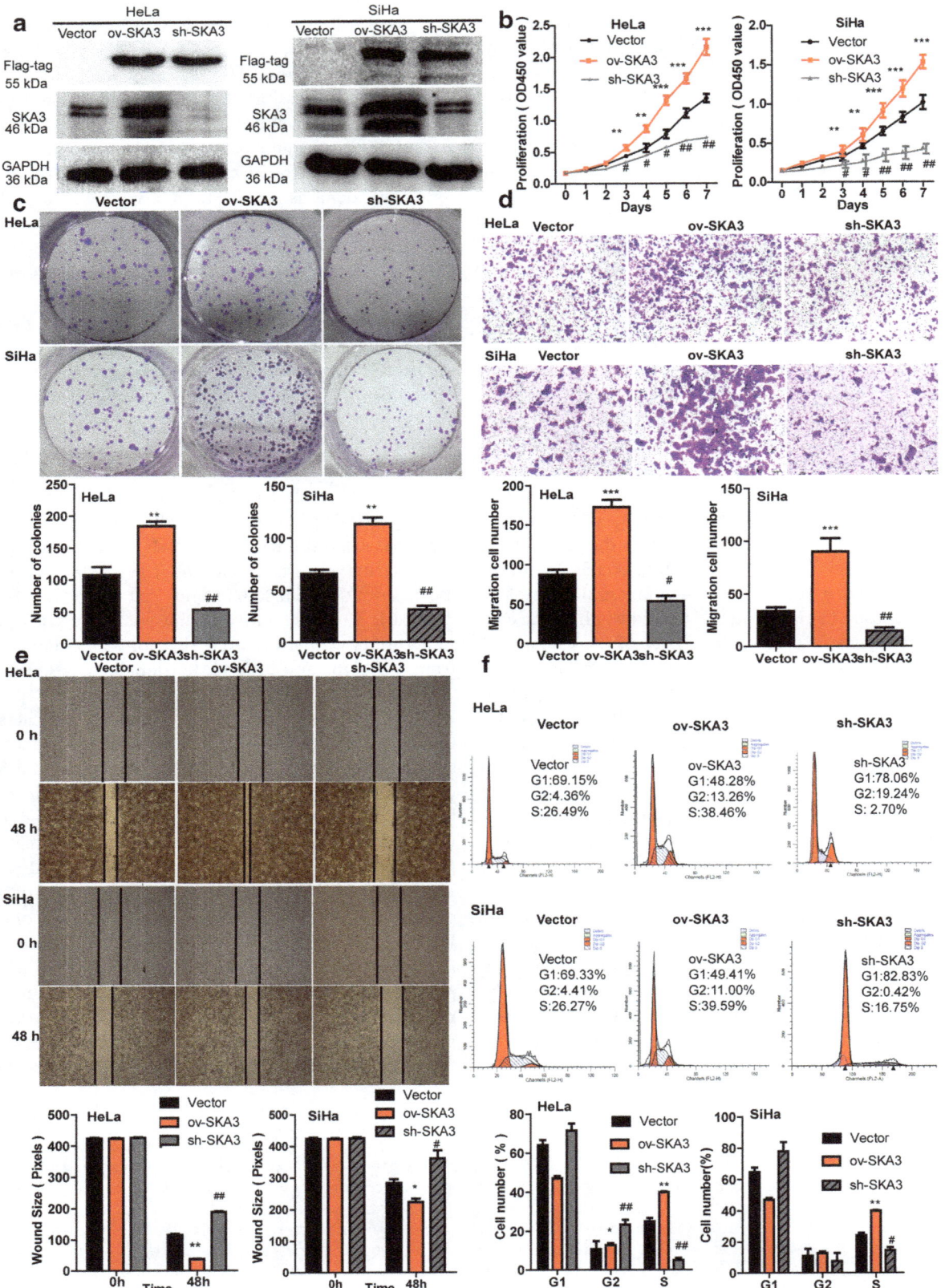

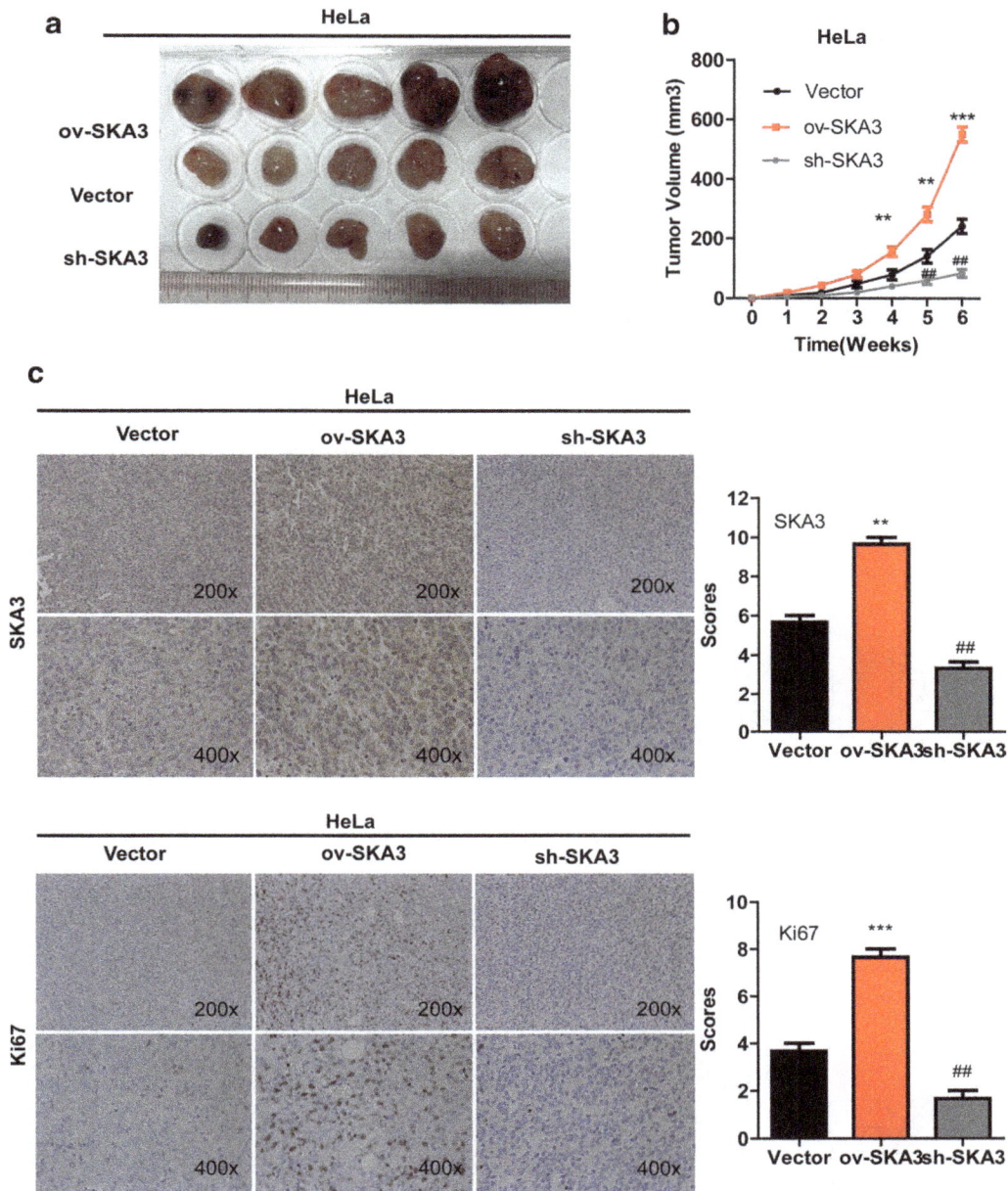

**Fig. 3** Overexpression of SKA3 accelerates CC tumor growth in vivo. **a** Representative picture of xenograft tumors formed. **b** Growth curves of xenograft tumors derived from HeLa cells with stable SKA3 overexpression, SKA3 knockdown and control plasmid expression. **c** Representative images of IHC staining for SKA3 and Ki67 in tumor sections (magnifications ×200). Data (mean ± SD; n = 6) were analyzed by Student's t test (*p < 0.05, **p < 0.01, over-SKA3 vs. control vector. #p < 0.05, ##p < 0.01, SKA3 knockdown vs. control vector)

was altered in vitro, we also performed IHC staining to examine regulation in vivo. Expression of CDK4 and cyclin D1 was increased in tumor sections with SKA3 overexpression (vs. control vector, **p < 0.01, Fig. 5c) but decreased in tumor sections with SKA3 knockdown. Taken together, our results show that SKA3

overexpression promoted cell cycle progression by activating the PI3K/Akt pathway.

### Blocking the PI3K–Akt pathway restored SKA3-induced cell proliferation and migration

To validate our predictions, we used the Akt inhibitor GSK690693 to block Akt activity in HeLa cells

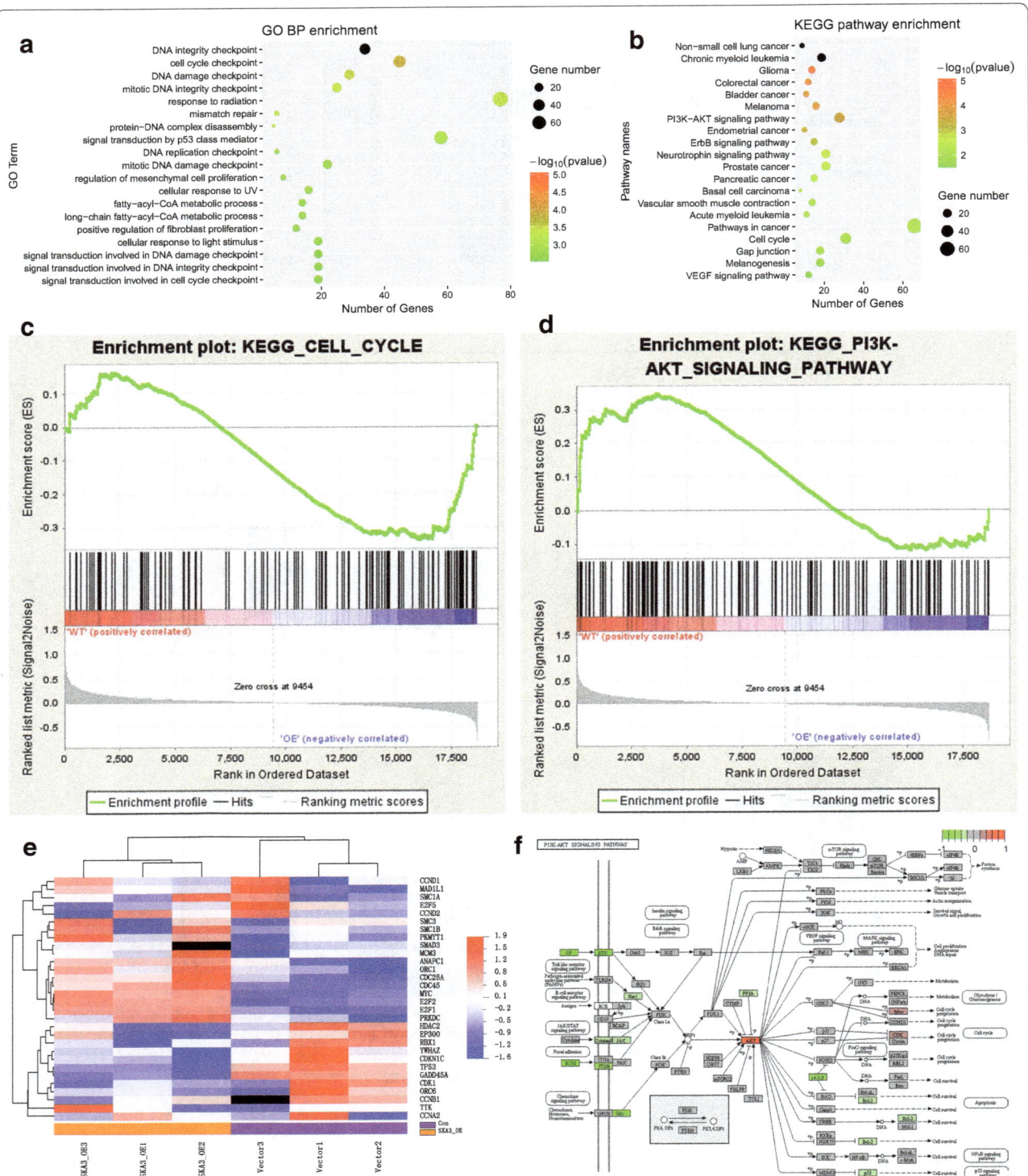

**Fig. 4** Overexpression of SKA3 facilitates the G1-S cell cycle transition and regulates the PI3K–Akt pathway in CC. **a** RNA-sequencing (RNA-Seq) analysis of genes in HeLa cells with stable SKA3 overexpression indicated involvement of the cell cycle. **b** KEGG pathway enrichment analysis (representative pathways) of genes in HeLa cells with stable SKA3 overexpression, including the PI3K–Akt pathway and cell cycle-associated genes. **c** Gene set enrichment analysis (GSEA) of HeLa cells with stable SKA3 overexpression for gene signatures of cell cycle- and **d** PI3K–Akt pathway-regulated genes. **e** Heat map of expression in the cell cycle gene set. **f** KEGG analysis of genes involved in the PI3K–Akt pathway and cell cycle

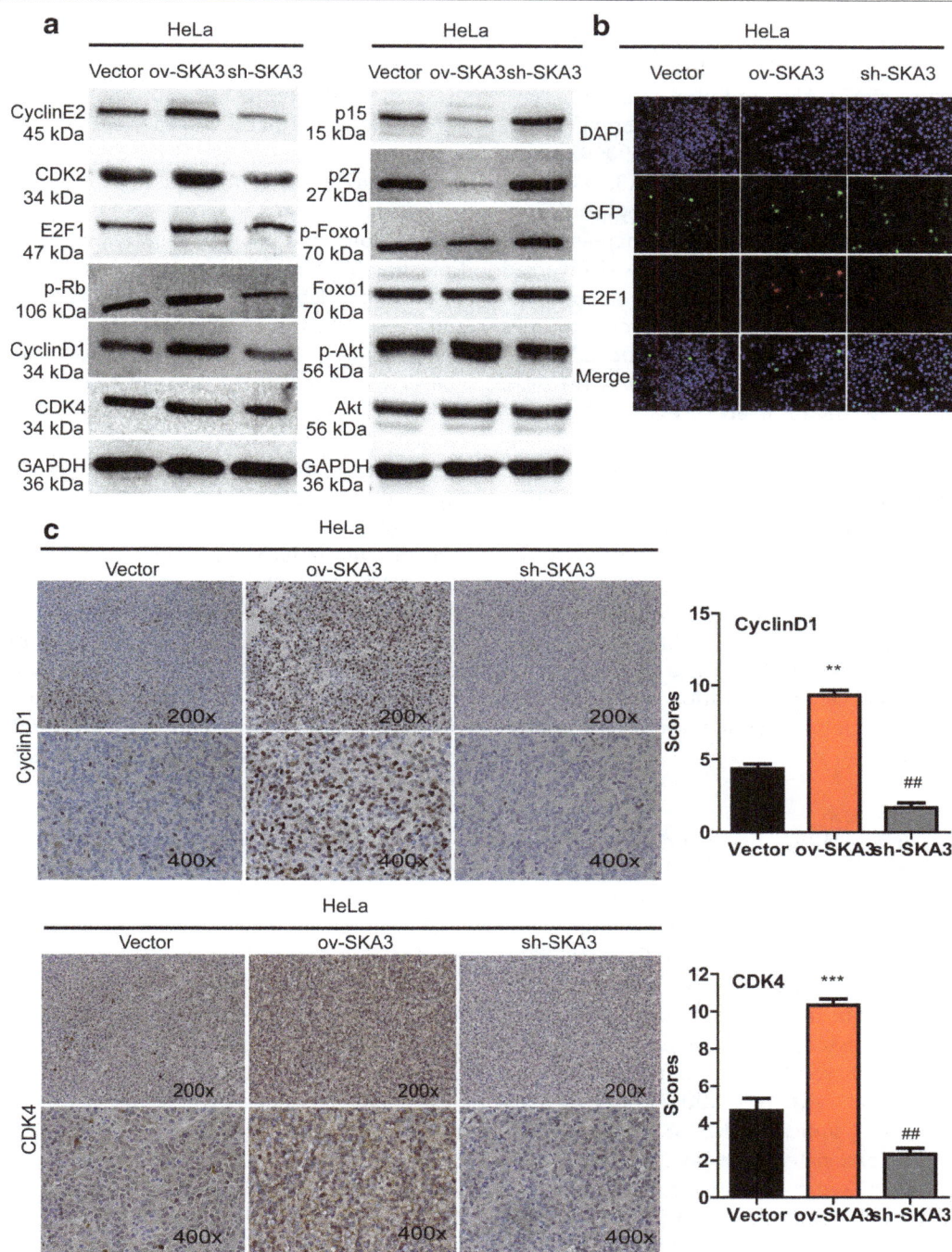

**Fig. 5** Overexpression of SKA3 promotes cell cycle progression by activating the PI3K–Akt pathway. **a** Representative western blot results of proteins related to the PI3K–Akt pathway and the cell cycle in HeLa cells with stable SKA3 overexpression, SKA3 knockdown and control plasmid expression. **b** Activity of E2F1 in HeLa cells with stable SKA3 overexpression, SKA3 knockdown and control plasmid expression by immunofluorescence. **c** Representative images of IHC staining for proteins related to the cell cycle (cyclin D1 and CDK4) in tumor sections with SKA3 overexpression, SKA3 knockdown and control plasmid expression (*p < 0.05, **p < 0.01, over-SKA3 vs. control vector. #p < 0.05, ##p < 0.01, SKA3 knockdown vs. control vector)

overexpressing SKA3. Cells were divided into 4 groups: stable vector expression, stable SKA3 overexpression, stable vector expression + Akt inhibitor and stable SKA3 overexpression + Akt inhibitor. CCK-8 assays showed that proliferation in HeLa cells overexpressing SKA3 was significantly inhibited by GSK690693 treatment from day 2 to day 7 (vs. over-SKA3, p < 0.001, Fig. 6a). In addition, clone formation assays indicated that SKA3 overexpression significantly increased the number of HeLa colonies, and this effect was reversed by GSK690693 (vs. SKA3 overexpression, #p < 0.05, ##p < 0.01, Fig. 6b, c). Besides, cell cycle analysis revealed that SKA3 overexpression significantly promoted the process of S phase, the effect was reversed by GSK690693 (vs. SKA3 overexpression, #p < 0.05, ##p < 0.01, Fig. 6d). We also examined proteins downstream of Akt and related to the cell cycle. Western blotting showed that levels of p-Akt, cyclin D1, CDK4, CDK2, p-Rb, and E2F1 were increased in HeLa cells overexpressing SKA3, and this induction was blocked by GSK690693 (Fig. 6e). Furthermore, E2F1 activity was increased in HeLa cells overexpressing SKA3, an effect that was reversed by GSK690693 (Fig. 6f). Consequently, our results show that SKA3 overexpression promotes cell HeLa cell proliferation and migration by enhancing cell cycle progression and activating the PI3K/Akt pathway.

## Discussion

Despite the use of the HPV vaccine and early detection methods, identifying new molecular mechanisms and novel target therapies is extremely important for CC treatment. Using an Oncomine dataset, we found that mRNA expression of SKA3 was higher in CC tissue than in normal tissue, thus, SKA3 may play a very important role in CC progression. In our study, the expression of SKA3 in CC patient tissue was higher than that in normal tissue, and similar results were found between CC cell lines and normal cells. In addition, survival data from a TCGA dataset indicated that SKA3 overexpression appears to be associated with poor survival in CC patients. Next, we aimed to investigate the function of SKA3 in CC, and the results suggested that SKA3 overexpression promotes HeLa cell proliferation, clone formation, migration and cell cycle progression and accelerates tumor growth in vivo. Mechanistically, we provided evidence that SKA3 promotes cell cycle progression via the PI3K–Akt pathway. Taken together, our results indicated that SKA3 may serve as a useful diagnostic and therapeutic target for CC and may be used to predict the prognosis of CC patients.

SKA3 localizes to the spindle and KT throughout mitosis and along spindle microtubules [30, 31] and has multiple functions in promoting mitotic progression [32], by phosphorylating Cdk1 in mitosis, binding to Ndc80C and recruiting the Ska complex to kinetochores [33]. Some studies have shown that SKA3 participates in cancer development. SKA3 depletion effectively blocks mitotic progression in asynchronously growing HeLa S3 cells [34]. An early study showed that SKA3 correlates with the progression of colorectal cancer, leading to higher chromosome instability (CIN) in tumors. Knockdown of SKA3 in CRC cells dramatically reduces cell growth rates, induces G2/M arrest and decreases migration and invasion [35]. In contrast, another study demonstrated that SKA3 overexpression significantly decreases migration in PC-3 [15]. In our study, as expected, the results showed that SKA3 overexpression promotes the cell proliferation, clone formation and migration in HeLa cells, which is partially consistent with the results found in CRC. Interestingly, we found no significant differences in cell apoptosis between HeLa cells with SKA3 overexpression/knockdown and cells expressing a control vector (p > 0.05). Nonetheless, our cell cycle data analysis showed that SKA3 promotes cell cycle progression mainly by facilitating the G1-S transition.

In addition, we constructed a xenograft tumor model by injecting HeLa cells overexpressing SKA3 or the control plasmid and found that expression of Ki67 was higher in tumors generated by HeLa cells overexpressing SKA3. Ki67 is a common proliferation marker, and the presence of tandem Ki67 in CC indicates a poor prognosis [36]. Our results suggest that SKA3 overexpression accelerates tumor growth and may serve as a predictor of poor prognosis in CC. To our knowledge, this is the first report that SKA3 can promote tumor growth of CC in vivo. We have thus shown that SKA3 promotes cell proliferation of CC both in vitro and in vivo.

(See figure on next page.)

**Fig. 6** An inhibitor of Akt blocked the cell proliferation abilities induced by SKA3 overexpression in HeLa cells. **a** The proliferation curves for HeLa cells with control vector expression, SKA3 overexpression, vector expression + inhibitor treatment and SKA3 overexpression + inhibitor treatment according to a CCK8 assay. **b** Representative images of clone formation in HeLa cells with control vector expression, SKA3 overexpression, vector expression + inhibitor treatment and SKA3 overexpression + inhibitor treatment. **c** Clone formation assay in HeLa cells with control vector expression, SKA3 overexpression, vector expression + inhibitor treatment and SKA3 overexpression + inhibitor treatment. **d** Representative cell cycle data were measured by flow cytometry in HeLa cells with control vector expression, SKA3 overexpression and SKA3 overexpression + inhibitor treatment. **e** Representative western blot analyses of proteins related to the PI3K–Akt pathway and the cell cycle in HeLa cells with control vector expression, SKA3 overexpression and SKA3 overexpression + inhibitor treatment. **f** Activity of E2F1 in HeLa cells with control vector expression, SKA3 overexpression and SKA3 overexpression + inhibitor treatment

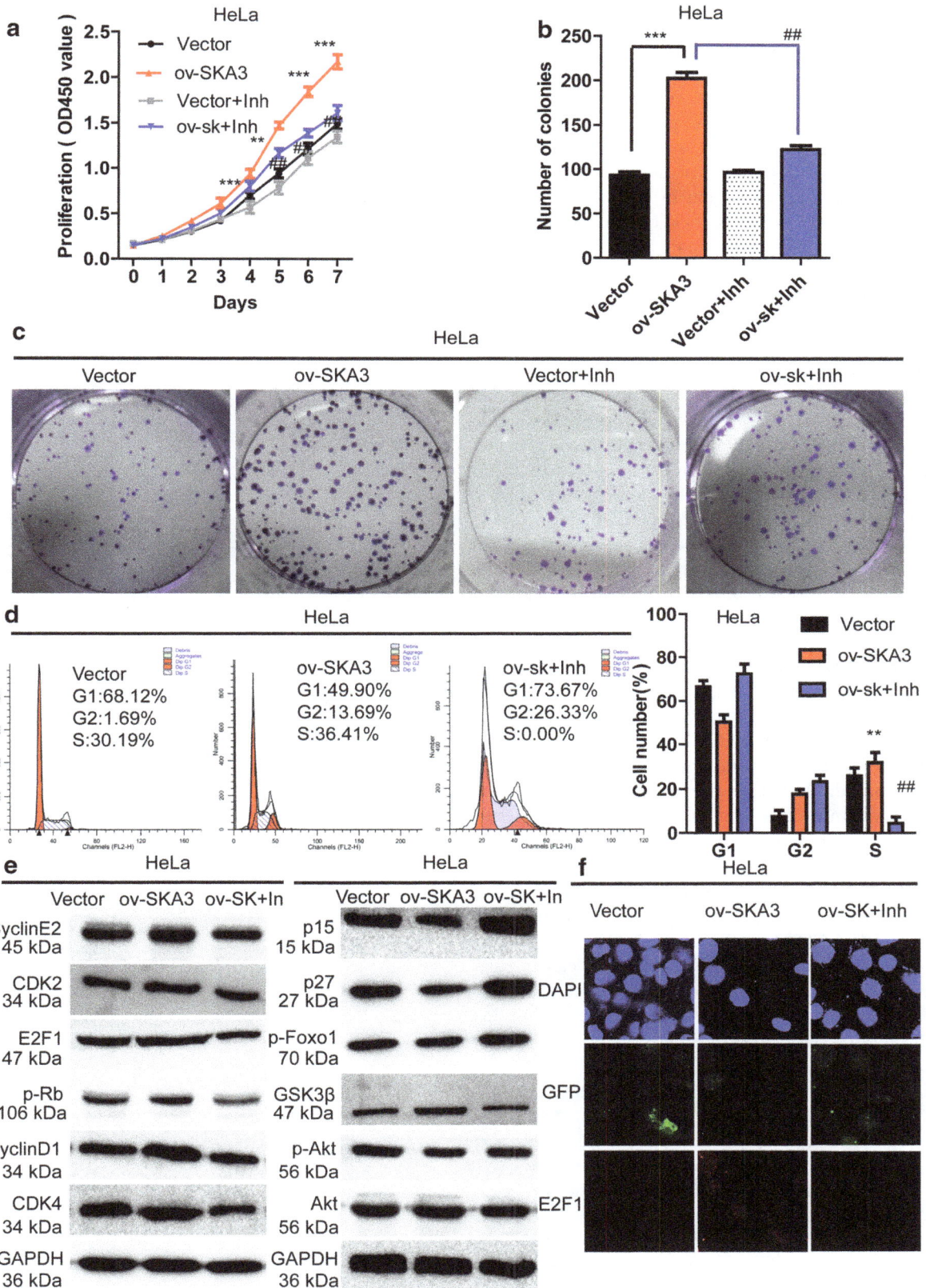

**a** HeLa

Vector
ov-SKA3
Vector+Inh
ov-sk+Inh

Proliferation ( OD450 value )

Days

**b** HeLa

Number of colonies

Vector   ov-SKA3   Vector+Inh   ov-sk+Inh

**c** HeLa

Vector          ov-SKA3          Vector+Inh          ov-sk+Inh

**d** HeLa

Vector
G1:68.12%
G2:1.69%
S:30.19%

ov-SKA3
G1:49.90%
G2:13.69%
S:36.41%

ov-sk+Inh
G1:73.67%
G2:26.33%
S:0.00%

HeLa

Vector
ov-SKA3
ov-sk+Inh

Cell number(%)

G1          G2          S

**e** HeLa                    HeLa                    **f** HeLa

Vector  ov-SKA3  ov-SK+In     Vector  ov-SKA3  ov-SK+In          Vector          ov-SKA3          ov-SK+Inh

CyclinE2    p15                                                   DAPI
45 kDa      15 kDa

CDK2        p27
34 kDa      27 kDa

E2F1        p-Foxo1                                               GFP
47 kDa      70 kDa

p-Rb        GSK3β
106 kDa     47 kDa

CyclinD1    p-Akt                                                 E2F1
34 kDa      56 kDa

CDK4        Akt
34 kDa      56 kDa

GAPDH       GAPDH
36 kDa      36 kDa

Furthermore, RNA-Seq was used to investigate the mechanism of SKA3 as a carcinogenic gene in CC, and the results revealed alterations in genes related to the cell cycle and the PI3K–Akt pathway were altered. The cell cycle is a complex and highly orchestrated process that involves numerous regulatory proteins [37]. Previous studies of the cell cycle in CC have mostly concentrated on G2/M phase [38, 39], whereas only a few studies have focused on the G1/S transition in CC [40]. Although a previous study showed that knockdown of SKA3 induced G2/M arrest in CRC cells, our results indicated that SKA3 promotes cell cycle progression in HeLa cells by enhancing the G1-S transition. Key cell cycle regulators that govern the progression of cells from G1 to S phase include Rb-E2F1, cyclin-dependent kinase (cdk) complexes and cdk inhibitors [41–43]. Additionally, western blotting results revealed that SKA3 overexpression up-regulated the level of cell cycle-related proteins such as cyclin D1, CDK4, CDK2, cyclin E2, and p-Rb and promoted the activity of E2F1. Mitogenic stimulation during G1 phase leads to sequential activation of cdk4/6-cyclin D and cdk2–cyclin E complexes, which hyperphosphorylate Rb and thereby cause the release of active E2F1 [44], which controls expression of downstream genes essential for transition from G1 to S [45]. These findings support our western blot results.

PI3K/Akt pathway is associated with characteristics of carcinogenesis and is frequently activated in numerous human cancer types, such as in non-small cell lung cancer [46], colorectal cancer [47], breast cancer [48] and prostate cancer [49]. In addition, a recent study showed that women with CC commonly display PI3K pathway alterations, indicating its potential value in the treatment of advanced and metastatic disease [50]. In the present study, western blotting results showed changes in the expression levels of genes downstream of the PI3K/Akt pathway. SKA3 overexpression up-regulated the level of p-Akt, which modulates cell cycle proteins such as cyclin D1, CDK4, CDK2, cyclin E2 and E2F1 while inhibiting the activity of foxo1, p15 and p27. In cancer cells, increased activation of p-Akt can promote cell growth by regulating cell cycle regulators, such as p21 and p27 [51], which supports our results. Furthermore, we blocked the PI3K/Akt signaling using an Akt inhibitor (GSK690693) in HeLa cells with stably overexpressing SKA3 or the control plasmid, which reversed cell proliferation and clone formation capacities induced by SKA3 overexpression. Additionally, western blotting demonstrated that the levels of p-Akt, cyclin E, CDK2, CDK4 and cyclin D1 were down-regulated, but those of foxo1, p15 and p27 up-regulated by the Akt inhibitor in HeLa cells. Thus, we propose that SKA3 overexpression promotes cervical

cancer cell proliferation and migration by regulating the cell cycle and the PI3K/Akt pathway, which might suggest a new strategy for finding novel targetable pathways in CC.

## Conclusion

In short, we suggest that SKA3 promotes cell proliferation and migration by promoting cell cycle progression and PI3K/Akt signaling pathway in CC. It may be a promising therapeutic candidate and prognostic indicator in CC.

## Additional file

**Additional file 1: Fig. S1.** Overexpression of SKA3 does not affect apoptosis in HeLa cells. (C) Representative apoptosis data, as measured by flow cytometry in (A) HeLa cells and (B) SiHa cells with stable SKA3 overexpression, SKA3 knockdown and control plasmid expression. All data (mean ± SD; n = 3) were analyzed by Student's t test (*p < 0.05, **p < 0.01, over-SKA3 vs. control vector. #p < 0.05, ##p < 0.01, SKA3 knockdown vs. control vector.

## Abbreviations

SKA3: spindle and kinetochore-associated complex subunit 3; CC: cervical cancer; IHC: immunohistochemistry; CDK: cyclin-dependent protein kinase; Rb: retinoblastoma.

## Authors' contributions

LL and LW participated in the study design and analysis of the data, RH and MW carried out most of the experiment and collected the results. WN provided ideas and analysed data and drafted the manuscript. RH was in charge of manuscript writing. All authors read and approved the final manuscript.

## Author details

[1] Shenzhen Hospital, Southern Medical University, No. 1333, Xinhu Road, Bao'an District, Shenzhen 518101, Guangdong, China. [2] School of Traditional Chinese Medicine, Southern Medical University, No. 1838, Guangzhou Avenue North, Baiyun District, Guangzhou 510515, Guangdong, China. [3] Zhujiang Hospital of Southern Medical University, No. 253, Industrial Avenue, Haizhu District, Guangzhou 510280, Guangdong, China. [4] The First Affiliated Hospital, Guangzhou University of Chinese Medicine, No.16 Baiyun Airport Road, Baiyun District, Guangzhou 510405, Guangdong, China. [5] Cancer Research Institute, Southern Medical University, No. 1838, Guangzhou Avenue North, Baiyun District, Guangzhou 510515, Guangdong, China. [6] Zhongshan Huangpu People's Hospital, No. 32, Long'an Street, Huangpu Town, Zhongshan 528429, Guangdong, China.

## Acknowledgements

Not applicable.

## Competing interests

The authors declare that they have no competing interests.

## Funding

This study was supported in part by the National Science Foundation of China (Program Nos. 81573729 and 81603472).

## References

1. Wu J, Chen M, Liang C, Su W. Prognostic value of the pretreatment neutrophil-to-lymphocyte ratio in cervical cancer: a meta-analysis and systematic review. Oncotarget. 2017;8(8):13400–12.
2. Siegel R, Naishadham D, Jemal A. Cancer statistics, 2013. CA Cancer J Clin. 2013;63(1):11–30.
3. Jemal A, Bray F, Center MM, Ferlay J, Ward E, Forman D. Global cancer statistics. CA Cancer J Clin. 2011;61(2):69–90.
4. Kuguyo O, Matimba A, Tsikai N, Magwali T, Madziyire M, Gidiri M, Dandara C, Nhachi C. Cervical cancer in Zimbabwe: a situation analysis. Pan Afr Med J. 2017;27:215.
5. Menvielle G, Richard JB, Ringa V, Dray-Spira R, Beck F. To what extent is women's economic situation associated with cancer screening uptake when nationwide screening exists? A study of breast and cervical cancer screening in France in 2010. Cancer Causes Control. 2014;25(8):977–83.
6. Klingelhutz AJ, Roman A. Cellular transformation by human papillomaviruses: lessons learned by comparing high- and low-risk viruses. Virology. 2012;424(2):77–98.
7. Mine KL, Shulzhenko N, Yambartsev A, Rochman M, Sanson GF, Lando M, Varma S, Skinner J, Volfovsky N, Deng T, Brenna SM, Carvalho CR, Ribalta JC, Bustin M, Matzinger P, Silva ID, Lyng H, Gerbase-DeLima M, Morgun A. Gene network reconstruction reveals cell cycle and antiviral genes as major drivers of cervical cancer. Nat Commun. 2013;4:1806.
8. Zhang Q, Li W, Kanis MJ, Qi G, Li M, Yang X, Kong B. Oncologic and obstetrical outcomes with fertility-sparing treatment of cervical cancer: a systematic review and meta-analysis. Oncotarget. 2017;8(28):46580–92.
9. Knoff J, Yang B, Hung CF, Wu TC. Cervical cancer: development of targeted therapies beyond molecular pathogenesis. Curr Obstet Gynecol Rep. 2014;3(1):18–32.
10. Liang H, Luo R, Chen X, Zhao Y, Tan A. miR-187 inhibits the growth of cervical cancer cells by targeting FGF9. Oncol Rep. 2017;38(4):1977–84.
11. Jeyaprakash AA, Santamaria A, Jayachandran U, Chan YW, Benda C, Nigg EA, Conti E. Structural and functional organization of the Ska complex, a key component of the kinetochore–microtubule interface. Mol Cell. 2012;46(3):274–86.
12. Sivakumar S, Daum JR, Tipton AR, Rankin S, Gorbsky GJ. The spindle and kinetochore-associated (Ska) complex enhances binding of the anaphase-promoting complex/cyclosome (APC/C) to chromosomes and promotes mitotic exit. Mol Biol Cell. 2014;25(5):594–605.
13. Zhang QH, Qi ST, Wang ZB, Yang CY, Wei YC, Chen L, Ouyang YC, Hou Y, Schatten H, Sun QY. Localization and function of the Ska complex during mouse oocyte meiotic maturation. Cell Cycle. 2012;11(5):909–16.
14. Jiao X, Hooper SD, Djureinovic T, Larsson C, Warnberg F, Tellgren-Roth C, Botling J, Sjoblom T. Gene rearrangements in hormone receptor negative breast cancers revealed by mate pair sequencing. BMC Genomics. 2013;14:165.
15. Lee M, Williams KA, Hu Y, Andreas J, Patel SJ, Zhang S, Crawford NP. GNL3 and SKA3 are novel prostate cancer metastasis susceptibility genes. Clin Exp Metastasis. 2015;32(8):769–82.
16. Evan GI, Vousden KH. Proliferation, cell cycle and apoptosis in cancer. Nature. 2001;411(6835):342–8.
17. Morgan DO. Cyclin-dependent kinases: engines, clocks, and microprocessors. Annu Rev Cell Dev Biol. 1997;13:261–91.
18. Bandi N, Vassella E. miR-34a and miR-15a/16 are co-regulated in non-small cell lung cancer and control cell cycle progression in a synergistic and Rb-dependent manner. Mol Cancer. 2011;10:55.
19. Bahrami A, Hasanzadeh M, ShahidSales S, Yousefi Z, Kadkhodayan S, Farazestanian M, Joudi MM, Gharib M, Mahdi HS, Avan A. Clinical significance and prognosis value of Wnt signaling pathway in cervical cancer. J Cell Biochem. 2017;118(10):3028–33.
20. Yousif NG, Sadiq AM, Yousif MG, Al-Mudhafar RH, Al-Baghdadi JJ, Hadi N. Notch1 ligand signaling pathway activated in cervical cancer: poor prognosis with high-level JAG1/Notch1. Arch Gynecol Obstet. 2015;292(4):899–904.
21. Wu X, Zhou J, Cai D, Li M. Matrine inhibits the metastatic properties of human cervical cancer cells via downregulating the p38 signaling pathway. Oncol Rep. 2017;38(2):1312–20.
22. Ji J, Zheng PS. Activation of mTOR signaling pathway contributes to survival of cervical cancer cells. Gynecol Oncol. 2010;117(1):103–8.
23. Xu CL, Wang JZ, Xia XP, Pan CW, Shao XX, Xia SL, Yang SX, Zheng B. Rab11-FIP2 promotes colorectal cancer migration and invasion by regulating PI3K/AKT/MMP7 signaling pathway. Biochem Biophys Res Commun. 2016;470(2):397–404.
24. Yin K, Wang L, Zhang X, He Z, Xia Y, Xu J, Wei S, Li B, Li Z, Sun G, Li Q, Xu H, Xu Z. Netrin-1 promotes gastric cancer cell proliferation and invasion via the receptor neogenin through PI3K/AKT signaling pathway. Oncotarget. 2017;8(31):51177–89.
25. Cui B, Zheng B, Zhang X, Stendahl U, Andersson S, Wallin KL. Mutation of PIK3CA: possible risk factor for cervical carcinogenesis in older women. Int J Oncol. 2009;34(2):409–16.
26. Liu P, Cheng H, Roberts TM, Zhao JJ. Targeting the phosphoinositide 3-kinase pathway in cancer. Nat Rev Drug Discovery. 2009;8(8):627–44.
27. Jiang E, Sun X, Kang H, Sun L, An W, Yao Y, Hu X. Dehydrocostus lactone inhibits proliferation, antiapoptosis, and invasion of cervical cancer cells through PI3K/Akt signaling pathway. Int J Gynecol Cancer. 2015;25(7):1179–86.
28. Schwarz JK, Payton JE, Rashmi R, Xiang T, Jia Y, Huettner P, Rogers BE, Yang Q, Watson M, Rader JS, Grigsby PW. Pathway-specific analysis of gene expression data identifies the PI3K/Akt pathway as a novel therapeutic target in cervical cancer. Clin Cancer Res. 2012;18(5):1464–71.
29. Wu J, Chen C, Zhao KN. Phosphatidylinositol 3-kinase signaling as a therapeutic target for cervical cancer. Curr Cancer Drug Targets. 2013;13(2):143–56.
30. Daum JR, Wren JD, Daniel JJ, Sivakumar S, McAvoy JN, Potapova TA, Gorbsky GJ. Ska3 is required for spindle checkpoint silencing and the maintenance of chromosome cohesion in mitosis. Curr Biol. 2009;19(17):1467–72.
31. Ohta S, Bukowski-Wills JC, Sanchez-Pulido L, Alves FL, Wood L, Chen ZA, Platani M, Fischer L, Hudson DF, Ponting CP, Fukagawa T, Earnshaw WC, Rappsilber J. The protein composition of mitotic chromosomes determined using multiclassifier combinatorial proteomics. Cell. 2010;142(5):810–21.
32. Sivakumar S, Gorbsky GJ. Phosphatase-regulated recruitment of the spindle- and kinetochore-associated (Ska) complex to kinetochores. Biol Open. 2017;6:1672–9.
33. Zhang Q, Sivakumar S, Chen Y, Gao H, Yang L, Yuan Z, Yu H, Liu H. Ska3 phosphorylated by Cdk1 binds Ndc80 and recruits Ska to kinetochores to promote mitotic progression. Curr Biol. 2017;27(10):1477–84.
34. Gaitanos TN, Santamaria A, Jeyaprakash AA, Wang B, Conti E, Nigg EA. Stable kinetochore-microtubule interactions depend on the Ska complex and its new component Ska3/C13Orf3. EMBO J. 2009;28(10):1442–52.
35. Chuang TP, Wang JY, Jao SW, Wu CC, Chen JH, Hsiao KH, Lin CY, Chen SH, Su SY, Chen YJ, Chen YT, Wu DC, Li LH. Over-expression of AURKA, SKA3 and DSN1 contributes to colorectal adenoma to carcinoma progression. Oncotarget. 2016;7(29):45803–18.
36. Stoenescu TM, Ivan LD, Stoenescu N, Azoicai D. Assessment tumor markers by immunohistochemistry (Ki67, p53 and Bcl-2) on a cohort of patients with cervical cancer in various stages of evolution. Rev Med Chir Soc Med Nat Iasi. 2011;115(2):485–92.
37. Mayank AK, Sharma S, Deshwal RK, Lal SK. LIMD1 antagonizes E2F1 activity and cell cycle progression by enhancing Rb function in cancer cells. Cell Biol Int. 2014;38(7):809–17.
38. Setiawati A, Setiawati A. Celecoxib, a COX-2 selective inhibitor, induces cell cycle arrest at the G2/M phase in HeLa cervical cancer cells. Asian Pac J Cancer Prev. 2016;17(4):1655–60.
39. Tian Q, Zang YH. Antiproliferative and apoptotic effects of the ethanolic herbal extract of *Achillea falcata* in human cervical cancer cells are mediated via cell cycle arrest and mitochondrial membrane potential loss. J BUON. 2015;20(6):1487–96.
40. Mou Z, Xu X, Dong M, Xu J. MicroRNA-148b acts as a tumor suppressor in cervical cancer by inducing G1/S-phase cell cycle arrest and apoptosis in a caspase-3-dependent manner. Med Sci Monit. 2016;22:2809–15.

40. Mou Z, Xu X, Dong M, Xu J. MicroRNA-148b acts as a tumor suppressor in cervical cancer by inducing G1/S-phase cell cycle arrest and apoptosis in a caspase-3-dependent manner. Med Sci Monit. 2016;22:2809–15.

41. Chellappan SP, Hiebert S, Mudryj M, Horowitz JM, Nevins JR. The E2F transcription factor is a cellular target for the RB protein. Cell. 1991;65(6):1053–61.

42. Bandara LR, La Thangue NB. Adenovirus E1a prevents the retinoblastoma gene product from complexing with a cellular transcription factor. Nature. 1991;351(6326):494–7.

43. Lundberg AS, Weinberg RA. Functional inactivation of the retinoblastoma protein requires sequential modification by at least two distinct cyclin-cdk complexes. Mol Cell Biol. 1998;18(2):753–61.

44. Rubin SM, Gall AL, Zheng N, Pavletich NP. Structure of the Rb C-terminal domain bound to E2F1-DP1: a mechanism for phosphorylation-induced E2F release. Cell. 2005;123(6):1093–106.

45. Giacinti C, Giordano A. RB and cell cycle progression. Oncogene. 2006;25(38):5220–7.

46. Zhou Y, Li S, Li J, Wang D, Li Q. Effect of microRNA-135a on cell proliferation, migration, invasion, apoptosis and tumor angiogenesis through the IGF-1/PI3K/Akt signaling pathway in non-small cell lung cancer. Cell Physiol Biochem. 2017;42(4):1431–46.

47. Zhao T, Li H, Liu Z. Tumor necrosis factor receptor 2 promotes growth of colorectal cancer via the PI3K/AKT signaling pathway. Oncol Lett. 2017;13(1):342–6.

48. Liu Y, Wang R, Zhang L, Li J, Lou K, Shi B. The lipid metabolism gene FTO influences breast cancer cell energy metabolism via the PI3K/AKT signaling pathway. Oncol Lett. 2017;13(6):4685–90.

49. Liu T, Gulinaer A, Shi X, Wang F, An H, Cui W, Li Q. Gene polymorphisms in the PI3K/AKT/mTOR signaling pathway contribute to prostate cancer susceptibility in Chinese men. Oncotarget. 2017;8(37):61305–17.

50. Bahrami A, Hasanzadeh M, Hassanian SM, ShahidSales S, Ghayour-Mobarhan M, Ferns GA, Avan A. The potential value of the PI3K/Akt/mTOR signaling pathway for assessing prognosis in cervical cancer and as a target for therapy. J Cell Biochem. 2017;118:4163–9.

51. Li D, Wei X, Ma M, Jia H, Zhang Y, Kang W, Wang T, Shi X. FFJ-3 inhibits PKM2 protein expression via the PI3K/Akt signaling pathway and activates the mitochondrial apoptosis signaling pathway in human cancer cells. Oncol Lett. 2017;13(4):2607–14.

# 6

# *Marsdenia tenacissima* extract induces apoptosis and suppresses autophagy through ERK activation in lung cancer cells

Yan-Na Jiao[1†], Li-Na Wu[2†], Dong Xue[1†], Xi-Juan Liu[2], Zhi-Hua Tian[2], Shan-Tong Jiang[1], Shu-Yan Han[1*] and Ping-Ping Li[1*]

## Abstract

**Background:** *Marsdenia tenacissima* is an herb medicine which has been utilized to treat malignant diseases for decades. The *M. tenacissima* extract (MTE) shows significant anti-proliferation activity against non-small cell lung cancer (NSCLC) cells, but the underlying mechanisms remain unclear. In this study, we explored the potential anti-proliferation mechanisms of MTE in NSCLC cells in relation to apoptosis as well as autophagy, which are two critical forms to control cancer cell survival and death.

**Methods:** The proliferation of H1975 and A549 cells was evaluated by MTT assay. Cell apoptosis was assessed by Annexin V and PI staining, Caspase 3 expression and activity. Autophagy flux proteins were detected by Western blot with or without autophagy inducer and inhibitor. Endogenous LC3-II puncta and LysoTracker staining were monitored by confocal microscopy. The formation of autophagic vacuoles was measured by acridine orange staining. ERK is a crucial molecule to interplay with cell autophagy and apoptosis. The role of ERK on cell apoptosis and autophagy influenced by MTE was determined in the presence of MEK/ERK inhibitor U0126.

**Results:** The significant growth inhibition and apoptosis induction were observed in MTE treated NSCLC cells. MTE induced cell apoptosis coexisted with elevated Caspase 3 activity. MTE also impaired autophagic flux by upregulated LC3-II and p62 expression. Autophagy inducer EBSS could not abolish the impaired autophagic flux by MTE, while it was augmented in the presence of autophagy inhibitor Baf A1. The autophagosome–lysosome fusion was blocked by MTE via affecting lysosome function as evidenced by decreased expression of LAMP1 and Cathepsin B. The molecule ERK became hyperactivated after MTE treatment, but the MEK/ERK inhibitor U0126 abrogated autophagy inhibition and apoptosis induction caused by MTE, suggested that ERK signaling pathways partially contributed to cell death caused by MTE.

**Conclusion:** Our results demonstrate that MTE caused apoptosis induction as well as autophagy inhibition in NSCLC cells. The activated ERK is partially associated with NSCLC apoptotic and autophagic cell death in response to MTE treatment. The present findings reveal new mechanisms for the anti-tumor activity of MTE against NSCLC.

**Keywords:** *Marsdenia tenacissima* extract (MTE), Apoptosis, Autophagy, ERK activation, NSCLC

*Correspondence: shuyanhan@bjmu.edu.cn; lppma123@sina.com
†Yan-Na Jiao, Li-Na Wu and Dong Xue contributed equally to this work
[1] Key Laboratory of Carcinogenesis and Translational Research (Ministry of Education/Beijing), Department of Integration of Chinese and Western Medicine, Peking University Cancer Hospital & Institute, No. 52 Fucheng Road, Haidian District, Beijing 100142, People's Republic of China
Full list of author information is available at the end of the article

## Background

Lung cancer remains one of the leading causes of cancer-related deaths worldwide. It can be divided into small-cell lung cancer (SCLC, 15%) and non-small cell lung cancer (NSCLC, 85%) according to the histologic features. In patients with advanced NSCLC who generally have a poor prognosis [1], new strategies to improve survival are urgently required.

Aberrant signal transduction pathways often occur in tumorigenesis and progress. Studies demonstrated that autophagy and apoptosis play central roles during lung cancer initiation and progression [2]. Fundamental cellular physiological activities such as apoptosis and autophagy are critical to control cell survival and cell death [2]. Apoptosis is one form of programmed cell death with the function of removing damaged cells. Resistance to apoptosis is regarded as one of the hallmarks of cancer [3], thus targeting apoptosis in cancer is a practicable therapy with the suggest of many studies [4].

Autophagy is a self-degradation process to keep constant supply of cellular energy [5]. The relationship between autophagy and cell death is subtle and intricate, and it may promote or inhibit cell death in different contexts. The role of autophagy in tumor initiation and progression is multifaceted and complicated. It has been reported that autophagy inhibits tumorigenesis in some circumstances but promotes carcinogenesis under most conditions [6]. Through upregulating autophagy, cancer cells can survive, growth and become aggressive under pressured microenvironment [6]. Therefore, it makes autophagy as an attractive therapeutic target for effective treatment of tumors including lung cancer [7, 8].

Traditional Chinese Medicine has been used extensively to treat diseases from ancient time. The stem of *Marsdenia tenacissima* (Roxb.) Wight et Arn. is mainly produced in Yunnan (China), and its medical use was firstly recorded in "Dian Nan Ben Cao", a medical literature written by Mao Lan in Ming Dynasty with the activity of expectorant, diuresis, eliminating heat and purging fire, lactating. *M. tenacissima* has long been used as a remedy to treat malignant diseases, tracheitis, and pneumonia in China [9, 10].

There is a great number of studies demonstrated that the water extract of *M. tenacissima* (MTE, trade name: Xiao-Ai-Ping injection) has anti-tumor effects in cell culture models, laboratory animal models and the clinics. (a) The cell culture models include gastric carcinoma cells (SGC-7901) [11], non-small cell lung cancer cells (H1975, H292, H460) [12], Burkitt lymphoma cells [13], human umbilical vein endothelial cells (HUVECs) [14, 15], hepatoma cells (HepG2) [14], esophageal cancer cells (KYSE150 and Eca-109) [16], etc. (b) Xenograft mouse models were generated from gastric cancer [11], hepatocellular carcinoma [17], lymphoma [13] and the chick embryo chorioallantoic membrane [14] etc. (c) The clinic trials were mainly conducted in advanced non-small cell lung cancer patients [18, 19]. Mechanisms accounting for the anti-tumor activities of MTE comprise of anti-angiogenesis [14], cell apoptosis induction [20] and cell cycle arrest [16]. However, the molecular mechanisms underlying the pharmacological action of MTE treatment resulting in cell death remains obscure and need further exploration.

Due to the vital role of apoptosis and autophagy in cell death, in the present study, we evaluated the influence of MTE on cell apoptosis and autophagy in NSCLC cell lines A549 and H1975. Meanwhile, the molecular mechanisms of MTE treatment shared by both apoptosis and autophagy were also explored and elucidated.

## Materials and methods

### Cell cultures and reagents

Human lung carcinoma cell lines A549 and H1975 (American Type Culture Collection, Manassas, VA, USA) were maintained in RPMI-1640 (GIBCO, Thermo Fisher, Hudson, NH, USA) supplemented with 10% fetal bovine serum, 100 U/ml penicillin and 100 μg/ml streptomycin in a humidified incubator at 37 °C under 5% $CO_2$/95% air. The reagents used in this study were: Earle's balanced salt solution (EBSS, Solarbio, H2020, Beijing, China), Bafilomycin A1 (Baf A1, B1793, Sigma-Aldrich, St. Louis, MO, USA), 3-(4,5-dimethyl-2-thiazolyl)-2,5-diphenyl-2-*H*-tetrazolium bromide (MTT, M2128, Sigma-Aldrich), 2-(4-amidinophenyl)-6-indolecarbamidine dihydrochloride (DAPI, D9542, Sigma-Aldrich), LysoTracker Red (L7528, Thermo Fisher), U0126 (S1102, Selleckchem, Houston, TX, USA). Antibodies of anti-LC3-II (L7543) was purchased from Sigma-Aldrich; anti-p62 (ab56416), anti-Cathepsin B (ab33538), and anti-Caspase 3 (ab32351) antibodies were purchased from Abcam (Cambridge, UK); anti-Poly (ADP-ribose) polymerase (PARP) (9542), anti-Lysosome-associated membrane protein 1 (LAMP1) (9091), anti-p-ERK1/2 (Thr202/Tyr204) (9101), anti- ERK1/2 (9102), anti-Bcl-2 alpha (2876) and anti-Bax (5023) were obtained from Cell Signal Technology (Beverly, MA, USA). Anti-β-actin (TDY041) was obtained from TDYbio (Beijing, China). Secondary antibodies including peroxidase-conjugated goat anti-mouse IgG (ZB2305), peroxidase-conjugated goat anti-rabbit IgG (ZB2301), and fluorescein-conjugated affiniPure goat anti-mouse IgG (ZF0312) were purchased from Beijing Zhongshan Golden Bridge Biotechnology Co. Ltd.

MTE (*M. tenacissima* extract, trade name: Xiao-Ai-Ping injection) (1 g crude/ml) was obtained from SanHome Pharmaceutical Co., Ltd (Nanjing, China).

The stem of *M. tenacissima* was collected from Yunnan, China. A voucher specimen (200907-T009-05) was deposited in the herbarium of SanHome Pharmaceutical Co., Ltd (NanJing, China) and was identified by Professor De-Kang Wu (Nanjing University of Chinese Medicine). The preparation of MTE is described as previously [21]. 1 kg powder of the stem of *M. tenacissima* was extracted with water for three times which is 1.5 h, 1 h and 0.8 h, respectively. The combined extracts were filtered, concentrated, and then precipitated with 8 times 85% ethanol at 4 °C for 24 h. The ethanol was recovered and new 85% ethanol was added to cause further precipitation. The ethanol in extract was recovered thoroughly and the insoluble precipitate was removed by filtration. Finally, the extract was concentrating to 200 ml. This condensed extract was dilute with water for injection, added 0.3% polysorbate 80, and adjust pH to 5.5–6.0 to get Xiao-Ai-Ping injection following the standard of State Food and Drug Administration (SFDA) of China.

### Cell viability assays

A549 or H1975 cells were suspended in complete RPMI-1640 medium and plated at a density of $5 \times 10^3$ cells/well in 96-well culture dishes (Costar, Cambridge, MA, USA). Following 24 h of culture, the medium was replaced with complete culture medium supplemented with various concentrations of drugs. On the collection time points, cells were incubated with MTT at 37 °C for 4 h, and the precipitate was dissolved in DMSO. Subsequently, the absorbance (optical density, OD) at 570 nm was measured using a microplate reader (Model 680; Bio-Rad Laboratories, Hercules, CA, USA) and cell viability was calculated according to the following formula: $(OD_{sample} - OD_{blank})/(OD_{control} - OD_{blank}) \times 100\%$.

### Western blot analysis

For immunoblot analysis, cells were harvested and lysed in RIPA lysis buffer (WB0002, TDYBio). Protein concentrations were determined using the BCA protein assay kit (Thermo Fisher). Protein samples (20 μg per lane) were separated on the 8–15% SDS–polyacrylamide gel electrophoresis (PAGE) and blotted onto polyvinylidene difluoride membranes (Immobilon-P, Millipore, Bedford, MA, USA). Following transfer, the membranes were blocked in 5% nonfat milk or bovine serum albumin (BSA) (for phosphorylated proteins) in phosphate-buffered saline (PBS) with 0.1% Tween-20, probed with primary antibodies overnight at 4 °C. After washing, the membranes were incubated with appropriate horseradish peroxidase-conjugated secondary antibodies. Visualization of the protein bands was accomplished using an Immobilon Western Chemiluminescent HRP substrate (Millipore). Image J software was used to calculate the expression of each protein, which was normalized by β-actin.

### Apoptosis analysis

Cell apoptosis was assayed by Annexin V and PI staining (AD10, Dojindo, Kumamoto, Japan). Cells were treated with different concentrations of MTE for 24 h, without or with MEK/ERK inhibitor U0126 (50 μM for A549, 20 μM for H1975). Then cells were collected and incubated with the buffer containing FITC-conjugated Annexin V and PI for 15 min at room temperature, and then analyzed by FACScan flow cytometry (Bection Dikinson, USA). Quantification of early apoptotic cells (Annexin V$^+$/PI$^-$ cells) and late apoptotic cells (Annexin V$^+$/PI$^+$ cells) was calculated by CellQuest software.

### Caspase 3 activity assay

The activity of Caspase 3 was determined using a kit from Beyotime Institute of Biotechnology (C1116, Beijing, China). The activity of Caspase 3 was based on its ability to change acetyl-Asp-Glu-Val-Asp p-nitroanilide (Ac-DEVD-pNA) into a yellow formazan product (p-nitroaniline (pNA)). An increase in absorbance at 405 nm was used to quantify Caspase 3 activity. After 24 h exposure, cells with various designated treatments were collected and rinsed with cold PBS, and then lysed by lysis buffer (60 μL) for 15 min on ice, respectively. Cell lysates were centrifuged at $16,000 \times g$ for 15 min at 4 °C. The detail analysis procedure was described in the manufacturer's protocol. The Caspase 3 activity was shown as fold change of enzyme activity compared to control. All the experiments were carried out in triplicates.

### Immunofluorescence, fluorescence, and confocal microscopy

Cells were seeded to cover glasses in 24-well plates and treated as indicated, fixed with 4% paraformaldehyde and permeabilized with 0.2% Triton X-100 (ST795, Beyotime). The cells were then blocked with 5% FBS for 1 h and exposed to anti-LC3-II (PM036, MBL, Nagoya, Japan) antibody overnight at 4 °C. After washing three times with PBS, cells were incubated with FITC-conjugated secondary antibody solution. After staining nuclei with DAPI, cells were observed under a confocal microscope (Leica, Welzler, Germany). For each group, the number of endogenous LC3-II puncta per cell was assessed in 100 cells, and statistical data were obtained from three independent experiments.

For LysoTracker staining, A549 or H1975 cells with stable expression of GFP-LC3 were cultured in confocal dishes and incubated for 90 min in complete RPMI-1640 medium supplemented with 500 nM LysoTracker Red.

The colocalization of LC3 and LysoTracker was analyzed by the confocal microscopy.

### Acridine orange (AO) staining

Autophagy is a lysosomal degradation pathway for cytoplasmic material and organelles. The acidic intracellular compartments were visualized by supravital AO staining. After the treatment with MTE (0, 20, 40 mg/ml) for 6 h, cells were washed with PBS and stained with 1 µg/ml AO (318337, Sigma-Aldrich) for 20 min at 37 °C. Subsequently, cells were analyzed under the confocal microscopy.

### Statistical analysis

All experiments were repeated at least three times and values are expressed as the mean ± standard error of mean (SEM). Student's t-test was used to determine the difference between two independent groups. All data were analyzed using SPSS statistical software 16.0 (SPSS Inc., Chicago, IL, USA). $P < 0.05$ was considered statistically significant difference between values.

### Results

#### MTE suppressed lung cancer cell proliferation in vitro

MTE is a Chinese medicine used to treat lung cancer, gastric cancer and other cancers with a good therapeutic efficacy. Firstly, we examined the IC50 (half maximal inhibitory concentration) in A549 and H1975 using MTT assay. The results demonstrated that MTE significantly inhibited NSCLC cells proliferation in a dose-dependent manner after 24, 48 and 72 h treatment. The IC50 values of A549 cells were 92.5 ± 4.3 mg/ml at 24 h, 69.0 ± 4.8 mg/ml at 48 h and 48.9 ± 5.1 mg/ml at 72 h, separately (Fig. 1a). The IC50 values of H1975

cells were 82.5 ± 4.9 mg/ml at 24 h, 56.3 ± 6.2 mg/ml at 48 h and 40.5 ± 3.0 mg/ml at 72 h, respectively (Fig. 1b). Such findings demonstrated that MTE can significantly suppress the growth of NSCLC cells.

#### MTE treatment induced apoptosis in lung cancer cells

To detect whether cell growth suppression after MTE treatment was through apoptosis, flow cytometry analysis was performed. As shown in Fig. 2a, b, NSCLC cells treated with various doses of MTE for 24 h caused cell apoptosis in a dose-dependent manner, especially in late-stage apoptosis. Briefly, MTE treatments led to cell late apoptotic rate from 7.5 ± 0.5% of control group to 10.6 ± 0.5% (20 mg/ml), 16.1 ± 0.7% (40 mg/ml) and 19.7 ± 0.4% (80 mg/ml) in A549 cells; from 2.9 ± 0.2% of control group to 8.4 ± 0.3% (20 mg/ml), 13.8 ± 0.6% (40 mg/ml) and 24.9 ± 1.5% (80 mg/ml) in H1975 cells. Meanwhile, the early apoptotic rate of cells in each group only ranged from 2.0 ± 1.1% to 3.3 ± 0.7% in A549, and from 1.1 ± 0.3% to 3.5 ± 1.3% in H1975.

Next, proteins associated with apoptosis were examined by Western blot. Treatment of MTE for 24 h decreased Caspase 3 zymogens expression (Fig. 2c) and increased Caspase 3 activities (Fig. 2d) in both cell lines. However, the cleaved PARP was raised in H1975 cells after MTE treatment, while only non-active PARP was reduced in A549 cells. In addition, mitochondrial associated apoptosis was involved in MTE-induced apoptosis, as evidenced by increased Bax and declined Bcl-2 protein expression (Additional file 1: Fig. S1A, B). These data indicated that cell apoptosis may contribute to cell growth suppression by MTE in NSCLC.

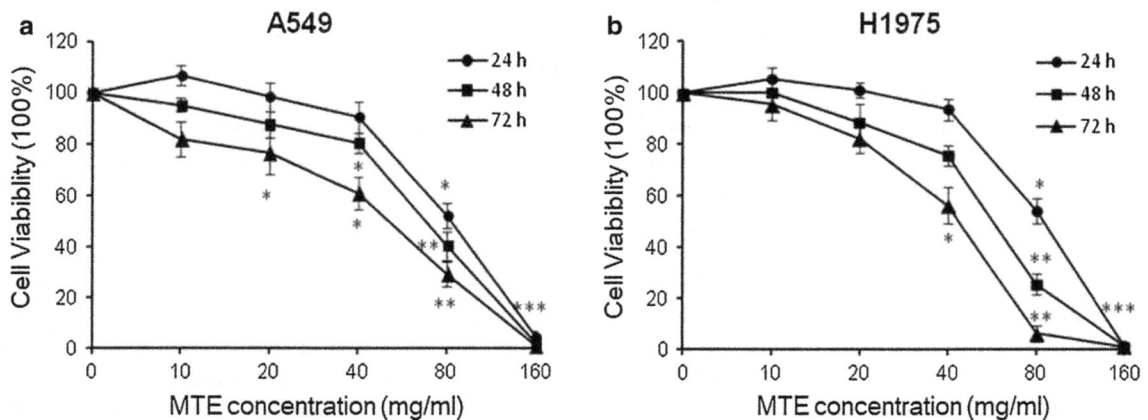

**Fig. 1** MTE suppressed lung cancer cell proliferation in vitro. MTT assay was performed to detect IC50 of MTE after 24, 48 and 72 h treatment in **a** A549 cells; **b** H1975 cells. Data were represented as mean ± SEM from three independent experiments. *$P < 0.05$, **$P < 0.01$, ***$P < 0.005$ vs control group

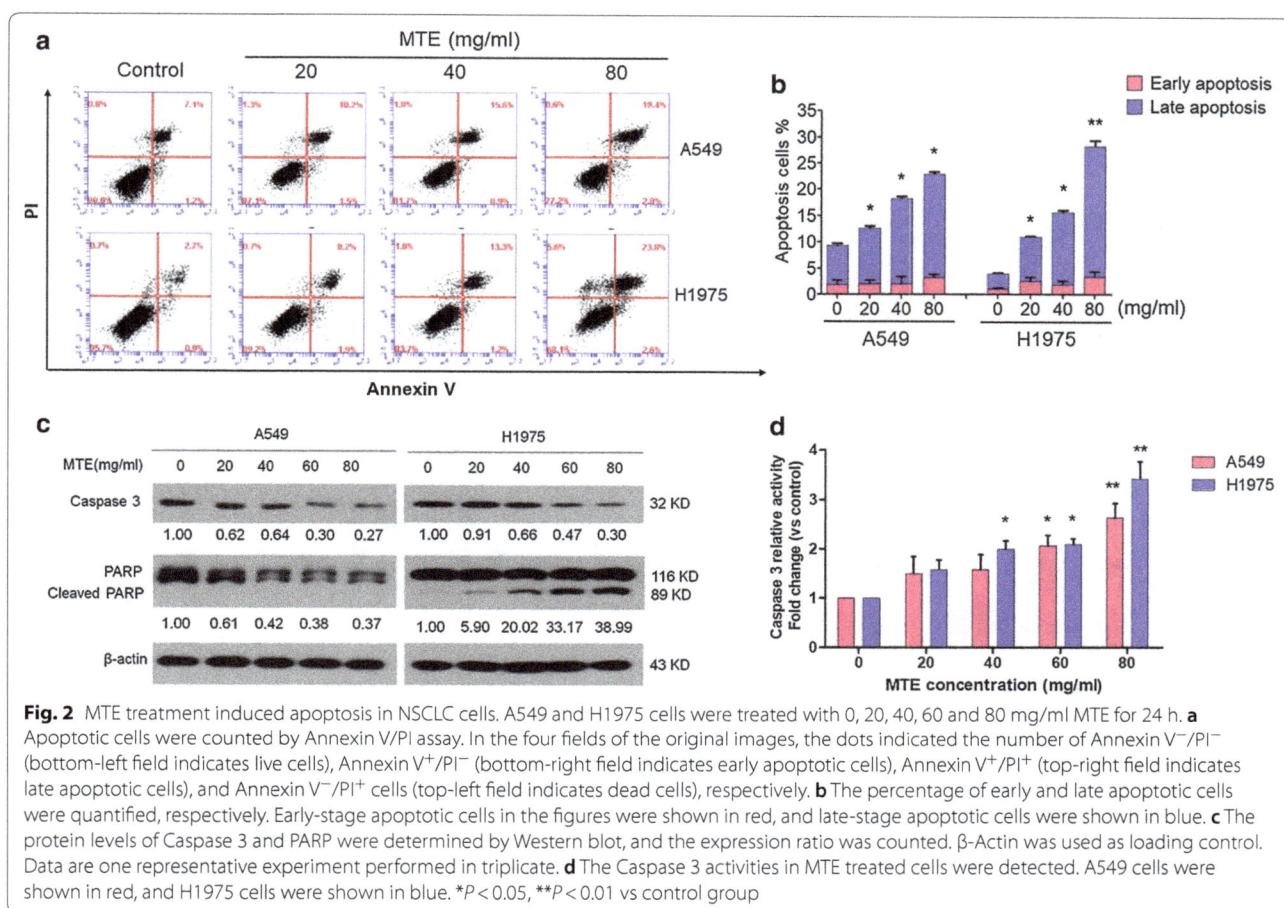

**Fig. 2** MTE treatment induced apoptosis in NSCLC cells. A549 and H1975 cells were treated with 0, 20, 40, 60 and 80 mg/ml MTE for 24 h. **a** Apoptotic cells were counted by Annexin V/PI assay. In the four fields of the original images, the dots indicated the number of Annexin V$^-$/PI$^-$ (bottom-left field indicates live cells), Annexin V$^+$/PI$^-$ (bottom-right field indicates early apoptotic cells), Annexin V$^+$/PI$^+$ (top-right field indicates late apoptotic cells), and Annexin V$^-$/PI$^+$ (top-left field indicates dead cells), respectively. **b** The percentage of early and late apoptotic cells were quantified, respectively. Early-stage apoptotic cells in the figures were shown in red, and late-stage apoptotic cells were shown in blue. **c** The protein levels of Caspase 3 and PARP were determined by Western blot, and the expression ratio was counted. β-Actin was used as loading control. Data are one representative experiment performed in triplicate. **d** The Caspase 3 activities in MTE treated cells were detected. A549 cells were shown in red, and H1975 cells were shown in blue. *$P < 0.05$, **$P < 0.01$ vs control group

## MTE treatment disrupted autophagic flux in NSCLC cells

Recent reports showed that cell apoptosis and autophagy are often affected by anticancer agents [22]. In order to investigate the effect of MTE on autophagy, firstly we monitored the classic autophagic marker LC3-II by Western blot. As shown in Fig. 3a, b, LC3-II increased in a dose- and time-dependent manner after MTE treatment in both A549 and H1975 cells, indicating MTE influenced the process of cell autophagy. MTE treatment also raised p62 protein level in a dose- and time-dependent manner (Fig. 3a, b). p62 is an adaptor protein that serves as a link between LC3 and ubiquitinated substrates; its increase suggested the substrate degradation was blocked and the autophagic flux was impaired after MTE treatment.

The autophagy flux after MTE treatment was further determined through the addition of autophagy inducer EBSS or inhibitor Baf A1. As shown in Fig. 3c (lane 6 vs lane 5), compared with EBSS alone, the co-treatment of MTE exerted an enhanced increase of LC3-II and p62 expression in A549 and H1975 cells, indicating MTE still suppressed cell autophagy even concurrent with EBSS treatment. Moreover, a synergistically impaired autophagy flux was observed with the combined treatment of MTE and Baf A1, which is an inhibitor to block the fusion of autophagosome with lysosome (Fig. 3c, lane 4 vs lane 3). In addition, we monitored LC3-II puncta in cells by immunofluorescence. In Fig. 3d, e, compared with control group, MTE treatment augmented the LC3-II puncta distribution in the presence or absence of EBSS or Baf A1, which is similar to the results of Western blot. These data suggested that the increased LC3-II and p62 in MTE treated NSCLC cells were due to suppression of autophagic flux in the late stage of autophagy.

## MTE suppressed autophagy by affecting lysosomal function

In order to further investigate the influence of MTE on the late stage of autophagy, we focused on the lysosomal function, which is critical for the maturation of autophagosomes and the degradation of their contents. The intralysosomal pH plays an important role in affecting the Cathepsin enzymatic activity and lysosomal functions. So, firstly we performed AO staining to visualize acidic vesicles after MTE treatment. AO is a fluorescent

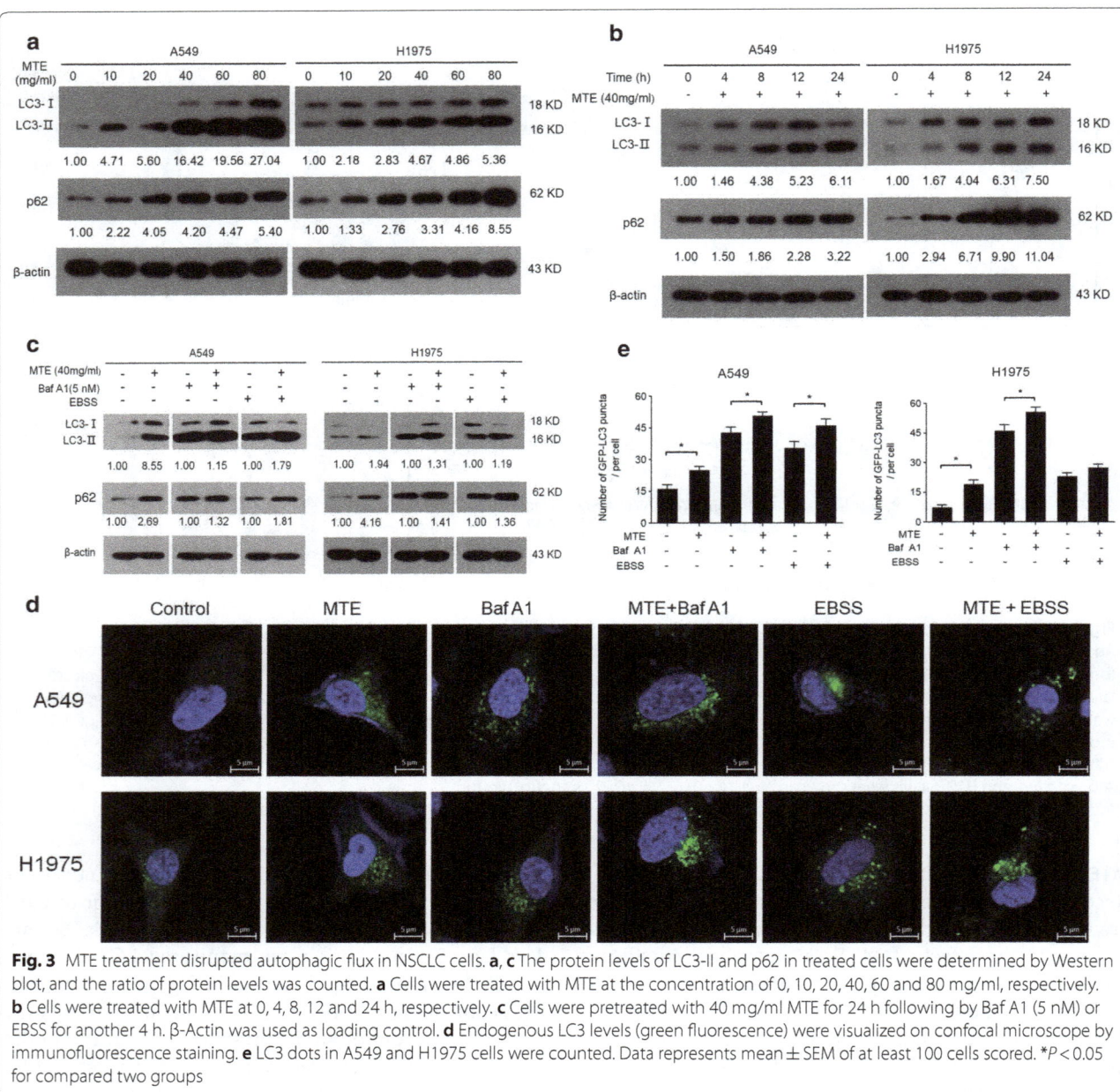

**Fig. 3** MTE treatment disrupted autophagic flux in NSCLC cells. **a, c** The protein levels of LC3-II and p62 in treated cells were determined by Western blot, and the ratio of protein levels was counted. **a** Cells were treated with MTE at the concentration of 0, 10, 20, 40, 60 and 80 mg/ml, respectively. **b** Cells were treated with MTE at 0, 4, 8, 12 and 24 h, respectively. **c** Cells were pretreated with 40 mg/ml MTE for 24 h following by Baf A1 (5 nM) or EBSS for another 4 h. β-Actin was used as loading control. **d** Endogenous LC3 levels (green fluorescence) were visualized on confocal microscope by immunofluorescence staining. **e** LC3 dots in A549 and H1975 cells were counted. Data represents mean ± SEM of at least 100 cells scored. *$P < 0.05$ for compared two groups

weak base that fluoresced bright red when accumulating in acidic compartments such as autolysosome and lysosome, whereas fluoresced bright green in cytoplasm and nucleolus [23]. As shown in Fig. 4a, b, MTE treatment for 6 h resulted in visible and increased bright red vacuoles compared with control groups both in A549 and H1975 cells, suggesting MTE treatment significantly decreased intralysosomal pH. Next, we tested whether MTE can affect lysosomal function through detecting LAMP1 and activated Cathepsin B by Western Blot. LAMP1 is located in lysosomal membrane involving in lysosomal motility,

and Cathepsin B is one of the most important proteases inside lysosome [24]. As shown in Fig. 4c, MTE treatment reduced LAMP1 and Cathepsin B protein expression with increased MTE concentration, confirming that MTE impaired lysosomal function.

Furthermore, we examined the fusion between autophagosome and lysosome by monitoring LysoTracker to detect its colocalization with the autophagosomal marker LC3 in GFP-LC3 stable cells. Presence of MTE in GFP-LC3 stable cells led to an increase of GFP-LC3/LysoTracker colocalization compared to control cells

(Fig. 4d for A549 and e for H1975, group 2 vs. group 1 in d–f). Such changes were similar to that cells treated with Baf A1 (Fig. 4d–f, group 4 vs. group 3). In EBSS treated A549 cells, GFP-LC3 punctation in MTE group was a little more colocalized with LysoTracker compare to control group, while no obvious change in H1975 cells (Fig. 4d–f, group 6 vs. group 5) was observed. Taken together, these results indicated that MTE impaired the fusion of autophagosome and lysosome, further confirming that MTE inhibits autophagy at the late stage in A549 and H1975 cells.

### ERK activation is required for apoptosis and autophagy regulation by MTE treatment

It has been reported that both autophagy and apoptosis are regulated by the MEK/ERK pathway [25, 26]. Thus, we examined whether this pathway accounts for MTE-caused cell apoptosis induction and autophagy inhibition. Western blot results in Fig. 5a, b (left panel) showed that MTE treatment upregulated phosphorylated ERK with a dose-dependent manner in both NSCLC cells. The role of ERK was further determined by using MEK/ERK inhibitor U0126, and we found that the activation of ERK by MTE was obviously attenuated via co-treatment with U0126 in A549 and H1975 cells (Fig. 5a, b, right panel). The above results showed that MTE activated MEK/ERK signaling in NSCLC.

Next, we examined the influence of ERK on autophagy associated molecules by MTE treatment. As shown in Fig. 5c, d, pre-treatment with U0126 deteriorated the autophagy inhibition caused by MTE, resulted in autophagy induction with increased LC3-II and decreased p62 in both cells. The function of lysosomes was damaged by MTE with down-regulated expression of LAMP1 and Cathepsin B. However, in presence of U0126, LAMP1 and Cathepsin B were upregulated, implying partly recovery of lysosomal function (Fig. 5c, d). These results demonstrated that MTE-caused autophagy inhibition was reversed by U0126, suggesting that MEK/ERK pathway contributed to the autophagy inhibition caused by MTE.

Finally, we evaluated the association between MTE-induced apoptosis and MEK/ERK pathway; and found

cell apoptosis, especially late-stage apoptosis was significantly decreased in the presence of U0126. As shown in Fig. 6a–d, MTE-caused late apoptotic A549 cells ranged from $4.5 \pm 0.7\%$ to $12.7 \pm 1.6\%$ in U0126 pretreated group, while it was $3.3 \pm 0.5\%$ to $18.6 \pm 0.8\%$ in no U0126 group. The ratio of MTE-induced late apoptotic H1975 cells was from $4.7 \pm 0.4\%$ to $13.5 \pm 1.3\%$ in U0126 pretreated group, compared with $2.5 \pm 0.5\%$ to $17.7 \pm 2.1\%$ in no U0126 group. There is no obvious difference for the early apoptotic cells in each group. The results suggested that MTE-induced apoptosis was dramatically attenuated by U0126. As shown in Fig. 6e, f, MTE treatment relieved the protein levels of zymogens of Caspase 3 in U0126 group compared with no U0126 group in both cell lines. Caspase 3 activity induced by MTE was decreased significantly after pretreated with U0126 (Fig. 6g, h). These data indicated that ERK activation is required for MTE-induced apoptosis.

### Discussion

Studies showed C21 steroidal glycosides are major components in *M. tenacissima*. Compounds such as Tenacigenoside A [13], 11α-O-benzoyl-12β-O-acetyl tenacigenin B [27], tenacissoside C, tenacissoside B, tenacissoside C, Tenacissoside I and marsdenoside K [28] etc. are demonstrated to possess anti-cancer activity. According to our previous HPLC–MS analysis, 13 compounds including most of compounds mentioned above were identified from MTE by HPLC–MS analysis [12]. In recent years, *M. tenacissima* has attracted extensive interest in cancer research area with multiple effects, such as inhibiting tumor growth and angiogenesis, reversing anti-tumor drug resistance [12, 14, 17]. However, the reasons why MTE treatment resulted in the inhibition on cancer cell growth still remain largely unknown. In the present study, we found MTE significantly induced cell apoptosis, suppressed cell autophagy through impairing lysosomes function in A549 and H1975 NSCLC cells. Our results also indicated that ERK may mediate autophagy inhibition and apoptosis induction effect of MTE in NSCLC cells.

Programmed forms of cell death pathway at least include apoptosis and autophagy. Apoptosis is a

(See figure on next page.)

**Fig. 4** MTE suppressed autophagy by affecting lysosomal function. **a** Acidic vacuolar compartment in cells treated MTE with 0, 20 and 40 mg/ml (red puncta) were measured by acridine orange staining. **b** Numbers of red puncta in A549 and H1975 cells treated as in (**a**) were counted. Data represents mean ± SEM of at least 100 cells scored (*P < 0.05). **c** The protein level of LAMP1, Cathepsin B in treated cells were detected by Western blot, and protein expression levels were counted. Cells were treated with 0, 10, 20, 40, 60, 80 mg/ml MTE for 24 h. β-Actin was used as a loading control. **d, e** Colocalization of GFP-LC3 (green) and LysoTracker (red) were visualized on confocal microscope. GFP-LC3 stable A549 (**d**) and H1975 (**e**) cells were pretreated with 40 mg/ml MTE for 24 h following by Baf A1 (5 nM) or EBSS for another 4 h, and then incubated with LysoTracker for 90 min to be observed by confocal microscope. **f** Numbers of yellow (merge of green and red) puncta in cells treated as in (**d, e**) were counted. Data represents mean ± SEM of at least 100 cells scored. *P < 0.05, **P < 0.01, ***P < 0.005 vs control

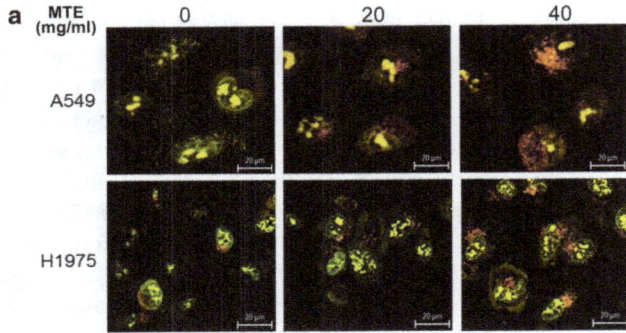

a

MTE (mg/ml): 0, 20, 40

A549

H1975

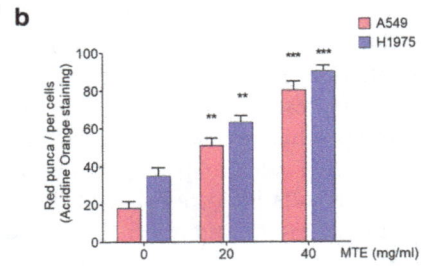

b

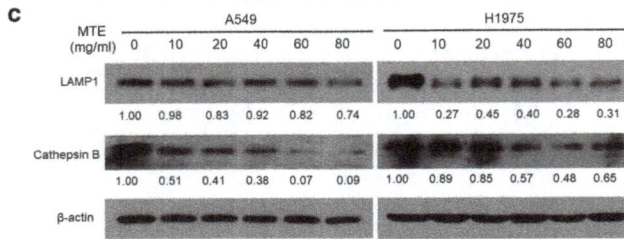

c

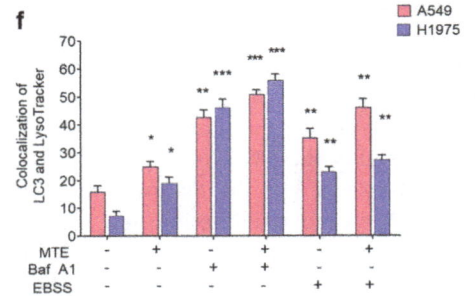

f

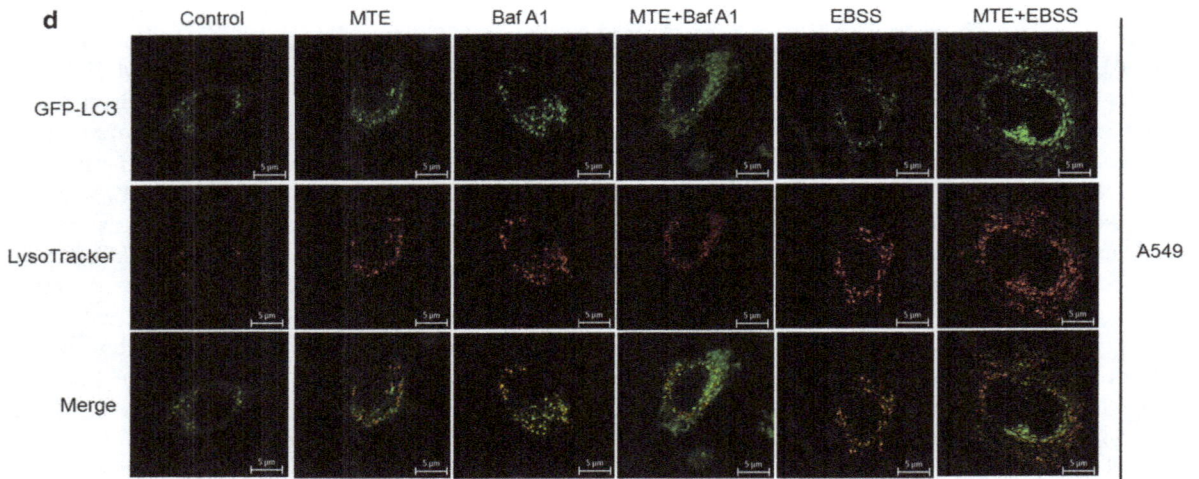

d

Control | MTE | Baf A1 | MTE+Baf A1 | EBSS | MTE+EBSS

GFP-LC3

LysoTracker

Merge

A549

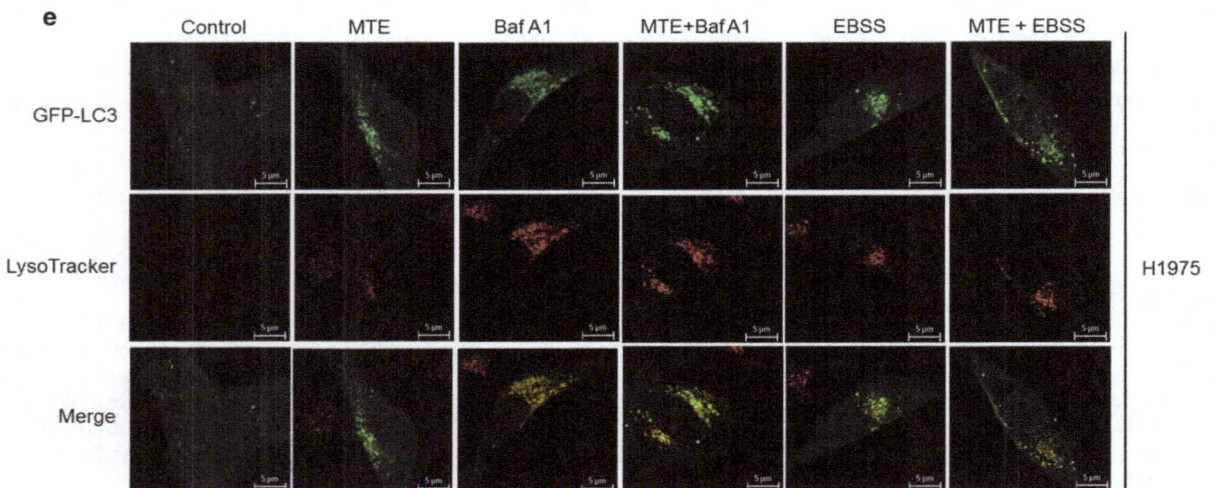

e

Control | MTE | Baf A1 | MTE+Baf A1 | EBSS | MTE + EBSS

GFP-LC3

LysoTracker

Merge

H1975

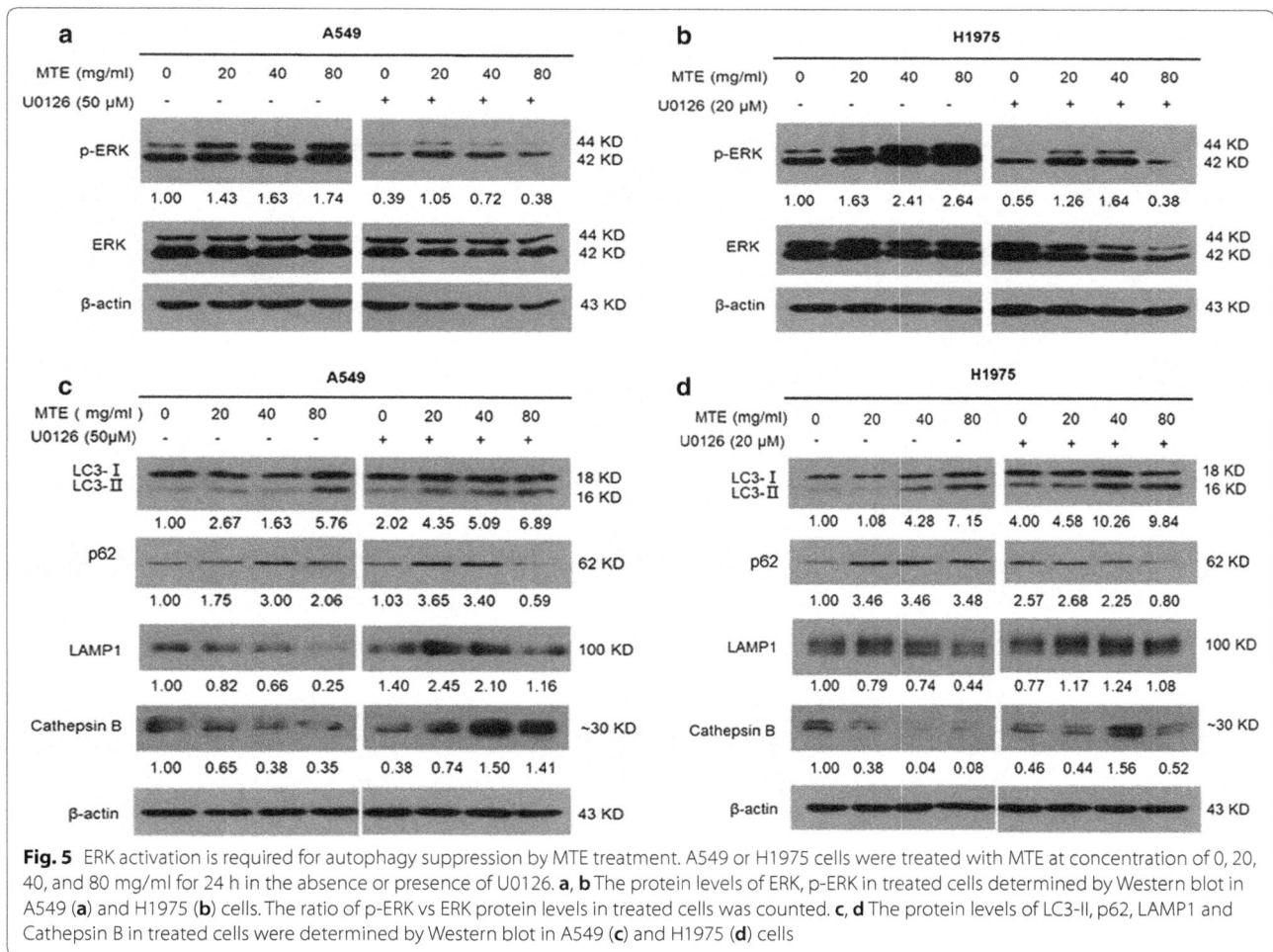

**Fig. 5** ERK activation is required for autophagy suppression by MTE treatment. A549 or H1975 cells were treated with MTE at concentration of 0, 20, 40, and 80 mg/ml for 24 h in the absence or presence of U0126. **a, b** The protein levels of ERK, p-ERK in treated cells determined by Western blot in A549 (**a**) and H1975 (**b**) cells. The ratio of p-ERK vs ERK protein levels in treated cells was counted. **c, d** The protein levels of LC3-II, p62, LAMP1 and Cathepsin B in treated cells were determined by Western blot in A549 (**c**) and H1975 (**d**) cells

physiological process to eliminate damaged, mutant or aged cells to maintain cellular homeostasis in normal tissue [29]. The inhibition of apoptosis is regarded as one of the hallmarks of cancer [3], and apoptosis-inducing has been exploited as an indispensable anticancer therapeutic strategy. Approaches targeting apoptotic pathway can result in cancer cell death, increasing sensitivity to current treatments or reversing drug resistance, thus may bring promising clinical benefits. Till now, different apoptosis targeted therapies have entered clinical trials for efficacy evaluation in various tumor types including lung cancer [30]. In the present study, MTE induced significant cell apoptosis in both A549 and H1975 cells along with Caspase 3 activation. Although cleaved PARP was not observed in A549 cells with MTE treatment, remarkable apoptotic cells presented after stained with Annexin V-FITC for flow cytometry analysis. The above results indicated that apoptosis-inducing may contribute to the cell death caused by MTE treatment.

Autophagy has complicated functions on cell death, as it may promote or inhibit cell death under certain circumstances. Although autophagy may offer tumor suppressive function in some conditions [31], it is mainly a cytoprotective process to facilitate cancer cells survive under stressful environments [32]. Studies showed that autophagy suppression in NSCLC cells resulted in cell proliferation suppression [33] and cell apoptosis increase [34]. In addition, constitutive activation of autophagy is also associated with anti-cancer therapeutic resistance [35], and inhibiting autophagy may overcome drug resistance in tumors [36]. Therefore, targeting autophagy is considered as a potential therapeutic strategy for cancer treatment.

LC3-II and p62 serve as marker of autophagic flux. The level of p62 increased when autophagy inhibition occurred; and decreased when autophagy is induced. In our study, MTE treatment caused accumulation of both LC3-II and p62, which means the substrate degradation was blocked and autophagic flux was

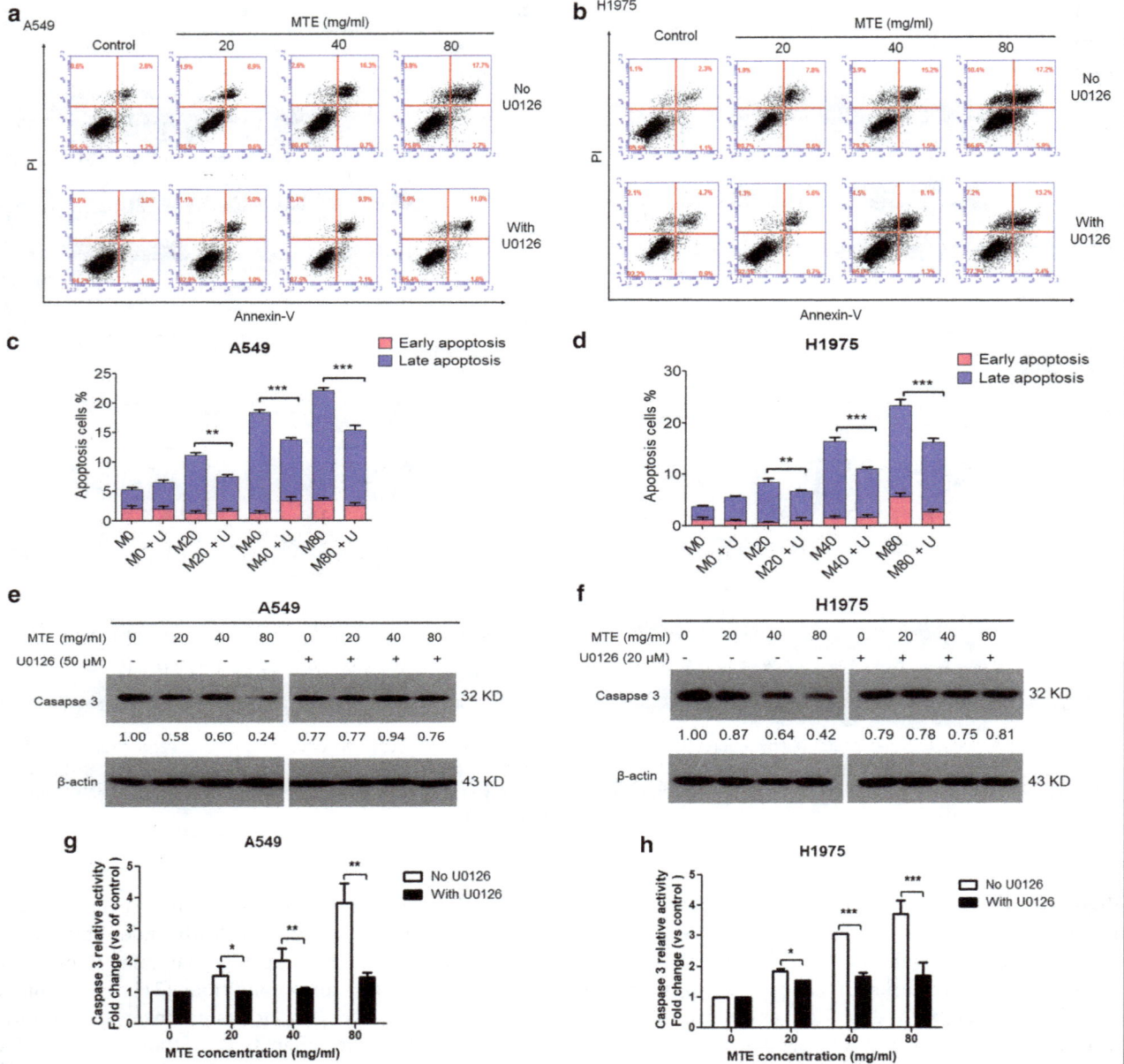

**Fig. 6** ERK activation is required for apoptosis induction by MTE treatment. **a, b** Apoptotic cells with indicated treatment were counted by Annexin V/PI assay. **c, d** The percentage of apoptotic cells with treatment was quantified. Early-stage apoptotic cells were shown in red, and late-stage apoptotic cells were shown in blue (M: MTE; U: U0126). **e, f** The protein level of Caspase 3 in treated cells was detected by Western blot, and the expression ratio was counted. Cells were treated with 20, 40, 80 mg/ml MTE for 24 h. **g, h** The caspase 3 activities in treated cells were detected. *$P < 0.05$, **$P < 0.01$, ***$P < 0.005$; Groups with U0126 vs groups without U0126

impaired. The autophagy inhibitory effect of MTE was further confirmed by adding autophagy inhibitor Baf A1 and autophagy inducer EBSS. Next, GFP-LC3 stable NSCLC cells labeled with LysoTracker showed MTE suppressed the fusion of lysosomes with autophagosome at the late stage. This effect was further confirmed by detecting lysosomal marker LAMP1 and lysosomal protease Cathepsin B, indicating MTE

impaired lysosomal function. Consistent with our results, other study demonstrated that inhibition of the fusion between lysosomes and autophagosomes leading to accumulated LC3-II and increased acidic vacuolar compartment [37]. Our results demonstrated that MTE can target both apoptosis and autophagy leading to NSCLC cells death. In fact, the molecular connections exist between apoptosis and autophagy, and some regulators are shared to maintain a subtle and complicated balance with each other [38–40]. ERK is a crucial molecule to control diverse cell responses including proliferation, migration, and differentiation [25]. High levels of ERK has been found in many malignant tumors, but ERK activation is not always correlated with cell survival protection, it can also interplay with cell death including apoptosis, autophagy, and senescence [25, 26]. Growing evidence demonstrated that activated ERK has positive contribution to cancer treatment, such as induced cell apoptosis and cell death [41, 42]. BPIQ, a synthetic quinoline analog, upregulated ERK phosphorylation leading to H1299 cell death, and this can be abrogated by ERK inhibitor [43]. In consistent with other studies, our results demonstrated that ERK activation plays important roles in drug-induced cancer cells apoptotic death.

Accumulated evidence demonstrated activated ERK is also involved in autophagic cell death [26]. 8-CEPQ, a novel quercetin derivative, inhibited colon cancer cell growth by inducing autophagic cell death through ERK activation [44]. Tan IIA induces autophagic cell death via activation of AMPK and ERK in KBM-5 cells, and ERK inhibitor PD184352 suppressed LC3-II expression induced by Tan IIA [45]. Rhuscoriaria induced autophagic cell death through p38 and ERK1/2 activation in breast cancer cells [46]. All the above studies link ERK activation with autophagic cell death. In our study, MEK/ERK inhibitor U0126 effectively abrogated the impaired autophagy flux caused by MTE. Taken together, our results revealed the effect of MTE on cell apoptosis-induction and autophagy-inhibition can partly ascribe to ERK activation.

## Conclusion

A Chinese herb preparation, MTE, induced significant cell apoptosis and impaired the fusion of lysosomes with autophagosome in NSCLC cells A549 and H1975. The molecule ERK, which links the crosstalk between apoptosis and autophagy, partly accounts for the underlying mechanisms of cell death caused by MTE. As cancer has complex networks of signaling pathways, thus multiple targeting autophagy and apoptosis by Chinese medicine may shed some light on the way for NSCLC cancer treatment.

## Additional file

**Additional file 1: Fig. S1.** Mitochondrial associated proteins were involved in MTE-induced apoptosis. (**A**, **B**) The protein level of Bcl-2 alpha and Bax in treated A549 cells (**A**) and H1975 cells (**B**) were detected by Western blot, and the ratio of protein levels treated was counted. Cells were treated with 0, 10, 20, 40, 60, 80 mg/ml MTE for 24 h.

## Abbreviations

SCLC: small-cell lung cancer; NSCLC: non-small cell lung cancer; MTE: water extract of *Marsdenia tenacissima*; EBSS: Earle's balanced salt solution; MTT: 3-(4,5-dimethyl-2-thiazolyl)-2,5-diphenyl-2-*H*-tetrazolium bromide; PARP: poly (ADP-ribose) polymerase; OD: optical density; PAGE: polyacrylamide gel electrophoresis; BSA: bovine serum albumin; PBS: phosphate-buffered saline; AO: acridine orange; SEM: standard error of mean; IC50: half maximal inhibitory concentration; Baf A1: Bafilomycin A1; DAPI: 2-(4-amidinophenyl)-6-indolecarbamidine dihydrochloride; LAMP1: lysosome-associated membrane protein 1.

## Authors' contributions

Study design (LNW, YNJ, DX, SYH, PPL); Biochemical experiments (YNJ, LNW, XJL, ZHT, STJ); Statistical analyses (YNJ, LNW, DX, XJL, ZHT, STJ, SYH); drafting the manuscript (LNW, YNJ, DX, SYH). All authors read and approved the final manuscript.

## Author details

[1] Key Laboratory of Carcinogenesis and Translational Research (Ministry of Education/Beijing), Department of Integration of Chinese and Western Medicine, Peking University Cancer Hospital & Institute, No. 52 Fucheng Road, Haidian District, Beijing 100142, People's Republic of China. [2] Key Laboratory of Carcinogenesis and Translational Research (Ministry of Education/Beijing), Central Laboratory, Peking University Cancer Hospital and Institute, Beijing 100142, People's Republic of China.

## Acknowledgements

We thank Prof. Yingyu Chen (Department of Immunology, Peking University School of Basic Medical Science; Key Laboratory of Medical Immunology, Ministry of Health, Peking University Health Sciences Center) for study design and materials help in autophagy.

## Competing interests

The authors declare that they have no competing interests.

## Funding

This research was supported by Beijing Municipal Natural Science Foundation (No. 7152034) and Beijing Municipal Health System Special Funds of High Level Medical Personnel Construction (Grant Number 2014

## References

1. Ali A, Goffin JR, Arnold A, Ellis PM. Survival of patients with non-small-cell lung cancer after a diagnosis of brain metastases. Curr Oncol. 2013;20(4):e300–6.
2. Liu G, Pei F, Yang F, Li L, Amin AD, Liu S, Buchan JR, Cho WC. Role of autophagy and apoptosis in non-small-cell lung cancer. Int J Mol Sci. 2017;18(2):367.
3. Hanahan D, Weinberg RA. The hallmarks of cancer. Cell. 2000;100(1):57–70.
4. Pore MM, Hiltermann TJ, Kruyt FA. Targeting apoptosis pathways in lung cancer. Cancer Lett. 2013;332(2):359–68.
5. Guo JY, Teng X, Laddha SV, Ma S, Van Nostrand SC, Yang Y, Khor S, Chan CS, Rabinowitz JD, White E. Autophagy provides metabolic substrates to maintain energy charge and nucleotide pools in Ras-driven lung cancer cells. Genes Dev. 2016;30(15):1704–17.
6. White E. The role for autophagy in cancer. J Clin Investig. 2015;125(1):42–6.
7. Chen N, Karantza V. Autophagy as a therapeutic target in cancer. Cancer Biol Ther. 2011;11(2):157–68.
8. Chude CI, Amaravadi RK. Targeting autophagy in cancer: update on clinical trials and novel inhibitors. Int J Mol Sci. 2017;18(6):1279.

9.  College JNM. Zhongyao dacidian (Encyclopedia of Chinese Materia Medica). Shanghai: Shanghai Science and Technology Press; 1977. p. 1976.

10. State Pharmacopoeia Committee. Chinese pharmacopoeia. Beijing: Medical Science and Technology Press; 2010. p. 986.

11. Li MQ, Shen JH, Xu B, Chen J. The mechanism of laboratory research for xiaoaiping treating SGC-7901 gastric carcinoma cellular strains. J Interven Radiol. 2001;10:228–31.

12. Han SY, Zhao MB, Zhuang GB, Li PP. *Marsdenia tenacissima* extract restored gefitinib sensitivity in resistant non-small cell lung cancer cells. Lung Cancer. 2012;75(1):30–7.

13. Li D, Li C, Song Y, Zhou M, Sun X, Zhu X, Zhang F, Zhou C, Huan Y, Xia S, et al. Marsdenia tenacissima extract and its functional components inhibits proliferation and induces apoptosis of human Burkitt leukemia/lymphoma cells in vitro and in vivo. Leuk Lymphoma. 2016;57(2):419–28.

14. Huang Z, Lin H, Wang Y, Cao Z, Lin W, Chen Q. Studies on the anti-angiogenic effect of *Marsdenia tenacissima* extract in vitro and in vivo. Oncol Lett. 2013;5(3):917–22.

15. Chen BY, Chen D, Lyu JX, Li KQ, Jiang MM, Zeng JJ, He XJ, Hao K, Tao HQ, Mou XZ, et al. Marsdeniae tenacissimae extract (MTE) suppresses cell proliferation by attenuating VEGF/VEGFR2 interactions and promotes apoptosis through regulating PKC pathway in human umbilical vein endothelial cells. Chin J Nat Med. 2016;14(12):922–30.

16. Fan W, Sun L, Zhou JQ, Zhang C, Qin S, Tang Y, Liu Y, Lin SS, Yuan ST. *Marsdenia tenacissima* extract induces G0/G1 cell cycle arrest in human esophageal carcinoma cells by inhibiting mitogen-activated protein kinase (MAPK) signaling pathway. Chin J Nat Med. 2015;13(6):428–37.

17. Jiang S, Qiu L, Li Y, Li L, Wang X, Liu Z, Guo Y, Wang H. Effects of *Marsdenia tenacissima* polysaccharide on the immune regulation and tumor growth in H22 tumor-bearing mice. Carbohyd Polym. 2016;137:52–8.

18. Wang WY, Zhou Y, Zhang XJ, Gao TH, Luo ZF, Liu MY. A random study of xiao-ai-ping injection combined with chemotherapy on the treatment of advanced non-small cell lung cancer. Chin Clin Oncol. 2009;14:936–8.

19. Huang ZQTH, Wang CY, Zhang HZ, Liu D, Zhou CZ, Liu X. Clinical research of combined xiaoaiping injection with chemotherapy on advanced non-small cell lung cancer. Chin Clin Oncol. 2007;12:97–9.

20. Chen BY, Chen D, Lyu JX, Li KQ, Jiang MM, Zeng JJ, Wang Z, et al. *Marsdeniae tenacissimae* extract (MTE) suppresses cell proliferation by attenuating VEGF/VEGFR2 interactions and promotes apoptosis through regulating PKC pathway in human umbilical vein endothelial cells. Chin J Nat Med. 2016;14:922–30.

21. Han SY, Zhao HY, Zhou N, Zhou F, Li PP. *Marsdenia tenacissima* extract inhibits gefitinib metabolism in vitro by interfering with human hepatic CYP3A4 and CYP2D6 enzymes. J Ethnopharmacol. 2014;151(1):210–7.

22. Qi QM, Xue YC, Lv J, Sun D, Du JX, Cai SQ, Li YH, Gu TC, Wang MB. Ginkgolic acids induce HepG2 cell death via a combination of apoptosis, autophagy and the mitochondrial pathway. Oncol Lett. 2018;15(5):6400–8.

23. Palmgren MG. Acridine orange as a probe for measuring pH gradients across membranes: mechanism and limitations. Anal Biochem. 1991;192(2):316–21.

24. Uchiyama Y. Autophagic cell death and its execution by lysosomal cathepsins. Arch Histol Cytol. 2001;64(3):233–46.

25. Mebratu Y, Tesfaigzi Y. How ERK1/2 activation controls cell proliferation and cell death: Is subcellular localization the answer? Cell Cycle. 2009;8(8):1168–75.

26. Cagnol S, Chambard JC. ERK and cell death: mechanisms of ERK-induced cell death–apoptosis, autophagy and senescence. FEBS J. 2010;277(1):2–21.

27. Ye B, Yang J, Li J, Niu T, Wang S. In vitro and in vivo antitumor activities of tenacissoside C from Marsdenia tenacissima. Planta Med. 2014;80(1):29–38.

28. Xue HL, et al. Effects of *Marsdenia tenacissima* extract on proliferation and apoptosis of hematologic neoplasm cell line cells. Sichuan Da Xue Xue Bao Yi Xue Ban. 2012;43(2):174–9 **(In Chinese)**.

29. Renehan AG, Booth C, Potten CS. What is apoptosis, and why is it important? BMJ. 2001;322(7301):1536–8.

30. Baig S, Seevasant I, Mohamad J, Mukheem A, Huri HZ, Kamarul T. Potential of apoptotic pathway-targeted cancer therapeutic research: where do we stand? Cell Death Dis. 2016;7:e2058.

31. Yoshida GJ. Therapeutic strategies of drug repositioning targeting autophagy to induce cancer cell death: from pathophysiology to treatment. J Hematol Oncol. 2017;10(1):67.

32. Rao S, Tortola L, Perlot T, Wirnsberger G, Novatchkova M, Nitsch R, Sykacek P, Frank L, Schramek D, Komnenovic V, et al. A dual role for autophagy in a murine model of lung cancer. Nat Commun. 2014;5:3056.

33. Kaminskyy VO, Piskunova T, Zborovskaya IB, Tchevkina EM, Zhivotovsky B. Suppression of basal autophagy reduces lung cancer cell proliferation and enhances caspase-dependent and -independent apoptosis by stimulating ROS formation. Autophagy. 2012;8(7):1032–44.

34. Xie WY, Zhou XD, Yang J, Chen LX, Ran DH. Inhibition of autophagy enhances heat-induced apoptosis in human non-small cell lung cancer cells through ER stress pathways. Arch Biochem Biophys. 2016;607:55–66.

35. Sui X, Chen R, Wang Z, Huang Z, Kong N, Zhang M, Han W, Lou F, Yang J, Zhang Q, et al. Autophagy and chemotherapy resistance: a promising therapeutic target for cancer treatment. Cell Death Dis. 2013;4:e838.

36. Kumar A, Singh UK, Chaudhary A. Targeting autophagy to overcome drug resistance in cancer therapy. Future Med Chem. 2015;7(12):1535–42.

37. Boya P, Gonzalez-Polo RA, Casares N, Perfettini JL, Dessen P, Larochette N, Metivier D, Meley D, Souquere S, Yoshimori T, et al. Inhibition of macroautophagy triggers apoptosis. Mol Cell Biol. 2005;25(3):1025–40.

38. Gorski SM, Chittaranjan S, Pleasance ED, Freeman JD, Anderson CL, Varhol RJ, Coughlin SM, Zuyderduyn SD, Jones SJ, Marra MA. A SAGE approach to discovery of genes involved in autophagic cell death. Curr Biol. 2003;13(4):358–63.

39. Levine B, Sinha S, Kroemer G. Bcl-2 family members: dual regulators of apoptosis and autophagy. Autophagy. 2008;4(5):600–6.

40. El Hasasna H, Athamneh K, Al Samri H, Karuvantevida N, Al Dhaheri Y, Hisaindee S, Ramadan G, Al Tamimi N, AbuQamar S, Eid A, et al. Rhus coriaria induces senescence and autophagic cell death in breast cancer cells through a mechanism involving p38 and ERK1/2 activation. Sci Rep. 2015;5:13013.

41. Nguyen TT, Tran E, Nguyen TH, Do PT, Huynh TH, Huynh H. The role of activated MEK-ERK pathway in quercetin-induced growth inhibition and apoptosis in A549 lung cancer cells. Carcinogenesis. 2004;25(5):647–59.

42. Kumari R, Chouhan S, Singh S, Chhipa RR, Ajay AK, Bhat MK. Constitutively activated ERK sensitizes cancer cells to doxorubicin: involvement of p53-EGFR-ERK pathway. J Biosci. 2017;42(1):31–41.

43. Fong Y, Wu CY, Chang KF, Chen BH, Chou WJ, Tseng CH, Chen YC, Wang HD, Chen YL, Chiu CC. Dual roles of extracellular signal-regulated kinase (ERK) in quinoline compound BPIQ-induced apoptosis and anti-migration of human non-small cell lung cancer cells. Cancer Cell Int. 2017;17:37.

44. Zhao Y, Fan D, Zheng ZP, Li ET, Chen F, Cheng KW, Wang M. 8-C-(E-phenylethenyl)quercetin from onion/beef soup induces autophagic cell death in colon cancer cells through ERK activation. Mol Nutr Food Res. 2017. https://doi.org/10.1002/mnfr.201600437.

45. Yun SM, Jung JH, Jeong SJ, Sohn EJ, Kim B, Kim SH. Tanshinone IIA induces autophagic cell death via activation of AMPK and ERK and inhibition of mTOR and p70 S6K in KBM-5 leukemia cells. Phytother Res. 2014;28(3):458–64.

46. El-Khattouti A, Selimovic D, Haikel Y, Hassan M. Crosstalk between apoptosis and autophagy: molecular mechanisms and therapeutic strategies in cancer. J Cell Death. 2013;6:37–55.

# 7

# TEAD4 overexpression promotes epithelial-mesenchymal transition and associates with aggressiveness and adverse prognosis in head neck squamous cell carcinoma

Wei Zhang[1†], Jin Li[1,2†], Yaping Wu[1,2], Han Ge[1], Yue Song[1], Dongmiao Wang[2], Hua Yuan[2], Hongbing Jiang[2], Yanling Wang[1*] and Jie Cheng[1,2*] [iD]

## Abstract

**Background:** Deregulated Hippo signaling has been uncovered to be intricately involved in tumorigenesis. Transcriptional factor TEADs serve as key mediators of Hippo signaling and have been increasingly appreciated as putative oncogenes driving cancer initiation and progression. However, its expression pattern and oncogenic role of TEAD4 in head and neck squamous cell carcinoma (HNSCC) remain largely unexplored.

**Methods:** TEAD4 mRNA expression in HNSCC was determined by data mining and analyses from TCGA dataset and four independent cohorts with transcriptional profiling data publically available. The protein abundance of TEAD4 was measured by immunohistochemistry in 105 primary HNSCC samples and associations between its expression and clinicopathological parameters and patient survival were evaluated. The oncogenic roles of TEAD4 was further determined by 4-nitroquinoline 1-oxide (4NQO)-induced animal model, both knockdown/overexpression assay and TGF-β1-induced epithelia-mesenchymal transition (EMT) in vitro.

**Results:** Both mRNA and protein abundance of TEAD4 were significantly increased in HNSCC as compared to its non-tumor counterparts. Overexpression of TEAD4 significantly associated with high pathological grade, cervical node metastasis, advanced clinical stage and reduced overall and disease-free survival. In the 4NQO-induced HNSCC mouse model, increased TEAD4 immunostaining was found associated with disease progression. TEAD4 knockdown significantly inhibited cell proliferation, migration and invasion, and induced cell apoptosis in HNSCC cells, while its overexpression resulted in opposite effects and EMT. Moreover, TEAD4 was critically involved in TGF-β1-induced EMT in HNSCC cells.

**Conclusions:** Our findings reveal that TEAD4 serves as a novel prognostic biomarker and putative oncogene for HNSCC by promoting cell proliferation, migration and invasion, and EMT.

**Keywords:** Head and neck squamous cell carcinoma, Hippo signaling, TEAD4, EMT, Prognostic biomarker

*Correspondence: wyl1280@163.com; leonardo_cheng@163.com
†Wei Zhang and Jin Li contributed equally to this study
[1] Jiangsu Key Laboratory of Oral Disease, Nanjing Medical University, 136 Hanzhong Road, Jiangsu 210029, People's Republic of China
[2] Department of Oral and Maxillofacial Surgery, Affiliated Stomatological Hospital, Nanjing Medical University, 136 Hanzhong Road, Nanjing 210029, People's Republic of China

## Background

Head and neck squamous cell carcinoma (HNSCC) is the sixth common cancer worldwide with more than 350,000 cancer-related deaths per year. Multiple etiological factors have been identified to critically contribute to this malignancy including smoking abuse, alcohol consumption, betel quid chew and human papillomavirus (HPV) infection [1]. Even though combined and multidisciplinary therapy against HNSCC have been established, the long-term survival rate of HNSCC patients has not been markedly improved in the past decades [2]. Major prognostic factors include invasive depth, cervical lymph node metastasis and advanced TNM stage [3]. Much efforts have been made to unveil the cellular and molecular mechanisms of HNSCC tumorigenesis [4]. However, the precise mechanisms under its initiation and development still remain fragmented. Thus, identification of new biomarkers and therapeutic targets for HNSCC is urgently needed for clinicians to improve the patients' prognosis.

The Hippo signaling pathway has increasingly been recognized as a key and indispensable mediator in tissue homeostasis, organ size control, metabolism, regeneration and tumorigenesis [5]. Defects in Hippo signaling and hyperactivation of its downstream effectors yes-associated protein (YAP) and transcriptional coactivator with PDZ-binding motif (TAZ) essentially contribute to cancer initiation, outgrowth, metastatic dissemination and therapeutic resistance [6, 7]. Pervasively activated YAP and TAZ in human malignancies accumulated in the nucleus where they drive gene transcription mainly by forming complexes with TEA domain DNA-binding family of transcription factors (TEADs) [8]. In mammal, there are four TEAD protein members, namely TEAD1–4. TEADs are broadly expressed but each member has tissue-specific expression pattern which suggests tissue-specific roles for each TEAD [9]. Previous studies have revealed important functions of TEAD members in various biological processed and human diseases [10, 11]. TEAD transcription factors are not only crucial for developmental process, but also play important roles in tumor initiation and progression [9, 11, 12]. TEADs promote cell proliferation, migration and invasion, epithelial-mesenchymal transition in several solid tumors including prostate, breast, colorectal and gastric cancers by binding with or without YAP/TAZ [13–15]. Previous reports largely focused on the expression and biological roles of YAP and TAZ during tumorigenesis [7, 16, 17]. However, the accurate biological functions of TEADs in human cancer are just beginning to disclose in selected contexts and remain yet unexplored in HNSCC.

Here, we sought to determine the expression of TEAD4 and its clinicopathological significance in human

HNSCC samples and chemical-induced HNSCC animal model. Moreover, we determined the tumorigenic roles of TEAD4 by functional assays in vitro and revealed the critical links between TEAD4 and EMT in HNSCC.

## Materials and methods

### Patients and tissue specimens

A total number of 105 patients with primary HNSCC (Jan. 2008 and Dec. 2014.) receiving radical resection of cancer at the Department of oral and maxillofacial surgery, Nanjing Medical University were enrolled. Written informed consent was obtained from these patients. Patient inclusion criteria were described as follows: (1) primary HNSCC with no prior chemotherapy or radiotherapy; (2) patients underwent radical tumor resection and neck lymph node dissection; (3) detailed demographic, clinical, pathological and follow-up data available. The archived tissue samples and haematoxylin–eosin stained sections of each patient were retrieved. The previous histological diagnosis as SCC were further histopathologically conformed according to the established histological criteria. Twenty samples of healthy oral mucosa were obtained from intraoral trauma surgery at the same period. This study protocol was reviewed and approved by the Research Ethic Committee of Nanjing Medical University.

### Cell lines and chemicals

A panel of HNSCC cell lines including Cal27, Fadu, SCC4, SCC25, HN4 and HN6 were used. Non-tumorigenic HOK and Cal27, Fadu, SCC4 and SCC25 were purchased from American Type Culture Collection (ATCC, Manassas, VA, USA). HN4 and HN6 cell lines were generous gifts from Prof. Wantao Chen from Shanghai Jiaotong University. Cancer cells were grown in DMEN/F12 (Invitrogen) supplemented with 10% FBS (Gibco) and 100 units/ml antibiotics, and maintained at 37 °C. For TGF-β1-induced EMT cell model in vitro, morphological changes and relevant markers expression were monitored in cells which were treated with recombinant human TGF-β1 (rhTGF-β1, 10 ng/ml, R&D Systems) for indicated times.

### Small interference RNA (siRNA) DNA constructs and transfection

The siRNA oligonucleotides including TEAD4 siRNA-1 (5′-CCGCCAAAUCUAUGACAAATT′, 5′-UUUGUC AUAGAUUUGGCGGTT′) TEAD4 siRNA-2 (5′-CGC UCUGUGAGUACAUGAUTT-3′, 5′-AUCAUGUAC UCACAGAGCGTT′) and control siRNA (5′-UUCUCC GAACGUGUCACGUTT-3′, 5′-ACGUGACACGUU CGGAGAATT-3′) were designed and purchased from GenePharma (Shanghai, China). Transfection of siRNA oligonucleotides with final concentration 100 nM was performed with Lipofectamine RNAiMAX (Life Technologies) according to the manufacturer's instruction. Then cells were harvested for further experiments 48 h after transfection unless otherwise specified.

The human TEAD4 overexpression construct tagged with single FLAG was generated by inserting the TEAD4 full-length cDNA template into plasmid GV141. Following transient transfection with TEAD4 overexpression plasmid, cells were harvested at 48 h for further experiments. Stable cell clones with TEAD4 overexpression were selected by appropriate antibiotics (G418, 500 ng/ml, Sigma) for 2 weeks after plasmid transfection.

### CCK-8 and colony formation assay

Cell proliferation and viability were assessed by absorbance using CCK-8 cell viability assay (Cell Counting Kit-8, Dojindo, Japan) per manufacturer's instructions. Cells were seeded in 96-well microplates at a density of $2 \times 10^3$ cells per well. Cells were incubated in new medium containing 10% CCK-8 reaction solution. After incubation for 2 h, the absorbance was measured on a spectrophotometer microplate reader (Multiskan MK3, Thermo) at a wavelength of 450 nm. Colony formation assay was performed as we previously reported [18].

### Cell apoptosis assessed by flow-cytometric assay

Cells were treated with trypsin (Gbico) and resuspended as single-cell suspension. Cells were stained with Annexin V:PE Apoptosis Detection Kit (BD Bioscience) and submitted to a FACSCalibur flow cytometer (BD Biosciences). Data were analyzed with CellQuest Pro software (BD Biosciences).

### In vitro cell invasion and wound healing assay

For wound-healing assays, cells were seeded at a density of $1 \times 10^6$ cell/well in six-well plates. Then we used a sterile 10 μl pipette tip to create an artificial wound on the confluent cell monolayer. The suspended cells were washed thoroughly with PBS, and cells were cultured in medium with 1% FBS (Gibco). The wounds were photographed at 0, 6, 12 and 24 h as indicated. Cell invasion were determined by a Matrigel transwell invasion assay. In brief, $1 \times 10^5$ viable cells were suspended in 200 μl of DMEN/F12 (Invitrogen) without serum and seeded into upper chamber precoated with Matrigel (BD Biosciences, USA). Complete medium with 10% serum was added to the lower chamber as chemoattractant. After incubation for 12 h, the non-invading cells were gently removed with a cotton swab, while those invaded cells adherent to the lower side of membrane were stained with a 0.1% crystal violet solution, photographed and counted as our revious reports [19, 20].

### Immunofluorescence assay

For immunofluorescence assays, cells were seeded on glass coverslips 18 h prior to experiment and fixed with 4% paraformaldehyde and washed thoroughly with PBS. After these, the cells were permeabilized in Triton X-100 (0.1% in PBS) for 1 h and washed thoroughly with PBS. Then cells were blocked with 3% bovine serum albumin (BSA) for 30 min at room temperature followed by incubation with primary antibodies against E-cadherin (1:200 dilution) and vimentin (1:150 dilution) overnight, respectively. Cells were further incubated with corresponding secondary antibodies and/or cytoskeleton actin/nuclear staining. Immunofluorescence was visualized under a Zeiss fluorescence microscope or confocal microscope.

### RNA extraction and real time RT-PCR

Total RNA was extracted from cells and subjected to reverse transcription and PCR reactions using Prime-ScriptTM RT-PCR kit (Takara) as described previously [19, 20]. Relative mRNA expression was quantified as compared to internal control GAPDH using comparative CT method. The primers were listed as follows: TEAD4 (forward: TCCACGAAGGTCTGCTCTTT, reverse: GTGCTTGAGCTTGTGGATGA) and GAPDH (forward: AGGTGAAGGTCGGAGTCAAC, reverse: AGTTGAGGTCAATGAAGGGG).

### Western blot analysis

Cells were harvested and lysed in ice-clod cell lysis buffer containing protease inhibitor cocktail (Invitrogen). The same amount of protein samples were electrophoresed through 10% SDS-PAGE and transferred to PVDF membranes (Bio-Rad). Following 5% non-fat milk or BSA blocking, these membranes were incubated at 4 °C overnight with primary antibodies TEAD4 (1:1000, ab58310, Abcam), E-cadherin (1:2000, #3195, Cell signaling), N-cadherin (1:1000, #13116, Cell signaling), vimentin (1:2000, #5741, Cell signaling), snail (1:1000, #3879, Cell signaling) and GAPDH (1:2000, sc-32233, Santa Cruz) followed by incubation with horseradish peroxidase(HRP)-conjugated secondary antibodies. Immunoreactive bands on the blots were detected by ECL chemiluminescence kit (Bio-Rad).

### 4-nitroquinoline 1-oxide (4NQO)-induced HNSCC animal model

In the 4NQO-induced HNSCC animal model, squamous cell carcinoma was initiated and progressed in tongue. This experimental was performed as our previous reports with minor modifications [21–23]. In brief, 6-week-old C57BL/6 mice were fed with drinking water containing 50 μg/mL 4NQO for consecutive 16 weeks and then given with normal water for another 8–10 weeks. Animals with normal water was used as controls. Lesions in tongue were visually inspected every week. Samples were harvested at 16, 20 and 24 weeks after chemical administration and subjected to histopathological analyses.

### Immunohistochemical staining and scoring

Immunohistochemical staining for TEAD4 was performed on 4 μm-thick slides from formalin-fixed paraffin-embedded samples using routine procedures as our previously reported [7]. Negative controls without primary TEAD4 antibody (1:200, GTX108750, GeneTex) incubation were included. Immunoreactivity was semi-quantitatively evaluated according to staining intensity and distribution using the immunoreactive score which was calculated as intensity score × proportion score as we reported previously [20, 24]. Intensity score was defined as 0, negative; 1, weak; 2, moderate; 3, strong, while the proportion score was defined as 0, negative; 1, < 10%; 2, 11–50%; 3, 51–80%; 4, > 80% positive cells. The total score ranged from 0 to 12. Accordingly, the immunoreactivity of each slide was categorized into three subgroups based on the final score: 0, negative; 1–4, low expression; 4–12, high expression as we reported before [20, 24].

### Data mining and analysis of TEAD4 mutation and expression in HNSCC via publicly available database

The original data concerning mutational landscape and mRNA expression of TEAD1–4 in HNSCC were retrieved from 3 publicly available databases including cBioPortal (http://www.cbioportal.org/) [25], TCGA (https://cancergenome.nih.gov/) and Oncomine (https://www.oncomine.org/) [26]. TEAD4 mRNA expression levels (log2-transformed) in HNSCC and normal counterparts were retrieved and statistically compared. The associations between expression status of TEAD4 mRNA (high or low using median value as cutoff) and patient survival were determined by Kaplan-Meir analysis.

### Statistical analysis

All quantitative data was presented as mean ± SD from two or three independent experiments and compared with Student's t-test or ANOVA with Bonferroni post hoc test unless otherwise specified. The correlations between TEAD4 expression and various clinicopathological parameters were evaluated by Chi square or Fisher exact test. Patient survival was estimated using Kaplan–Meier method and compared with Log-rank test. The prognostic analyses were performed by univariate and multivariate Cox regression models to determine the individual clinicopathological variables with patient overall survival. P values less than 0.05 (two-sided) were considered statistically significant. All statistical analyses

were performed using GraphPad Prism 8 or SPSS 21.0 software.

## Results

### Aberrant upregulation of TEAD4 mRNA in HNSCC via bioinformatics analyses

We have previously identified genetic variants of Hippo pathway genes (YAP1 rs11225163, TEAD1 rs7944031 and TEAD4 rs1990330) and revealed that Hippo effector TAZ significantly associated with unfavorable survival in cutaneous melanoma and primary OSCC [7, 27, 28]. Given the increasingly appreciated roles of TEADs during tumorigenesis, we initially sought to explore the mRNA expression patterns of TEAD 1–4 in HNSCC using the publicly available TCGA dataset. As shown in Fig. 1a–d, TEAD2 and 4 were significantly upregulated in HNSCC samples as compared to their non-tumor counterparts, while TEAD1 and TEAD3 were markedly downregulated in cancerous samples relative to non-tumor samples. Moreover, four independent HNSCC patients cohorts from Oncomine database such as Peng's [29], Ginos' [30], Cromer's [31] and Ye's [32] cohorts were identified and utilized to measure TEAD4 mRNA expression. As shown in Fig. 1e–h, significantly higher abundance of TEAD4 mRNA was observed in HNSCC samples compared to their non-tumor counterparts. Several lines of evidence have revealed that TEAD4 is frequently amplified and/or aberrantly overexpressed in multiple cancers and associates with unfavorable prognosis [14, 15, 33]. Data integration and interrogation using cBioPortal platform indicated that total frequency of TEAD4 genetic alteration in HNSCC was rare, less than 2.5% in total patients. To identify potential associations between TEAD4 mRNA expression and clinicopathological parameters, we compared its abundance among diverse subgroups based on pathological grade and clinical stage, respectively. However, as shown in Additional file 1: Figure S1, the abundance of TEAD4 mRNA was comparable without significant difference among different subgroups stratified by pathological grade and clinical stage. In addition, there was no significant associations between TEAD4 mRNA expression and patient overall survival in TCGA-HNSCC cohort, when the median value of TEAD4 mRNA was used as cutoff to stratify patients into low and high TEAD4-expressing subgroups (Additional file 1: Figure S1).

### Overexpression of TEAD4 correlates with aggressive clinicopathological parameters in HNSCC

To further determine expression pattern of TEAD4 in HNSCC, we next performed immunohistochemical staining of TEAD4 in 105 primary HNSCC samples. The detailed demographic and clinicopathological parameters

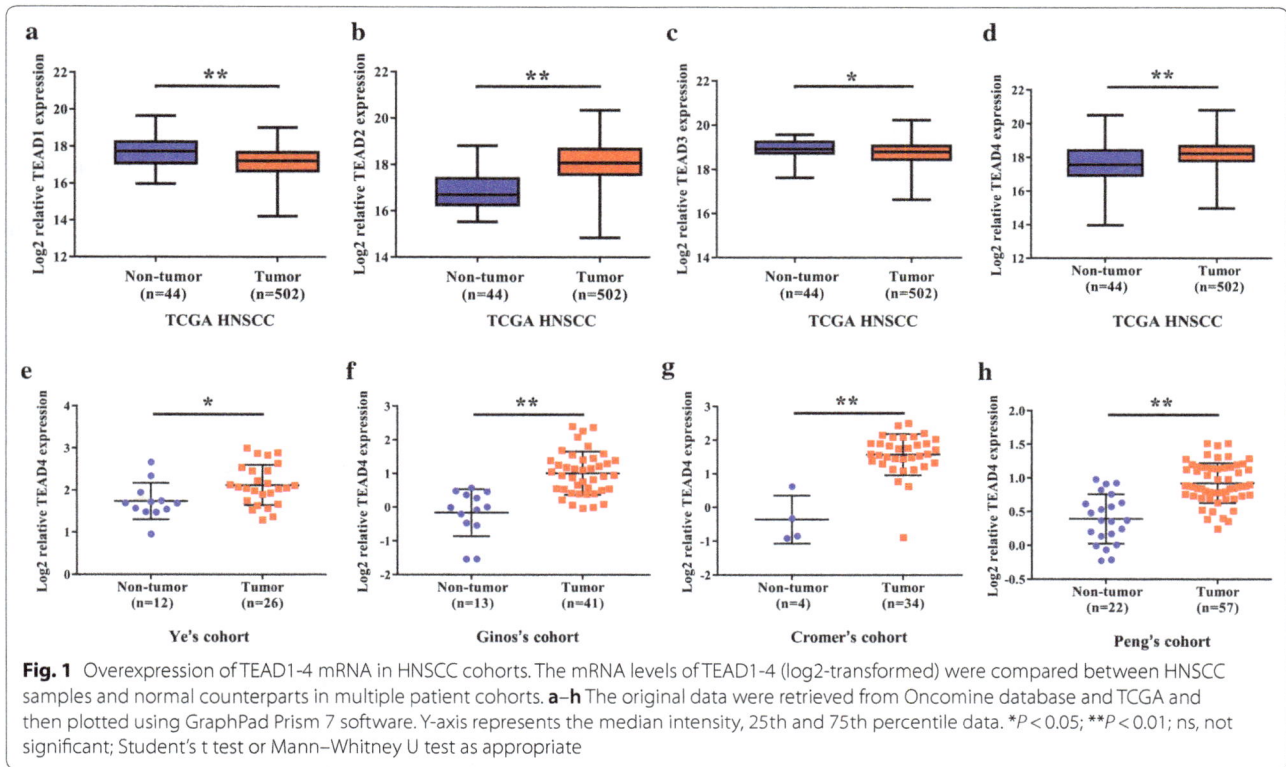

**Fig. 1** Overexpression of TEAD1-4 mRNA in HNSCC cohorts. The mRNA levels of TEAD1-4 (log2-transformed) were compared between HNSCC samples and normal counterparts in multiple patient cohorts. **a–h** The original data were retrieved from Oncomine database and TCGA and then plotted using GraphPad Prism 7 software. Y-axis represents the median intensity, 25th and 75th percentile data. *$P < 0.05$; **$P < 0.01$; ns, not significant; Student's t test or Mann–Whitney U test as appropriate

of these patients were listed in Table 1. In brief, 63 males and 42 females were enrolled with mean age 59.5 years. The follow-up durations ranged from 6 to 78 months (mean 39.5 months). Until the last follow-up, 77 (73.3%) patients remained alive with disease-free, 5 (4.8%) still alive but with recurrences and/or cervical nodal metastases, 23 (21.9%) died due to post-surgical recurrence, metastases or other unrelated diseases.

As shown in Fig. 2, rare positive staining of TEAD4 was observed in most healthy oral mucosa samples and a minority of HNSCC samples, whereas positive nuclear TEAD4 staining was detected in a fraction of HNSCC samples. TEAD4 expression patterns in HNSCC and normal oral epithelial were categorized according to immunohistochemistry scores. Consequently, TEAD4 protein abundance can be classified into low (55) or high expression (50) in HNSCC samples while negative (7), low (9) or high expression (4) in normal oral epithelial samples, indicative of aberrant TEAD4 overexpression in HNSCC ($P < 0.0001$, Chi square test). The detailed correlations between TEAD4 protein expression and clinicopathological parameters were further listed in Table 1. There was no significant associations between TEAD4 expression and gender, age, smoking, alcohol drinking and tumor size.

However, high TEAD4 expression positively associated with advanced pathological grade, cervical node metastasis and advanced clinical stage with $P$-value 0.034, 0.0214 and 0.0397, respectively.

## Overexpression of TEAD4 significantly associated with reduced survival in HNSCC patients

Next, we utilized Kaplan–Meier survival analyses to determine the association between TEAD4 expression and patient prognosis. As shown in Fig. 3, patients with high TEAD4 expression had significantly reduced overall survival and disease-free survival compared with those with low TEAD4 expression (log-rank test, $P = 0.0102$, 0.0066). Moreover, we applied both univariate and multivariate survival analyses to further evaluate the prognostic value of TEAD4 expression in HNSCC. In line with Kaplan–Meier survival analysis, the univariate regression assay revealed that TEAD4 expression was significantly associated with patient survival ($P = 0.009$). Furthermore, after adjusting for other demographic and clinicopathological parameters, TEAD4 expression was identified as an independent factor for patients' survival ($P = 0.028$), along with the established prognostic factor, the clinical stage ($P = 0.050$, Table 2).

**Table 1 The associations between TEAD4 expression and multiple clinicopathological parameters in HNSCC samples**

| Clinicopathological parameters | Cases | TEAD4 | | P-values |
|---|---|---|---|---|
| | | Low* | High | |
| Gender | 105 | 55 | 50 | |
| Male | 63 | 33 | 30 | > 0.9999 |
| Female | 42 | 22 | 20 | |
| Age | | | | |
| ≤60 | 43 | 22 | 21 | 0.8453 |
| >60 | 62 | 33 | 29 | |
| Smoking | | | | |
| No | 74 | 37 | 37 | 0.5232 |
| Yes | 31 | 18 | 13 | |
| Alcohol use | | | | |
| No | 83 | 42 | 41 | 0.6319 |
| Yes | 22 | 13 | 9 | |
| Tumor size | | | | |
| T1–T2 | 74 | 42 | 32 | 0.2011 |
| T3–T4 | 31 | 13 | 18 | |
| Pathological grade | | | | |
| I | 58 | 37 | 21 | *0.0340* |
| II | 34 | 13 | 21 | |
| III | 13 | 5 | 8 | |
| Cervical node metastasis | | | | |
| N(0) | 71 | 43 | 28 | *0.0214* |
| N(+) | 34 | 12 | 22 | |
| Clinical stage | | | | |
| I | 19 | 11 | 8 | *0.0397* |
| II | 30 | 21 | 9 | |
| III | 25 | 8 | 17 | |
| IV | 31 | 15 | 16 | |

* Both of patients with low and negative TEAD4 staining are stratified into low TEAD4 category for simplicity. The number in italic indicate statistical significance with P-values less than 0.05

## Increased TEAD4 expression in chemical-induced HNSCC tumorigenesis

Having revealed aberrant overexpression of TEAD4 in a fraction of HNSCC, we wondered whether it played a role during HNSCC development. To address this, we utilized a well-established chemical-induced HNSCC animal model to characterize the expression pattern during HNSCC initiation and progression (Fig. 4A). In this model, lesions like hyperplasia, dysplasia, carcinoma in situ and invasive SCC were routinely found in the tongue, which resembles the pathological process of HNSCC. Thus, whole tongue was harvested at 16th, 20th and 24th week after 4NQO administration, which was subjected to histological analysis. As shown in Fig. 4B–I, immunohistochemical staining in these samples indicated significant strong nuclear staining of TEAD4 in

carcinoma in situ and invasive carcinoma, while negative or low staining in normal tongue mucosa and epithelial with hyperplasia. Positive TEAD4 staining was commonly observed in carcinoma (87.5%, 7/8), but much less in samples with healthy mucosa (12.5%, 1/8), hyperplasia (25.0%, 2/8) or dysplasia/carcinoma in situ (37.5%, 3/8). Moreover, in line with the IHC findings, we found that the mRNA levels of TEAD4 in pre-stored carcinoma samples were significantly upregulated by qRT-PCR (Fig. 4J). Collectively, our findings from this well-established chemical-induced HNSCC model indicated that TEAD4 might serve as a putative oncogene driving HNSCC development.

## TEAD4 promotes cell proliferation, migration, invasion and EMT in HNSCC cells

Considering that our clinical results supported a potential pro-tumorigenic role of TEAD4 in HNSCC, we next aimed to delineate its oncogenic roles driving HNSCC initiation and progression by siRNA-mediated loss-of-function approach. To address this, we first measured the abundance of TEAD4 in a panel of HNSCC cell lines and found that TEAD4 protein was significantly overexpressed in all HNSCC cell lines examined compared to immortalized oral epithelial cell (HOK) (Fig. 5a). Due to the relatively higher endogenous TEAD4 in Cal27 and Fadu cells, we next selected them for knockdown experiments. After 2 independent siRNAs targeting human TEAD4 were introduced into Cal27 and Fadu cells, the consequent changes of TEAD4 expression and cell phenotype were monitored. As shown in Fig. 5b, TEAD4 protein was significantly reduced in Cal27 and Fadu cells following siRNA transfection. Both results from CCK-8 viability assay and colony formation assay showed significantly lower proliferation rate upon TEAD4-siRNA transfection (Fig. 5c, d). Additionally, annexin V-PI flow cytometric assay revealed that the proportions of apoptotic cells in siTEAD4-treated cells were significantly increased from 5.5 to 15.1% in Cal27, from 7.6 to 24.4% in Fadu, respectively (Fig. 5e, f). Furthermore, the migratory and invasive potentials of cells were also measured using wound healing and transwell invasion assay after TEAD4 knockdown, respectively. As shown in Fig. 5g, h, the migratory and invasive abilities of cells following TEAD4 knockdown were significantly reduced.

To further confirm the tumorigenic roles of TEAD4 in HNSCC, we subcloned the full-length human TEAD4 cDNA with an N-terminal Flag tag into plasmid and generated stable TEAD4 overexpressing cells in HN6 (relatively low endogenous TEAD4) after antibiotics selection. As expected, TEAD4 protein was significantly increased in HN6 and HEK293T cells following plasmid transfection (Fig. 6a). We next utilized

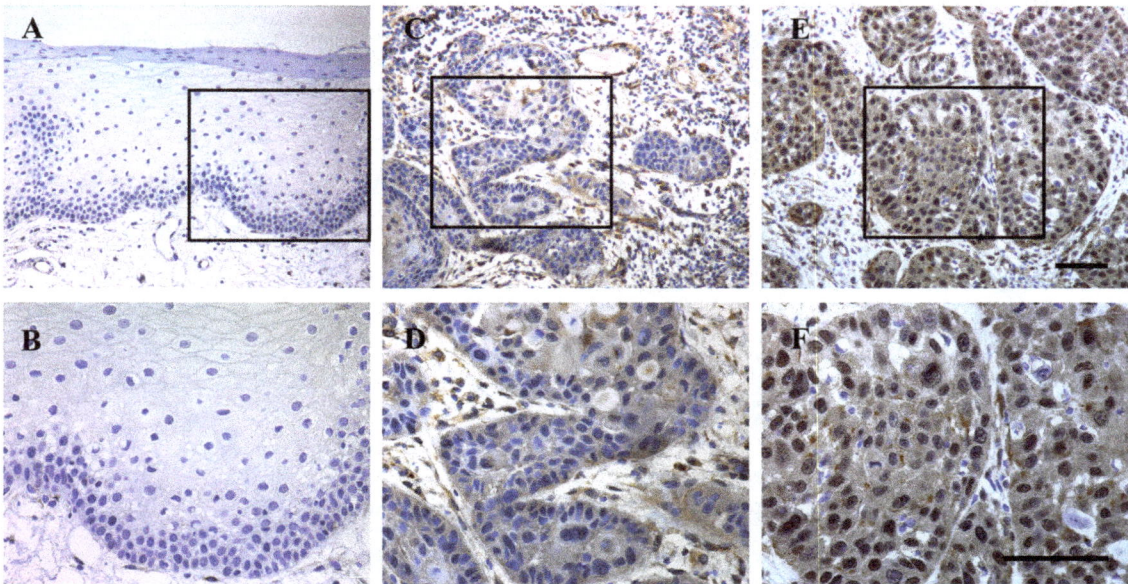

**Fig. 2** Immunohistochemical staining of TEAD4 in human HNSCC samples. **A**, **B** Representative negative staining of TEAD4 in normal oral epithelial; **C**, **D** representative low expression of TEAD4 in primary human HNSCC sample; **E**, **F** representative high expression of TEAD4 in primary human HNSCC sample. Nuclei are counterstained with hematoxylin. The areas marked by black box in the **A**, **C**, **E** images (upper panel) were shown in larger magnification as **B**, **D**, **F** images (lower panel), respectively. Scale bar: 100 μm

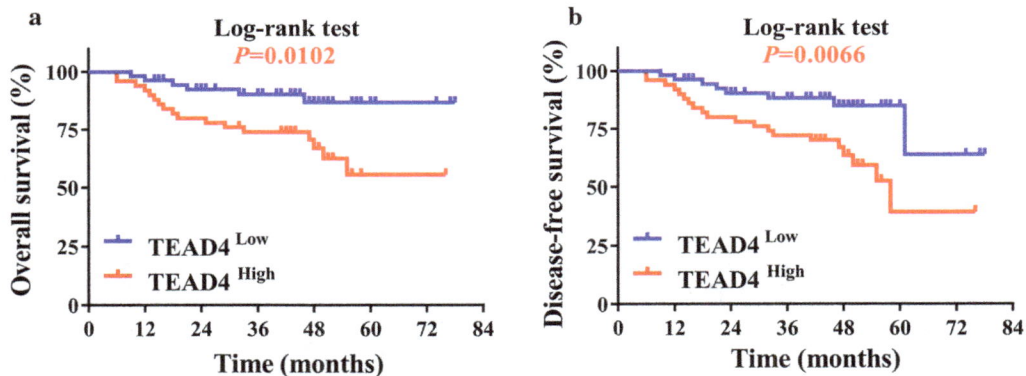

**Fig. 3** High TEAD4 expression positively associates with reduced overall survival in HNSCC patients. Overall survival (**a**) and disease-free survival (**b**) analyses of patients stratified with high or low expression of TEAD4 were estimated by Kaplan–Meier method and compared with Log-rank test

the HN6 cells with stable TEAD4 overexpression for subsequent experiments. Overexpression of TEAD4 accelerated cell proliferation in HN6 (Fig. 6b, c) as evidenced by results from CCK-8 and colony formation assay, which was consistent with the well-established pro-proliferative function of TEAD4. Interestingly, as shown in Fig. 6d, TEAD4-overexpressing cells became elongated, scattering distributed with fibroblast-like appearance, while control cells remained typical cobblestone morphology with tight adhesion. Moreover,

remarkably enhanced migration and invasion abilities were observed in TEAD4-overexpressing cells (Fig. 6e, f). These morphological and functional changes induced by TEAD4 suggested that TEAD4 might be capable of promoting EMT in HNSCC cells. To confirm this notion, we further determined the levels of EMT-related markers by western blot and immunofluorescence assays. As shown in Fig. 6g, h, downregulation of E-cadherin and upregulation of N-cadherin, Vimentin and Snail were detected upon TEAD4 overexpression,

**Table 2  Univariate and multivariate survival analyses (proportional hazards method) for patients with primary HNSCC**

| Variable | Univariate survival analysis | | | Multivariate survival analysis | | |
|---|---|---|---|---|---|---|
| | Hazard ratio | 95% CI | P-value | Hazard ratio | 95% CI | P-value |
| Gender (male, female) | 0.701 | 0.299–1.645 | 0.415 | | | N/A |
| Smoking (No, Yes) | 0.958 | 0.409–2.243 | 0.922 | | | N/A |
| Alcohol use (No, Yes) | 0.651 | 0.255–1.660 | 0.369 | | | N/A |
| Age (≤60, >60) | 0.995 | 0.429–2.307 | 0.991 | 0.944 | 0.405–2.202 | 0.895 |
| Tumorsize (T1–T2, T3–T4) | 0.591 | 0.261–1.336 | 0.206 | 2.010 | 0.535–7.547 | 0.301 |
| Pathological grade (I, II–III) | 0.587 | 0.260–1.327 | 0.200 | 0.909 | 0.366–2.261 | 0.838 |
| Cervical nodal metastasis (N0, N+) | 0.540 | 0.238–1.225 | 0.140 | 1.816 | 0.483–6.832 | 0.377 |
| Clinical stage (I–II, III–IV) | 0.311 | 0.123–0.788 | *0.014* | 0.194 | 0.038–0.998 | *0.050* |
| TEAD4 expression (low, high) | 0.029 | 0.115–0.732 | *0.009* | 0.344 | 0.133–0.893 | *0.028* |

The numbers in italic indicate statistical significance with *P*-values less than 0.05

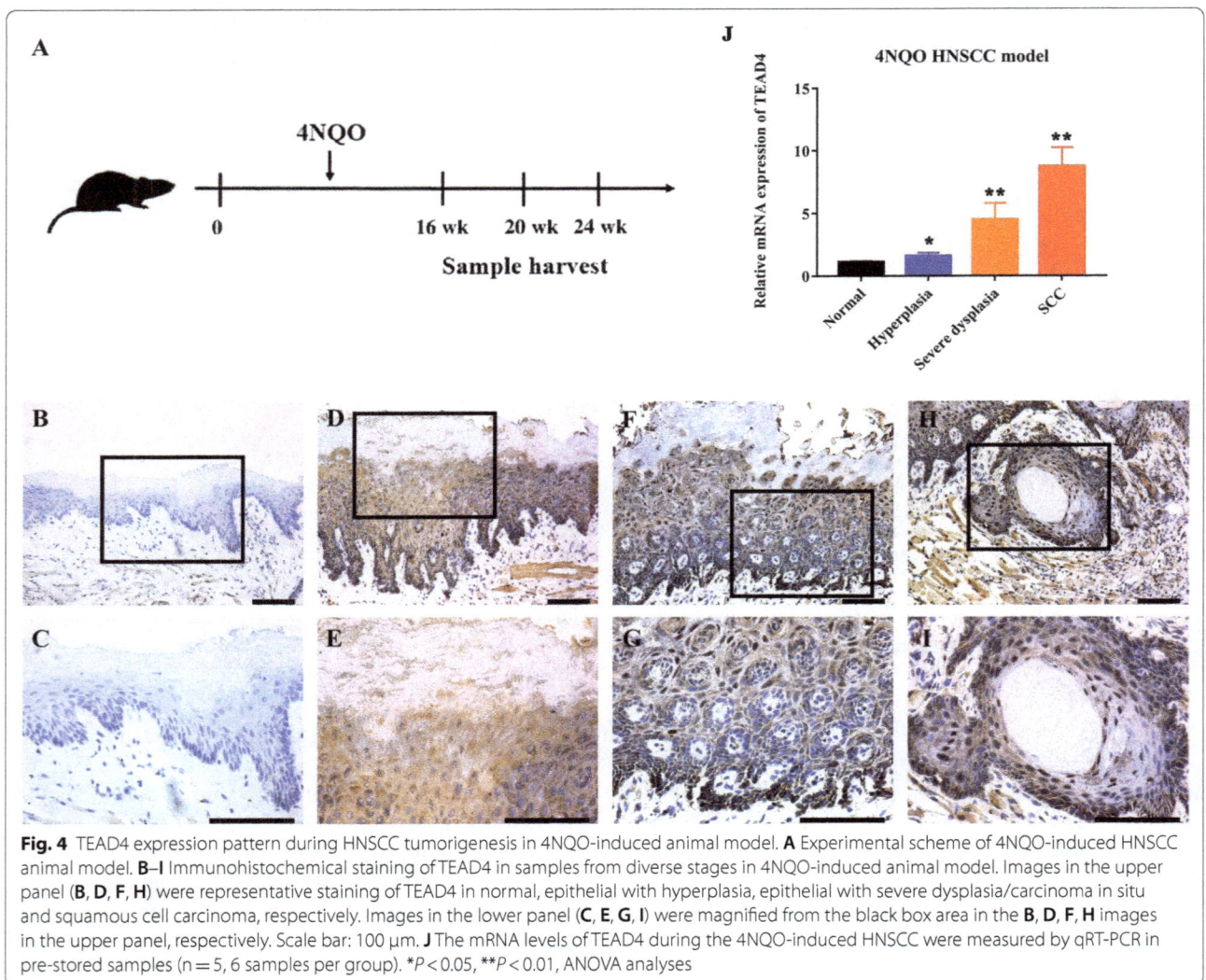

**Fig. 4** TEAD4 expression pattern during HNSCC tumorigenesis in 4NQO-induced animal model. **A** Experimental scheme of 4NQO-induced HNSCC animal model. **B–I** Immunohistochemical staining of TEAD4 in samples from diverse stages in 4NQO-induced animal model. Images in the upper panel (**B, D, F, H**) were representative staining of TEAD4 in normal, epithelial with hyperplasia, epithelial with severe dysplasia/carcinoma in situ and squamous cell carcinoma, respectively. Images in the lower panel (**C, E, G, I**) were magnified from the black box area in the **B, D, F, H** images in the upper panel, respectively. Scale bar: 100 μm. **J** The mRNA levels of TEAD4 during the 4NQO-induced HNSCC were measured by qRT-PCR in pre-stored samples (n = 5, 6 samples per group). *P < 0.05, **P < 0.01, ANOVA analyses

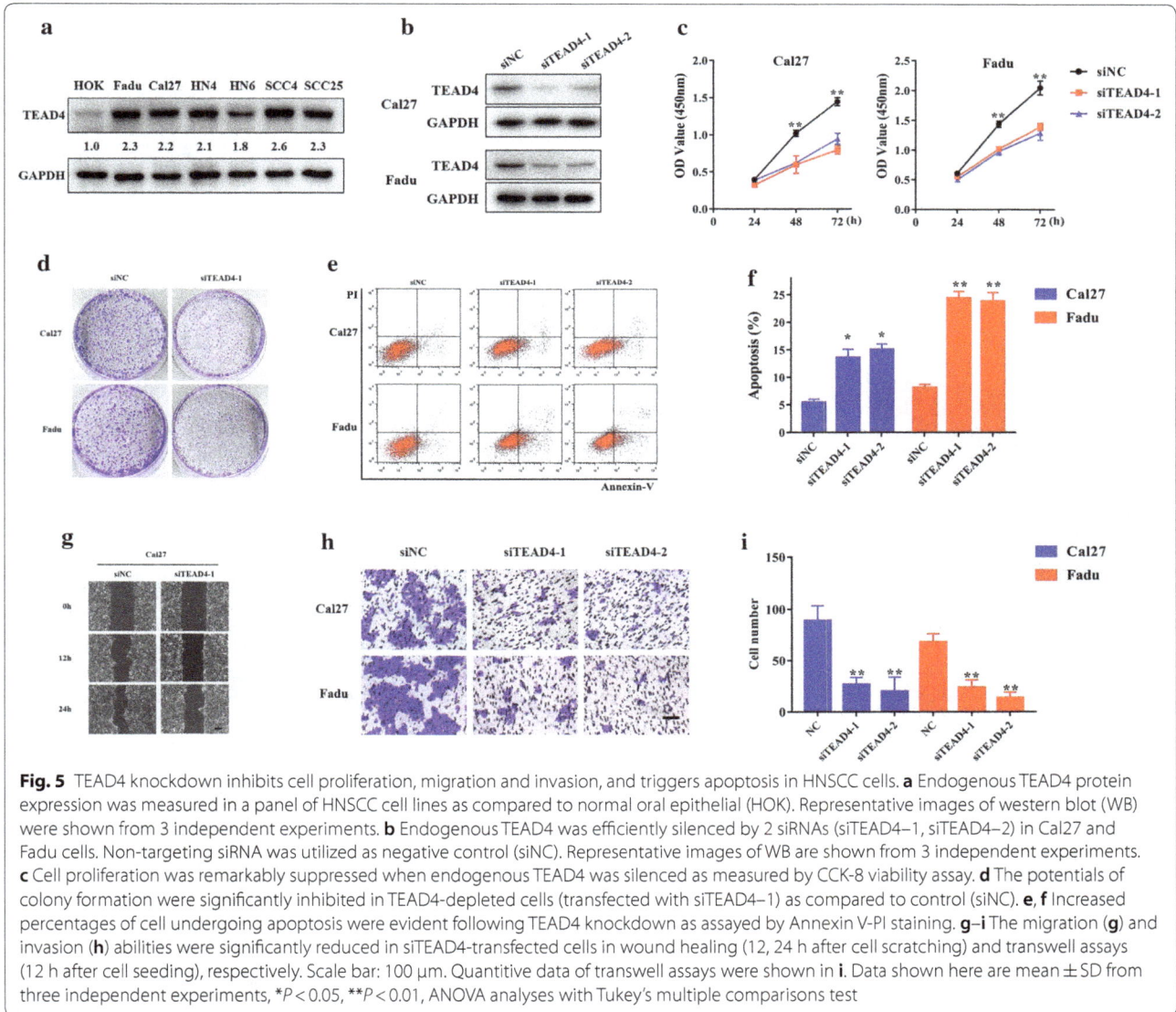

**Fig. 5** TEAD4 knockdown inhibits cell proliferation, migration and invasion, and triggers apoptosis in HNSCC cells. **a** Endogenous TEAD4 protein expression was measured in a panel of HNSCC cell lines as compared to normal oral epithelial (HOK). Representative images of western blot (WB) were shown from 3 independent experiments. **b** Endogenous TEAD4 was efficiently silenced by 2 siRNAs (siTEAD4–1, siTEAD4–2) in Cal27 and Fadu cells. Non-targeting siRNA was utilized as negative control (siNC). Representative images of WB are shown from 3 independent experiments. **c** Cell proliferation was remarkably suppressed when endogenous TEAD4 was silenced as measured by CCK-8 viability assay. **d** The potentials of colony formation were significantly inhibited in TEAD4-depleted cells (transfected with siTEAD4–1) as compared to control (siNC). **e, f** Increased percentages of cell undergoing apoptosis were evident following TEAD4 knockdown as assayed by Annexin V-PI staining. **g–i** The migration (**g**) and invasion (**h**) abilities were significantly reduced in siTEAD4-transfected cells in wound healing (12, 24 h after cell scratching) and transwell assays (12 h after cell seeding), respectively. Scale bar: 100 μm. Quantitive data of transwell assays were shown in **i**. Data shown here are mean ± SD from three independent experiments, *$P < 0.05$, **$P < 0.01$, ANOVA analyses with Tukey's multiple comparisons test

which strongly suggested EMT following TEAD4 introduction in vitro.

## TEAD4 is involved in TGF-β1-induced EMT in HNSCC

Accumulating evidence indicates that EMT-mediated metastatic spread dictates patients survival in various solid cancers including HNSCC [34]. Both gain-of-function and loss-of-function in vitro assays suggested the potential roles of TEAD4 involving EMT and invasion of HNSCC. Thus, we next aimed to further verify the EMT-inducing role of TEAD4 in HNSCC. To address this, we firstly utilized two independent siRNAs to knockdown endogenous TEAD4 and revealed upregulation of E-cadherin and downregulation of Vimentin, N-cadherin and Snail following TEAD4 silencing in Cal27 and Fadu cells,

which was well consistent with EMT-mediated marker changes (Fig. 7a). Next, we employed the well-established TGF-β1-induced EMT cell model [35] and found that both TEAD4 mRNA and protein expression significantly increased with TGF-β1-treated time in Cal27 (Fig. 7b). In addition, when cells were treated siTEAD4 alone or together with TGF-β1 for 48 h, immunofluorescence assay indicated that TGF-β1 exposure resulted in more cells with positive vimentin staining but less with positive E-cadherin staining, and TEAD4 knockdown by siRNA largely abolished these effects of TGF-β1 in vitro (Fig. 7c). Moreover, TGF-β1-induced EMT marker changes as measured by western blot assay were largely abolished upon TEAD4 depletion (Fig. 7d). In line with these marker changes, TGF-β1-induced enhancement

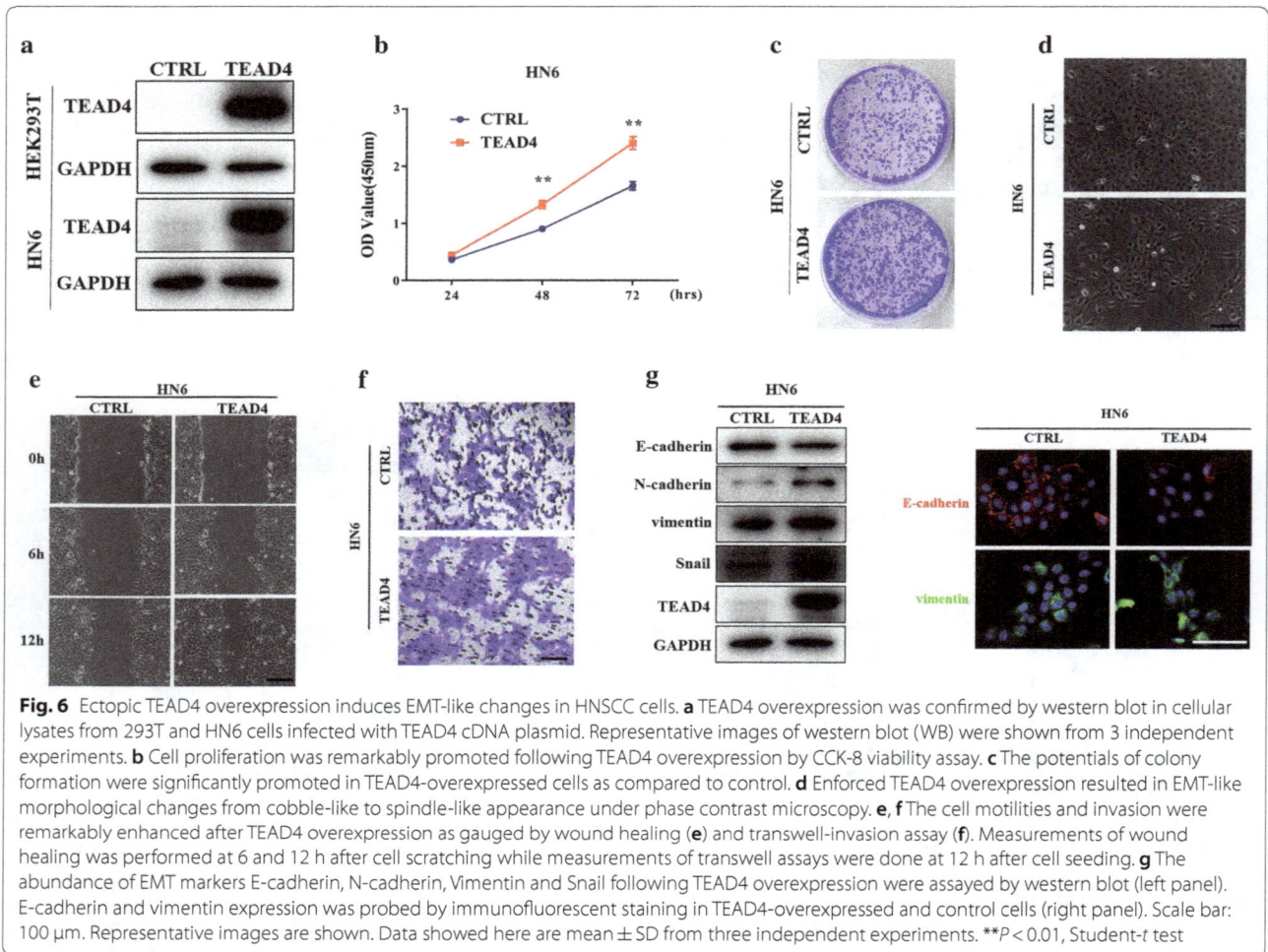

**Fig. 6** Ectopic TEAD4 overexpression induces EMT-like changes in HNSCC cells. **a** TEAD4 overexpression was confirmed by western blot in cellular lysates from 293T and HN6 cells infected with TEAD4 cDNA plasmid. Representative images of western blot (WB) were shown from 3 independent experiments. **b** Cell proliferation was remarkably promoted following TEAD4 overexpression by CCK-8 viability assay. **c** The potentials of colony formation were significantly promoted in TEAD4-overexpressed cells as compared to control. **d** Enforced TEAD4 overexpression resulted in EMT-like morphological changes from cobble-like to spindle-like appearance under phase contrast microscopy. **e, f** The cell motilities and invasion were remarkably enhanced after TEAD4 overexpression as gauged by wound healing (**e**) and transwell-invasion assay (**f**). Measurements of wound healing was performed at 6 and 12 h after cell scratching while measurements of transwell assays were done at 12 h after cell seeding. **g** The abundance of EMT markers E-cadherin, N-cadherin, Vimentin and Snail following TEAD4 overexpression were assayed by western blot (left panel). E-cadherin and vimentin expression was probed by immunofluorescent staining in TEAD4-overexpressed and control cells (right panel). Scale bar: 100 μm. Representative images are shown. Data showed here are mean ± SD from three independent experiments. **$P < 0.01$, Student-$t$ test

of invasiveness were significantly impaired following TEAD4 knockdown (Fig. 7e). Finally, we extracted the original HNSCC dataset from TCGA platform and applied a generic gene signature of EMT to score the EMT status of these samples which was a versatile tool for objective and systematic investigation of EMT roles and dynamics in cancer progression [36]. Our results from EMT scoring revealed that TEAD4 expression was positively correlated with EMT score in HNSCC (Fig. 7f). Collectively, these results supported the critical roles of TEAD4 involved in TGF-β1-induced EMT in HNSCC, although the underlying regulatory network still required further delineation.

## Discussion

Until now, deregulated Hippo signaling pathway has been demonstrated to be intricately associated with tumorigenesis and serves as viable therapeutic targets with translational potentials [6]. TEAD4 functions as a key member of Hippo signaling mediating transcriptional

output via forming complex with YAP or TAZ. Several lines with evidence have revealed that TEAD4 has oncogenic roles and prognostic significance underlying multiple cancer contexts [14, 15, 37, 39]. In the present study, we utilized the HNSCC samples, animal model and in vitro cellular assay to delineate the expression pattern, prognostic roles and tumorigenic functions of TEAD4 in HNSCC. Our findings revealed that TEAD4 served as a novel putative oncogene to promote HNSCC tumorigenesis and as a novel prognsotic biomarker for HNSCC.

Previous studies have revealed that TEAD4 is usually amplificated and/or overexpressed in multiple cancers including atypical teratoid/rhabdoid tumor, serous ovarian carcinoma, colorectal cancer, lung adenocarcinoma, gastric cancer and OSCC [14, 15, 33, 38–40]. In line with this, both bioinformatics analyses from multple independent patient cohorts and immunohistochemistry in primary HNSCC samples revealed aberrant overexpression of TEAD4 in a large subset of patients examined. Moreover, results from 4NQO-induced HNSCC model

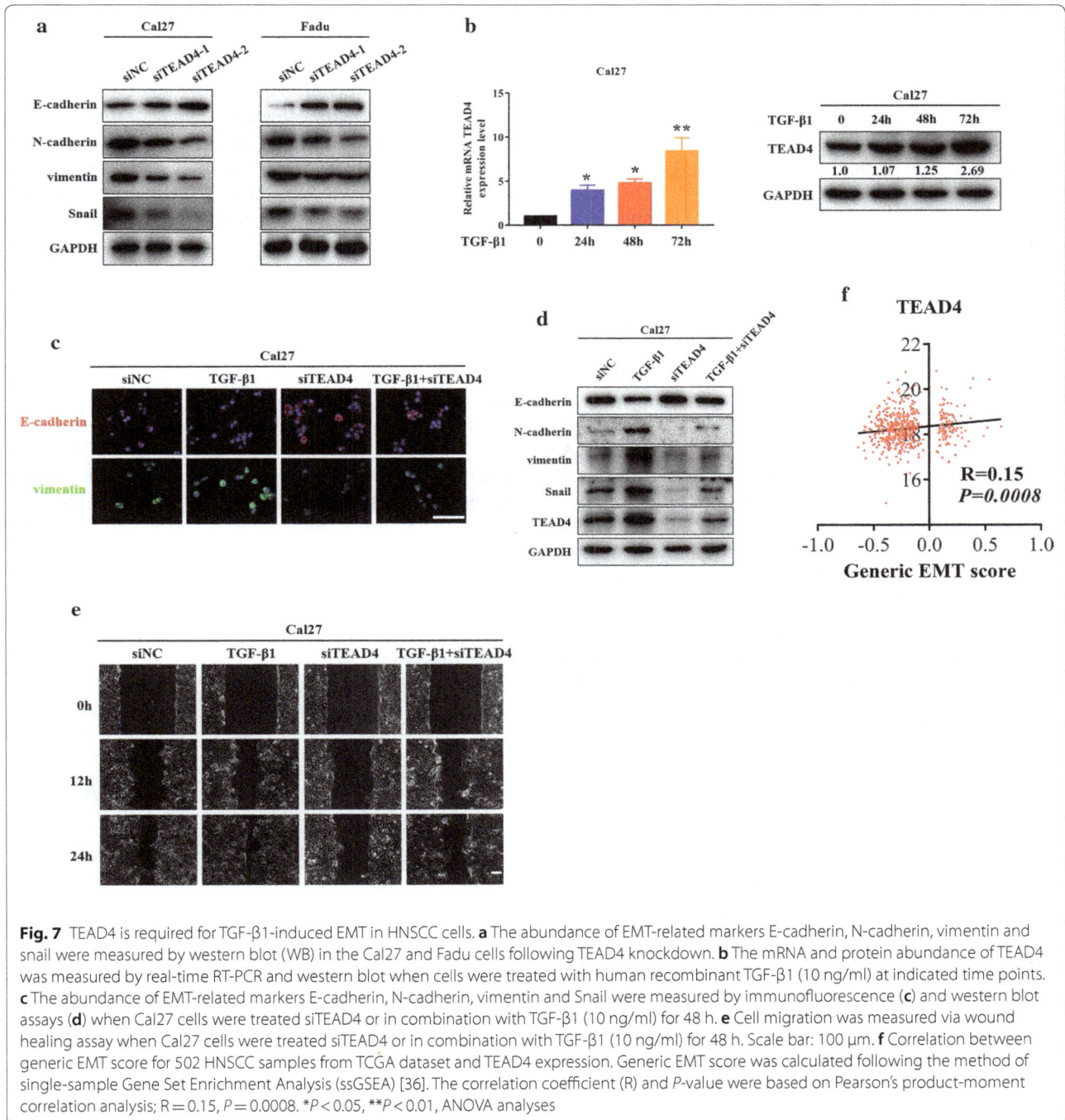

**Fig. 7** TEAD4 is required for TGF-β1-induced EMT in HNSCC cells. **a** The abundance of EMT-related markers E-cadherin, N-cadherin, vimentin and snail were measured by western blot (WB) in the Cal27 and Fadu cells following TEAD4 knockdown. **b** The mRNA and protein abundance of TEAD4 was measured by real-time RT-PCR and western blot when cells were treated with human recombinant TGF-β1 (10 ng/ml) at indicated time points. **c** The abundance of EMT-related markers E-cadherin, N-cadherin, vimentin and Snail were measured by immunofluorescence (**c**) and western blot assays (**d**) when Cal27 cells were treated siTEAD4 or in combination with TGF-β1 (10 ng/ml) for 48 h. **e** Cell migration was measured via wound healing assay when Cal27 cells were treated siTEAD4 or in combination with TGF-β1 (10 ng/ml) for 48 h. Scale bar: 100 μm. **f** Correlation between generic EMT score for 502 HNSCC samples from TCGA dataset and TEAD4 expression. Generic EMT score was calculated following the method of single-sample Gene Set Enrichment Analysis (ssGSEA) [36]. The correlation coefficient (R) and P-value were based on Pearson's product-moment correlation analysis; R = 0.15, P = 0.0008. *P < 0.05, **P < 0.01, ANOVA analyses

showed that TEAD4 expression increased along with disease initiation and progression from hyperplasia to invasive carcinoma. Although TEAD4 amplification was identified in selected cancers [33, 38], genetic amplification of TEAD4 was not prominent as evidenced by the fact that less than 2.5% HNSCC samples harbored genetic alternations of TEAD4, thus largely precluding

the possibility of genetic amplification of TEAD4 responsible for its overexpression in most HNSCC samples. Together, these findings gave strong support to the idea that TEAD4 as a bona fide oncogene promotes HNSCC tumorigenesis, although the precise molecular mechanisms underlying its overexpression await further elucidation. To the best of our knowledge, this might be the first study to reveal the abnormal overexpression pattern of TEAD4 in HNSCC.

Several previous reports have proposed important clinical relevance of TEAD4 overexpression in human cancer [14, 15, 39]. For example, elevated TEAD4 expression significantly associated with advanced stage, distant metastasis and poor outcome in colorectal cancer [14]. Consistantly, our data from primary HNSCC samples revealed that TEAD4 overexpression significantly associated with high pathological grade, cervical node metastasis and advanced clinical stage. Moreover, results from Kaplan–Meier survival and univariate/multivariate Cox-regression analyses showed that TEAD4 overexpression significantly associated with reduced survival and served as an independent prognostic predictor for patients' survival. However, we failed to reveal positive correlations between TEAD4 mRNA level and clinical grades, pathological stages as well as overall survival from TCGA-HNSCC dataset. We reasoned that it's conceivable due to prominent heterogeneity of HNSCC and different strategies for patient stratification between TCGA-HNSCC cohort and our cohort. Inconsistency between mRNA and protein expression of TEAD4 might also account for this discrepancy. Of course, larger amount of patients with HNSCC from multiple centers is needed to establish the prognostic significance of TEAD4 and its clinical benefits of TEAD4 as a novel biomarker for patient stratification.

Previous reports have demonstrated that TEAD4 is critically involved in tumorigenesis by promoting cell proliferation, metastasis, EMT and suppressing apoptosis [14, 15, 37, 40]. For example, impaired cell proliferation and induction of G1 cell cycle arrest were observed in OSCC cell upon TEAD4 knockdown [40]. TEAD4 silencing markedly attenuated cell migration and invasiveness in lung adenocarcinoma [41]. In addition, increased nuclear TEAD4 expression promoted EMT and metastasis in colorectal cancer while its knockdown induced mesenchymal-epithelial transition and decreased cell mobility in vitro and metastasis in vivo [14]. Consistent with these above-mentioned findings, our results indicate that TEAD4 has multiple tumorigenic roles by modulating cell proliferation, apoptosis, migration and invasion in HNSCC cells. Noticeably, our results also indicated that TEAD4 promoted invasion and motility by facilitating EMT in HNSCC as evidenced by morphological alternations and EMT marker changes upon TEAD4 depletion and overexpression, its critical role during TGF-β1-induced EMT as well as positive association between TEAD4 expression and cervical node metastasis. Multiple downstream targets including vimentin and FSCN1 have been identified to mediate EMT induced by TEAD4 in colorectal cancer and gastric cancer [14,

42]. Moreover, Liu et al. [43] have reported that TEAD4 and AP1 co-occupy on active enhancer or promoter and drive a core set of downstream targets like CDH2 (encoding N-cadherin) to coordinate cancer cell migration and invasion. However, the downstream targets responsible for TEAD4-induced EMT in HNSCC remains unknown and requires further exploration. In addition, further studies are still needed to unravel the intricate crosstalk between TEAD4 and TGF-β pathway behind EMT and metastasis in HNSCC. Collectively, our findings together with others strongly suggest that TEAD4 probably functions as a putative pro-tumorigenic gene via enhancing cancer cell proliferation, migration and invasion in HNSCC.

## Conclusion

In conclusion, our findings revealed the expression pattern, prognostic and tumorigenic roles of TEAD4 and identified TEAD4 as a novel biomarker with diagnostic and prognostic significance in HNSCC and as a putative oncogenic mediator underlying HNSCC initiation and progression. Our findings suggest that selective targeting of TEAD4 by genetic or chemical approach might hold translational promise against HNSCC.

## Additional file

**Additional file 1: Figure S1.** A: Relative expression of TEAD4 mRNA (Log2-transformed) was compared TCGA-HNSCC subgroups stratified by pathological grades. NS denotes not significant difference between groups. Y-axis represents the median intensity, 25th, and 75th percentile data. B: Relative expression of TEAD4 mRNA (Log2-transformed) was compared in TCGA-HNSCC subgroups stratified by clinical stage. Y-axis represents the median intensity, 25th, and 75th percentile data. C: Overall survival analyses of TCGA-HNSCC patients with high or low expression of TEAD4 mRNA (median value as cutoff) were estimated by Kaplan-Meier method and compared with Log-rank test.

### Abbreviations
HNSCC: head neck squamous cell carcinoma; TEADs: the TEAD transcription factor; 4NQO: 4-nitroquinoline 1-oxide-induced HNSCC animal model; EMT: epithelial-mesenchymal transition.

### Authors' contributions
WZ, JL and YW performed the experimental study, data collection and analysis and manuscript writing. WZ, HG and YS carried out the most experiments. DW, HY and HJ performed histological and statistical analyses. JC and YW conceived and supervised the whole project. All authors read and approved the final manuscript.

### Acknowledgements
Not applicable.

### Competing interests
The authors declare that they have no competing interests.

**Funding**

This work is financially supported, in whole or in part, by National Natural Science Foundation of China (81572669, 81602386, 81602378), Natural Science Foundation of Jiangsu Province (BK20151561, BK20161564, BK20161024), A Project Funded by the Priority Academic Program Development of Jiangsu Higher Education Institutions (2014-37), Natural Scientific Research Project for College in Jiangsu Province (16KJB320002), Cooperative Project of Southeast University and Nanjing Medical University (2242017K3DN20) and Project from Nanjing Municipal Committee of Science and Technology (201803044).

**References**

1. Siegel RL, Miller KD, Jemal A. Cancer statistics, 2017. CA Cancer J Clin. 2017;67(1):7–30.

2. Miller KD, Siegel RL, Lin CC, Mariotto AB, Kramer JL, Rowland JH, Stein KD, Alteri R, Jemal A. Cancer treatment and survivorship statistics, 2016. CA Cancer J Clin. 2016;66(4):271–89.

3. Rapidis AD, Gullane P, Langdon JD, Lefebvre JL, Scully C, Shah JP. Major advances in the knowledge and understanding of the epidemiology, aetiopathogenesis, diagnosis, management and prognosis of oral cancer. Oral Oncol. 2009;45(4–5):299–300.

4. Cancer Genome Atlas N. Comprehensive genomic characterization of head and neck squamous cell carcinomas. Nature. 2015;517(7536):576–82.

5. Moroishi T, Hansen CG, Guan KL. The emerging roles of YAP and TAZ in cancer. Nat Rev Cancer. 2015;15(2):73–9.

6. Harvey KF, Zhang X, Thomas DM. The Hippo pathway and human cancer. Nat Rev Cancer. 2013;13(4):246–57.

7. Li Z, Wang Y, Zhu Y, Yuan C, Wang D, Zhang W, Qi B, Qiu J, Song X, Ye J, et al. The Hippo transducer TAZ promotes epithelial to mesenchymal transition and cancer stem cell maintenance in oral cancer. Mol Oncol. 2015;9(6):1091–105.

8. Zhao B, Ye X, Yu J, Li L, Li W, Li S, Yu J, Lin JD, Wang CY, Chinnaiyan AM, et al. TEAD mediates YAP-dependent gene induction and growth control. Genes Dev. 2008;22(14):1962–71.

9. Lin KC, Park HW, Guan KL. Regulation of the Hippo pathway transcription factor TEAD. Trends Biochem Sci. 2017;42(11):862–72.

10. Yagi R, Kohn MJ, Karavanova I, Kaneko KJ, Vullhorst D, DePamphilis ML, Buonanno A. Transcription factor TEAD4 specifies the trophectoderm lineage at the beginning of mammalian development. Development. 2007;134(21):3827–36.

11. Pobbati AV, Hong W. Emerging roles of TEAD transcription factors and its coactivators in cancers. Cancer Biol Ther. 2013;14(5):390–8.

12. Home P, Saha B, Ray S, Dutta D, Gunewardena S, Yoo B, Pal A, Vivian JL, Larson M, Petroff M, et al. Altered subcellular localization of transcription factor TEAD4 regulates first mammalian cell lineage commitment. Proc Natl Acad Sci U S A. 2012;109(19):7362–7.

13. Knight JF, Shepherd CJ, Rizzo S, Brewer D, Jhavar S, Dodson AR, Cooper CS, Eeles R, Falconer A, Kovacs G, et al. TEAD1 and c-Cbl are novel prostate basal cell markers that correlate with poor clinical outcome in prostate cancer. Br J Cancer. 2008;99(11):1849–58.

14. Liu Y, Wang G, Yang Y, Mei Z, Liang Z, Cui A, Wu T, Liu CY, Cui L. Increased TEAD4 expression and nuclear localization in colorectal cancer promote epithelial-mesenchymal transition and metastasis in a YAP-independent manner. Oncogene. 2016;35(21):2789–800.

15. Zhou Y, Huang T, Zhang J, Wong CC, Zhang B, Dong Y, Wu F, Tong JHM, Wu WKK, Cheng ASL, et al. TEAD1/4 exerts oncogenic role and is negatively regulated by miR-4269 in gastric tumorigenesis. Oncogene. 2017;36(47):6518–30.

16. Hiemer SE, Zhang L, Kartha VK, Packer TS, Almershed M, Noonan V, Kukuruzinska M, Bais MV, Monti S, Varelas X. A YAP/TAZ-regulated molecular signature is associated with oral squamous cell carcinoma. Mol Cancer Res. 2015;13(6):957–68.

17. Zanconato F, Forcato M, Battilana G, Azzolin L, Quaranta E, Bodega B, Rosato A, Bicciato S, Cordenonsi M, Piccolo S. Genome-wide association between YAP/TAZ/TEAD and AP-1 at enhancers drives oncogenic growth. Nat Cell Biol. 2015;17(9):1218–27.

18. Wu Y, Diao P, Li Z, Zhang W, Wang D, Wang Y, Cheng J. Overexpression of WD repeat domain 5 associates with aggressive clinicopathological features and unfavorable prognosis in head neck squamous cell carcinoma. J Oral Pathol Med. 2018;47(5):502–10.

19. Li Z, Wang Y, Yuan C, Zhu Y, Qiu J, Zhang W, Qi B, Wu H, Ye J, Jiang H, et al. Oncogenic roles of Bmi1 and its therapeutic inhibition by histone deacetylase inhibitor in tongue cancer. Lab Invest. 2014;94(12):1431–45.

20. Li ZW, Wang YL, Qiu J, Li Q, Yuan CP, Zhang W, Wang DM, Ye JH, Jiang HB, Yang JR, et al. The polycomb group protein EZH2 is a novel therapeutic target in tongue cancer. Oncotarget. 2013;4(12):2532–49.

21. Chen D, Wu M, Li Y, Chang I, Yuan Q, Ekimyan-Salvo M, Deng P, Yu B, Yu Y, Dong J, et al. Targeting BMI1(+) cancer stem cells overcomes chemoresistance and inhibits metastases in squamous cell carcinoma. Cell Stem Cell. 2017;20(5):621–634 e626.

22. Li J, Liang F, Yu D, Qing H, Yang Y. Development of a 4-nitroquinoline-1-oxide model of lymph node metastasis in oral squamous cell carcinoma. Oral Oncol. 2013;49(4):299–305.

23. Wang Y, Zhu Y, Wang Q, Hu H, Li Z, Wang D, Zhang W, Qi B, Ye J, Wu H, et al. The histone demethylase LSD1 is a novel oncogene and therapeutic target in oral cancer. Cancer Lett. 2016;374(1):12–21.

24. Liu LK, Jiang XY, Zhou XX, Wang DM, Song XL, Jiang HB. Upregulation of vimentin and aberrant expression of E-cadherin/beta-catenin complex in oral squamous cell carcinomas: correlation with the clinicopathological features and patient outcome. Mod Pathol. 2010;23(2):213–24.

25. Cerami E, Gao J, Dogrusoz U, Gross BE, Sumer SO, Aksoy BA, Jacobsen A, Byrne CJ, Heuer ML, Larsson E, et al. The cBio cancer genomics portal: an open platform for exploring multidimensional cancer genomics data. Cancer Discov. 2012;2(5):401–4.

26. Rhodes DR, Kalyana-Sundaram S, Mahavisno V, Varambally R, Yu J, Briggs BB, Barrette TR, Anstet MJ, Kincead-Beal C, Kulkarni P, et al. Oncomine 3.0: genes, pathways, and networks in a collection of 18,000 cancer gene expression profiles. Neoplasia. 2007;9(2):166–80.

27. Yuan H, Liu H, Liu Z, Zhu D, Amos CI, Fang S, Lee JE, Wei Q. Genetic variants in Hippo pathway genes YAP1, TEAD1 and TEAD4 are associated with melanoma-specific survival. Int J Cancer. 2015;137(3):638–45.

28. Wei Z, Wang Y, Li Z, Yuan C, Zhang W, Wang D, Ye J, Jiang H, Wu Y, Cheng J. Overexpression of Hippo pathway effector TAZ in tongue squamous cell carcinoma: correlation with clinicopathological features and patients' prognosis. J Oral Pathol Med. 2013;42(10):747–54.

29. Peng CH, Liao CT, Peng SC, Chen YJ, Cheng AJ, Juang JL, Tsai CY, Chen TC, Chuang YJ, Tang CY, et al. A novel molecular signature identified by systems genetics approach predicts prognosis in oral squamous cell carcinoma. PLoS ONE. 2011;6(8):e23452.

30. Ginos MA, Page GP, Michalowicz BS, Patel KJ, Volker SE, Pambuccian SE, Ondrey FG, Adams GL, Gaffney PM. Identification of a gene expression signature associated with recurrent disease in squamous cell carcinoma of the head and neck. Cancer Res. 2004;64(1):55–63.

31. Cromer A, Carles A, Millon R, Ganguli G, Chalmel F, Lemaire F, Young J, Dembele D, Thibault C, Muller D, et al. Identification of genes associated with tumorigenesis and metastatic potential of hypopharyngeal cancer by microarray analysis. Oncogene. 2004;23(14):2484–98.

32. Ye H, Yu T, Temam S, Ziober BL, Wang J, Schwartz JL, Mao L, Wong DT, Zhou X. Transcriptomic dissection of tongue squamous cell carcinoma. BMC Genomics. 2008;9:69.

33. Suzuki M, Kondo A, Ogino I, Arai H, Tomita T, Sredni ST. Overexpression of TEAD4 in atypical teratoid/rhabdoid tumor: new insight to the pathophysiology of an aggressive brain tumor. Pediatr Blood Cancer. 2017;64(7):e26398.

34. Valastyan S, Weinberg RA. Tumor metastasis: molecular insights and evolving paradigms. Cell. 2011;147(2):275–92.

35. Zavadil J, Bottinger EP. TGF-beta and epithelial-to-mesenchymal transitions. Oncogene. 2005;24(37):5764–74.

36. Tan TZ, Miow QH, Miki Y, Noda T, Mori S, Huang RY, Thiery JP. Epithelial-mesenchymal transition spectrum quantification and its efficacy in deciphering survival and drug responses of cancer patients. EMBO Mol Med. 2014;6(10):1279–93.

37. Zhang Q, Fan H, Zou Q, Liu H, Wan B, Zhu S, Hu Y, Li H, Zhang C, Zhou L, et al. TEAD4 exerts pro-metastatic effects and is negatively regulated by

miR6839-3p in lung adenocarcinoma progression. J Cell Mol Med. 2018. https://doi.org/10.1111/jcmm.13634.

38.  Nowee ME, Snijders AM, Rockx DA, de Wit RM, Kosma VM, Hamalainen K, Schouten JP, Verheijen RH, van Diest PJ, Albertson DG, et al. DNA profiling of primary serous ovarian and fallopian tube carcinomas with array comparative genomic hybridization and multiplex ligation-dependent probe amplification. J Pathol. 2007;213(1):46–55.

39.  Tang JY, Yu CY, Bao YJ, Chen L, Chen J, Yang SL, Chen HY, Hong J, Fang JY. TEAD4 promotes colorectal tumorigenesis via transcriptionally targeting YAP1. Cell Cycle. 2018;17(1):102–9.

40.  Takeuchi S, Kasamatsu A, Yamatoji M, Nakashima D, Endo-Sakamoto Y, Koide N, Takahara T, Shimizu T, Iyoda M, Ogawara K, et al. TEAD4-YAP interaction regulates tumoral growth by controlling cell-cycle arrest at the G1 phase. Biochem Biophys Res Commun. 2017;486(2):385–90.

41.  Zhang Q, Fan H, Zou Q, Liu H, Wan B, Zhu S, Hu Y, Li H, Zhang C, Zhou L, et al. TEAD4 exerts pro-metastatic effects and is negatively regulated by miR6839-3p in lung adenocarcinoma progression. J Cell Mol Med. 2018;22(7):3560–71.

42.  Lim B, Park JL, Kim HJ, Park YK, Kim JH, Sohn HA, Noh SM, Song KS, Kim WH, Kim YS, et al. Integrative genomics analysis reveals the multilevel dysregulation and oncogenic characteristics of TEAD4 in gastric cancer. Carcinogenesis. 2014;35(5):1020–7.

43.  Liu X, Li H, Rajurkar M, Li Q, Cotton JL, Ou J, Zhu LJ, Goel HL, Mercurio AM, Park JS, et al. Tead and AP1 coordinate transcription and motility. Cell Rep. 2016;14(5):1169–80.

# 8

# M3 muscarinic acetylcholine receptors regulate epithelial–mesenchymal transition, perineural invasion, and migration/metastasis in cholangiocarcinoma through the AKT pathway

Yujie Feng[1*], Xiao Hu[1], Guangwei Liu[2], Lianfang Lu[1], Wei Zhao[1], Fangzhen Shen[3], Kai Ma[1], Chuandong Sun[1], Chengzhan Zhu[1] and Bingyuan Zhang[1*]

## Abstract

**Background:** Cholangiocarcinoma is a highly malignant tumor type that is not sensitive to radiotherapy or chemotherapy due to aggressive perineural invasion and metastasis. Unfortunately, the mechanisms underlying these processes and the signaling factors involved are largely unknown. In this study, we analyzed the role of M3 muscarinic acetylcholine receptors (M3-mAChR) in cell migration, perineural invasion, and metastasis during cholangiocarcinoma.

**Methods:** We assessed 60 human cholangiocarcinoma tissue samples and 30 normal biliary tissues. Immunohistochemical staining was used to detect M3-mAChR expression and the relationship between expression and clinical prognosis was evaluated. The biological functions of M3-mAChR in cholangiocarcinoma cell migration, perineural invasion, and epithelial–mesenchymal transition (EMT) were investigated using the human cholangiocarcinoma cell lines FRH0201 and RBE in conjunction with various techniques, including agonist/antagonist treatment, RNA interference, M3-mAChR overexpression, dorsal root ganglion co-culturing, immunohistochemistry, western blotting, etc.

**Results:** M3-mAChR were highly expressed in cholangiocarcinoma tissue and expression was closely related to differentiation and lymphatic metastasis, affecting patient survival. Treatment with the M3-mAChR agonist pilocarpine and M3-mAChR overexpression significantly promoted migration and perineural invasion, while the M3-mAChR antagonist atropine blocked these effects. Similarly, M3-mAChR knock-down also weakened cell migration and perineural invasion. The expression of phosphatase and tensin homolog, AKT, E-cadherin, vimentin, and Snail, which are components of the phosphatidylinositol 3-kinase/AKT signaling pathway and EMT, were altered by pilocarpine, and these effects were again blocked by atropine. Notably, AKT knock-down decreased M3-mAChR expression and reversed the downstream effects of this receptor.

**Conclusions:** M3-mAChR are involved in tumor cell migration, perineural invasion, and EMT during cholangiocarcinoma, and these effects are modulated via the AKT signaling pathway.

**Keywords:** Cholangiocarcinoma, M3 muscarinic acetylcholine receptors, Perineural invasion, Epithelial–mesenchymal transition, AKT

*Correspondence: fengyj1943@163.com; bingyuanzhang@126.com
[1] Department of Hepatobiliary and Pancreatic Surgery, The Affiliated Hospital of Qingdao University, No. 16 Jiangsu Road, Qingdao 266003, Shandong, China
Full list of author information is available at the end of the article

## Background

Cholangiocarcinoma, which originates from biliary epithelial cells, is a type of malignant tumor that is characterized by low diagnostic rates and high fatality rates [1]. Concealed pathogenesis, lack of early diagnostic markers, and low sensitivity to conventional radiotherapy and chemotherapy treatments are the crucial reasons underlying the poor prognosis of cholangiocarcinoma patients. Currently, surgical resection is the only effective treatment method for this disease. Moreover, recent studies have found that perineural invasion is a common biological characteristic of cholangiocarcinoma and is closely related to postoperative recurrence rates and prognoses [2].

Cholangiocarcinoma undergoes perineural invasion early in development and involves tumor cells surrounding the nerve fibers, entering the perineurium, and spreading via local infiltration and metastasis. Recent studies have shown that the biliary system is rich in autonomic nerves, and biliary tract malignancy occurs near the celiac plexus; thus, tumor cells are more likely to invade the surrounding nerve plexus, causing perineural invasion [3]. Another study reconstructed the perineural invasion and metastasis processes that occur during cholangiocarcinoma by computer-assisted three-dimensional (3D) analysis and formed 3D images of cholangiocarcinoma to display existing small vessels, lymph vessels, and nerve fibers around the tumor [4]. They concluded that tumor cells survive independently in spaces around the nerves, including in the small vessels and small lymph vessels. Accordingly, perineural invasion was found to be the fifth self-existent route of metastasis following direct invasion and metastasis, implantation metastasis, lymphatic metastasis, and blood metastasis of abdominal tumors. Metastasis occurs in the nerve fibers via jumping, meaning that cholangiocarcinoma can either invade and metastasize to the liver through the perineural space or metastasize to the retroperitoneal ganglions. This is also why cholangiocarcinoma is difficult to cure.

As an important digestive organ, the biliary system regulates biliary secretion and excretion and is surrounded by vagus nerves, which can interact with the liver vascular system and inevitably affect the pathophysiology of the biliary epithelium [5]. However, while these systems interact and affect the health and function of each other, for the cancer cells to spread from the primary site, they must develop migratory and invasive properties. Epithelial-to-mesenchymal transition (EMT) is a phenomenon in which epithelial cells lose their original polarity and transform into Leydig cells. EMT is comprised of a series of intricate biological and biochemical changes that cause the cell to lose its differentiated epithelial-like state and gain a more mesenchymal-like phenotype. Moreover,

the EMT is closely related to tumorigenesis, local invasion, distant metastasis, and tumor resistance [6–9] and appears to play a distinct role in cholangiocarcinoma [10]. The various processes involved in cholangiocarcinoma, including perineural invasion, metastasis, and EMT, likely require complex signaling pathway function as well as a host of independent factors, many of which have not been elucidated.

Muscarinic acetylcholine receptors (mAChRs) are members of the G protein-coupled receptor family and include five receptor subtypes (M1, M2, M3, M4, and M5) [11]. The M3-mAChR are mainly distributed in the digestive tract glands and vascular smooth muscles and modulate glandular secretion and smooth muscle relaxation. Various studies have also shown that M3-mAChR play an important role in the proliferation and invasion of cancer cells [12–14]. However, the role of M3-mAChR in cholangiocarcinoma has not been evaluated.

In this study, we investigated the function of M3-mAChR during perineural invasion, metastasis, and EMT in cholangiocarcinoma. To our knowledge, this is the first time M3-mAChR-mediated regulation has been explored in cholangiocarcinoma.

## Methods

### Patients and tissue specimens

We collected paraffin-embedded biliary pathology tissues obtained during surgical resection at the Affiliated Hospital of Qingdao University from December 2008 to December 2013. The samples included 60 cholangiocarcinoma tissues and 30 normal biliary tissues (from patients with choledochocysts and liver transplantation). Patient data was also collected. None of the patients had undergone radiotherapy or chemotherapy/drugs treatment before the operation. All procedures in this study that involved human participants were performed in accordance with the 1964 Helsinki declaration and its later amendments. The protocol was approved by the Ethics Committee of The Affiliated Hospital of Qingdao University. Informed consent was obtained from all individual participants included in the study.

### Immunohistochemistry

The paraffin-embedded biopsy tissue specimens were cut into 4-μm-thick sections and deparaffinized. The sections were pretreated and incubated with primary anti-M3 mAChR antibodies (1:1000; Abcam, Cambridge, UK) overnight at 4 °C according to the manufacturer's instructions. Then, the sections were incubated with secondary antibodies for 30 min, stained with diaminobenzidine, and finally, counterstained with hematoxylin. The stained sections were then imaged (400×; OLYMPUS, Tokyo,

Japan). Positive staining in the basement membrane was manifested as a brownish-yellow color.

For statistical analysis, 10 random fields of the tumor were selected in each section, and 100 cells from each field were counted. The samples were then graded according to the proportion of positive cells to the total number of cells. When the percentage of positively stained cholangiocarcinoma cells was less than 25%, the result was considered negative. Alternatively, when the percentage was between 25 and 55% or more than 55%, the staining was described as positive and strongly positive, respectively.

### Cell lines, culture conditions and reagents

The cholangiocarcinoma cell lines FRH0201 and RBE were purchased from the Shanghai Cell Bank of the Chinese Academy of Sciences. The cell lines were all authenticated. The cells were grown and cultivated in RPMI-1640 medium supplemented with 10% newborn calf serum (Thermo Scientific Hyclone, USA) in an incubator containing 5% $CO_2$ at 37 °C. M3-mAChR agonist pilocarpine and M3-mAChR antagonist atropine were purchased from Sigma-Aldrich (Taufkirchen, Germany).

### Constructing the lentivirus vector for RNAi and receptor overexpression

The most effective M3-targeting small hairpin RNA (shRNA) sequences (5′-GCAGTGACAGTTGGAACA ACA-3′) were transfected into the cultured cells using Lipofectamine 2000 Reagent (Invitrogen, Carlsbad, CA, USA). M3-NC (5′-TTCTCCGAACGTGTCACGT-3′) was used to generate the negative (scrambled) control lentiviral vectors. Lentivirus was added to the cells according to the manufacturer's recommended protocol.

The high-copy plasmid pcDNA 3 1(+) (Invitrogen, Carlsbad, CA, USA) harbouring the complete cDNA of the human mAchR3 was performed according to the manufacturer's protocol using a commercially available kit (Qiagen, Hilden, Germany).

### RNAi treatment

FRH0201-M3 cells were transfected with siAKT (5′-TTGTACGCAGAGAGAATAACT-3′), using the Lipofectamine transfection reagent (Invitrogen) for 48 h. Retrovirus packaging and transfection were conducted according to the manufacturer's instructions.

### Quantitative real-time polymerase chain reaction (qRT-PCR)

Total RNA was extracted from cultured cells using TRIzol reagent in a one-step method according to the manufacturer's instructions. Primer design was performed using Primer5 software with sequences for human M3-mAChR obtained from GenBank. The following primers were used in this study:M3-mAChR (forward, 5′-CACAATAACAGTACAACCTCGCC-3′ and reverse, 5′-GCCAGGATGCCCGTTAAGAAA-3′). internal control GAPDH (forward, 5′-GCACCGTCA AGGCTGAGAAC-3′ and reverse, 5′-TGGTGAAGA CGCCAGTGGAT-3′. M3-mAChR gene expression was quantitated using the $2^{-\Delta\Delta Ct}$ method. The data are presented as the fold change compared to the specified controls using an average result of three independent experiments. Differences were considered biologically relevant when the fold change was > 2.0 or < 0.5 [15].

### Western blot analysis

Whole cell lysates were prepared using RIPA lysis buffer and protease inhibitor (keyGEN, Nanjing, China), and the protein concentrations were determined using a BCA kit (Thermo Scientific™). A total of 50 µg of protein was loaded into each well of a sodium dodecyl sulfate polyacrylamide gel electrophoresis (SDS-PAGE) gel, and the proteins were separated. After the proteins were transferred to a polyvinylidene difluoride membrane, the membranes were blocked with 5% nonfat dried milk for 2 h. Next, the membranes were incubated overnight with primary antibodies targeting M3-mAChR, phosphatase and tensin homolog (PTEN), AKT, E-cadherin, vimentin, and Snail (all purchased from Santa Cruz Biotechnology, Santa Cruz, CA, USA) at 4 °C. The membranes were then incubated with secondary antibodies for 2 h at room temperature. Finally, the protein bands were visualized using enhanced chemiluminescence, and their intensity was quantified.

### Migration assay

For the transwell migration assays, $10^5$ cells were seeded in 100 µL of serum-free Dulbecco's modified Eagle's medium in fibronectin-coated polycarbonate membrane inserts in a transwell apparatus. The diameter of the membrane micropores was 8 µm. A total of 600 µL of RPMI-1640 culture medium with 10% serum was added to the lower wells. After culturing cells for 36 h at 37 °C, the transwell chambers were removed and washed with phosphate-buffered saline three times. Cells that had not invaded were removed using aseptic cotton buds, and the chambers were then fixed in 4% formalin solution for 20 min. Next, cells on the chambers were stained with 0.1% crystal violet for 15 min and then imaged under an optical microscope. Cells in 10 fields were counted (400× magnification). The experiment was performed in triplicate.

### Dorsal root ganglion isolation and ex vivo culture

As described in a previous study [16], newborn Kunming mice (24 h old) were disinfected using 75% ethyl alcohol, sacrificed by cervical dislocation, and fixed in the prone position. The mediodorsal skin was cut using sterile eye scissors to expose the muscles of the back. Taper eye scissors were then used to cut an opening and expose the spinal cord, which was excised and washed with normal saline several times, until the dorsal root ganglion (DRG) could be observed. Next, the DRG was carefully removed using smooth microforceps and washed once in normal saline. The washed DRG was then transferred into a 24-well plate, and thawed Matrigel (BD Biosciences, Franklin Lake, NJ, USA) was added to completely cover it. The Matrigel-coated DRG was then incubated at 37 °C for 30 min until coagulation. Notably, all of these procedures involving the care and use of laboratory animals were performed in accordance with the principles and standards set forth in the Principles for Use of Animals (National Guide for Grants and Contracts).

### DRG immunohistochemical staining

#### Nissl staining to observe the state of nerve cell viability

Remove the neurons from which the culture solution was discarded, and wash it with 0.01 mol/L PBS three times for 5 min each time. Then 4% paraformaldehyde was fixed at room temperature for 1 h, and washed with 0.01 mol/L PBS for 3 times for 5 min each time followed by 0.1% toluidine blue dyeing at 37 °C for 10 min. After the final 95% ethanol separation, the cells were dehydrated in 50%–100% gradient ethanol for 3–5 min each time. The xylene was transparent and the gel was sealed, and then the neuron viability was observed under a microscope.

#### Neurofilament protein (NF) immunocytochemical staining of DRG

Co-infiltrate and purify the cultured DRG, discard the culture solution and wash it with 0.0 l mol/L PBS for 3 times for 5 min each time; 4% paraformaldehyde was fixed at room temperature for 1 h, washed with PBS; 0.3% $H_2O_2$ methanol was added., placed for 10 min to remove endogenous catalase, washed with PBS and moved to a wet box. Add 10% sheep serum to the coverslip, add 3 drops per well, and incubate in a 37 °C oven for 30 min; after aspirating the blocking solution, l:200 rabbit anti-mouse NF antibody (Beyotime, Shanghai, China) 3 drops per tablet, at 4 °C refrigerator save. Immediately after the PBS cleaning, add goat anti-rabbit IgG (1:200 biotinylated, Beyotime, Shanghai, China) on the coverslip, 3 drops per well, incubate in a 37 °C oven, and wash with PBS after 30 min. Add the ready-to-use ABC solution onto the coverslip and incubate in a 37 °C oven for 30 min; wash with PBS, add DAB coloring solution for

8–10 min, then rinse again with PBS. Finally, dehydrated in 50% concentration gradient ethanol, about 5 min each time, xylene was transparent and the gel was sealed, and then the axon extension of each group was observed under a microscope.

### Co-culturing of DRG segments and RBE cells

For co-culturing, untreated RBE cells in the logarithmic growth phase were added to each well of the 24-well plate containing a Matrigel-coated DRG at a concentration of $2.5 \times 10^4$ cells/well in 500 μL of medium (RPMI-1640 containing serum). The DRGs were treated as follows: MOCK (medium + RBE cells), ShM3 (medium + ShM3-treated RBE cells), PILO [medium + RBE cells + pilocarpine (1.0 mM)]; ATR [medium + RBE cells + atropine (0.1 mM)], and PILO + ATR [medium + RBE cells + pilocarpine (1.0 mM) + atropine (0.1 mM)]. Cell adhesion to the DRG nerve fibers was observed using an inverted microscope every 4 h. After 72 h, the number of cholangiocarcinoma cells adhering to nerve fibers was quantified.

### General matrix metalloproteinase (MMP) activity assay

The general activity of MMP enzymes was determined using an assay kit (ab112146, Abcam, Cambridge, MA, USA) according to the manufacturer's protocol. In brief, experimental cells were seeded into triplicate wells of 6-well plates and allowed to attach overnight, then starved with serum free media for another 18 h. A kinetic measurement was then performed for the MMP activity by taking medium samples at 5 min intervals over a 1 h period after starting the reaction by using a microplate reader with a filter set of Ex/Em = 490/525 nm.

### Statistical analysis

Statistical analyses were performed using SPSS 17.0 software. Each value in the present study was obtained from at least three independent experiments. Data are presented as the mean ± standard error of the mean (SEM). Survival analyses and cumulative recurrence rates were assessed using the Kaplan–Meier method and the log-rank test. The difference between two groups was evaluated with the Student's $t$-test and was considered statistically significant when $P < 0.05$.

## Results

### Clinicopathological features and patient demographics

All of the cases of cholangiocarcinoma (n = 60; 43 men, 17 women; median age, 56 years; range, 30–82 years) were diagnosed as adenocarcinoma. Of these, 46 cases (76.67%) had lymphatic metastasis, while 14 (23.33%) did not. A total of 18 cases (30%) of high differentiation and 42 cases (70%) of moderate or low differentiation were observed. Furthermore, after classification the tumors according to the Union International Control Cancer TNM staging system [17], 16 cases (26.67%) were found to be stage I-II, while 44 cases (73.33%) were stage III-IV. Finally, we found that 53 cases (88.33%) of them had perineural invasion and the remaining 7 cases (11.67%) without perineural invasion.

### M3-mAChR is highly expressed in cholangiocarcinoma and plays an important role in metastasis and prognosis in cholangiocarcinoma patients

Using immunohistochemistry, we observed M3-mAChR to be highly expressed in histopathological sections from cholangiocarcinoma tissues, but was found at lower levels in normal biliary tissues, with positive rates of 90% (54/60) and 3.33% (1/30), respectively ($P < 0.01$; Fig. 1a, b). In the positive tissues, M3-mAChR expression was mainly distributed in granules or sheets located in the cytoplasm near the cell membrane. In addition, perineural invasion was observed in the cholangiocarcinoma tissues at a positive rate of 91.7% (55/60; Fig. 1c, d).

Notably, M3-mAChR expression appears to be significantly correlated with the level of differentiation ($P < 0.05$), with the positive rate of M3-mAChR expression

in III–IV staged tumors being higher than that in I–II staged tumors ($P < 0.01$). Similarly, expression was also correlated with lymphatic metastasis ($P < 0.05$), being higher in histopathological sections of cholangiocarcinoma with lymph node metastasis ($P < 0.01$). We also found that M3-mAChR expression is significantly associated with perineural invasion ($P < 0.01$; Table 1). The survival time of cholangiocarcinoma patients with high M3-mAChR expression was also distinctly shorter than that of patients with low M3-mAChR expression. Moreover, the survival time of cholangiocarcinoma patients was shorter when perineural invasion had occurred than in patients without perineural invasion (Fig. 1e, f). There were no connections between M3-mAChR expression and patient age, sex, tumor location ($P > 0.05$). Collectively, these results show that M3-mAChR plays an important role in the invasion and metastasis of cholangiocarcinoma and affects treatment and prognosis.

### M3-mAChR mediate migration in cultured cholangiocarcinoma cells

Preliminary studies showed that both FRH0201 and RBE cells express M3-mAChR, although expression was higher in RBE cells than in FRH0201 cells (Fig. 2a,

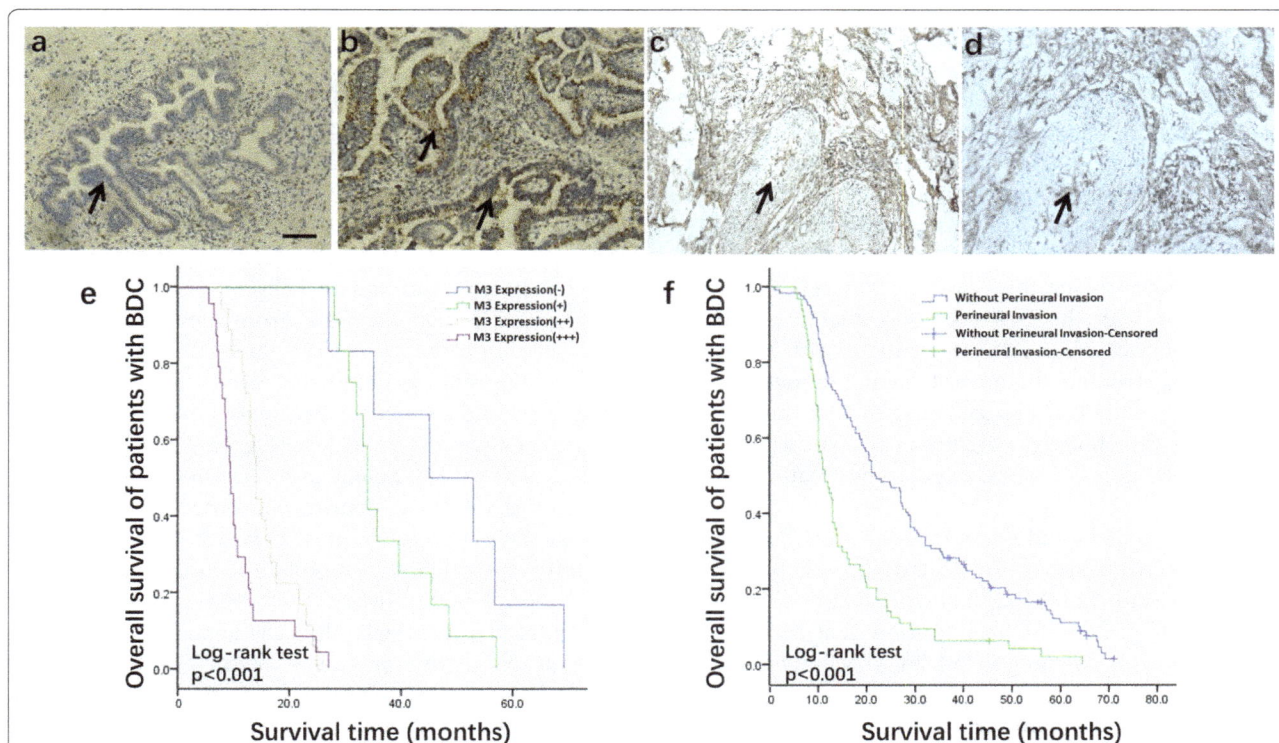

**Fig. 1** **a** Normal biliary duct gland tissues had regular shapes (arrow; ×200). **b** Gland tissues of in the cholangiocarcinoma patients were enlarged and disordered (arrow; ×200). **c** and **d** Intermediate cholangiocarcinoma invasion of nerve fibers (arrows; **c**: ×200 and **d**: ×400). **e** Cholangiocarcinoma patient survival is related to M3-mAChR expression. **f** Survival times of patients with cholangiocarcinoma with or without perineural invasion. Scale bars, 200 μm

**Table 1  Clinicopathological features of patients with cholangiocarcinoma and correlations with M3 expression**

| Factor | n | M3 expression | | | | | P value |
|---|---|---|---|---|---|---|---|
| | | (−) | (+) | (++) | (+++) | Positive rate (%) | |
| Sex | | | | | | | |
| Male | 43 | 5 | 6 | 14 | 18 | 88.89 | 0.500 |
| Female | 17 | 1 | 6 | 4 | 6 | 93.33 | |
| Age | | | | | | | |
| <59 | 23 | 2 | 5 | 7 | 9 | 91.30 | 0.962 |
| ≥59 | 37 | 4 | 7 | 11 | 15 | 89.19 | |
| Differentiation of tumors | | | | | | | |
| High | 18 | 3 | 4 | 5 | 6 | 83.33 | 0.308 |
| Middle and poorly | 42 | 3 | 8 | 13 | 18 | 92.86 | |
| Lymph node metastasis | | | | | | | |
| Yes | 46 | 1 | 8 | 15 | 22 | 97.83 | 0.001 |
| No | 14 | 5 | 4 | 3 | 2 | 64.29 | |
| TNM stage | | | | | | | |
| I–II | 16 | 5 | 5 | 3 | 3 | 68.75 | 0.002 |
| III–IV | 44 | 1 | 7 | 15 | 21 | 97.73 | |
| Tumor location | | | | | | | |
| Hilar | 19 | 2 | 3 | 6 | 6 | 88.23 | 0.756 |
| Middle and distal | 41 | 4 | 9 | 12 | 18 | 90.70 | |
| Perineural invasion | | | | | | | |
| Yes | 53 | 3 | 10 | 16 | 24 | 94.34 | 0.007 |
| No | 7 | 3 | 2 | 2 | 0 | 57.14 | |

Correlations were estimated by Fisher's exact test. Significant when p < 0.05

b). Notably, in RBE and FRH0201 cells treated with the M3-mAChR agonist pilocarpine, we observed an increase in the quantity of migrating cells compared with that of the untreated control group (Fig. 2c, d), suggesting that the M3-mAChR agonist significantly promoted the invasive characteristics of the cholangiocarcinoma cells. Moreover, while there was no difference between cells treated with the M3-mAChR antagonist atropine and control cells, when cells were treated with both pilocarpine and atropine, the quantity of migrating cells was reduced (Fig. 2b, c). These data suggest that the invasive capacity of the cholangiocarcinoma cells was decreased owing to antagonism of the pilocarpine-treated cells by atropine.

To further understand the role of M3-mAChR in cholangiocarcinoma cells, we transfected RBE cells with lentiviral vectors carrying shM3 to downregulate M3-mAChR expression (Fig. 3a). Our results show that M3-mAChR expression was downregulated in shM3-treated RBE cells, and the number of migrating cells was reduced. Furthermore, treatment with pilocarpine increased the invasive capacity of the shM3-treated RBE cells (Fig. 3b). In contrast, in FRH0201 cells, M3-mAChR expression was increased by transfecting the cells with an M3-mAChR plasmid, and this overexpression mediated an increase

in cholangiocarcinoma cell invasion (Fig. 3b). Moreover, downregulation of M3-mAChR expression largely blocked invasion.

### Perineural invasion is regulated by M3-mAChR

To investigate the role of M3-mAChR in perineural invasion of cholangiocarcinoma cells, we used an ex vivo DRG model. When the DRG from newborn Kunming mice were cultured alone (Fig. 4a-1–3), the Nissl bodies became granular after being dyed, showing obvious staining around the perinuclear region, but little staining around the edges of the nucleus (Fig. 4a–7). After Gomori staining and neurofilament protein immunohistochemical staining (NF IHC), neuritis was observed growing up from the DRG periphery, most of which showed branching and were generally present in a radial arrangement (Fig. 4a-6). Notably, when the DRG was co-cultured with untreated RBE cells, the cells appear to invade the DRG and the surrounding nerve fibers (Fig. 4b). Furthermore, when pilocarpine was added to the co-cultures, the quantity of RBE cells invading the DRG and surrounding nerve fibers was increased, suggesting that pilocarpine promotes perineural invasion during cholangiocarcinoma. The effects of pilocarpine were decreased by co-treatment with atropine, which decreased the number of

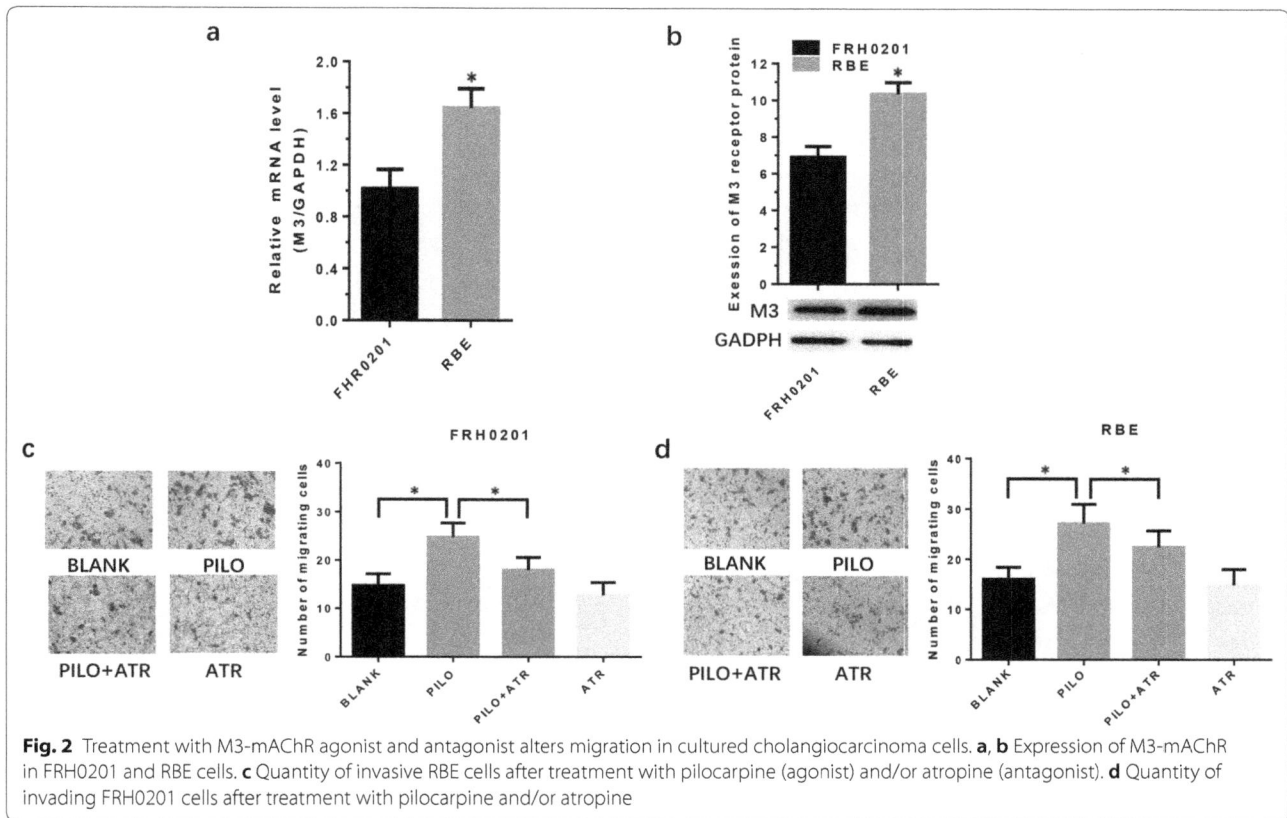

**Fig. 2** Treatment with M3-mAChR agonist and antagonist alters migration in cultured cholangiocarcinoma cells. **a**, **b** Expression of M3-mAChR in FRH0201 and RBE cells. **c** Quantity of invasive RBE cells after treatment with pilocarpine (agonist) and/or atropine (antagonist). **d** Quantity of invading FRH0201 cells after treatment with pilocarpine and/or atropine

RBE cells invading the DRG (Fig. 4b). Notably, atropine alone did not significantly affect the level of perineural invasion compared with that in the control group, which is consistent with our earlier cell culture data.

Furthermore, when the DRG were co-cultured with shM3-treated RBE cells, we found that although the shM3-treated RBE cells still invade the DRG, the quantity of invading cells was reduced compared with that in the untreated RBE group. Treating these DRG-shM3-RBE co-cultured cells with pilocarpine, the number of invading cells was increased (Fig. 4c). Conversely, when FRH0201 cells overexpressing M3-mAChR were co-cultured with DRG, the number of cells invading the DRG increased compared with that in the untreated FRH0201 group. Treatment these DRG-M3-FRH0201 co-cultured cells with pilocarpine, the number of invading cells was further increased (Fig. 4c). These results show that M3-mAChR expression in cholangiocarcinoma cells regulate perineural invasion.

### M3-mAChR participate in AKT-mediated EMT in cholangiocarcinoma

Through this experiment we found that pilocarpine can induce the increase of M3-mAChR protein levels in cholangiocarcinoma, and atropine blocked these changes. So

we believe that pilocarpine interacts with M3-mAChR and acts through M3-mAChR.

As EMT plays a key role in cholangiocarcinoma metastasis, we examined the effects of M3-mAChR agonist and antagonist treatment on the expression of EMT factors related to the PI3K/AKT pathway in RBE cells. Our results showed that pilocarpine treatment decreases the expression of PTEN and the epithelial cell marker E-cadherin, but increases the expression AKT and the Leydig cell marker vimentin. The expression of Snail, which induces EMT, was also increased. Notably, atropine blocked these changes (Fig. 5a, b). Similarly, shM3-mediated disruption of receptor expression in the RBE cells also resulted in increased expression of PTEN and E-cadherin and decreased expression of AKT, vimentin, and Snail. In contrast, upregulation of M3-mAChR in FRH0201 cells decreased PTEN and E-cadherin expression and increased AKT, vimentin, and Snail expression (Fig. 5c, d).

To better understand the role of M3-mAChR in AKT-mediated EMT, we knocked down AKT expression in FRH0201 cells overexpressing M3-mAChR. This disruption resulted in the downregulation of M3-mAChR, Snail, and vimentin expression, whereas the expression of PTEN and E-cadherin was upregulated (Fig. 6).

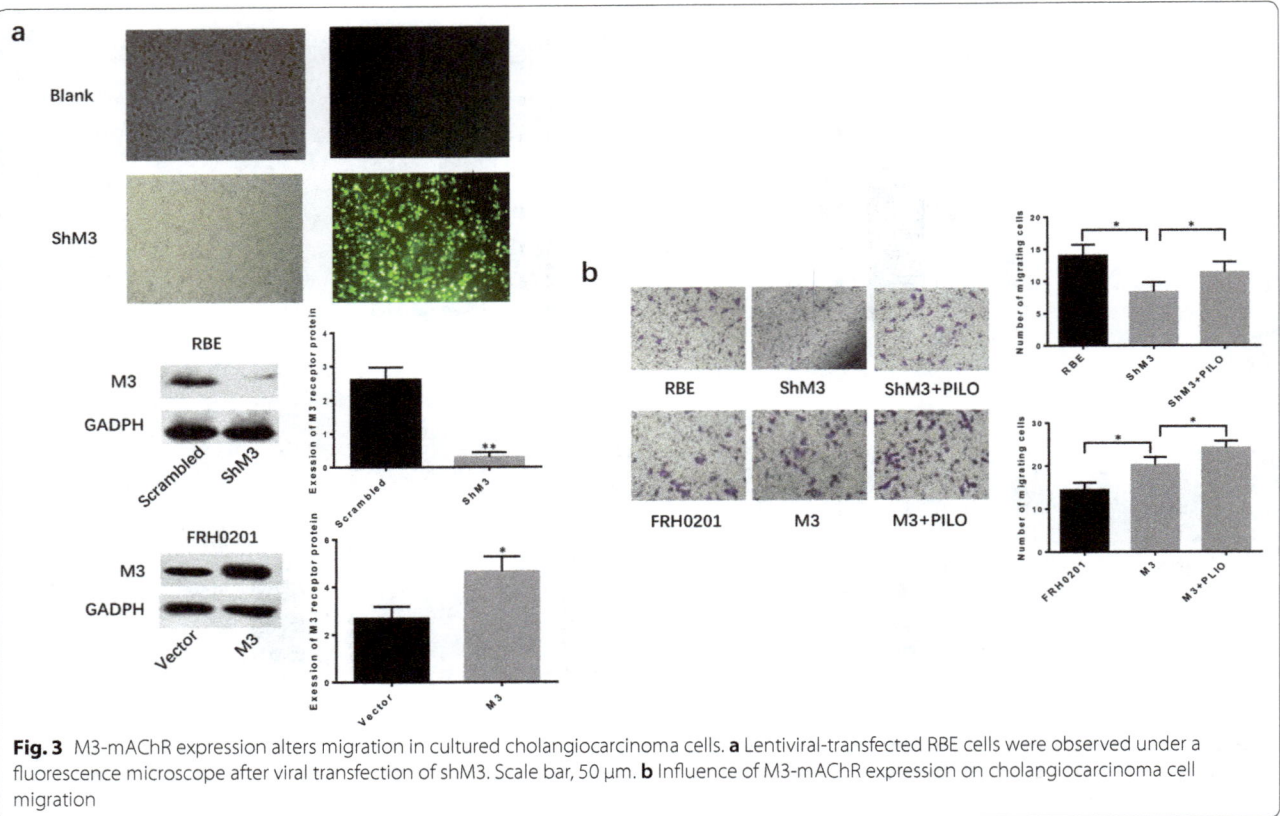

**Fig. 3** M3-mAChR expression alters migration in cultured cholangiocarcinoma cells. **a** Lentiviral-transfected RBE cells were observed under a fluorescence microscope after viral transfection of shM3. Scale bar, 50 μm. **b** Influence of M3-mAChR expression on cholangiocarcinoma cell migration

Moreover, when AKT was downregulated, the levels of invasion and perineural invasion were significantly decreased. We also found that down-regulating the expression of AKT can reduce the activity of MMP in cholangiocarcinoma cells. Taken together, these results showed that the AKT pathway plays a significant role in M3-mAChR-mediated invasion and perineural invasion in cholangiocarcinoma.

## Discussion

As an important digestive organ, the biliary system is responsible for biliary secretion and excretion and is surrounded by vagus nerves that can affect and be affected by processes occurring in the biliary cells. Notably, acetyl choline acts is the main neurotransmitter in this system, and acetyl choline receptors, including nicotinic acetylcholine receptors and mAchRs, play an important functional role during signaling. mAChRs are G protein-coupled receptors that regulate adenylate cyclase, ion channels, and phosphatidylinositol lipid turnover, thus modulating various biological reactions [18, 19].

Studies have shown that the M3-mAChR is widely expressed in digestive tract tumors and may play an important role in the proliferation, differentiation, and progression of cancer [13, 14, 20–22]. Our results show that the M3-mAChR is highly expressed in cholangiocarcinoma and is closely related to the differentiation and clinical stages of the tumor as well as the presence of lymphatic metastasis. Indeed, poor cholangiocarcinoma differentiation was associated with high M3-mAChR expression. In III-IV cancers, the positive rate of M3-mAChR expression in cholangiocarcinoma was notably higher than that observed in I–II cancers, and the expression of M3-mAChR in cholangiocarcinoma patients with concomitant lymphatic metastasis was also increased. Thus, the pattern and correlation of M3-mAChR expression with survival indicate an important function for this receptor in the occurrence and development of cholangiocarcinoma along with patient prognosis.

In 1998, Wessler et al. [23] proposed the concept of the non-neuronal acetylnergic system, which is based on the non-neuronal acetylcholine system, and includes its synthetase, transporter, inactivation enzyme, and functional receptors. Functional abnormalities in this non-neuronal acetylnergic system have been related to various diseases, including inflammation, atherosclerosis, local and systemic infection, and cancer [24]. Many recent studies have also examined the interactions between neurotransmitters and tumors, particularly tumors exhibiting

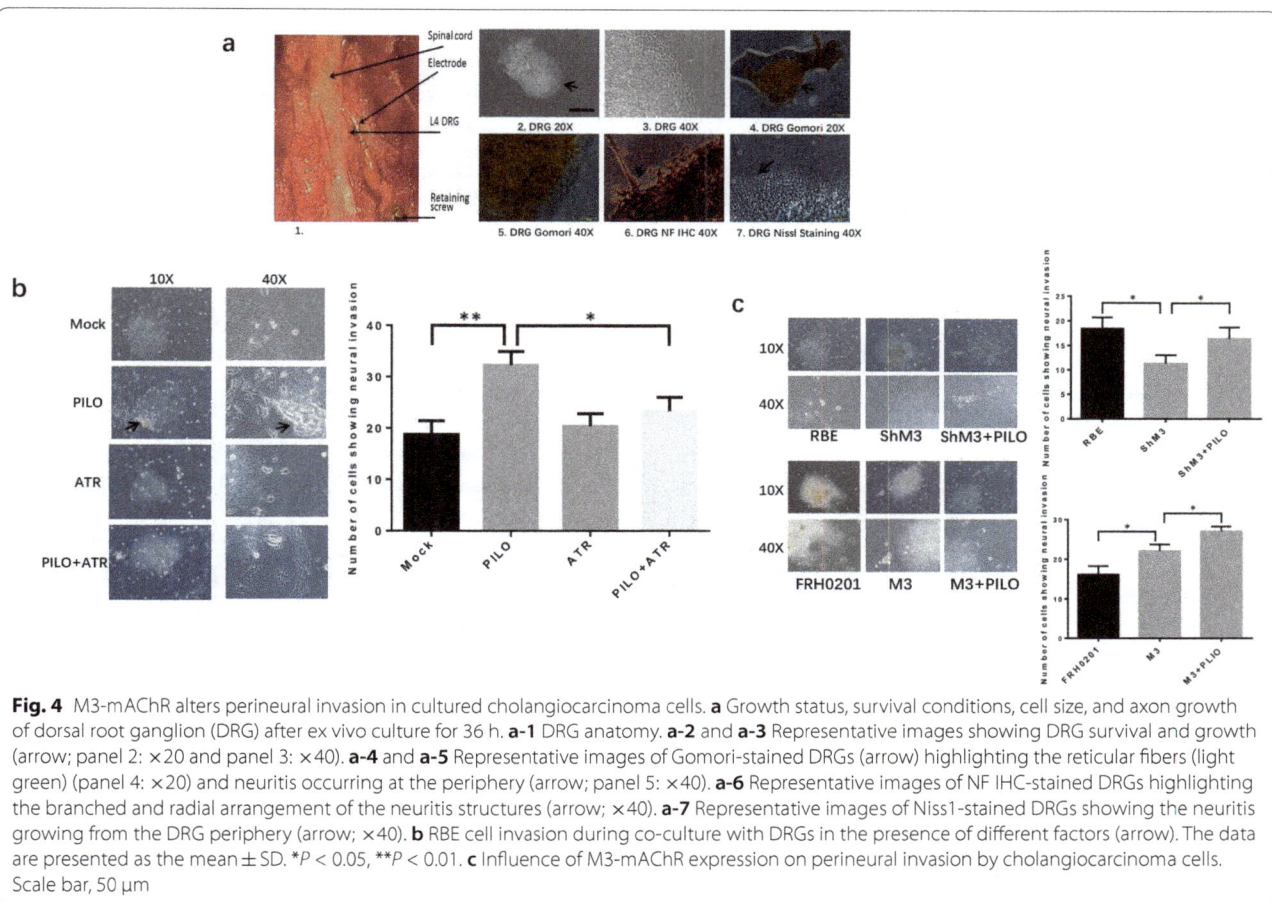

**Fig. 4** M3-mAChR alters perineural invasion in cultured cholangiocarcinoma cells. **a** Growth status, survival conditions, cell size, and axon growth of dorsal root ganglion (DRG) after ex vivo culture for 36 h. **a-1** DRG anatomy. **a-2** and **a-3** Representative images showing DRG survival and growth (arrow; panel 2: ×20 and panel 3: ×40). **a-4** and **a-5** Representative images of Gomori-stained DRGs (arrow) highlighting the reticular fibers (light green) (panel 4: ×20) and neuritis occurring at the periphery (arrow; panel 5: ×40). **a-6** Representative images of NF IHC-stained DRGs highlighting the branched and radial arrangement of the neuritis structures (arrow; ×40). **a-7** Representative images of Niss1-stained DRGs showing the neuritis growing from the DRG periphery (arrow; ×40). **b** RBE cell invasion during co-culture with DRGs in the presence of different factors (arrow). The data are presented as the mean ± SD. *$P < 0.05$, **$P < 0.01$. **c** Influence of M3-mAChR expression on perineural invasion by cholangiocarcinoma cells. Scale bar, 50 μm

perineural invasion, such as cholangiocarcinoma [25–27]. In fact, abnormal neurotransmitter expression and/or receptor signaling in tumors greatly affects tumor proliferation, differentiation, and metastasis, with receptor agonists increasing these characteristics and receptor antagonists blocking them [28, 29]. In a previous study, we found that the M3-mAChR agonist pilocarpine promoted the proliferation of cholangiocarcinoma cells, increased M3-mAChR expression in cholangiocarcinoma, and enhanced the effects of M3-mAChR; all of which were blocked by treatment with the antagonist atropine [12]. In the present study, we not only verified these changes, but we also found that M3-mAChR regulate the migration and metastasis of cholangiocarcinoma cells. Our data show that when M3-mAChR expression is downregulated via receptor knock-down, the migratory capacity of the affected cholangiocarcinoma cells was low. However, when treated with the M3-mAChR agonist pilocarpine, migration was increased. A similar effect was also observed when M3-mAChR was overexpressed in cholangiocarcinoma cells. However, it appears that these enhanced effects can be blocked using atropine,

highlighting the potential use of this or other antagonists in clinical treatment.

Cholangiocarcinoma is one of the deadliest malignant tumors because of the high levels of local invasion and metastasis and the insensitivity of the cells to radiotherapy and chemotherapy. The early occurrence of perineural invasion and metastasis in cholangiocarcinoma has also been shown to affect mortality rate [30]. In addition to its role in migration, we also found that high M3-mAChR expression (via overexpression) promotes perineural invasion, whereas low M3-mAChR expression (via receptor knock-down) was associated with lower levels of perineural invasion. Similar results were also observed using pilocarpine and atropine. These findings suggest that decreasing M3-mAChR expression via knock-down or antagonist treatment may limit perineural invasion of cholangiocarcinoma tumors in the clinical setting.

To understand how M3-mAChR regulate migration, perineural invasion, and metastasis in cholangiocarcinoma, we evaluated the expression and function of various factors and signaling pathways. EMT is widely known

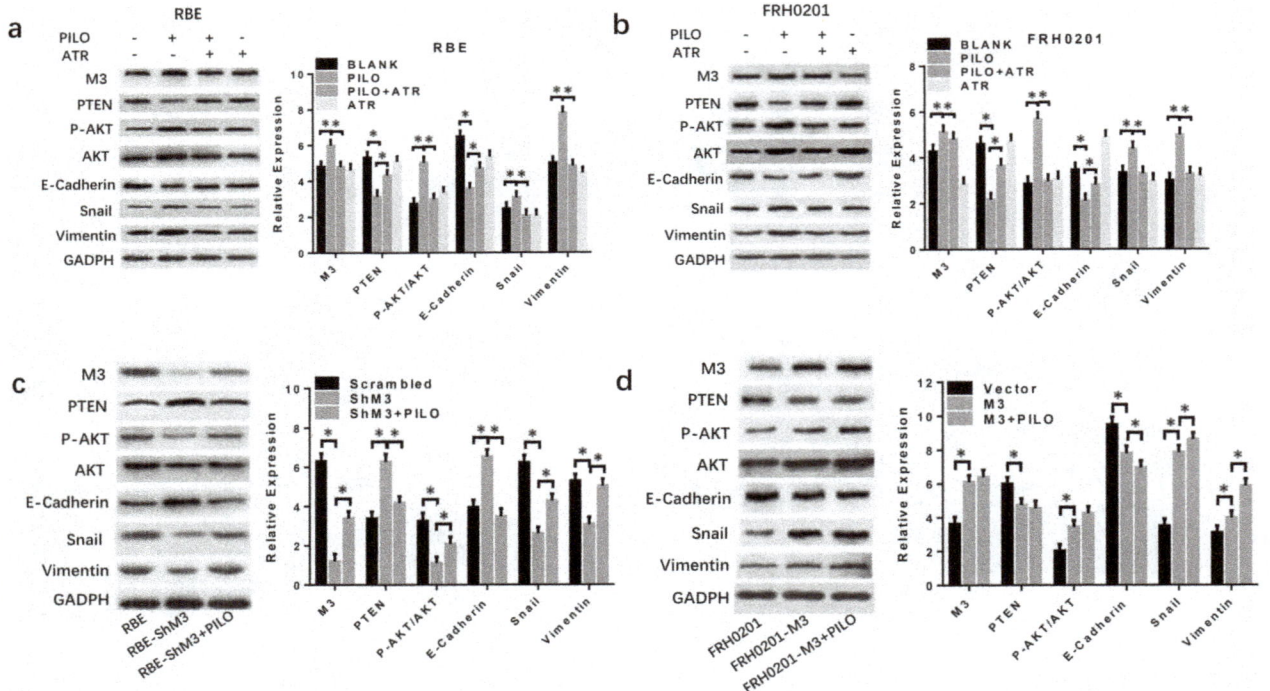

**Fig. 5** M3-mAChR agonist and antagonist influence cholangiocarcinoma cell EMT through the PTEN/AKT pathway. **a–d** Western blots showing the expression of the indicated EMT markers. The quantitated data are presented as the mean ± SD. *$P < 0.05$, **$P < 0.01$

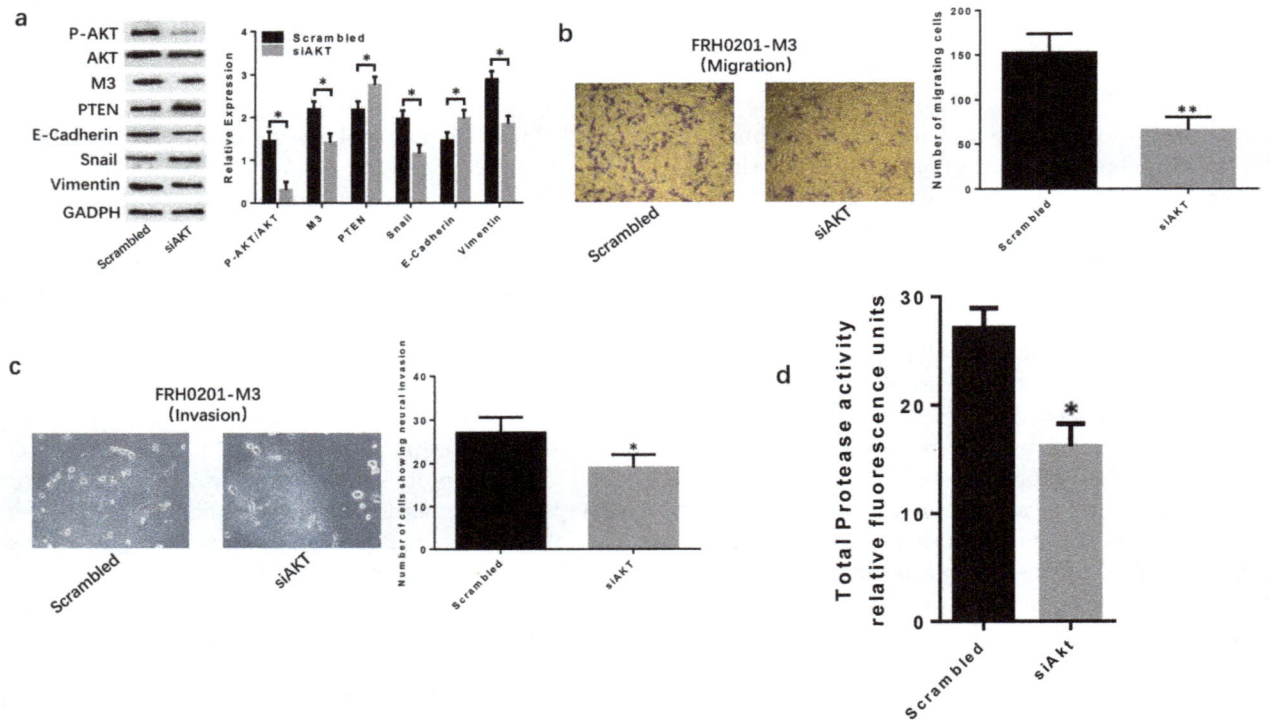

**Fig. 6** M3-mAChR participate in AKT-mediated EMT in cholangiocarcinoma. **a** Western blots showing the expression of the indicated EMT markers. **b** Influence of AKT knock-down on the invasiveness of FRH0201-M3 cells. **c** Influence of AKT knock-down on the perineural invasion of FRH0201 cells. **d** Influence of AKT knock-down on MMP activity. The quantitated data are presented as the mean ± SD. *$P < 0.05$, **$P < 0.01$

to play an essential role in metastasis and confers noninvasive cells with invasive and aggressive features [7], leading to the occurrence and progression of epithelial cell tumors [17]. The phosphatidylinositol-3-kinase (PI3K)/Akt signaling pathway plays an important role in regulating cell proliferation and EMT of malignant cells [31–33]. Our results show that downregulation of M3-mAChR expression in cholangiocarcinoma cells also decreases the expression of PTEN and the epithelial cell marker E-cadherin, while increasing that of AKT and the Leydig cell marker vimentin. These results demonstrate that downregulation of M3-mAChR blocks EMT, whereas upregulation of M3-mAChR transforms cholangiocarcinoma cells into Leydig cells, leading to invasion and metastasis. Additionally, the expression of Snail, an important factor promoting EMT, was also increased after M3-mAChR downregulation, which could subsequently activate other deviant signaling pathways.

The serine/threonine kinase AKT (also known as protein kinase B), which contains a panel of three isoforms (AKT1, AKT2 and AKT3) in mammals, is a key communicator of PI3 K signaling. Further, knockdown of AKT in FRH0201 cells overexpressing M3-mAChR which resulted in the downregulation of M3-mAChR, Snail, and vimentin expression, whereas the expression of PTEN and E-cadherin was upregulated. AKT may have negative feedback in the regulation of M3-mAChR. Moreover, when AKT was downregulated, the levels of invasion and perineural invasion were significantly decreased. We also found that down-regulating the expression of AKT can reduce the activity of MMP in cholangiocarcinoma cells which may be the cause of the decline in invasiveness. The AKT pathway appears to play a particularly prominent role in M3-mAChR signaling as downregulation of this factor significantly decreased migration, metastasis, and perineural invasion.

## Conclusions

In this study, we evaluated the changes in M3-mAChR expression in human tissue samples and in cultured tumor cells in addition to investigating the effects of these changes on migration/metastasis, perineural invasion, and EMT in cholangiocarcinoma. Our results demonstrate that M3-mAChR regulate EMT through the AKT pathway and subsequently affect perineural invasion and metastasis during cholangiocarcinoma pathogenesis. While additional work, particularly the validation of these findings in animal models of the disease, is required, this study is the first to indicate a distinct role for M3-mAChR-mediated regulation in multiple aspects of cholangiocarcinoma. Furthermore, our data also highlight a theoretical basis for blocking perineural invasion and metastasis during cholangiocarcinoma using antagonists. Taken together, this study provides essential insight into the mechanisms and potential treatment options of cholangiocarcinoma.

## Abbreviations

M3 mAChRs: M3 muscarinic acetylcholine receptors; EMT: epithelial–mesenchymal transition; PNI: perineural invasion; PTEN: phosphatase and tensin homolog; AKT: protein kinase B; shRNA: small hairpin RNA; DRG: dorsal root ganglio; PILO: pilocarpine; ATR: atropine; PI3K: phosphatidylinositol-3-kinase.

## Authors' contributions

FYJ and ZBY designed the experiments; FYJ, HX and LGW performed the experiments; LLF and ZW collected the data; MK and FYJ analyzed the data; SFZ and SCD provided the human samples; FYJ and ZCZ wrote the manuscript. All authors read and approved the final manuscript.

## Author details

[1] Department of Hepatobiliary and Pancreatic Surgery, The Affiliated Hospital of Qingdao University, No. 16 Jiangsu Road, Qingdao 266003, Shandong, China. [2] Department of Outpatient, The Affiliated Hospital of Qingdao University, No. 16 Jiangsu Road, Qingdao 266003, Shandong, China. [3] Department of Oncology, The Affiliated Hospital of Qingdao University, No. 16 Jiangsu Road, Qingdao 266003, Shandong, China.

## Acknowledgements

Not applicable.

## Competing interests

The authors declare that they have no competing interests.

## Funding

This work was supported by a Grant from the National Natural Science Foundation (81272362).

## References

1.  Razumilava N, Gores GJ. Cholangiocarcinoma. Lancet. 2014;383(9935):2168–79.
2.  Nakagohri T, Asano T, Kinoshita H, Kenmochi T, Urashima T, Miura F, Ochiai T. Aggressive surgical resection for hilar-invasive and peripheral intrahepatic cholangiocarcinoma. World J Surg. 2003;27(3):289–93.
3.  Murakawa K, Tada M, Takada M, Tamoto E, Shindoh G, Teramoto K, Matsunaga A, Komuro K, Kanai M, Kawakami A, Fujiwara Y, Kobayashi N, Shirata K, Nishimura N, Okushiba S, Kondo S, Hamada J, Katoh H, Yoshiki T, Moriuchi T. Prediction of lymph node metastasis and perineural invasion of biliary tract cancer by selected features from cDNA array data. J Surg Res. 2004;122(2):184–94.
4.  Maxwell P, Hamilton PW, Sloan JM. Three-dimensional reconstruction of perineural invasion in carcinoma of the extrahepatic bile ducts. J Pathol. 1996;180(2):142–5.
5.  Natsis K, Paraskevas G, Papaziogas B, Agiabasis A. "Pes anserinus" of the right phrenic nerve innervating the serous membrane of the liver: a case report (anatomical study). Morphologie. 2004;88(283):203–5.
6.  Yazumi S, Ko K, Watanabe N, Shinohara H, Yoshikawa K, Chiba T, Takahashi R. Disrupted transforming growth factor-beta signaling and deregulated growth in human biliary tract cancer cells. Int J Cancer. 2000;86(6):782–9.
7.  Zhang KJ, Wang DS, Zhang SY, Jiao XL, Li CW, Wang XS, Yu QC, Cui HN. The E-cadherin repressor slug and progression of human extrahepatic hilar cholangiocarcinoma. J Exp Clin Cancer Res. 2010;29:88.
8.  Yoshida GJ. Emerging role of epithelial–mesenchymal transition in hepatic cancer. J Exp Clin Cancer Res. 2016;35(1):141.
9.  Du R, Wu S, Lv X, Fang H, Wu S, Kang J. Overexpression of brachyury contributes to tumor metastasis by inducing epithelial–mesenchymal transition in hepatocellular carcinoma. J Exp Clin Cancer Res. 2014;33:105.

10. Vaquero J, Guedj N, Clapéron A, Nguyen Ho-Bouldoires TH, Paradis V, Fouassier L. Epithelial–mesenchymal transition in cholangiocarcinoma: from clinical evidence to regulatory networks. J Hepatol. 2017;66(2):424–41.

11. Caulfield MP, Birdsall NJ. International union of pharmacology. XVII. Classification of muscarinic acetylcholine receptors. Pharmacol Rev. 1998;50(2):279–90.

12. Feng YJ, Zhang BY, Yao RY, Lu Y. Muscarinic acetylcholine receptor M3 in proliferation and perineural invasion of cholangiocarcinoma cells. Hepatobiliary Pancreat Dis Int. 2012;11(4):418–23.

13. Raufman JP, Samimi R, Shah N, Khurana S, Shant J, Drachenberg C, Xie G, Wess J, Cheng K. Genetic ablation of M3 muscarinic receptors attenuates murine colon epithelial cell proliferation and neoplasia. Cancer Res. 2008;68(10):3573–8.

14. Ukegawa JI, Takeuchi Y, Kusayanagi S, Mitamura K. Growth-promoting effect of muscarinic acetylcholine receptors in colon cancer cells. J Cancer Res Clin Oncol. 2003;129(5):272–8.

15. Livak KJ, Schmittgen TD. Analysis of relative gene expression data using real-time quantitative PCR and the 2(-Delta Delta C(T)) method. Methods. 2001;25(4):402–8.

16. Na'ara S, Gil Z, Amit M. In vitro modeling of cancerous neural invasion: the dorsal root ganglion model. J Vis Exp. 2016;110:e52990.

17. Hwang S, Lee YJ, Song GW, Park KM, Kim KH, Ahn CS, Moon DB, Lee SG. Prognostic impact of tumor growth type on 7th AJCC staging system for intrahepatic cholangiocarcinoma: a single-center experience of 659 cases. J Gastrointest Surg. 2015;19(7):1291–304.

18. Gilman AG. G proteins and dual control of adenylate cyclase. Cell. 1984;36(3):577–9.

19. Malbon CC. G proteins in development. Nat Rev Mol Cell Biol. 2005;6(9):689–701.

20. Park YS, Cho NJ. Enhanced proliferation of SNU-407 human colon cancer cells by muscarinic acetylcholine receptors. BMB Rep. 2008;41(11):803–7.

21. Frucht H, Jensen RT, Dexter D, Yang WL, Xiao Y. Human colon cancer cell proliferation mediated by the M3 muscarinic cholinergic receptor. Clin Cancer Res. 1999;5(9):2532–9.

22. Wegener C, Hamasaka Y, Nässel DR. Acetylcholine increases intracellular Ca²⁺ via nicotinic receptors in cultured PDF-containing clock neurons of Drosophila. J Neurophysiol. 2004;91(2):912–23.

23. Wessler I, Kirkpatrick CJ, Racké K. Non-neuronal acetylcholine, a locally acting molecule, widely distributed in biological systems: expression and function in humans. Pharmacol Ther. 1998;77(1):59–79.

24. Grando SA, Kawashima K, Kirkpatrick CJ, Kummer W, Wessler I. Recent progress in revealing the biological and medical significance of the non-neuronal cholinergic system. Int Immunopharmacol. 2015;29(1):1–7.

25. Schuller HM, Porter B, Riechert A. Beta-adrenergic modulation of NNK-induced lung carcinogenesis in hamsters. J Cancer Res Clin Oncol. 2000;126(11):624–30.

26. Drell TL 4th, Joseph J, Lang K, Niggemann B, Zaenker KS, Entschladen F. Effects of neurotransmitters on the chemokinesis and chemotaxis of MDA-MB-468 human breast carcinoma cells. Breast Cancer Res Treat. 2003;80(1):63–70.

27. Masur K, Niggemann B, Zanker KS, Entschladen F. Norepinephrine-induced migration of SW480 colon carcinoma cells is inhibited by beta-blockers. Cancer Res. 2001;61(7):2866–9.

28. Radu A, Pichon C, Camparo P, Antoine M, Allory Y, Couvelard A, Fromont G, Hai MT, Ghinea N. Expression of follicle-stimulating hormone receptor in tumor blood vessels. N Engl J Med. 2010;363(17):1621–30.

29. Leu FP, Nandi M, Niu C. The effect of transforming growth factor beta on human neuroendocrine tumor BON cell proliferation and differentiation is mediated through somatostatin signaling. Mol Cancer Res. 2008;6(6):1029–42.

30. Shen FZ, Zhang BY, Feng YJ, Jia ZX, An B, Liu CC, Deng XY, Kulkarni AD, Lu Y. Current research in perineural invasion of cholangiocarcinoma. J Exp Clin Cancer Res. 2010;29:24.

31. Wang C, Mao ZP, Wang L, Wu GH, Zhang FH, Wang DY, Shi JL. Long non-coding RNA MALAT1 promotes cholangiocarcinoma cell proliferation and invasion by activating PI3 K/Akt pathway. Neoplasma. 2017;64(5):725–31.

32. Choi Y, Ko YS, Park J, Choi Y, Kim Y, Pyo JS, Jang BG, Hwang DH, Kim WH, Lee BL. HER2-induced metastasis is mediated by AKT/JNK/EMT signaling pathway in gastric cancer. World J Gastroenterol. 2016;22(41):9141–53.

33. Xu W, Yang Z, Lu N. A new role for the PI3K/Akt signaling pathway in the epithelial–mesenchymal transition. Cell Adh Migr. 2015;9(4):317–24.

# 9

# RelB plays an oncogenic role and conveys chemo-resistance to DLD-1 colon cancer cells

Xiaojun Zhou[1†], Zhili Shan[1†], Hengying Yang[1], Jingjing Xu[2], Wenjing Li[3] and Feng Guo[4*]

## Abstract

**Background:** Nuclear transcription factor kappa B (NF-κB) subunits exhibit crucial roles in tumorigenesis and chemo-sensitivity. Recent studies suggest that RelB, the key subunit of the alternative NF-κB pathway, plays a critical role in the progression of diverse human malignancies. However, the significance of RelB in colorectal cancer (CRC) remains unclear. Here, we systematically explored the functions of the alternative NF-κB subunit RelB in colon cancer cells and its underlying mechanism.

**Methods:** Stably transfected RelB-shRNA DLD-1 cells were established using Lipofectamine 2000. NF-κB DNA-binding capability was quantified using an ELISA-based NF-κB activity assay. Cell growth was monitored by an x-Celligence system. Cell proliferation was analyzed by a CCK-8 and a Brdu proliferation assay. Response to 5-FU was assessed by an x-Celligence system. Cell apoptosis and cell cycle was detected using flow cytometry analyses. Cell migration and invasion abilities were detected by an x-Celligence system, Transwell inserts, and wound-healing assays. RelB expression and its clinical significance were analyzed using the CRC tissue microarray. The expression of NF-κB signaling subunits, AKT/mTOR signaling molecules, cell cycle related proteins, MMP2, MMP9, and Integrin β-1 were measured by Western blotting analyses.

**Results:** The RelB-silencing inhibited cell growth of DLD-1 cells. The RelB-silencing exerted the anti-proliferative by downregulation of AKT/mTOR signaling. The RelB-silencing caused $G_0$–$G_1$ cell cycle arrested likely due to decreasing the expression of Cyclin D1 and CDK4, concomitant with increased expression of p27$^{Kip1}$. The RelB-silencing enhanced cytotoxic effect of 5-FU and induced cell accumulation in S-phase. The RelB-silencing impaired the migration and invasion potential of DLD-1 cells, which was related to downregulation of MMP2, MMP9, and Integrin β-1. Importantly, the RelB expression was correlated with depth of tumor invasion, lymph node metastasis, metastasis stage, and pTNM stage. High-RelB expression was significantly correlated with poor overall survival in CRC patients.

**Conclusion:** Our studies here provided evidence that RelB plays an oncogenic role and conveys chemo-resistance to 5-FU. RelB can be considered as an independent indicator of prognosis in CRC.

**Keywords:** RelB, Colorectal cancer, Migration and invasion, Chemo-sensitivity, Cell cycle, Prognostic factor

## Background

Colorectal cancer (CRC) is a leading cause of morbidity and mortality worldwide, and is a multistep genetic disorder. It ranks the third most common cancer among both men and women in the United States [1]. In China, CRC is the fifth leading cause of cancer deaths among both men and women [2]. Despite the achievements in the diagnosis and treatment of CRC acquired in recent years, the overall 5-year survival rate is still unfavored [3]. The development of CRC is a complex process, involving inactivation of several tumor suppressor genes and activation of proto-oncogenes. The main factors affecting the prognosis of CRC are metastasis, relapse, and chemo-resistance [4]. Therefore, a lot of efforts are desired to illuminate of the molecular mechanism underlying the CRC progression and metastasis, and to develop effective therapeutic target for CRC.

*Correspondence: 550045590@qq.com
†Xiaojun Zhou and Zhili Shan contributed equally to this work
4 Department of Oncology, Nanjing Medical University Affiliated Suzhou Hospital, Baita West Road 16, Suzhou 215001, China
Full list of author information is available at the end of the article

The nuclear transcription factor kappa B (NF-κB) has been identified as a nuclear factor binding to the kappa light chain enhancer in B cells in 1986 [5]. The NF-κB family includes RelA (p65), RelB, c-Rel, NF-κB1 (p50 and its precursor p105), and NF-κB2 (p52 and its precursor p100) [6]. NF-κB can be activated through the classical (canonical) and the alternative (or non-canonical) signaling pathways [7]. The classical NF-κB pathway involves activation of the IκB kinase (IKK) complex (composed of IKKα, IKKβ, and IKKγ subunits), leading to phosphorylation of IκB proteins. This pathway usually regulates the nuclear translocation activity of p50/RelA and p50/c-Rel heterodimers. In the alternative pathway, the NF-κB inducing kinase (NIK) activates IKKα, then leading to the phosphorylation and proteasome-mediated partial degradation of p100 to generate p52, resulting in the formation of RelB/p52 complexes. RelB/p52 heterodimers then translocate to the nucleus and activate target genes [8]. The role of the classical NF-κB activity has been extensively studied in a variety of human malignancies [9]. Many studies have focused on the function of the classical NF-κB pathway in CRC. In CRC, the NF-κB pathway plays a critical role in cancer related processes including cell proliferation, apoptosis, and metastasis [10]. The role of chronic inflammation in CRC is undisputed and the NF-κB pathway may serve as the link between inflammation and the tumorigenesis of colon epithelium [11]. Previous study shows that IKKβ-mediated NF-κB activity has a key role in the development of colitis-associated cancer using a mouse model of colitis-associated CRC [12]. Overexpression of the NIK- and IKK-β-binding protein (NIBP) can increase CRC metastases via classical NF-κB activity, which further upregulates matrix metallopeptidase 2 (MMP2) and matrix metallopeptidase 9 (MMP9) [13]. The classical NF-κB activity has also been implicated in the chemo-resistance and proteasome inhibition targeting NF-κB in CRC [14].

RelB is the main subunit of the alternative NF-κB signaling pathway, triggering effective transcription activation upon heterodimerizing with p52 [15]. Previous studies using the $RelB^{-/-}$ mice have shown that RelB exerts crucial roles on numerous biological processes including lymphoid organogenesis, B cell maturation, T-cell homeostasis, and immune response. The lack of RelB cannot be functionally compensated by other NF-κB subunits [16–18]. Increasing studies have focused on the role of the alternative NF-κB activity, represented by RelB, in the tumourigenesis. The mRNA level of RelB is correlated with bladder cancer pathological, clinical stage, and lymph node metastasis [19]. The level of nuclear RelB expression correlates with prostate cancer patient's Gleason score, suggesting that RelB is involved in prostate cancer progression [20]. RelB expression exhibits opposing effects of ascorbic acid in prostatic cancer and normal cells. RelB exerts a radio-protective role in aggressive prostate cancer cells through the induction of the manganese superoxide dismutase (*MnSOD*) gene [21]. Our previous studies have demonstrated that the RelB-silencing significantly attenuates the migration and invasion abilities of DU145 prostate cancer cells via the reduction of Integrin β-1 (ITGB1) [22]. Enhancer of zeste homology 2 (EZH2) can promote the transcriptional activation of RelB, driving self-renewal and tumor-initiating cell phenotype of triple-negative breast cancer cells [23]. Moreover, RelB is an independent prognostic factor for patients with non-small cell lung cancer (NSCLC). RelB promotes cell migration and invasion, and conveys radio-resistance to the NSCLC cells [24, 25]. Collectively, accumulated reports indicate that RelB functions importantly in the progression and chemo-sensitivity of various solid tumors.

The exact molecular mechanism of RelB in CRC remains unclear. The study here was aiming to define the significance of RelB in colon cancer cells. Our results indicated that RelB affected many cellular behaviors of DLD-1 colon cancer cells including proliferation, migration, invasion, and chemo-sensitivity. The expression of RelB was correlated with CRC clinical stage, tumor differentiation, and lymph node metastasis. RelB could be considered as an independent prognostic biomarker for CRC patients. Taken together, we provided evidences that RelB played an oncogenic role in CRC.

## Materials and methods
### Cell lines and culture condition
The human colon cancer cell lines DLD-1, HT-29, and Caco-2 were purchased from Shanghai Chinese Academy. All cells were cultured in RPMI-1640 media containing 10% fetal bovine serum (FBS, Gibco, USA), 100 U/ml penicillin, and 100 μg/ml streptomycin in a humidified atmosphere of 37 °C containing 5% $CO_2$.

### Cell transfection
The short hairpin RNA (shRNA) specifically targeting the human *RelB* gene was designed and constructed by Invitrogen (Beijing, China). The sequences of RelB-shRNA are 275–293: 5′-GCACAGATGAATTGGAGAT-3′. The shRNA-RelB was subcloned into the pSilencer3.1-H1-neo plasmid (Cat Nr. 5770, Thermo Scientific™, China), which was linearized by restriction endonucleases HindIII and BamHI. DLD-1 colon cancer cells were pre-cultured to 60–80% confluence in 24-well plates and transfected using Lipofectamine 2000 (Cat Nr. 12566014, Thermo Scientific™, China) for 6 h. To obtain stably transfected clones, cells were selected in the medium

containing G418 (800 ng/µl, Cat Nr. E859-5G, Amresco, USA).

## Western blot analysis and antibodies

Cells were collected and then lysed with a modified radioimmune precipitation assay (RIPA) buffer containing a protease inhibitor cocktail. Total protein and cytoplasmic/nuclear fractions were extracted, and denatured. Protein extracts were separated on 8–12% SDS-PAGE gels and further semi-electrically transferred into nitrocellulose membranes. After being blocked with 5% skim milk for 1 h at room temperature (RT), the membranes were incubated with appropriate primary antibodies (Abs) overnight at 4 °C. After washing with TBS-T buffer, the membranes were incubated with appropriate secondary Abs for 1 h at RT and scanned with an Odyssey® infrared imaging system (LI-COR Biosciences, USA). Both primary and secondary Abs used in this study were diluted according to the manufacturer's instructions. Band density was normalized to either β-actin or Lamin A/C expression. Abs against NF-κB p65 (C-20, sc-372), RelB (C-19, sc-226), c-Rel (N, sc-70), NF-κB p105/50 (H-119, sc-7178), NF-κB p100/52 (K-27, sc-298), IKBα (H-4), IKKα (B-8),and Lamin A/C (H-110, sc-20681) were purchased from Santa Cruz Biotechnology, lnc. Phospho-Akt Pathway Antibody Sampler Kit (#9916), Cell Cycle Regulation Sampler Kit (#9932) were purchased from Cell Signaling Technology, Inc. Abs against IKKβ (#2684), Phospho-IKKβ (#2694), Phospho-GSK-3β (#5558), Phospho-mTOR (#2971), Phospho-p70 S6 Kinase (#9205), MMP2 (D8N9Y), MMP9 (D603H), and Integrin β-1 (D2E5) were purchased from Cell Signaling Technology, Inc. β-actin Ab (AT0001) was purchased from Abgent (Suzhou, China). IRDye 680CW (#926-32222) and IRDye 800CW (#926-32210) secondary Abs were purchased from LI-COR Biosciences.

## RNA extraction and quantitative real-time PCR (qRT-PCR)

Total RNA was isolated using TRIzol reagent (Tiangen Biotech Co., Ltd., Beijing, China). RNA yield and purity were determined by Nanodrop-1000 spectrophotometer (Thermo Fisher Scientific, China). The absorbance ratio (A260/280) of all samples ranged from 1.8 to 2.0. Total RNA (2 µg) was reverse-transcribed into cDNA using Moloney Murine Leukemia Virus (M-MLV) (Cat Nr. 28025013, Promega, China) according to the manufacturer's instructions. cDNA was then amplified by qRT-PCR assay though a SYBR Green PCR kit (Applied Biosystems, Shanghai, China) with a LightCycler 480 System (Roche, China). The mRNA expression level was calculated via Pfaffl method using β-actin as the internal control. Primers

for qRT-PCR were designed using Primer-BLAST (Pubmed) and synthesized from Invitrogen.

## NF-κB DNA-binding capability assay

NF-κB DNA-binding capability was quantified using a Trans^AM NF-κB family transcription factor assay kit (Cat Nr. #43296, Active Motif, Carlsbad, CA, USA). Briefly, 5 µg of nuclear extracts were incubated in a 96-well plate coated with immobilized NF-κB consensus oligonucleotides (5′-GGGACTTTCC-3′) for 1 h at RT. Then captured complexes were incubated with individual NF-κB antibodies (1:1000) for 1 h, and subsequently with HRP-conjugated secondary antibody (1:1000) for 1 h. After colorimetric reaction, the absorbance was read as optical density (OD) value at 450 nm.

## Cell growth assay

The cell growth rates were detected by an x-Celligence RTCA instrument (Roche Diagnostics, China). In this assay, cells were seeded in an E-plate at a density of 5000 cells per well in 100 µl RPMI-1640 media containing 10% FBS. Impedance of cells for indicated times were continuously monitored by the system for 72 h and the value was measured as 'cell index'. The data were analyzed by RTCA software 1.2. The x-Celligence system was also used to examine the effects of 5-Fluorouracil (5-FU, Cat Nr. F6627, Sigma Chemical) on cell growth. Cells were pro-cultured in an E-plate (5000 cells per well) in 100 µl RPMI-1640 media containing 10% FBS for 24 h. And cells were then treated with different concentrations of 5-FU (0–200 µM). Impedance of cells for indicated times were continuously monitored by the system for 48 h and the value was measured as 'normalized cell index'. The dosage of 5-FU for 50% inhibition of proliferation (IC50) was analyzed by the RTCA software 1.2.

## CCK-8 assay

Cell proliferation was also measured using a Cell Counting Kit-8 (CCK-8, Dojindo, Kumomoto, Japan) assay. In the assay, cells were cultured in 96-well plates (3000 cells/well) and tested at the indicated times according to the manufacturer's instructions. The absorbance of 450 nm was measured to calculate cell growth rates. Each experiment was repeated in triplicate.

## Brdu cell proliferation assay

Brdu cell proliferation assay kit (Cat Nr. 2750, Merck Millipore, Germany) was used to examine the cellular proliferation. In brief, cells were cultured in 96-well plates for 24 h and 10 µl Brdu was added for 5 h' incubation. Then, the Brdu-labeled cells were fixed, and DNA was denatured. The cells were then incubated with peroxidase-conjugated anti-Brdu antibody for 1 h at RT. The immune complex was detected using a tetramethyl benzidine substrate reaction, and OD value at 450 nm was measured using spectrophotometer microplate reader (Biotek, USA). Each experiment was repeated in triplicate.

### Colony formation assay

For the colony formation assay, 1000 cells were seeded in 6-cm dishes, cultured in a humidified atmosphere of 37 °C containing 5% $CO_2$ for 2 weeks, and then stained with Giemsa. Colonies containing more than 50 cells were counted, and the efficiency was calculated as a percentage of inoculated cells. Each experiment was repeated in triplicate.

### Cell apoptosis assay

Cells were cultured in 6-well plates for 0, 24, 48, and 72 h and were stained with AnnexinV together with propidium iodide (PI) using APC-AnnexinV Binding apoptosis assay kit (Cat Nr. 22837, AATBioquest, USA). Cells were incubated for 15 min at RT in the dark. Cell apoptosis was examined by a FACSCalibur™ cytometer (BD Biosciences, USA).

### Cell cycle assay

Cells were harvested and fixed with 70% ethanol overnight at 4 °C. Subsequently, the single cell suspensions were prepared to stain with PI (Cat Nr. P4170, Sigma, Germany) containing RNaseA (Cat Nr. 12091-021, Invitrogen, USA) according to the manufacturer's instructions. Cell cycle ($2 \times 10^4$ cells) was measured by a FACSCalibur™ cytometer. The percentage of cells in the $G_0$–$G_1$, S, and G2-M phases was calculated by ModFit LT cell cycle analysis software.

### Cell migration and invasion assay using an x-Celligence system

Cells were seeded into the upper chamber in a CIM-plate assembled with the serum-free RPMI-1640 media. 200 µl RPMI-1640 media containing 10% FBS was added to each well of the lower chamber. For cell invasion assay, the Matrigel (Cat Nr. 356234, BD Biosciences, China) was diluted (1:40) using serum-from RPMI-1640 media. Wells of the upper chamber were pre-coated with Matrigel (30 µl) for 4 h. Cell migration or invasion through Matrigel towards the lower chamber was continuously monitored by an x-Celligence system, and data were collected and analyzed by RTCA software 1.2.

### Cell migration and invasion assay using a Transwell system

Cell migration and invasion assays were also performed using 24-well Transwell plates (Falcon cell culture inserts,

8-µm pore size, BD Biosciences, USA). To eliminate the influences of cell proliferation on cell migration and invasion, the cells were pre-treated with Mitomycin C (1M, CAS 50-07-7, Santa Cruz Biotechnology) for 1 h. For the migration assay, cells ($5 \times 10^4$) were seeded into the upper chamber of Transwell inserts containing serum-free RPMI-1640 media. 600 µl of RPMI-1640 media with 10% FBS was added as the chemotactic factor into the lower chamber. For the invasion assays, cells ($10 \times 10^4$) were seeded into the upper chamber of Transwell inserts pre-coated with 50 µl Matrigel. Upon incubation at 37 °C for 24 h, cells remaining on the upper surface were removed by swabs. Cells on the filter surface were fixed with 4% paraformal dehydrate for 20 min, and stained with 0.1% crystal violet for 15 min. Then the numbers of migratory or invasive cells were counted and photographed with a light System microscope IX71 (Olympus, Japan).

### Wound-healing assay

Artificial homogeneous wounds were created using a 200-µl micropipette tip and washed three times with PBS. Cells were then cultured with RPMI-1640 media supplemented with 10% FBS and photographed at 0, 24, 48, and 72 h with a light System microscope IX71 (Olympus, Japan).

### Clinical samples

The expression of RelB in CRC tissue was determined using tissue microarray [TMA, Lot Nr. XT16-027, Shanghai Outdo Biotech Company from the National Human Genetic Resources Sharing Service Platform (2005DKA21300)]. Use of patient samples and clinical data in this study was approved by the Ethics Committee of Shanghai Outdo Biotech Company. TMA consists of 87 paired CRC and para-carcinoma tissues. All patients underwent operation from November 2009 to May 2010. Patients' follow-up information was obtained from 2009 to 2015. The final follow-up date was July 2015.

### Immunohistochemistry (IHC)

The sections of TMA were blocked by hydrogen peroxide and serum, and then incubated with primary Abs of RelB (1:200 dilutions). PBS was used as negative control for primary Abs. Staining and processing were performed with the GTVision™ III Detection System/Mo&Rb (Cat Nr. GK500705, Shanghai) according to the manufacturer's instructions. IHC-staining results were analyzed by two experienced pathologists under a microscope BX51 (Olympus, Japan). The scores were as follows: 0 for no staining; 1+ for light; 2+ for moderate; 3+ for strong. The distribution of positive staining was scored as the percentages of labeled cells for five groups: 0: no staining; 1: < 25% staining; 2: 26–50% staining; 3: 51–75% staining;

and 4: 75–100% staining. The product of the intensity and extent grades $\geq 4$ of positive cells was considered as high-expression, and the score of 0–3 of positive cells was regarded as low-expression.

### Statistical analysis
All analyses were analyzed by SPSS 24.0 and GraphPad Primer5 software. The measured data of normal distribution were expressed as mean $\pm$ SD, and differences between groups were examined by Student's $t$-test. A Pearson's Chi square or Fisher's exact test was used to analyze the correlation between RelB expression and clinic-pathological characteristics. Kaplan–Meier test were used for survival analysis. Multivariate Cox proportional risk models were performed to value the effect of RelB expression levels on disease-specific survival. A value of $p < 0.05$ was considered statistical significant. * for $p < 0.05$, ** for $p < 0.01$, *** for $p < 0.001$.

## Results

### Introduction of RelB-shRNA into DLD-1 colon cancer cells
The endogenous expression of all NF-κB subunits in the whole-cell extracts was examined by Western blotting analysis in the three colon cancer cell lines including DLD-1, HT-29, and Caco-2. As shown in Fig. 1a, the expression levels of each NF-κB subunits were quite different among the three colon cancer cell lines. All the NF-κB subunits could be detected in the DLD-1 cells albeit at different levels. The expression of RelA, RelB, p105, and p50 could be detected in the HT-29 cells, while the expression of c-Rel, p100, and p52 not detected. All the NF-κB subunits except of c-Rel could be detected in the Caco-2 cells.

To investigate the function of RelB on the biological cellular behaviors of colon cancer cells, the DLD-1 cells with high RelB expression were preferred for the following experiments. The DLD-1 cells were transfected with plasmid carrying either RelB-shRNA or control-shRNA respectively. Cells were cultured in the presence of G418 until monoclones formed. The expression of RelB in the DLD-1 monoclones was examined by both qRT-PCR and Western blotting analysis and the representative results were present here. As shown in Fig. 1b, the mRNA

expression of *RelB* was decreased about twofold in the DLD-1-siRelB cells (transfected with the RelB-shRNA plasmid) compared with that in the DLD-1-sictrl cells (transfected with the control-shRNA plasmid). Similarly, the RelB expression at protein level was much lower in the DLD-1-siRelB cell compared with that in the DLD-1-sictrl cells (Fig. 1c).

To examine whether the RelB-silencing affected the NF-κB signaling, the Western blotting analysis was performed. As shown in Fig. 1d, the expression of RelA, p50, p105, and c-Rel in both cytoplasmic extracts (CE) and nuclear extracts (NE) stayed unchanged, while the expression of p100 and p52 was also reduced in CE and NE in the DLD-1 cells lacking the expression of RelB. The expression of certain upstream molecules of the NF-κB signaling, such as IKKβ and phosphorate-IKKβ, was not influenced by the RelB-silencing in the DLD-1 cells (Fig. 1e). To further investigate the effects of the RelB-silencing on NF-κB DNA-binding capability, an ELISA-based NF-κB activity assay was performed. Compared to that in the DLD-1-sictrl cells, the average RelB DNA-binding capability in NE of the DLD-1-siRelB cells was considerably reduced ($p < 0.01$). Meanwhile, the average p52 DNA-binding capability was slightly reduced, albeit with no statistical significance. The average DNA-binding capabilities of RelA, p50, and c-Rel in the DLD-1-siRelB and DLD-1-sictrl cells were comparable (Fig. 1f). In addition, the mRNA levels of important genes regulated by the alternative NF-κB signaling were examined by qRT-PCR. As shown in Fig. 1g, the mRNA expression of the *MMP2* (3.4-fold, $p < 0.01$), *MMP9* (1.5-fold, $p < 0.05$), *CyclinD1* (1.7-fold, $p < 0.01$), and *ITGB1* (1.3-fold, $p < 0.05$) genes was decreased at different levels in the DLD-1-siRelB cells compared with that in the DLD-1-sictrl cells. Collectively, these results indicated that a successful RNA-interference of the *RelB* gene was created in the DLD-1 cells.

### RelB affects the DLD-1 cell growth
In order to explore the effects of the RelB-silencing on cell growth, the cellular growth was continuously monitored by a real-time x-Celligence system using E-plates. As shown in Fig. 2a, the cell growth curves of

(See figure on next page.)
**Fig. 1** Establishment of RelB-silencing DLD1 cells. **a** Western blotting analysis of the protein expression of NF-κB subunits in DLD-1, HT-29, and Caco-2 cells. The level of each protein was normalized against Actin. **b** Relative RelB mRNA expression levels were detected using qRT-PCR. β-Actin normalized gene expression, measured in triplicates was displayed. **c** Western blotting analysis for protein levels of RelB expression. Protein expression was normalized against Actin. **d** RelB-silencing affects the expression of other individual NF-κB subunits. Western blotting analysis of the protein expression in cytoplasmic and nuclear extracts was normalized against Actin and Lamin A/C, respectively. **e** Western blotting analysis of the protein expression of IKKβ, p-IKKβ, IKBα, and IKKα in siRelB and sictrl cells. Protein levels were normalized against Actin. **f** The DNA-binding activity of nuclear extracts was detected and quantified using a Trans^AM NF-κB family transcription factor assay kit. **g** The mRNA expression levels of specific target genes downstream of NF-κB pathway were detected using qRT-PCR. β-Actin normalized gene expression, measured in triplicates was displayed. Data are shown as mean $\pm$ SD form three individual experiments. *$p < 0.05$; **$p < 0.01$; ***$p < 0.001$

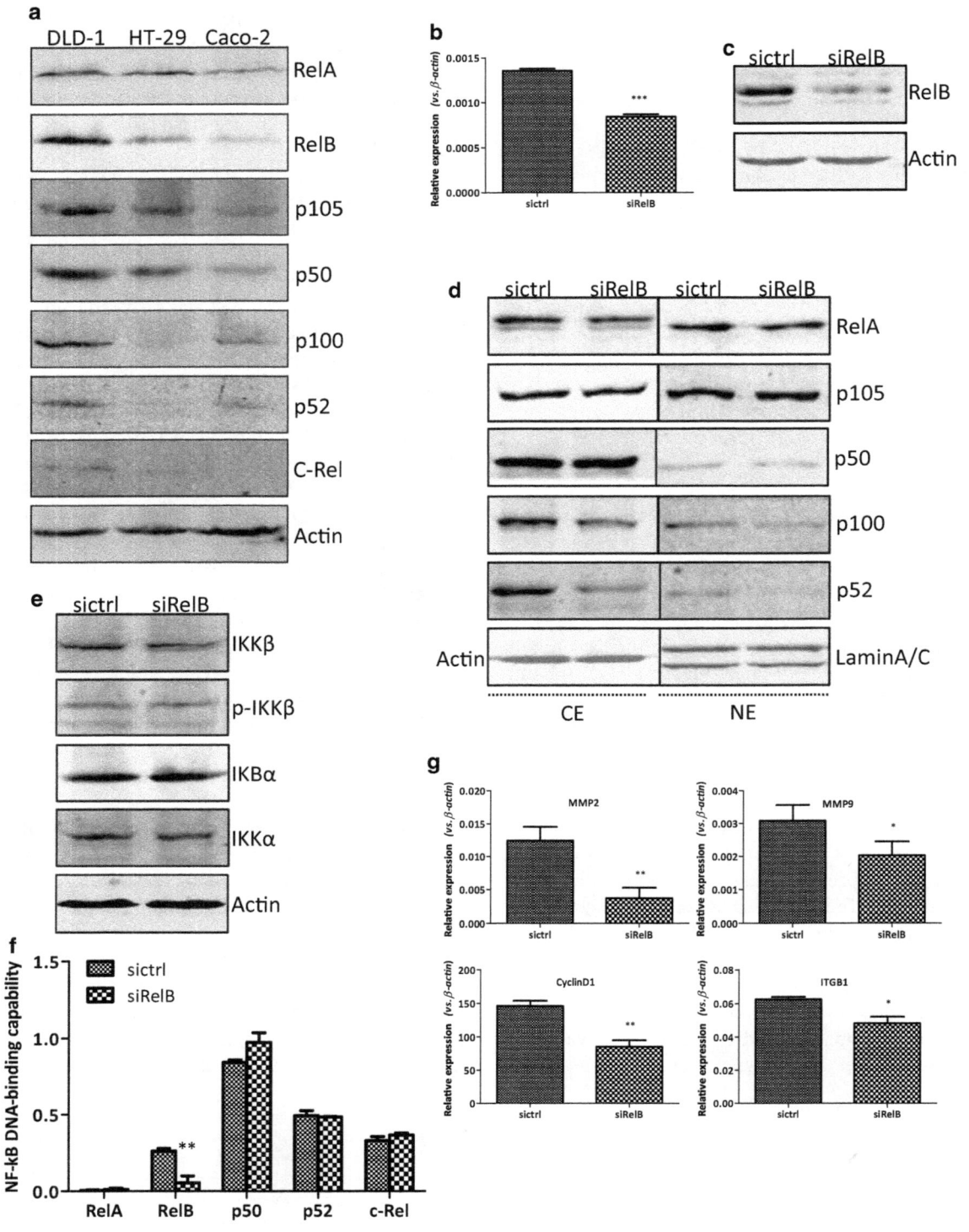

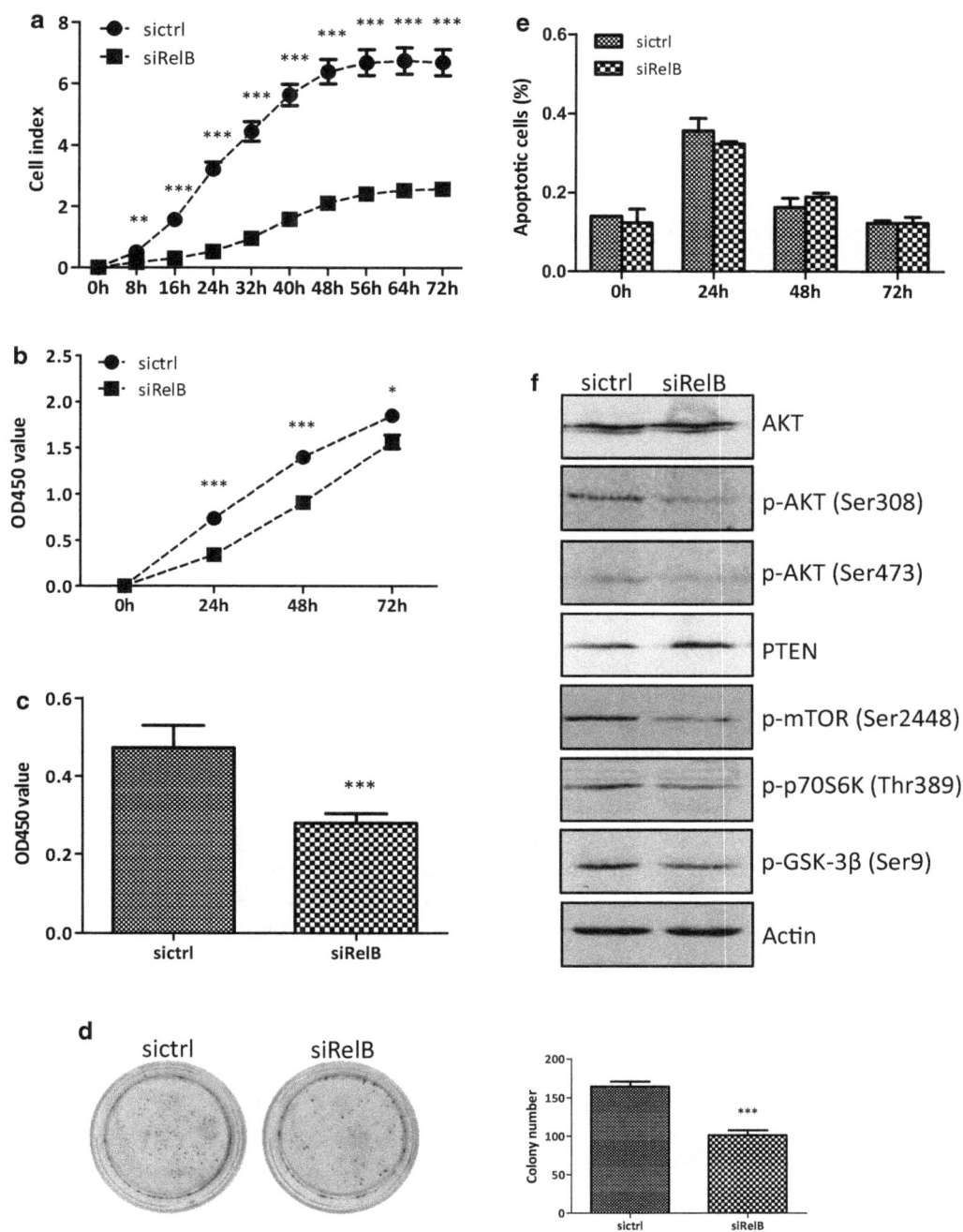

**Fig. 2** RelB-silencing inhibits the DLD-1 cell growth. **a** The cell growth rates were monitored by a real-time x-Celligence system for 72 h. **b** Cell proliferation was detected by CCK-8 assay. OD450 was measured using spectrophotometer microplate reader at 24, 48, and 72 h. **c** Cell proliferation was detected by Brdu assay. OD450 was measured after transfection with siRNA for 24 h. **d** Cell proliferation was evaluated by colony formation assay. 1000 cells were seeded in 6-cm dishes and cultured for 2 weeks. Colonies containing > 50 cells were counted. **e** Cell apoptosis assay was examined by Flow cytometry at 0, 24, 48, and 72 h. **f** Western blotting analysis of the protein expression of total AKT, p-AKT$^{Ser473}$, p-AKT$^{Ser308}$, p-mTOR$^{Ser2448}$, p-p70S6K$^{Thr389}$, PTEN, and p-GSK-3β$^{Ser9}$ in siRelB and sictrl cells. Protein levels were normalized against Actin. *$p < 0.05$; **$p < 0.01$; ***$p < 0.001$

the DLD-1-siRelB and DLD-1-sictrl cells were clearly separated during the 72 h's continuous monitoring. The DLD-1-siRelB cells grew much slower than the DLD-1-sictrl cells. There were statistically significant differences between the two established cell lines after culturing for 8 h and later ($p < 0.01$ at 8 h time point, $p < 0.001$ from 16 h). Cell proliferation was examined by a CCK-8 assay (Fig. 2b). The OD450 values of the DLD-1-sictrl cells were $0.73 \pm 0.01$, $1.40 \pm 0.05$, and $1.85 \pm 0.07$, while the values of the DLD-1-siRelB cells were $0.34 \pm 0.00$, $0.90 \pm 0.04$, and $1.56 \pm 0.08$ at 24, 48 and 72 h, respectively. The OD450 values were clearly decreased in the DLD-1-siRelB cells, and there were statistically significant differences between the two cell lines at 24 h ($p < 0.001$), 48 h ($p < 0.001$), and 72 h ($p < 0.05$). A Brdu assay was carried out to examine the cellular proliferation as well. The OD450 value of the DLD-1-siRelB cells ($0.28 \pm 0.01$) was lower than that of the DLD-1-sictrl cells ($0.47 \pm 0.03$) at 24 h ($p < 0.01$, Fig. 2c). The results got from the Brdu assay were in line with the CCK-8 assay data. In colony formation assay, colonies containing at least 50 cells from the DLD-1-sictrl cells were $165 \pm 4$, while $101 \pm 4$ colonies from the DLD-1-siRelB cells (Fig. 2d). The colony formation efficiency of the DLD-1-siRelB cells (10.1%) was fewer than that of the DLD-1-sictrl cells (16.5%, $p < 0.01$). Taken together, these data clearly demonstrated that the RelB-silencing in the DLD-1 cells affected cell proliferation.

RelB has been reported to function in the spontaneous or radiotherapy-induced apoptosis in tumor cells.. As shown in Fig. 2e, the percentages of spontaneous apoptosis were quite low, $0.32 \pm 0.00\%$, $0.19 \pm 0.00\%$, and $0.12 \pm 0.00\%$ in the DLD-1-siRelB group, and $0.36 \pm 0.02\%$, $0.16 \pm 0.01\%$, and $0.12 \pm 0.00\%$ in the DLD-1-sictrl group at 24, 48 and 72 h, respectively. There were no significant differences between the two established cell lines at all time points. Therefore, RelB unlikely affected spontaneous apoptosis; rather, RelB promoted the cellular proliferation of the DLD-1 cells, which further quickened the cell growth.

Protein kinase B (AKT, as known as PKB)/mammalian target of rapamycin (mTOR) signaling pathway regulates various biological processes including cell proliferation, survival, and angiogenesis. To verify whether the signaling was influenced in the DLD-1 cells lacking RelB expression, Western blotting assay was performed to examine the important molecules in the signaling. As shown in Fig. 2f, the total AKT stayed unchanged. The expression of phosphor-AKT (Thr308) and phosphor-AKT (Ser473) in the DLD-1-siRelB cells were evidently reduced compared to that of the DLD-1-sictrl cells. Phosphate and tension homology deleted on chromosome ten (PTEN), a negative regulator of the AKT signaling, was

induced in the DLD-1-siRelB cells. mTOR is a key kinase downstream of AKT. The phosphorylation of mTOR at Ser2448, regulated directly by AKT and leading to the activation of mTOR, was deduced in the DLD-1-siRelB cells. Ribosomal protein S6 kinase beta-1 (S6K1, known as p70S6 K), a downstream target of mTOR signaling, was also deduced in the DLD-1-siRelB cells. Glycogen syntheses kinase 3β (GSK-3β) could be inactivated by phosphorylation of serine at residue 9, triggered by the AKT and mitogen-activated protein kinase (MAPK) signaling pathways. The diminished phosphorylation of GSK-3β at Ser9, leading to GSK-3β activation, was observed in the DLD-1-siRelB cells. Take together, the data here showed that the AKT/mTOR signal pathway was inactivated by the RelB-silencing in the DLD-1 cells, which contributed to the impaired cell proliferation.

### RelB affects 5-FU response

5-FU is a powerful chemo-therapeutic agent used wildly in treating diverse solid tumors, including CRC [26]. To examine whether the RelB-silencing affected the 5-FU efficacy on the DLD-1 colon cancer cells, the cell growth was monitored by the x-Celligence system. Both the DLD-1-sictrl and DLD-1-siRelB cells were treated with different concentrations of 5-FU (0, 1, 5, 10, 25, 50, 100, and 200 μM) for 48 h. The cell growth rate of the DLD-1-sictrl and DLD-1-siRelB cells upon treated with 5-FU was decreased in a dose-dependent manner (Fig. 3a, b). The IC50 of 5-FU for the DLD-1-siRelB cells was 113 μM (95% CI 95–138 μM), for the DLD-1-sictrl cells was 1202 μM (95% CI 403–11258 μM). The IC50 of 5-FU for the DLD-1-siRelB cells was significantly lower compared with that of the control cells, and there was statistically significant difference ($p < 0.001$, Fig. 3c). The results suggested that of the RelB-silencing enhanced the sensitivity to 5-FU of the DLD-1 colon cancer cells.

Cell cycle distribution was examined by PI-staining which was followed by flow cytometry analyses. The distributions of $G_0$–$G_1$, S, and $G_2$-M phase in the DLD-1-sictrl cells were $41.69 \pm 0.41\%$, $27.65 \pm 0.06\%$, and $31.15 \pm 0.47\%$, while those in the DLD-1-siRelB cells were $57.65 \pm 0.36\%$, $28.89 \pm 0.71\%$, and $13.16 \pm 1.30\%$, respectively (Fig. 3d). Cell cycle progression of the DLD-1-siRelB cells was notably arrested in the $G_0$–$G_1$ phase ($p < 0.001$). Cyclin D1 can form a complex with and function as a regulatory subunit of cyclin-dependent kinase 4 (CDK4) or cyclin-dependent kinase 6 (CDK6), whose activity is required for cell cycle progression through the $G_1$ phase. Cyclin-dependent kinase inhibitor 1B (p27Kip1) binds to and prevents the activation of Cyclin D1-CDK4 complexes, and thus controls the cell cycle progression at $G_1$ phase. As shown in Fig. 3e, both Cyclin D1 and CDK4 were clearly decreased while p27[Kip1] was

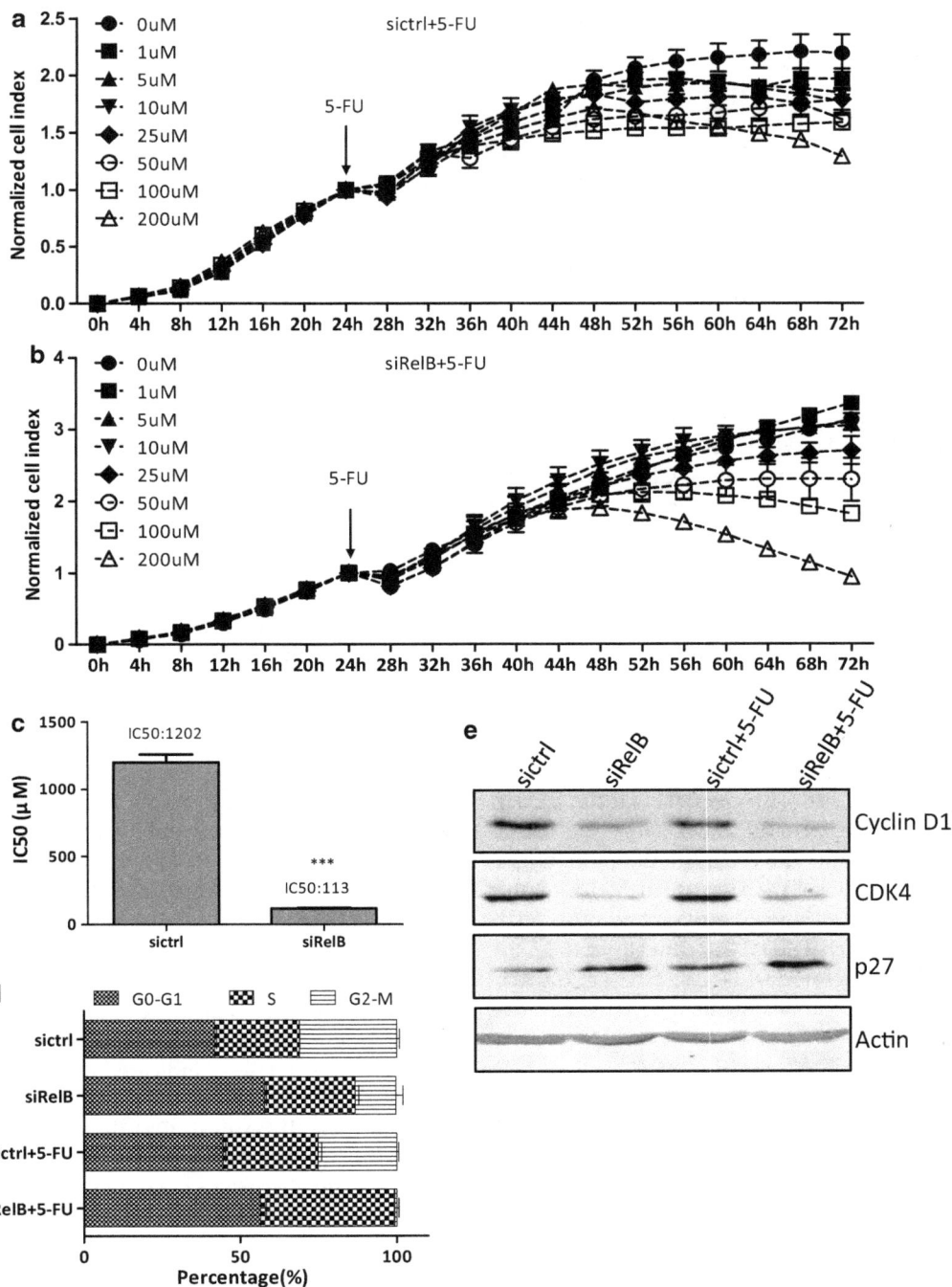

**Fig. 3** RelB-silencing enhances cytotoxic effect of 5-FU toward DLD-1 cells. **a**, **b** X-Celligence system was used to examine the effects of 5-FU on cell growth. Cells were pro-cultured in an E-plate (5000 cells per well) for 24 h and then different concentrations of 5-FU (0, 1, 5, 10, 50, 100, 200 μM) were added. Impedance of cells for indicated times were continuously monitored by the system for 72 h and the value was measured as 'normalized cell index'. **c** The dosage of 5-FU for IC50 was analyzed at the time of treated with 5-FU for 48 h. **d** Cell cycle assay determined by flow cytometry. The distribution of the $G_0$–$G_1$, S, and G2-M phase were displayed in the table. **e** Western blotting analysis of the expression of cell cycle related-proteins. Protein levels were normalized against Actin.$*p < 0.05$; $**p < 0.01$; $***p < 0.001$

increased in the DLD-1-siRelB cells. RelB likely affected several cell-cycle regulatory molecules, especially Cyclin D1, CDK4, and p27$^{Kip1}$, which contributed together to the $G_0$–$G_1$ arrest.

Expose to 5-FU (113 μM) for 48 h, the distributions of $G_0$–$G_1$, S, and $G_2$-M phase in the DLD-1-sictrl cells were $44.43 \pm 0.44\%$, $30.31 \pm 0.70\%$, and $25.26 \pm 0.30\%$, while those in the DLD-1-siRelB cells were $56.35 \pm 1.04\%$, $42.94 \pm 0.70\%$, and $0.71 \pm 0.40\%$ (Fig. 3d). Importantly, treated with 5-FU caused cell accumulation in the S phase in both cell lines, from 27.65% to 30.31% ($p < 0.05$) in the DLD-1-sictrl cells, from 28.89% to 42.94% ($p < 0.001$) in the DLD-1-siRelB cells. The induction of the cell arrest in the S-phase was significant in the DLD-1-siRelB cells upon treated with 5-FU (14.05% vs. 2.66%, $p < 0.001$). In both DLD-1-sictrl and DLD-1-siRelB cells with or without 5-FU treatment, the expression of CDK4 and p27$^{Kip1}$ stayed unchanged. However, the expression of Cyclin D1 was slightly decreased (Fig. 3e).

### RelB promotes cell migration and invasion

To investigate whether RelB played a role in cell migration in the DLD-1 cells, cells were continuously monitored by the x-Celligence system using CIM-plate for 24 h. As shown in Fig. 4a, the DLD-1-siRelB cells migrated dramatically slower than the DLD-1-sictrl cells. There were statistically significant differences between the two established cell lines from 12 to 24 h ($p < 0.05$ at 12 h, $p < 0.01$ at 15 h, $p < 0.001$ at 18, 21, and 24 h). Transwell inserts were also used to examine the role of RelB on the migration abilities of DLD-1 cells. Cells which had migrated the inserts were counted and photographed after 24 h. The number of migrated DLD-1-siRelB cells was $52 \pm 7$, less than that of the migrated DLD-1-sictrl cells, $206 \pm 18$ ($p < 0.001$, Fig. 4b). Wound healing assay was also carried out, and photographs were taken under microscope at 0, 24, 48, and 72 h, respectively. The DLD-1-siRelB cells migrated from the edge of the scratch toward the scratch centre much slower than the DLD-1-sictrl cells (Fig. 4c). Taken together, these results suggested that the RelB-silencing hampered the migratory ability of DLD-1 cells.

The invasion ability was detected also used the real-time x-Celligence system with CIM-plate pre-coated with Matrigel. As shown in Fig. 4d, the DLD-1-siRelB cells invaded the Matrigel much slower than the DLD-1-sictrl cells. There were statistically differences between the two established cell lines from 15 to 24 h ($p < 0.01$ at 15 h, $p < 0.001$ at 18, 21, and 24 h). Transwell inserts, pre-coated with Matrigel, were also used to investigate whether RelB affected the invasive ability of DLD-1 cells. The number of invaded DLD-1-siRelB cells was $56 \pm 9$, significantly fewer than that of the invaded DLD-1-sictrl cells, $157 \pm 6$ ($p < 0.001$, Fig. 4e). The RelB-silencing

markedly impaired the cell invasion capacity of DLD-1 cells.

A variety of molecules are involved in regulating cellular migration and invasion of cancer cells, including the MMPs. As shown in Fig. 4f, the protein expression of MMP2 and MMP9 in the DLD-1-siRelB was clearly decreased compared with that of the DLD-1-sictrl cells. The mRNA levels of the *MMP2* and *MMP9* genes were reduced as well (Fig. 1g). Meanwhile, the decreased Integrin β1 expression was observed in the DLD-1-siRelB cells. These results suggested that RelB promoted the DLD-1 cell migration and invasion abilities, likely due to regulating the expression of MMP2, MMP9, and Integrin β-1.

### Relationship between RelB and clinic-pathological features of CRC patients

To assess the putative clinical significance of RelB expression in CRC patients, RelB expression was identified in CRC tissues and adjacent colorectal mucosa of 93 patients by IHC staining. Representative images of RelB expression in CRC and adjacent non-neoplastic tissues were present in Fig. 5a. RelB could be detected in both the nucleus and cytoplasm fractions of CRC cells. The expression of RelB was highly expressed in the CRC tissue while the expression of RelB was barely detected in the adjacent colorectal mucosa. According to the RelB expression, 93 patients were divided into two groups, RelB-high (53/93, 56.9%) and RelB-low (40/93, 43.1%).

As shown in Table 1, the clinico-pathological association study demonstrated that the expression of RelB was positively correlated with depth of tumor invasion ($p = 0.018$), lymph node metastasis ($p < 0.001$), metastasis stage ($p = 0.031$), and pTNM stage ($p = 0.001$). The expression of RelB was not correlated with age, gender, site of origin, or differentiation status of CRC patients. Kaplan–Meier analyses indicated that CRC patients with high-RelB expression were significantly correlated with a poorer overall survival (OS) than those with low-RelB expression. ($p = 0.006$, Fig. 5b).

Univariate survival analyses indicated that tumor differentiation ($p < 0.001$), N stage ($p = 0.001$), M stage ($p = 0.001$), pTNM stage ($p < 0.001$), and RelB expression ($p = 0.002$) had statistical significances (Table 2). Multivariate Cox regression analyses indicated that tumor differentiation and RelB expression had statistical significances, with hazard ratio (HR) of 2.115 for tumor differentiation (95% CI 1.044–4.286, $p = 0.038$) and 2.996 for RelB (95% CI 1.848–6.047, $p = 0.002$). These analyses indicated that poor tumor differentiation and high RelB expression were independent factor for shorter OS in CRC patients.

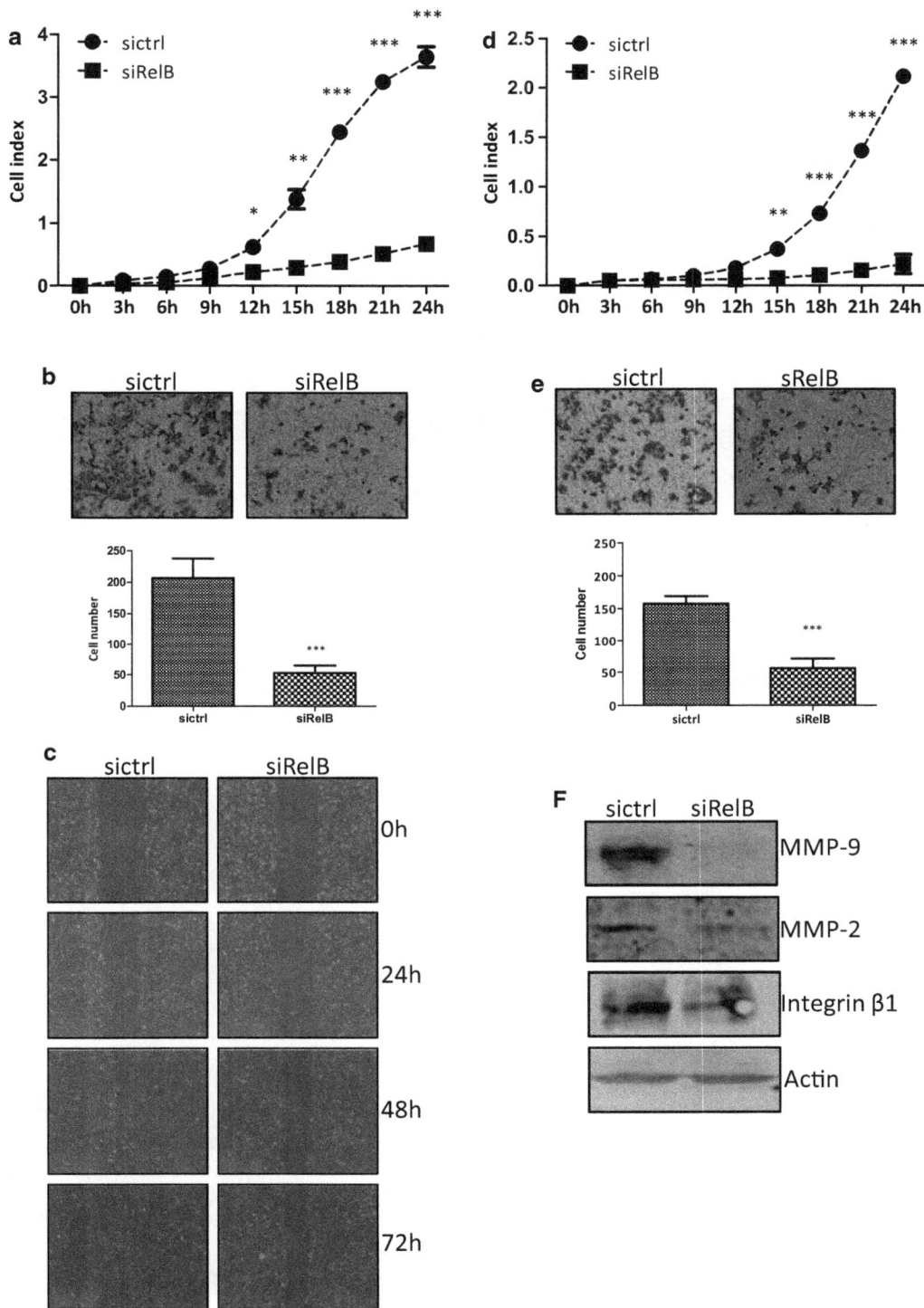

**Fig. 4** RelB-silencing hampers the migration and invasion abilities of DLD-1 cells. **a** The migration abilities of the two established cells were assessed by a real-timex-Celligence system for 24 h. **b** Representative images and data of a Transwell migration assay. The number of migratory cells were counted and photographed at 24 h. **c** Cell migration ability assessed by wound healing assay at 0, 24, 48, and 72 h. **d** The invasion abilities of the two established cells were detected by a real-time x-Celligence system using CIM-plate pre-coated with Matrigel (1:40) and Cell invasion was continuous monitored for 24 h. **e** Representative images and data of a Transwell invasion assay. Transwell chambers were pre-coated with Matrigel (1:8) and the number of invasive cells were counted and photographed at 24 h. **f** Western blotting analysis of the protein expression of MMP9, MMP2, and ITGB1 in siRelB and sictrl cells. Protein levels were normalized against Actin.*$p < 0.05$; **$p < 0.01$; ***$p < 0.001$

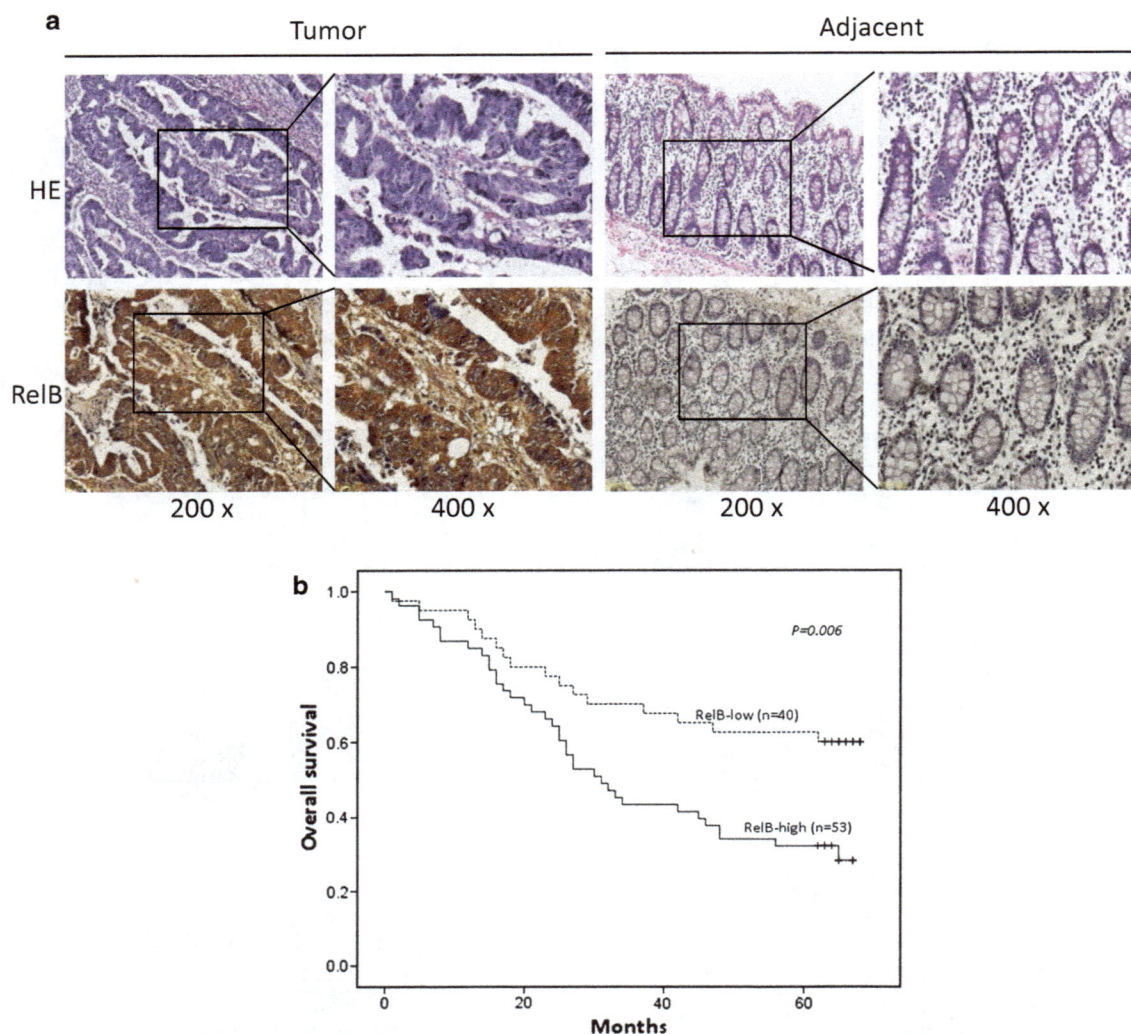

**Fig. 5** Clinical significance of RelB expression in CRC tissues. **a** Representative images of RelB expression in CRC tissues and adjacent colorectal mucosas were shown by IHC (×200 and ×400). **b** Kaplan–Meier curves that depict the 5-year overall survival in CRC patients. Patients were divided into two groups according to the RelB expression with significantly different prognosis (n = 93, p = 0.006). RelB-low represented the RelB low expression group; RelB-high represented the RelB high expression group

## Discussion

The NF-κB signaling pathway is involved in multiple steps of carcinogenesis, such as initiation, proliferation, survival, metastasis, and chemo-resistance [6]. Chronic inflammation is considered as an important carcinogenic mechanism leading to the occurrence of CRC and the NF-κB family members have been served as the bridge between inflammation and the tumourigenesis of colon epithelium [11, 27]. Studies have demonstrated that activation of targets of the NF-κB signaling pathway promote CRC metastasis and connect the inflammatory processes to carcinogenesis [10]. Many efforts have been made to develop NF-κB inhibitors, such as drugs targeting IKKs

[28]. However, these drugs have many off-target effects on other signaling pathways. Thus, targeting specific NF-κB signaling component may help to overcome these obstacles [8]. RelB is involved in the initiation, progression, and chemo-resistance of several solid tumors including prostate, breast, endometrium, bladder, laryngeal, and non-small cell lung cancer [29–32].

The functions of RelB in DLD-1 colon cancer have not been addressed. The RelB-silencing slowed down the DLD-1 cell growth. The retarded cell growth in vitro in the absence of RelB expression was largely due to the reduced cell proliferation, which was attributed to the decreased phosphor-AKT and phosphor-mTOR. These

**Table 1 Relationship between RelB expression and clinico-pathological characteristics**

| Characteristics | Total N = 93 | RelB expression | | p value |
|---|---|---|---|---|
| | | High N = 53 | Low N = 40 | |
| Age (years) | | | | |
| ≤ 60 | 34 | 18 | 16 | 0.549 |
| > 60 | 59 | 35 | 24 | |
| Gender | | | | |
| Male | 52 | 28 | 24 | 0.491 |
| Female | 41 | 25 | 16 | |
| Site | | | | |
| Right | 34 | 19 | 15 | 0.915 |
| Left | 53 | 29 | 24 | |
| Unknown | 6 | 5 | 1 | |
| Differentiation | | | | |
| Well | 2 | 1 | 1 | 0.332 |
| Moderate | 73 | 39 | 34 | |
| Poor | 18 | 13 | 5 | |
| Depth of tumor invasion | | | | |
| T1 | 0 | 0 | 0 | 0.018* |
| T2 | 5 | 1 | 4 | |
| T3 | 64 | 32 | 32 | |
| T4 | 16 | 13 | 3 | |
| Unknown | 8 | 1 | 7 | |
| Lymph nodes | | | | |
| N0 | 51 | 21 | 30 | < 0.001*** |
| N1 | 28 | 22 | 6 | |
| N2 | 9 | 9 | 0 | |
| Unknown | 5 | 1 | 4 | |
| Metastasis | | | | |
| Yes | 4 | 4 | 0 | 0.031* |
| No | 89 | 49 | 40 | |
| pTNM stage | | | | |
| I | 4 | 1 | 3 | 0.001*** |
| II | 41 | 14 | 27 | |
| III | 35 | 29 | 6 | |
| IV | 4 | 4 | 0 | |
| Unknown | 9 | 5 | 4 | |

A value of $p < 0.05$ was considered statistical significant. * $p < 0.05$, ** $p < 0.01$, *** $p < 0.001$

observations pinpointed that RelB affected DLD-1 cell proliferation by regulating the AKT/mTOR signaling pathway. AKT, a serine/threonine-specific protein kinase, regulates cell proliferation and survival via phosphorylating and activating or inactivating downstream molecules. The results here are similar to previous finding that emphasizes the role of the alternative NF-κB pathway in cell proliferation, regulated by the AKT/mTOR signaling pathway [33]. In SPC-A1 lung cancer cells, cell proliferation is suppressed by the RelB-silencing. The volume and weight of subcutaneous tumors established by the subcutaneous xenograft model using the RelB-silencing SPC-A1 cells are also reduced [25]. Increased RelB expression enhances endometrioid adenocarcinoma (EEC) cell growth by regulating cell proliferation, leading to endometrial cell tumourigenicity [32]. The regulation between RelB and the AKT signaling requires further investigations. STI571, a tyrosine kinase inhibitor, enhances RelB nuclear translocation in LnCaP prostatic cancer cells. STI571 can inhibit the PI3K-AKT-IKKα pathway in PC-3 prostatic cancer cells by decreasing the phosphorylation of AKT at Ser473 [34].

RelB is reported as a crucial positive regulator of cell survival in multiple tumors, such as multiple myeloma, chronic lymphocytic leukemia, and prostatic cancer [22, 35–37]. However, different from previous reports, the RelB-silencing did not affect the survival of DLD-1 colon cancer cells. The constantly present RelA activity in the DLD-1 cells, in the presence of RelB-silencing, is certainly a potent survival regulator.

The cell cycle was significantly arrested in the $G_0$–$G_1$ phase in the DLD-1 cells lacking RelB expression, which was caused by decreased expression levels of Cyclin D1 and CDK4 together with up-regulated expression of $p27^{KIP1}$. Cyclin D1 is expressed relatively early in the cell cycle and is essential for DNA synthesis. Studies demonstrate that NF-κB induces cell proliferation by regulating key cell-cycle regulatory genes including Cyclin D1 and CDKs [38]. It has been also shown that the RelB-silencing results in the arrest of EEC cells at the $G_1$ phase via inhibiting Cyclin D1 [32]. Therefore, our results are consistent with the previous studies that the RelB-silencing caused $G_0$–$G_1$ arrest in the DLD-1 cells and inhibited cell proliferation. GS-3β mediated phosphorylation of Cyclin D1 plays a central role in the $G_1$-to-S-phase cell-cycle transition [39]. The phosphorylation of GSK-3β, triggered by the AKT signaling pathway and led to GSK-3β inactivation, was clearly decreased in the DLD-1-siRelB cells.

5-Fluorouracil is one of the most commonly used chemotherapy drug for CRC. However, drug resistance is always acquired in CRC cells after 5-FU treatment [40]. Pharmacological targeting of NF-κB, such as inhibitor of the IKKβ to block NF-κB activation potentiate the cytotoxic effect of 5-FU [41]. Recent studies show that inhibiting NF-κB signaling may be an effective strategy to reverse 5-FU resistance in CRC [42]. Whether RelB regulates the chemo-sensitivity of CRC cells to 5-FU has not been reported. In this study, the RelB-silencing enhanced cytotoxic effects of 5-FU on the DLD-1 cells. To further explore the possible mechanism, the cell cycle of the DLD-1 cells treated with 5-FU was examined. The RelB-silencing induced cell cycle accumulation in $G_0$–$G_1$

**Table 2 Univariate and multivariate analyses of OS in patients with CRC**

| Characteristics | Univariate analysis | | Multivariate analysis | |
|---|---|---|---|---|
| | HR (95%) CI | p value | HR (95%) CI | p value |
| Age (≥ 60 vs. < 60) | 1.525 (0.838–2.776) | 0.167 | | |
| Gender (male vs. female) | 0.835 (0.487–1.432) | 0.512 | | |
| Site (right vs. left) | 0.738 (0.415–1.312) | 0.738 | | |
| Differentiation (poor vs. well, moderate) | 3.034 (1.664–5.533) | < 0.001*** | 2.115 (1.044–4.286) | 0.038* |
| T stage (T4 vs. T2, T3) | 1.574 (0.804–3.079) | 0.186 | | |
| N stage (N1, N2 vs. N0) | 2.725 (1.550–4.793) | 0.001*** | | |
| M stage (M1 vs. M0) | 2.725 (1.550–4.793) | 0.001*** | | |
| pTNM stage (III, IV vs. I, II) | 2.916 (1.635–5.201) | < 0.001*** | | |
| RelB expression (high vs. low) | 2.657 (1.438–4.907) | 0.002** | 2.996 (1.484–6.047) | 0.002** |

A value of p < 0.05 was considered statistical significant. * p < 0.05, ** p < 0.01, *** p < 0.001

phase, and caused S-phase arrest after treatment with 5-FU. The RelB-silencing enhanced cytotoxic effects to 5-FU, by increasing the cell accumulation in S-phase. Many studies show that RelB plays an important role in terms of sensitivity to chemotherapy [43]. Treated with 5-FU induces S-phase arrest, which is related with upregulation of p27 and downregulation of Cyclin D1 [44]. Cyclin D1 is needed to allow the cells progress from $G_1$ to S phase. With high level of Cyclin D1, cells can prevent 5-FU to be incorporated into the DNA [45]. Overexpression of Cyclin D1 protects CRC cells against 5-FU treatment [46]. Our results showed that there were more cells arrested in the S-phase in the absence of RelB after treated with 5-FU, likely due to reduction of Cyclin D1. Thus, the results suggested that the RelB-silencing enhanced 5-FU response by decreasing Cyclin D1 expression.

Metastasis is a main feature of advanced malignancies, and is an important factor in affecting the patient's prognosis. A variety of molecular regulators are implicated to regulate the migration and invasion of cancer cells. Integrin β1, belonging to the family of heterodimeric transmembrane cell surface receptors, has multiple functions in cell adhesion and migration [47]. A recent study shows that miR-30e-5p overexpression inhibits CRC cell adhesion, migration, and invasion by decreasing Integrin β1 [48]. Loss of Integrin β1 expression in CRC shows poor survival and correlates with advanced clinical stage and lymph node metastasis [49, 50]. Previous studies show that the RelB-silencing suppresses migration and invasion abilities of DU145 prostatic cancer cells and SPC-A1 lung cancer cells by decreasing the expression of Integrin β1 [22, 25]. Our results are similar to previous findings, indicating that RelB regulates cell migration and invasion abilities in the DLD-1 cells. MMP2 and MMP9 are the representative members of MMPs. Tumor cells can alter

extracellular matrix by overexpression of MMPs to promote invasion. Studies show that high expression levels of MMP2 in CRC tissues are correlated with reduced survival. The mRNA expression levels of MMP2 and MMP9 in CRC tissues are higher than that of normal mucosa [51, 52]. Recent studies shows tumor necrosis factor-like weak inducer of apoptosis (TWEAK) increases MMP9 expression to promote glioma cell invasion by activating the non-canonical NF-κB signaling pathway. RelB can promote invasion in glioma cells without affecting the activity of RelA and the classical NF-κB signaling [53]. Bioinformatics analysis also suggests that MMPs family genes are positively correlated with RelB in glioma tumorigenesis [54]. Moreover, Curcumin can inhibit colon cancer cell invasion by suppressing NF-κB-mediated transcriptional activation MMP9 [55]. NIK- and IKKβ-binding protein (NIBP) increases the CRC metastatic potential by activating the NF-κB pathway and increasing MMP2 and MMP9 expression [13]. Our results showed that the RelB-silencing suppressed the migration and invasion abilities of DLD-1 cells. The expression of MMP2 and MMP9, both at protein and mRNA levels, was decreased in the DLD-1-siRelB cells. The results here are consistent with previous studies, suggesting that RelB plays a role in the cell migration and invasion in DLD-1 cells by regulating the MMP2 and MMP9 expression.

In present study, we found that RelB expression was positively related to depth of tumor invasion, lymph node metastasis, metastasis stage, and pTNM stage. Therefore, the results indicated that RelB played a significant role in the metastasis of CRC, concomitant with in vitro experimental results. Furthermore, multivariate Cox regression analyses revealed that high expression of RelB was a poor prognostic marker in CRC, indicating that RelB can be considered as an independent prognostic factor. The TNM staging system is currently used to assess the prognosis of patients with CRC. For rectal cancer patients who undergo neo-adjuvant chemo-radiation, it is sometime unable to detect enough lymph nodes. Then TNM staging system is not always accurate. New biological markers of prognosis such as RelB may supplement its disadvantages.

## Conclusions

Our findings add an understanding to the unexplored functions of NF-κB subunit, RelB, in CRC. RelB significantly affects cell proliferation, cell migration and invasion, and chemo-sensitivity to 5-FU treatment via cell cycle alteration in DLD-1 cells. Moreover, RelB may function as a potential prognostic indicator of CRC patients. Therefore, RelB may represent a new strategy to CRC therapy. Our present study has several limitations. We used only one colon cancer cell line and did not perform any in vivo expression experiments, which will be performed in our future studies.

### Abbreviations
CRC: colorectal cancer; NF-κB: nuclear transcription factor kappa B; NIK: NF-κB inducing kinase; NIBP: NIK- and IKK-β binding protein; EZH2: enhancer of zeste homology 2; 5-FU: 5-fluorouracil; NSCLC: non-small cell lung cancer; FBS: fetal bovine serum; shRNA: short hairpin RNA; Abs: antibodies; qRT-PCR: quantitative real-time PCR; CCK-8: Cell Counting Kit-8; PI: propidium iodide; PBS: phosphate-buffered saline; TMA: tissue microarray; IHC: immunohistochemistry; SD: standard deviation; OS: overall survival; CE: cytoplasmic extract; NE: nuclear extract; OD450: optical density at 450 nm; IC50: 50% inhibition of proliferation; MMPs: matrix metalloproteinase family; HR: hazard ratio; TWEAK: tumor necrosis factor-like weak inducer of apoptosis.

### Authors' contributions
FG designed the research; XJZ, ZLS, HYY, JJX, and WJL performed the research; FG, XJZ, and ZLS analyzed the data; FG, ZLS, and XJZ wrote the manuscript. All authors read and approved the final manuscript.

### Author details
[1] Department of General Surgery, The First Affiliated Hospital of Soochow University, Suzhou 215006, China. [2] Center for Clinical Laboratory, The First Affiliated Hospital of Soochow University, Suzhou 215006, China. [3] Department of Clinical Laboratory, Nanjing Medical University Affiliated Suzhou Hospital, Suzhou 215006, China. [4] Department of Oncology, Nanjing Medical University Affiliated Suzhou Hospital, Baita West Road 16, Suzhou 215001, China.

### Acknowledgements
Not applicable.

### Competing interests
The authors declare that they have no competing interests.

### Funding
This study was supported by the Project of Invigorating Health Care through Science, Technology and Education, Jiangsu Provincial Medical Youth Talent (Grant Number: QNRC2016725), and the Suzhou Natural Science Foundation (Grant Number: SS201875).

### References
1. Siegel R, Miller K, Jemal A. Cancer statistics, 2018. CA Cancer J Clin. 2018;68(1):7–30.
2. Chen W, Zheng R, Baade PD, Zhang S, Zeng H, Bray F, Jemal A, Yu XQ, He J. Cancer statistics in China, 2015. CA Cancer J Clin. 2016;66(2):115–32.
3. Siegel RL, Miller KD, Fedewa SA, Ahnen DJ, Meester RGS, Barzi A, Jemal A. Colorectal cancer statistics, 2017. CA Cancer J Clin. 2017;67(3):177–93.
4. Tsilimigras D, Ntanasis-Stathopoulos I, Bagante F, Moris D, Cloyd J, Spartalis E, Pawlik T. Clinical significance and prognostic relevance of KRAS, BRAF, PI3K and TP53 genetic mutation analysis for resectable and unresectable colorectal liver metastases: a systematic review of the current evidence. Surg Oncol. 2018;27(2):280–8.
5. Sen R, Baltimore D. Inducibility of kappa immunoglobulin enhancer-binding protein Nf-kappa B by a posttranslational mechanism. Cell. 1986;47(6):921–8.
6. Kaltschmidt B, Greiner J, Kadhim H, Kaltschmidt C. Subunit-specific role of NF-κB in cancer. Biomedicines. 2018;6(2):44–57.
7. Colombo F, Zambrano S, Agresti A. NF-κB, the importance of being dynamic: role and insights in cancer. Biomedicines. 2018;6(2):45–58.
8. Tegowski M, Baldwin A. Noncanonical NF-κB in cancer. Biomedicines. 2018;6(2):66–86.
9. Imbert V, Peyron J. NF-κB in hematological malignances. Biomedicines. 2017;5(2):27–42.
10. Patel M, Horgan PG, McMillan DC, Edwards J. NF-kappaB pathways in the development and progression of colorectal cancer. Transl Res. 2018;197:43–56.
11. Porta C, Ippolito A, Consonni F, Carraro L, Celesti G, Correale C, Grizzi F, Pasqualini F, Tartari S, Rinaldi M, et al. Protumor steering of cancer inflammation by p50 NF-κB enhances colorectal cancer progression. Cancer Immunol Res. 2018;6(5):578–93.
12. Greten F, Eckmann L, Greten T, Park J, Li Z, Egan L, Kagnoff M, Karin M. IKKbeta links inflammation and tumorigenesis in a mouse model of colitis-associated cancer. Cell. 2004;118(3):285–96.
13. Qin M, Liu S, Li A, Xu C, Tan L, Huang J, Liu S. NIK- and IKKβ-binding protein promotes colon cancer metastasis by activating the classical NF-κB pathway and MMPs. Tumour Biol. 2016;37(5):5979–90.
14. Anthony N, Baiget J, Berretta G, Boyd M, Breen D, Edwards J, Gamble C, Gray A, Harvey A, Hatziieremia S, et al. Inhibitory kappa B kinase α (IKKα) inhibitors that recapitulate their selectivity in cells against isoform-related biomarkers. J Med Chem. 2017;60(16):7043–66.
15. Baud V, Collares D. Post-translational modifications of RelB NF-kappaB subunit and associated functions. Cells. 2016;5(2):22–32.
16. Grinberg-Bleyer Y, Caron R, Seeley J, De Silva N, Schindler C, Hayden M, Klein U, Ghosh S. The alternative NF-κB pathway in regulatory T cell homeostasis and suppressive function. J Immunol. 2018;200(7):2362–71.
17. Weih F, Carrasco D, Durham S, Barton D, Rizzo C, Ryseck R, Lira S, Bravo R. Multiorgan inflammation and hematopoietic abnormalities in mice with a targeted disruption of RelB, a member of the NF-kappa B/Rel family. Cell. 1995;80(2):331–40.
18. Guo F, Tanzer S, Busslinger M, Weih F. Lack of nuclear factor-kappa B2/p100 causes a RelB-dependent block in early B lymphopoiesis. Blood. 2008;112(3):551–9.
19. Shen M, Duan X, Zhou P, Zhou W, Wu X, Xu S, Chen Y, Tao Z. Lymphotoxin β receptor activation promotes bladder cancer in a nuclear factor-κB-dependent manner. Mol Med Rep. 2015;11(2):783–90.
20. Lessard L, Bégin L, Gleave M, Mes-Masson A, Saad F. Nuclear localisation of nuclear factor-kappaB transcription factors in prostate cancer: an immunohistochemical study. Br J Cancer. 2005;93(9):1019–23.
21. Wei X, Xu Y, Xu F, Chaiswing L, Schnell D, Noel T, Wang C, Chen J, St Clair D, St Clair W. RelB expression determines the differential effects of ascorbic acid in normal and cancer cells. Cancer Res. 2017;77(6):1345–56.
22. Wang J, Yi S, Zhou J, Zhang Y, Guo F. The NF-κB subunit RelB regulates the migration and invasion abilities and the radio-sensitivity of prostate cancer cells. Int J Oncol. 2016;49(1):381–92.

23. Lawrence C, Baldwin A. Non-canonical EZH2 transcriptionally activates RelB in triple negative breast cancer. PLoS ONE. 2016;11(10):e0165005.

24. Qin H, Zhou J, Zhou P, Xu J, Tang Z, Ma H, Guo F. Prognostic significance of RelB overexpression in non-small cell lung cancer patients. Thorac Cancer. 2016;7(4):415–21.

25. Qin H, Zhou J, Xu J, Cheng L, Tang Z, Ma H, Guo F. The nuclear transcription factor RelB functions as an oncogene in human lung adenocarcinoma SPC-A1 cells. Cancer Cell Int. 2018;18(1):88–101.

26. Tejpar S, Yan P, Piessevaux H, Dietrich D, Brauchli P, Klingbiel D, Fiocca R, Delorenzi M, Bosman F, Roth A. Clinical and pharmacogenetic determinants of 5-fluorouracil/leucovorin/irinotecan toxicity: results of the PETACC-3 trial. Eur J Cancer. 2018;99:66–77.

27. Vaiopoulos A, Papachroni K, Papavassiliou A. Colon carcinogenesis: learning from NF-kappaB and AP-1. Int J Biochem Cell Biol. 2010;42(7):1061–5.

28. Awasthee N, Rai V, Chava S, Nallasamy P, Kunnumakkara A, Bishayee A, Chauhan S, Challagundla K, Gupta S. Targeting IkappaB kinases for cancer therapy. Semin Cancer Biol. 2018. https://doi.org/10.1016/j.semcancer.2018.02.007.

29. Zhu HC, Qiu T, Dan C, Liu XH, Hu CH. Blockage of RelB expression by gene silencing enhances the radiosensitivity of androgen independent prostate cancer cells. Mol Med Rep. 2015;11(2):1167–73.

30. Mineva N, Wang X, Yang S, Ying H, Xiao Z, Holick M, Sonenshein G. Inhibition of RelB by 1,25-dihydroxyvitamin D3 promotes sensitivity of breast cancer cells to radiation. J Cell Physiol. 2009;220(3):593–9.

31. Giopanou I, Lilis I, Papaleonidopoulos V, Marazioti A, Spella M, Vreka M, Papadaki H, Stathopoulos G. Comprehensive evaluation of nuclear factor-κB expression patterns in non-small cell lung cancer. PLoS ONE. 2015;10(7):e0132527.

32. Ge QL, Liu SH, Ai ZH, Tao MF, Ma L, Wen SY, Dai M, Liu F, Liu HS, Jiang RZ, et al. RelB/NF-kappaB links cell cycle transition and apoptosis to endometrioid adenocarcinoma tumorigenesis. Cell Death Dis. 2016;7(10):e2402.

33. Chen Q, Costa M. PI3K/Akt/mTOR signaling pathway and the biphasic effect of arsenic in carcinogenesis. Mol Pharmacol. 2018;94(1):784–92.

34. Holley A, Xu Y, St Clair D, St Clair W. RelB regulates manganese superoxide dismutase gene and resistance to ionizing radiation of prostate cancer cells. Ann N Y Acad Sci. 2010;1201:129–36.

35. Xu J, Zhou P, Wang W, Sun A, Guo F. RelB, together with RelA, sustains cell survival and confers proteasome inhibitor sensitivity of chronic lymphocytic leukemia cells from bone marrow. J Mol Med. 2014;92(1):77–92.

36. Demchenko YN, Glebov OK, Zingone A, Keats JJ, Bergsagel PL, Kuehl WM. Classical and/or alternative NF-kappaB pathway activation in multiple myeloma. Blood. 2010;115(12):3541–52.

37. Vallabhapurapu S, Noothi S, Pullum D, Lawrie C, Pallapati R, Potluri V, Kuntzen C, Khan S, Plas D, Orlowski R, et al. Transcriptional repression by the HDAC4-RelB-p52 complex regulates multiple myeloma survival and growth. Nat Commun. 2015;6:8428–42.

38. Joyce D, Albanese C, Steer J, Fu M, Bouzahzah B, Pestell R. NF-kappaB and cell-cycle regulation: the cyclin connection. Cytokine Growth Factor Rev. 2001;12(1):73–90.

39. Manning B, Toker A. AKT/PKB signaling: navigating the network. Cell. 2017;169(3):381–405.

40. Chen L, She X, Wang T, He L, Shigdar S, Duan W, Kong L. Overcoming acquired drug resistance in colorectal cancer cells by targeted delivery of 5-FU with EGF grafted hollow mesoporous silica nanoparticles. Nanoscale. 2015;7(33):14080–92.

41. Lagadec P, Griessinger E, Nawrot M, Fenouille N, Colosetti P, Imbert V, Mari M, Hofman P, Czerucka D, Rousseau D, et al. Pharmacological targeting of NF-kappaB potentiates the effect of the topoisomerase inhibitor CPT-11 on colon cancer cells. Br J Cancer. 2008;98(2):335–44.

42. Wang Z, Zhao X, Wang W, Liu Y, Li Y, Gao J, Wang C, Zhou M, Liu R, Xu G, et al. ZBTB7 evokes 5-fluorouracil resistance in colorectal cancer through the NF-κB signaling pathway. Int J Oncol. 2018;53(5):2102–10.

43. Fabre C, Mimura N, Bobb K, Kong S, Gorgun G, Cirstea D, Hu Y, Minami J, Ohguchi H, Zhang J, et al. Dual inhibition of canonical and noncanonical NF-κB pathways demonstrates significant antitumor activities in multiple myeloma. Clin Cancer Res. 2012;18(17):4669–81.

44. Choi J, Yoon J, Won Y, Park B, Lee Y. Chloroquine enhances the chemotherapeutic activity of 5-fluorouracil in a colon cancer cell line via cell cycle alteration. APMIS. 2012;120(7):597–604.

45. Meiyanto E, Septisetyani EP, Larasati YA, Kawaichi M. Curcumin analog pentagamavunon-1 (PGV-1) sensitizes Widr cells to 5-fluorouracil through inhibition of NF-kappaB activation. Asian Pac J Cancer Prev. 2018;19(1):49–56.

46. Qin A, Yu Q, Gao Y, Tan J, Huang H, Qiao Z, Qian W. Inhibition of STAT3/cyclinD1 pathway promotes chemotherapeutic sensitivity of colorectal caner. Biochem Biophys Res Commun. 2015;457(4):681–7.

47. Sun Q, Zhou C, Ma R, Guo Q, Huang H, Hao J, Liu H, Shi R, Liu B. Prognostic value of increased integrin-beta 1 expression in solid cancers: a meta-analysis. Onco Targets Ther. 2018;11:1787–99.

48. Laudato S, Patil N, Abba M, Leupold J, Benner A, Gaiser T, Marx A, Allgayer H. P53-induced miR-30e-5p inhibits colorectal cancer invasion and metastasis by targeting ITGA6 and ITGB1. Int J Cancer. 2017;141(9):1879–90.

49. Langan R, Mullinax J, Ray S, Raiji M, Schaub N, Xin H, Koizumi T, Steinberg S, Anderson A, Wiegand G, et al. A pilot study assessing the potential role of non-CD133 colorectal cancer stem cells as biomarkers. J Cancer. 2012;3:231–40.

50. Liu Q, Gao X, Chang W, Gong H, Fu C, Zhang W, Cao G. Expression of ITGB1 predicts prognosis in colorectal cancer: a large prospective study based on tissue microarray. Int J Clin Exp Pathol. 2015;8(10):12802–10.

51. Vinnakota K, Zhang Y, Selvanesan B, Topi G, Salim T, Sand-Dejmek J, Jönsson G, Sjölander A. M2-like macrophages induce colon cancer cell invasion via matrix metalloproteinases. J Cell Physiol. 2017;232(12):3468–80.

52. Collins H, Morris T, Watson S. Spectrum of matrix metalloproteinase expression in primary and metastatic colon cancer: relationship to the tissue inhibitors of metalloproteinases and membrane type-1-matrix metalloproteinase. Br J Cancer. 2001;84(12):1664–70.

53. Cherry E, Lee D, Jung J, Sitcheran R. Tumor necrosis factor-like weak inducer of apoptosis (TWEAK) promotes glioma cell invasion through induction of NF-κB-inducing kinase (NIK) and noncanonical NF-κB signaling. Mol Cancer. 2015;14(1):9–21.

54. Shen F, Guo Q, Hu Q, Zeng A, Wu W, Yan W, You Y. RelB, a good prognosis predictor, links cell-cycle and migration to glioma tumorigenesis. Oncol Lett. 2018;15(4):4404–10.

55. Tong W, Wang Q, Sun D, Suo J. Curcumin suppresses colon cancer cell invasion via AMPK-induced inhibition of NF-κB, uPA activator and MMP9. Oncol Lett. 2016;12(5):4139–46.

# 10

# Somatic mutations in renal cell carcinomas from Chinese patients revealed by whole exome sequencing

Jie Wang[1], Zhijun Xi[1*], Jianzhong Xi[2*], Hanshuo Zhang[3], Juan Li[2], Yuchao Xia[4] and Yuanxue Yi[4]

## Abstract

**Background:** While the somatic mutation profiles of renal cell carcinoma (RCC) have been revealed by several studies worldwide, the overwhelming majority of those were not derived from Chinese patients. The landscape of somatic alterations in RCC from Chinese patients still needs to be elucidated to determine whether discrepancies exist between Chinese patients and sufferers from other countries and regions.

**Methods:** We collected specimens from 26 Chinese patients with primary RCC, including 15 clear cell renal cell carcinoma (ccRCC) samples, 5 papillary renal cell carcinoma (PRCC) samples and 6 chromophobe renal cell carcinoma (ChRCC) samples. Genomic DNAs were isolated from paired tumor-normal tissues and subjected to whole exome sequencing (WES). Immunohistochemistry analysis was performed to detect the programmed death ligand 1 (PD-L1) expression in tumor tissues.

**Results:** A total of 1920 nonsynonymous somatic variants in exons and 86 mutations at splice junctions were revealed. The tumor mutation burden of ccRCC was significantly higher than that of ChRCC ($P < 0.05$). For both ccRCC and PRCC, the most frequent substitution in somatic missense mutations was T:A > A:T, which was different from that recorded in the COSMIC database. Among eight significantly mutated genes in ccRCC in the TCGA database, six genes were verified in our study including *VHL* (67%), *BAP1* (13%), *SETD2* (13%), *PBRM1* (7%), *PTEN* (7%) and *MTOR* (7%). All the mutations detected in those genes had not been reported in ccRCC before, except for alterations in *VHL* and *PBRM1*. Regarding the frequently mutated genes in PRCC in our study, *DEPDC4* (p.E293A, p.T279A), *PNLIP* (p.N401Y, p.F342L) and *SARDH* (p.H554Q, p.M1T) were newly detected gene mutations predicted to be deleterious. As the most recurrently mutated gene in ChRCC in the TCGA dataset, *TP53* (p.R81Q) was somatically altered only in one ChRCC case in this study. The HIF-1 signaling pathway was the most affected pathway in ccRCC, while the PI3K-Akt signaling pathway was altered in all of the three RCC types. Membranous PD-L1 expression was positive in tumor cells from 6/26 (23%) RCC specimens. The PD-L1-positive rate was higher in RCC samples with the somatically mutated genes *CSPG4*, *DNAH11*, *INADL* and *TMPRSS13* than in specimens without those ($P < 0.05$).

**Conclusions:** Using WES, we identified somatic mutations in 26 Chinese patients with RCC, which enriched the racial diversity of the somatic mutation profiles of RCC subjects, and revealed a few discrepancies in molecular characterizations between our study and published datasets. We also identified numerous newly detected somatic mutations, which further supplements the somatic mutation landscape of RCC. Moreover, 4 somatically mutated genes,

*Correspondence: xizhijun@hsc.pku.edu.cn; jzxi@pku.edu.cn
[1] Department of Urology, Peking University First Hospital and Institute of Urology, National Research Center for Genitourinary Oncology, No 8, Xishiku Street, Xicheng District, Beijing, China
[2] Department of Biomedical Engineering, College of Engineering, Peking University, No 5, Yiheyuan Road, Haidian District, Beijing, China
Full list of author information is available at the end of the article

including *CSPG4*, *DNAH11*, *INADL* and *TMPRSS13*, might be promising predictive factors of PD-L1-positive expression in RCC tumor cells.

**Keywords:** Renal cell carcinoma, Whole exome sequencing, Somatic mutation, Gene, PD-L1

## Background

Renal cell carcinoma (RCC) is one of the most common human malignancies, with an estimated 63,990 new cases and 14,400 deaths occurring annually in the United States [1]. In China, RCC is not reported among the top 10 cancer incidences and mortalities [2]. Among the different histological subtypes of RCC, clear cell renal cell carcinoma (ccRCC) is the most common type, followed by papillary renal cell carcinoma (PRCC) and chromophobe renal cell carcinoma (ChRCC). The molecular profiles of those three common subtypes of RCC have been studied using next generation sequencing (NGS) in a multitude of research projects such as The Cancer Genome Atlas (TCGA) and other projects from Japan, the European Union and France.

In ccRCC, *VHL* is the gene most frequently altered by germline and somatic mutations. According to TCGA analysis, *VHL*, *PBRM1*, *BAP1* and *SETD2* are the four most frequently somatically mutated genes in human ccRCC, all of which are typically mutated in combination with the loss of chromosome 3p, followed by *KDM5C*, *PTEN*, *MTOR* and *TP53* [3]. PRCC consists of two subtypes, type 1 and 2, based on distinct histological and genetic characteristics. In the TCGA database, several significantly mutated genes have been identified, including *MET*, *SETD2*, *NF2*, *KDM6A*, *SMARCB1*, *FAT1*, *BAP1*, *PBRM1*, *STAG2*, *NFE2L2* and *TP53*. Notably, somatic mutations in *MET* are mainly found in type 1 PRCC, whereas type 2 PRCC is primarily associated with somatic mutations in *SETD2*, *BAP1* and *PBRM1*, all of which are also frequently mutated in human ccRCC. Furthermore, *TFE3* and *TFEB* gene fusion and loss of *CNKD2A* have been shown to be dominant in type 2 PRCC [4]. In contrast to ccRCC and PRCC, ChRCC mainly manifests copy number variations of chromosomes, while relatively few somatic mutations are shown. *TP53* is the most recurrently somatically mutated gene in the TCGA dataset, followed by *PTEN* [5].

Up to now, the overwhelming majority of genomic datas of RCC have originated from the USA and European countries. As a consequence, most specimens have been collected from Caucasian and black patients, while very few Asian patients have been included. In the cBioPortal for Cancer Genomics (http://www.cbioportal.org), only 98 ccRCC samples from Japanese patients have been investigated. According to the International Cancer Genome Consortium (ICGC) Data Portal (https://dcc.icgc.org), only 10 Chinese donors are available in kidney cancer projects. The discrepancy between the somatic mutation profiles of RCC from Chinese patients and the published data still requires elucidation.

As a biomarker of response to the immune checkpoint inhibitor, PD-L1 expression in tumor cells was shown to correlate with the efficacy of immunotherapy involving programmed death 1 (PD-1)/PD-L1 inhibitors in many cancers. A recent study indicated that a longer progression-free survival was achieved with nivolumab plus ipilimumab than with sunitinib among advanced RCC patients with $\geq$ 1% PD-L1 expression but not among those with < 1% PD-L1 expression. Furthermore, PD-L1 was shown to serve as a predictive factor in terms of response and overall survival benefit from the nivolumab plus ipilimumab combination or nivolumab monotherapy as second-line treatment [6]. However, the association between PD-L1 expression and somatic mutations in RCC has not been widely investigated.

In this study, we aimed to uncover the somatic alterations in RCC from Chinese patients diagnosed with primary RCC including ccRCC, PRCC and ChRCC by using WES, as well as tried to find some correlations between somatic mutations and PD-L1 expression.

## Methods

### Patients and samples

Cancerous and paracancerous tissues were collected from patients with RCC who underwent either radical nephrectomy or partial nephrectomy at the Department of Urology of Peking University First Hospital. These tissues were promptly frozen in liquid nitrogen during the surgery and then stored at − 80 °C in our departmental tissue bank. A total of 26 RCC specimens with paired tumor-normal freshly frozen tissues were included in the present study, including 15 ccRCC specimens, 5 PRCC specimens and 6 ChRCC specimens. The pathological characteristics of these specimens were confirmed by pathologists. The study was approved by the Biomedical Research Ethics Committee of Peking University First Hospital, and written informed content was acquired from all enrolled patients.

### DNA extraction and WES

Genomic DNA (gDNA) was extracted from those tissues using TIANamp Genomic DNA Kit (Tiangen, China) according to the manufacturer's instructions. The quality and quantity of the DNA were evaluated using the Qubit 3 Fluorometer (Invitrogen, United States), the Agilent 2100 Bioanalyzer (Agilent, United States) and agarose gel electrophoresis. The library was prepared using NEBNext DNA Library Prep Master Mix Set for Illumina (New England BioLabs, United States). Briefly: 200 ng of gDNA from each specimen was fragmented. The barcoded fragments were purified by XP beads and hybridized to the "capture library" containing specially designed probes. Subsequently, the hybridized DNA fragments were captured using streptavidin-coated beads, and the captured libraries were amplified with indexing primers and then purified. The quantity and quality of the final library were evaluated by the Qubit 3 Fluorometer and Agilent 2100 Bioanalyzer respectively. Meanwhile, qPCR was used to quantify each index-tagged library. At last, sequencing was performed on the Illumina Hiseq 2000 platform. The tumor tissue sequencing depth was set to 200×, and the paracancerous tissue sequencing depth was set to 100×.

### Data analysis

The short reads were first aligned to the hg19 reference genome using the Burrows Wheeler Aligner (BWA). The alignments were then recalibrated and filtered by the Genome Analysis Toolkit (GATK) [7]. MuTect2 was then applied to identify somatic mutations by comparing tumors against paracancerous tissues. Somatic variants were further filtered if the sequencing depth was below 10×, the coverage was below 5 reads or the mutation frequency was below 1%.

All somatic variants were annotated by Annovar [8]. The functional impacts of missense mutations were predicted by SIFT, PolyPhen2 HDIV, PolyPhen2 HVAR, LRT, MutationTaster, MutationAssessor, and FATHMM. The variants were considered deleterious mutations if they were scored by at least two algorithms as deleterious. Missense mutations that were not scored by those algorithms were classified as "unavailable" and excluded from the analysis. Other variants, including nonsense, frameshift and canonical ± 1 or ± 2 splice site mutations, were deemed pathogenic. This classification is consistent with the standards and guidelines of the American College of Medical Genetics (ACMG) [9].

The lollipop plot and oncoprint diagram were created using the Mutation Mapper and Oncoprint tools respectively [10, 11]. The tumor mutation burden (TMB), an emerging biomarker of immunotherapy responses, was calculated for each case [12]. The major signaling pathways associated with RCC in which genes were somatically mutated were analysed using the Kyoto Encyclopedia of Genes and Genomes (KEGG) database (http://www.genome.jp/kegg/pathway.html) [13].

### Immunohistochemistry and PD-L1 quantification

After all haematoxylin and eosin (H&E) tumor slides were reviewed by two pathologists, the corresponding formalin-fixed and paraffin-embedded blocks from the 26 RCC specimens were prepared into slides. All tumor slides were de-paraffinized and stained for PD-L1 using standard IHC techniques. The optimal dilution of the PD-L1 Rabbit mAb (E1L3 N; Cell Signaling Technology, Danvers, Massachusetts) was 1:200. All stained slides were assessed by two pathologists who were blinded to the clinical outcomes. The PD-L1 immunoreactivity in tumor cells was scored as follows: strong positive (++ to +++), > 5% stained cells with moderate or strong staining; weakly positive (+), 1–5% stained cells with any intensity; negative (−), < 1% stained cells.

### Statistical analysis

Correlations between the histological subtypes of RCC and the TMB were evaluated by the Mann–Whitney U test, and associations between PD-L1 expression and somatically altered genes were analysed via the Fisher's exact test. $P < 0.05$ was considered statistically significant. SPSS 23.0 (USA) was employed to perform all the tests.

## Results

### Clinical and pathological characteristics of patients

In this study, 26 RCC cases consisted of 15 ccRCC cases, 6 ChRCC cases and 5 PRCC cases. In total, 9 females and 17 males were included. The median age was 59. All the patients suffered from primary RCC and none manifested distant or lymphatic metastasis. Details of clinical and pathological characteristics of the 26 patients with RCC are listed in Table 1.

### Summary of somatic mutations

In total, 1920 somatic nonsynonymous variants in exons and 86 mutations at splice junctions were revealed. Among all the somatic nonsynonymous variants, 1689 missense mutations, 139 stop-gain mutations, 84 frameshift mutations and 8 stop-loss mutations were identified. The TMB of ccRCC was significantly higher than that of ChRCC as revealed by the Mann–Whitney U test (P < 0.05), while the TMB of PRCC was not significantly different from that of ccRCC or ChRCC (P > 0.05) (Fig. 1). The TMB showed no statistical correlations with tumor grade, stage or size (P > 0.05).

In 15 ccRCC cases, we identified 1024 missense mutations, 81stop-gain mutations, 50 frameshift mutations, 48 splice mutations and 6 stop-loss mutations (Fig. 2a). Among all the missense mutations with available annotation information, 724 variants (72%) were predicted to be deleterious, and 277 mutations (28%) were predicted

**Table 1  clinical and pathological information of RCC patients**

| Sample ID | Gender | Age at Diagnosis | Surgical Approach | Histological Subtype | Laterality | Tumor Grade | TNM Stage | Tumor Stage |
|---|---|---|---|---|---|---|---|---|
| 1 | M | 44 | LSRN | ccRCC | Left | G3 | T3aN0M0 | III |
| 3 | M | 33 | LSPN | ccRCC | Left | G1 | T1aN0M0 | I |
| 4 | M | 60 | LSRN | ccRCC | Left | G2 | T1aN0M0 | I |
| 5 | F | 52 | LSPN | ccRCC | Left | G1 | T1aN0M0 | I |
| 6 | M | 59 | LSPN | ccRCC | Left | G1 | T1aN0M0 | I |
| 7 | F | 59 | LSRN | ChRCC | Right | NA | T1bN0M0 | I |
| 8 | F | 70 | LSPN | ccRCC | Right | G1 | T1aN0M0 | I |
| 9 | F | 58 | LSRN | ccRCC | Right | G2 | T3aN0M0 | III |
| 10 | M | 49 | LSRN | ccRCC | Right | G2 | T2aN0M0 | II |
| 11 | M | 70 | LSRN | ccRCC | Right | G1 | T1bN0M0 | I |
| 12 | M | 76 | LSRN | ccRCC | Right | G3 | T3bN0M0 | III |
| 13 | M | 46 | LSPN | ccRCC | Left | G3 | T1aN0M0 | I |
| 14 | M | 63 | LSRN | ccRCC | Right | G2 | T1bN0M0 | I |
| 15 | M | 52 | LSRN | ccRCC | Left | G1 | T1bN0M0 | I |
| 25 | F | 43 | ORN | ChRCC | Left | NA | T2bN0M0 | II |
| 36 | M | 38 | LSRN | ccRCC | Left | G3 | T1aN0M0 | I |
| 38 | M | 60 | LSRN | ccRCC | Left | G1 | T1bN0M0 | I |
| 39 | F | 24 | LSRN | ChRCC | Right | NA | T1bN0M0 | I |
| 78 | M | 54 | LSRN | ChRCC | Left | NA | T3aN0M0 | III |
| 82 | F | 76 | LSPN | PRCC (II) | Right | G3 | T1aN0M0 | I |
| 98 | F | 63 | LSPN | ChRCC | Left | NA | T1aN0M0 | I |
| 114 | M | 65 | LSRN | ChRCC | Right | NA | T1bN0M0 | I |
| 129 | M | 52 | LSRN | PRCC (II) | Right | G2 | T3aN0M0 | III |
| 130 | F | 78 | LSRN | PRCC (II) | Right | G2 | T1bN0M0 | I |
| 131 | M | 72 | LSPN | PRCC (II) | Right | G2 | T1aN0M0 | I |
| 137 | M | 38 | LSPN | PRCC (I) | Right | G2 | T1aN0M0 | I |

M, male; F, female; LSRN, laparoscopic radical nephrectomy; LSPN, laparoscopic partial nephrectomy; ORN, open radical nephrectomy; NA, not available

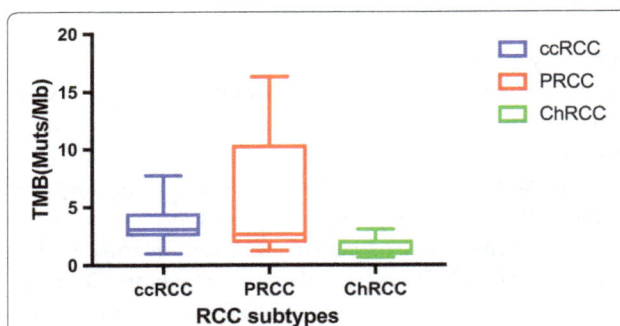

**Fig. 1** The box plot showing that the distribution of TMB in different RCC subtypes

to be neutral or benign (Fig. 2b). The most frequent substitution in somatic missense mutations was exposed to be T:A > A:T, which was also the least common type in ChRCC cases (Fig. 3). In total, 13 mutated genes had a mutation frequency above 20%, each of which was

altered in at least three samples (Fig. 4a). Consistent with previous studies, the most commonly mutated gene was *VHL* (10/15) in our study. These mutations contained five missense mutations (p.P86L, p.R120G, p.S80N, p.V130L, p.F136V), three frameshift deletions (p.G127fs, p.N141fs, p.N90fs) and two stop-gain mutations (p.E70X, p.Q145X). Those variants in *VHL* were located in the commonly known region of the VHL protein domain, all of which had been reported in the TCGA or COSMIC database (Fig. 5). Among the 12 most commonly mutated genes, only *CDC42EP1* had not been reported in ccRCC previously. In the *CDC42EP1* gene, the somatic missense mutation (S260P) was detected in three cases, which was not located in the protein domain for *CDC42EP1* and was predicted to be benign.

Regarding 5 PRCC cases, 537 missense mutations, 56 stop-gain mutations, 31 frameshift mutations, 34 splice mutations and 2 stop-loss mutations were detected (Fig. 2c). Among the 528 missense mutations with available annotation information, 375 variants (71%) were

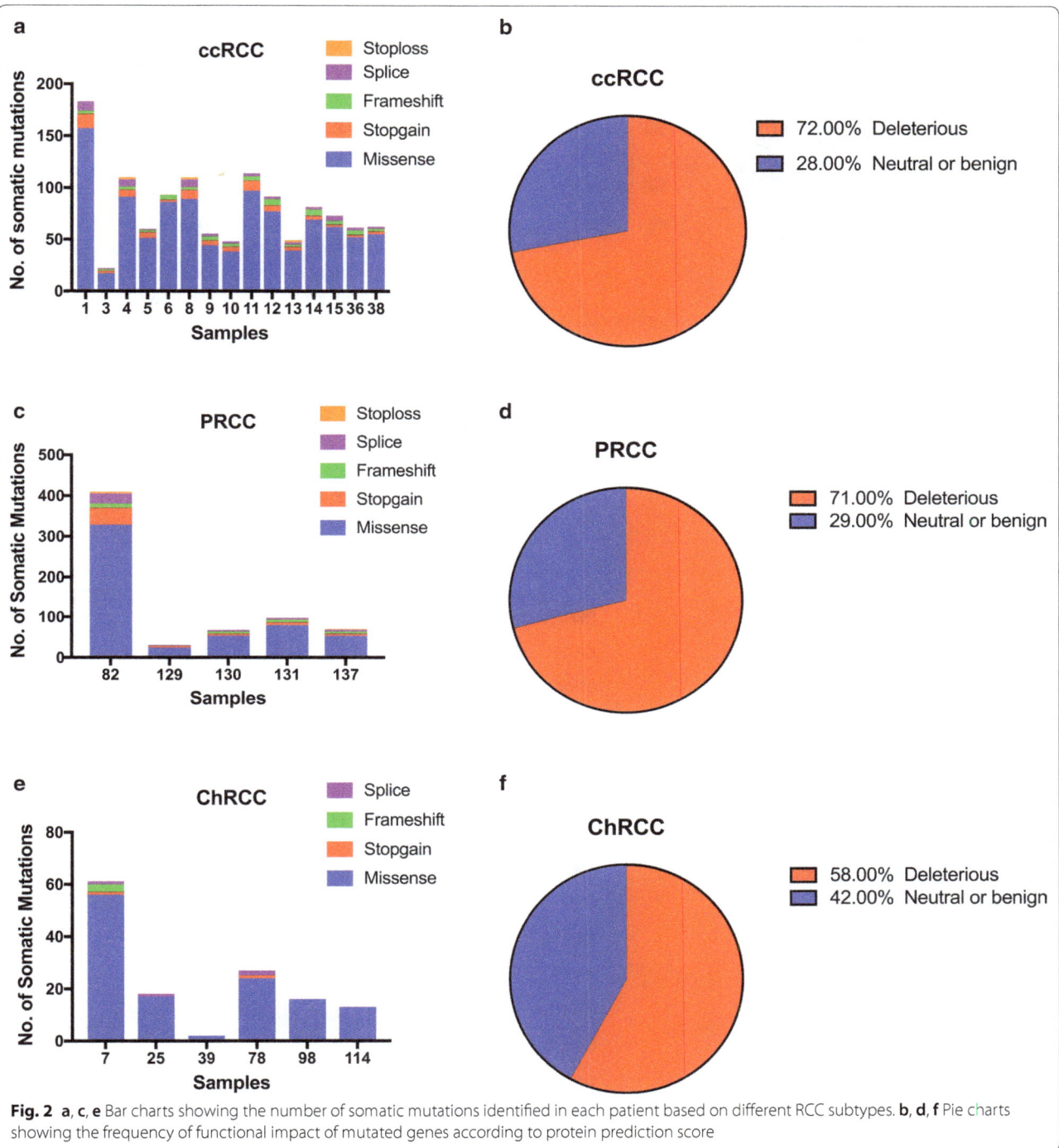

**Fig. 2** **a**, **c**, **e** Bar charts showing the number of somatic mutations identified in each patient based on different RCC subtypes. **b**, **d**, **f** Pie charts showing the frequency of functional impact of mutated genes according to protein prediction score

predicted to be deleterious and 153 mutations (29%) were forecasted to be neutral or benign (Fig. 2d). Like in the ccRCC cases, the most common substitution in missense mutations was T:A > A:T (Fig. 3). In total, 19 mutated genes were detected at a frequency above 40%, and each mutated gene was identified in at least two cases (Fig. 4b).

*PER3* was the most commonly mutated gene observed in 3 PRCC cases (50%), which was also mutated in 4 ccRCC cases (27%). None of the variants detected in *PER3* were located in its protein domain and they were all predicted to be neutral or benign. Among the remaining frequently mutated genes, *DEPDC4* (p.E293A, p.T279A), *PNLIP*

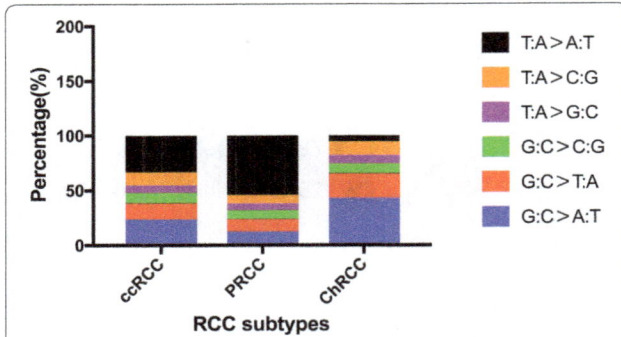

**Fig. 3** Bar charts showing that the percentage of different substitutions in missense mutations according to distinct RCC subtypes

(p.N401Y, p.F342L) and *SARDH* (p.H554Q, p.M1T) had not been reported to correlate with PRCC before, and they were all predicted to be deleterious.

In the 6 ChRCC cases, 128 missense mutations, 2 stop-gain mutations, 3 frameshift mutations and 4 splice mutations were identified (Fig. 2e). Among the 124 missense mutations that had been annotated successfully, 72 variants (58%) were predicted to be deleterious, and 52 mutations (42%) were thought to be neutral or benign (Fig. 2f). The most recurrent substitution in missense mutations was G:C > A:T, which was distinct from that in ccRCC and PRCC cases (Fig. 3). Only 3 genes (*KRTAP4–8*, *MUC16*, *ZNF814*) were mutated at a frequency of 33%, and each gene mutation was uncovered in two cases (Fig. 4c). It's worth noting that the *ZNF814* gene was also mutated in 4 ccRCC cases and 2 PRCC cases. Among all these mutations in *ZNF814* gene, p.P323H, p.R322K and p.G320E presented as a fixed combination occurring in three RCC types. Furthermore, p.P323H and p.G320E in *ZNF814* were predicted to be deleterious, while p.R322K was predicted to be benign. The *KRTAP4–8* gene had not been reported to be somatically altered in ChRCC previously. Among the 4 missense mutations in *KRTAP4–8*,

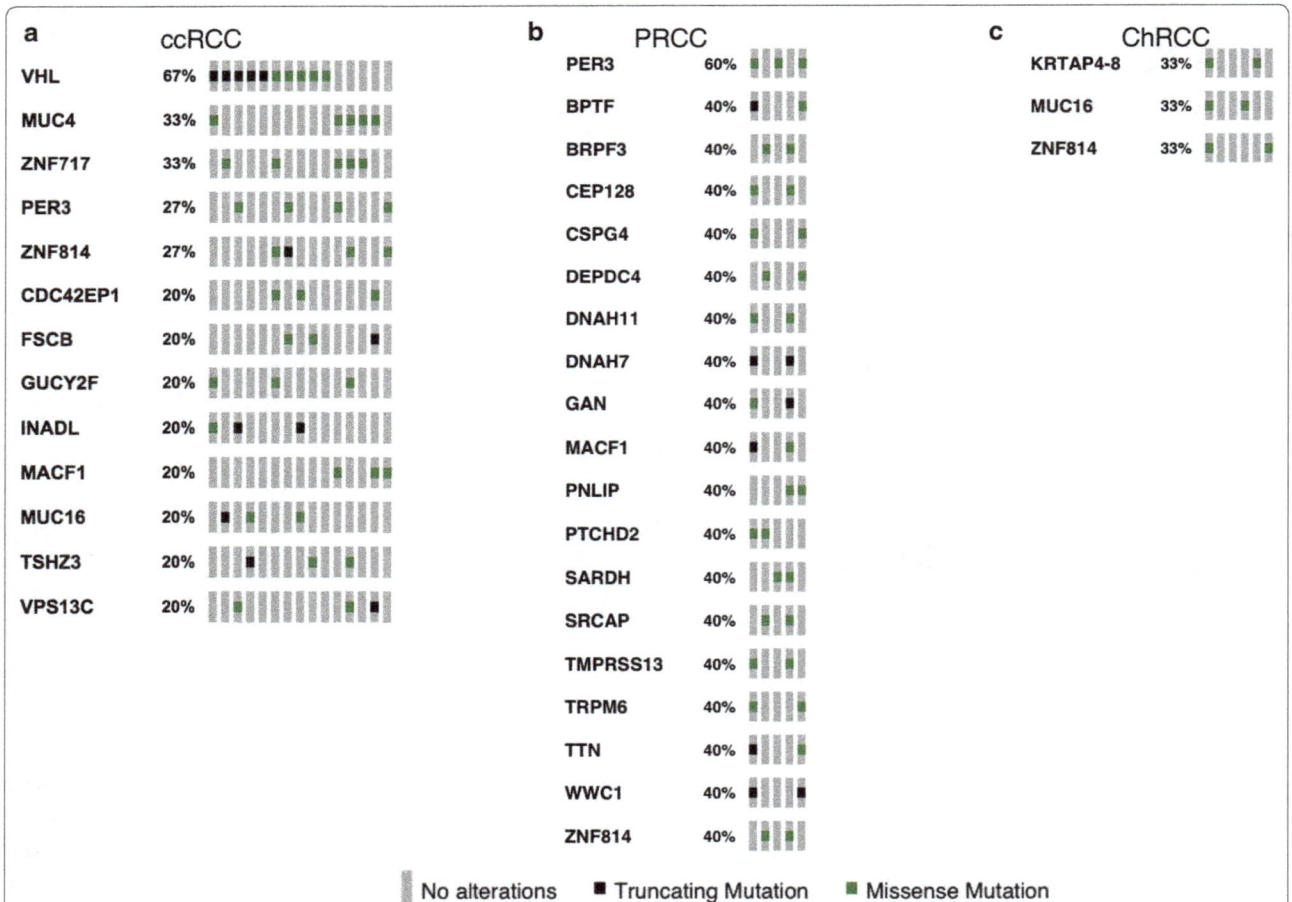

**Fig. 4** Oncoprint diagram **a** showing the mutated genes in at least three patients with ccRCC. Oncoprint diagram **b** and **c** illustrating the altered genes in at least two patients with PRCC and ChRCC respectively

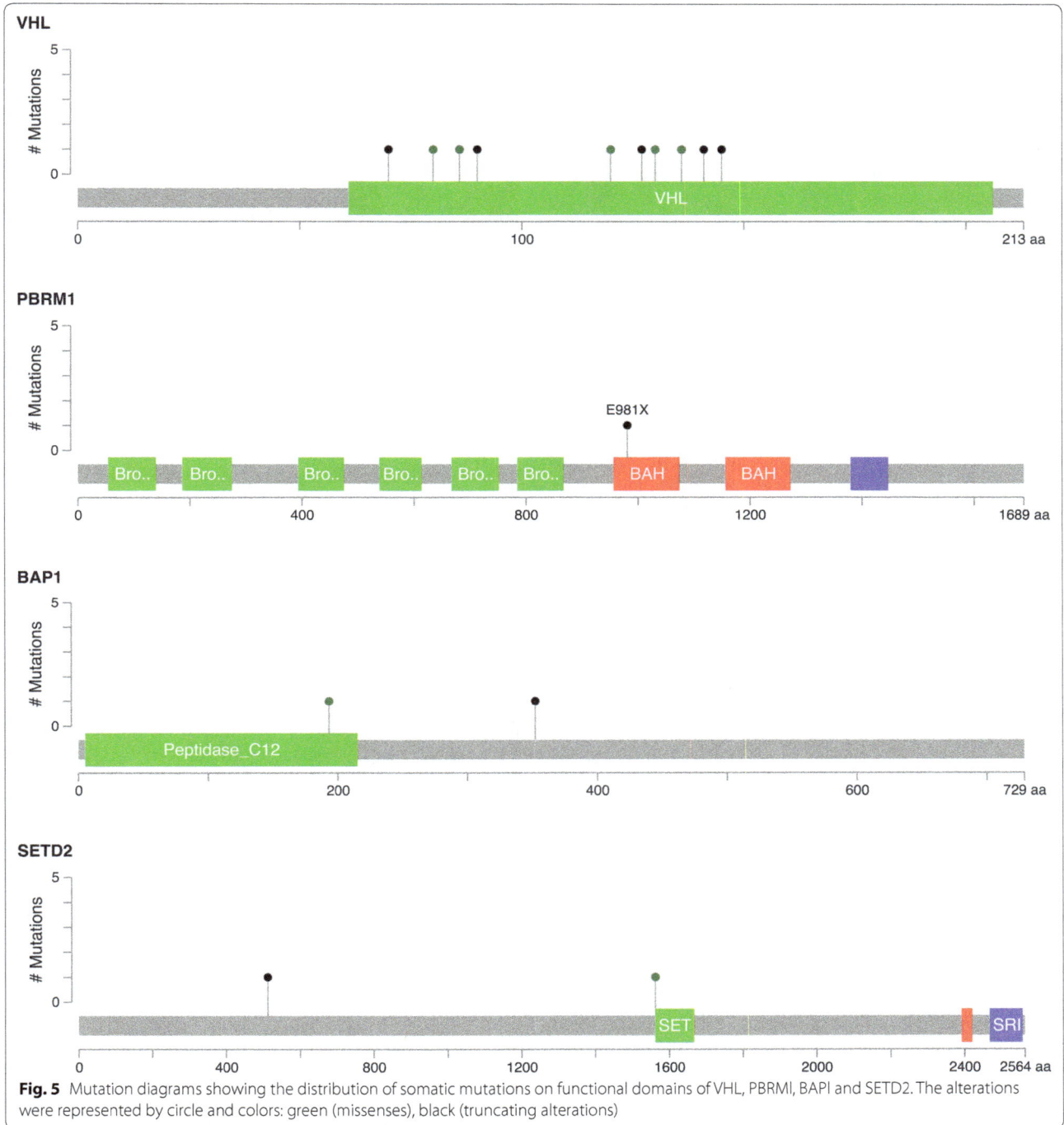

**Fig. 5** Mutation diagrams showing the distribution of somatic mutations on functional domains of VHL, PBRMI, BAPI and SETD2. The alterations were represented by circle and colors: green (missenses), black (truncating alterations)

p.V71M and p.S68R were forecasted to be deleterious, while p.H91R and p.K76R were predicted to be benign.

### Comparison with public databases

In the COSMIC database, the most frequent substitution in missense mutations in ccRCC is G:C > A:T, which is different from what we found in this study (T:A > A:T).

Among the top 8 frequently mutated genes (*VHL, PBRM1, BAP1, SETD2, KDM5C, PTEN, MTOR, TP53*) in ccRCC in the COSMIC database, which also represent the eight most significantly mutated genes in the TCGA database, six were verified in our study, including *VHL* (67%), *PBRM1* (7%), *BAP1* (13%), *SETD2* (13%), *PTEN* (7%) and *MTOR* (7%) (Fig. 6). It's worth noting that the

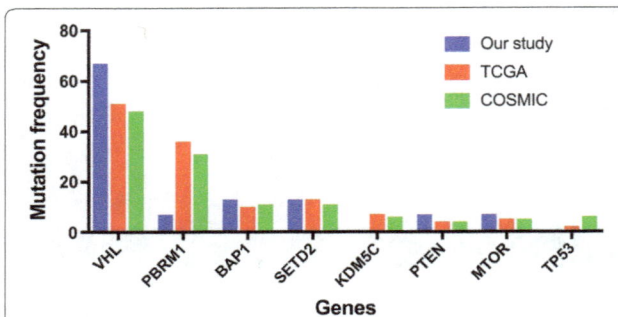

**Fig. 6** The bar chart showing that discrepancies of the mutation frequency of eight significantly mutated genes (*VHL, PBRMI, BAPI, SETD2, KDM5C, PTEN, MTOR, TP53*) between our study and two public datasets (TCGA and COSMIC)

amino acid alterations p.P352fs and p.H193Q in *BAP1*, p.W1562C and p.S512X in *SETD2*, p.V343fs in *PTEN* and p.R882S in *MTOR* had not been reported previously in ccRCC, all of which were considered to be deleterious in this study. Figure 5 shows the distribution of somatic mutations identified in this study in functional domains for *VHL, PBRM1, BAP1* and *SETD2*.

For PRCC, the most recurrently mutated gene is *MET* in the COSMIC database (6%), which is also the most significantly mutated gene evaluated by MutSigCV in the TCGA database (7.45%). However, no mutations in *MET* gene was detected in our study. Notably, *PBRM1* gene that was mutated in one ccRCC case was also altered in one PRCC case (type 2), which was reported to be mutated at a frequency of 2% in the COSMIC database and 3.9% in the TCGA database. Moreover, in accordance with ccRCC, the most common substitution in missense mutations in PRCC in the COSMIC database is G:C > A:T, which is distinct from what we found in this study (T:A > A:T).

Both in the TCGA and COSMIC database, *TP53* is the most frequently mutated gene in ChRCC, with mutation frequencies of 30.77 and 11% respectively, which was also verified in one ChRCC case in this study. Moreover, the amino acid alteration p.R81Q in *TP53* had not been reported before and was predicted to be deleterious. In the COSMIC database, the most frequent substitution in missense mutations in ChRCC is G:C > A:T, which is consistent with our finding.

### Major signaling pathways altered in RCCs

The somatically mutated genes discovered in this study were used to evaluate the impact on the major signaling pathways associated with RCC, including the PI3K-Akt, mTOR, p53, HIF-1, Hippo, MAPK signaling pathways and the SWI/SNF complex [3, 4, 14]. According to our analysis, the HIF-1 signaling pathway (12/15) was the

most affected pathway in ccRCC, in which *VHL* was the most frequently mutated gene (67%), followed by the PI3K-Akt signaling pathway (10/15). The PI3K-Akt signaling pathway (4/5) was the most influenced pathway in PRCC, followed by the Hippo signaling pathway (3/5) and the p53 signaling pathway (2/5). In ChRCC, a few mutated genes were identified as components of the signaling pathways mentioned above, including the PI3K-Akt (3/6), MAPK (2/6) and HIF-1 (2/6) signaling pathway. Notably, the *TP53* gene that was only mutated in one ChRCC case was involved both in the PI3K-Akt and MAPK signaling pathway, which was reported to be the most recurrently mutated gene in the TCGA database [5] (Additional file 1: Table S1).

### Association between PD-L1 expression and somatic mutations

Membranous PD-L1 expression was positive in tumor cells from 6/26 (23%) RCC specimens, including 3 ccRCC samples, 2 PRCC samples and 1 ChRCC sample (Fig. 7). Only case 82 showed strong positivity (+++) in tumor cells for PD-L1 expression, in which the TMB (16.33 Muts/Mb) was the highest among 26 RCC cases, while the other 5 cases showed weak positivity (+). However, we didn't find any statistical correlation between the TMB and PD-L1 expression (P > 0.05). In total, six genes were somatically mutated in two of the three PD-L1-positive ccRCC cases, including *VHL, INADL, MUC4, RAD21, CSPG4* and *BAP1*. Both of the two PD-L1-positive PRCC cases contained somatic alterations in six other genes, namely, *MACF1, DNAH7, DNAH11, TMPRSS13, CEP128* and *GAN*. In addition, *TMPRSS13* was also somatically mutated in one ccRCC case. Fisher's exact test revealed that somatic mutations in *CSPG4, DNAH11, INADL* and *TMPRSS13* were significantly associated with PD-L1-positive expression in RCC tumor cells. Among the 26 RCC cases, the PD-L1-positive rate in tumor cells was higher in samples with the 4 somatically mutated genes, including *CSPG4, DNAH11, INADL* and *TMPRSS13*, than in samples without those (P > 0.05).

### Discussion

In recent years, the landscape of genomic somatic alterations in RCC has been depicted by several research projects including the TCGA, supported by multiple countries, which could be helpful for studying oncogenesis and new treatment strategies. However, racial differences might also contribute to the diversity of genomic somatic aberrations in tumors. For instance, in a study focusing on racial differences in the sequencing results of hereditary malignancies, Caswell and colleagues reported that a higher proportion of whites than nonwhites carried deleterious *CHEK2* mutations [15]. It's well known

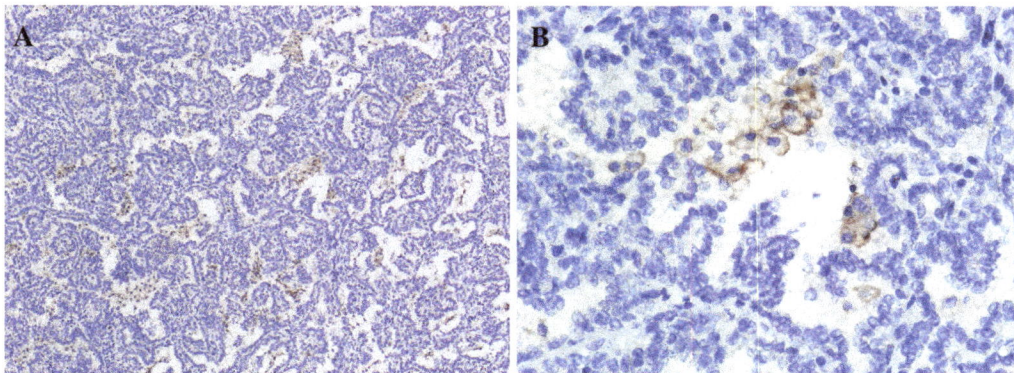

**Fig. 7** Immunohistochemical staining of PD-LI in RCC specimens . PD-LI membranous staining was identified in tumor cells. **A** ×10 magnification; **B** ×40 magnification

that the vast majority of somatic mutation profiles associated with ccRCC, PRCC and ChRCC were unmasked by foreign researchers. The subjects were mainly Caucasian and black patients. Only 10 Chinese patients with ccRCC have been evaluated using WES before [16]. These data can be acquired via the ICGC data portal. The discrepancies and similarities of the somatic mutation landscapes in ccRCC, PRCC and ChRCC between Chinese patients and sufferers from other countries and regions still need to be elucidated with a larger sample size. In this study, we performed WES on paired fresh-frozen tissues obtained from 26 RCC cases.

In previous investigations, *VHL* was always reported to be the most frequently mutated gene in ccRCC. As revealed in a study about WES performed on 106 ccRCC specimens from Tokyo [14], *VHL* gene was somatically mutated at a frequency of 40.57%. According to the TCGA database [3], the mutation frequency of *VHL* was 51.42%, which was much lower (20%) in the WES study performed on 10 Chinese patients with ccRCC [16]. In our study on 15 paired tumor-normal ccRCC samples from Chinese patients, the mutation frequency of *VHL* was 66.67%, which was much higher than that in the WES study performed on 10 Chinese with ccRCC previously. The big difference in the mutation frequency of *VHL* between those two Chinese studies is probably due to the distinct sample amount, diverse sequencing platforms and different sample source centers. In this study, all of the somatic mutations in *VHL* were located in the known domain for *VHL* and determined to be deleterious to protein function. In other words, the function of VHL protein (pVHL) was altered or even lost. As a part of the ubiquitin-mediated proteolysis pathway, the pVHL plays an important role in the degradation of several cellular proteins containing hypoxia-induced factors (HIF). HIF includes two subunits, namely, HIF1α and HIF2α,

which participates in the transcription of some genes regulating metabolism and angiogenesis [17, 18]. Hence, the absence of pVHL function can result in the accumulation of HIF, which can contribute to the dysregulation of signaling pathways associated with metabolism, inflammation and angiogenesis, accelerating oncogenesis consequently [19]. Considering these published ideas together, we can speculate that the deleterious mutations in *VHL* identified in our study might play a leading role in the oncogenesis of ccRCC. However, loss of *VHL* activity is unable to induce ccRCC by itself, as there are some other ingredients cooperating with that towards the oncogenesis of ccRCC. Amrita and colleagues demonstrated that the deficiencies of *Vhl* and *Pbrm1* in the mouse kidney can lead to multifocal ccRCC with a tendency of metastasis [20]. Sabine and colleagues showed that the combined deletion of *Vhl*, *Trp53* and *Rb1* targeted in renal epithelial cells in mice caused ccRCC, which shared molecular markers and mRNA expression with human ccRCC [21].

As the second most frequently mutated gene in ccRCC both in the TCGA and COSMIC databases, *PBRM1* is located at chromosome 3p21 encoding the BAF180 protein, which is a vital component of the PBAF SWI/SNF chromatin remodeling complex [22]. In this study, only a stop-gain mutation (p.E981X) in *PBRM1* was detected in one ccRCC case, which had been reported previously. Compared with the data documented in the TCGA (30.6%) and COSMIC datasets (31%), the mutation frequency of *PBRM1* in ccRCC in this study was relatively lower (6.7%). Varela and partners disclosed truncating mutations in *PBRM1* at a frequency of 41% in 227 ccRCC cases [23]. The discrepancy in the mutation frequency of *PBRM1* in ccRCC between our study and previous studies might result from racial differences in the subjects. Moreover, the smaller sample amount in our study might also contribute to that, which should be taken into consideration. Therefore, additional analysis with a larger sample size still needs to confirm the data reported herein. Nowadays, it has been generally accepted that *PBRM1* acts as a tumor suppressor gene in the kidney and plays a critical role in the pathogenesis and progression of ccRCC [19]. It had been demonstrated that loss of *Vhl* and *Pbrm1* in mouse kidney could generate ccRCC [24]. As revealed in our study, *PBRM1* and *VHL* were somatically mutated in the same ccRCC case. Consequently, we speculated that somatically altered *PBRM1* and *VHL* genes worked cooperatively for the oncogenesis of ccRCC in our study. More recently, another study showed that depressed *PBRM1* and *VHL* expression was associated with elevated tumor aggressiveness [25]. In addition, the *PBRM1* mutation was also identified in one type 2 PRCC case in this study, which was consistent with the previous finding that mutated *PBRM1* was mainly associated with type 2 PRCC [4].

Apart from *VHL* and *PBRM1*, there are some other genes significantly mutated in ccRCC based on the TCGA and COSMIC datasets, such as *SETD2* and *BAP1*, which are both located at chromosome 3p21. For *BAP1*, a missense mutation (p.H193Q) and a frameshift-deletion (p.P352fs) were found in two different ccRCC cases in this study. Regarding *SETD2*, we also identified two somatic mutations in two distinct ccRCC cases consisting of a missense mutation (p.W1562C) and a stop-gain mutation (p.S512X). All of those mutations in *SETD2* and *BAP1* had not been reported before and were predicted to be deleterious. Serving as tumor suppressor genes in ccRCC, *BAP1* and *SETD2* mutations were related to worse cancer-specific survival [26]. In the TCGA database, only mutations in *BAP1* were reported to be associated with poor survival outcome [3]. Miura and colleagues unraveled in their research that deficiency of *BAP1* protein expression at metastatic sites indicated poor progression in patients with ccRCC [27]. Unfortunately, no prognostic information was available in our study. Thus, ccRCC patients who were confirmed to have *BAP1* and *SETD2* mutations should be followed up regularly. Further research with a larger sample size focusing on Chinese ccRCC patients, mainly concerning about the progression and prognosis of patients with altered *BAP1* and *SETD2*, should be considered.

It has been widely known that *TP53* is the most frequently mutated gene in ChRCC, with a frequency of 30.77% according to the TCGA dataset, which was only somatically mutated in one ChRCC case in this study and predicted to be deleterious. While Casuscelli and partners unraveled that *TP53* was mutated at a frequency of 58% in 38 metastatic ChRCC cases, which was much higher than that unmasked by the TCGA project and our

study. In addition, those researchers found that mutations in *TP53* and *PTEN* and imbalanced chromosome duplication in primary ChRCC were associated with worse survival [28]. In contrast, all the specimens in our study were harvested from patients with no metastasis. It seemed that metastasis might underlie the discrepancy in the reported TP53 mutation frequencies. Thus, we hypothesised that somatically mutated *TP53* might serve as an important factor contributing to the aggressiveness of ChRCC. However, more further studies should be performed to confirm this hypothesis.

The PI3K/AKT/mTOR signaling pathway has been demonstrated to be highly involved in a variety of cancer types by contributing to the regulation of a series of cellular mechanisms, including proliferation, angiogenesis, metastasis and survival [29]. It was also reported that the PI3K/AKT/mTOR signaling pathway was significantly altered and activated in ccRCC [3, 14], playing a dominant role in the tumorigenesis in distal tubules of rats and human beings [30]. In our study, a multitude of somatically mutated genes associated with the PI3K/AKT signaling pathway were identified in all the three RCC types, while none of the mutated genes was involved in the mTOR signaling pathway. As an important therapeutical target, mTOR inhibitors, such as everolimus, have been recommended for the treatment of patients with metastatic ccRCC. To the best of our knowledge, investigations concerning about mTOR inhibitors and metastatic RCC have been launched to search for predictive factors among the components of the PI3K/AKT/mTOR signaling pathway [31]. However, in order to better use mTOR inhibitors for the treatment of metastatic RCC, further more studies focusing on the correlation between the PI3K/AKT/mTOR signaling pathway and RCC are still required.

Currently, PD-L1 expression in tumor cells has become a predictor of the response to immunotherapy with PD-1/PD-L1 inhibitors among diverse cancers including RCC [6]. In this study, among the 26 RCC cases, PD-L1-positive rate in tumor cells was significantly higher in specimens with 4 somatically mutated genes, including *CSPG4*, *DNAH11*, *INADL* and *TMPRSS13*, than in samples without those (P < 0.05). None of those gene mutations were reported to correlate with PD-L1 expression in RCC tumor cells previously. In other words, those altered genes could serve as predictors of the PD-L1-positive expression in RCC tumor cells. Consequently, it could be speculated that those four somatically mutated genes might become the potential targeted genes for predicting responses to immunotherapy with PD-1/PD-L1 inhibitors in RCC. Nevertheless, whether those four mutated genes can influence the expression of PD-L1 in RCC is in need of further investigation. Previous studies had revealed that PD-L1 expression had an association with poor overall survival in ccRCC [32], while the TCGA database indicated that only mutations in *BAP1* were associated with poor survival in ccRCC [3]. Both of somatically mutated *BAP1* and PD-L1 expression were demonstrated to correlate with the poor prognosis of ccRCC patients. As revealed in this study, *BAP1* was altered in only two ccRCC specimens, both of which exhibited PD-L1-positive in tumour cells. Those two mutations in *BAP1* were predicted to be deleterious. Therefore, we hypothesised that somatically altered *BAP1* might serve as a critical ingredient contributing to the PD-L1 expression in ccRCC tumor cells, and most likely work in concert with PD-L1 in tumor cells contributing to the aggressiveness of ccRCC. The interaction between somatic mutations in *BAP1* and PD-L1 expression in ccRCC needs to be further elucidated in additional studies.

## Conclusion

We identified somatic mutations in RCC from 26 Chinese patients using WES, which enriched the racial diversity of the somatic mutation profiles of RCC subjects. Several discrepancies in molecular characterizations were elucidated, such as the significant difference in the most frequent substitution in somatic missense mutations between our study and published databases. We also detected numerous novel somatic mutations in this study, which further supplements the somatic mutation profiles of RCC. Moreover, our study revealed that 4 somatically mutated genes, including *CSPG4*, *DNAH11*, *INADL* and *TMPRSS13*, might act as promising predictive factors of PD-L1-positive expression in RCC tumor cells.

## Abbreviations

RCC: renal cell carcinoma; ccRCC: clear cell renal cell carcinoma; PRCC: papillary renal cell carcinoma; ChRCC: chromophobe renal cell carcinoma; NGS: next generation sequencing; WES: whole exome sequencing; TCGA: The Cancer Genome Atlas; ICGC: International Cancer Genome Consortium; TMB: tumor mutation burden; gDNA: genomic DNA; BWA: Burrows Wheeler Aligner; GATK: Genome Analysis Toolkit; ACMG: American College of Medical Genetics; KEGG: Kyoto Encyclopedia of Genes and Genomes; pVHL: VHL protein; HIF: hypoxia-induced factor; PD-L1: programmed death ligand 1; PD-1: programmed death 1.

## Authors' contributions

ZX and JX conceived and designed the project; HZ and JL provided technical support; YX and YY contributed to the analysis and diagram; JW collected and processed the samples, provided clinical counseling and wrote the manuscript. All authors read and approved the final manuscript.

## Author details

[1] Department of Urology, Peking University First Hospital and Institute of Urology, National Research Center for Genitourinary Oncology, No 8, Xishiku Street, Xicheng District, Beijing, China. [2] Department of Biomedical Engineering, College of Engineering, Peking University, No 5, Yiheyuan Road, Haidian District, Beijing, China. [3] Beijing Genex Health Technology Co., Ltd., Beijing, China. [4] Chongqing Institute of Innovation and Entrepreneurship for Precision Medicine, Chongqing, China.

## Acknowledgements
Not applicable.

## Competing interests
The authors declare that they have no competing interests.

## Funding
The study was funded by the National Natural Science Foundation of China (Grant No. 81272829).

## References

1. Siegel RL, Miller KD, Jemal A. Cancer statistics, 2017. Cancer J Clin. 2017;67:7–30.
2. Chen WQ, Li H, Sun KX, et al. Report of cancer incidence and mortality in China, 2014. Zhonghua Zhong Liu Za Zhi. 2018;40:5–13.
3. Cancer Genome Atlas Research N. Comprehensive molecular characterization of clear cell renal cell carcinoma. Nature. 2013;499:43–9.
4. Cancer Genome Atlas Research N. Comprehensive molecular characterization of papillary renal-cell carcinoma. N Engl J Med. 2013;499:43–9.
5. Davis CF, Ricketts CJ, Wang M, et al. The somatic genomic landscape of chromophobe renal cell carcinoma. Cancer Cell. 2014;26:319–30.
6. Motzer RJ, Tannir NM, McDermott DF, et al. Nivolumab plus Ipilimumab versus sunitinib in advanced renal-cell carcinoma. N Engl J Med. 2018;378:1277–90.
7. Van der Auwera GA, Carneiro MO, Hartl C, et al. From FastQ data to high confidence variant calls: the Genome Analysis Toolkit best practices pipeline. Curr Protoc Bioinform. 2013;43:11.
8. Wang K, Li M, Hakonarson H. ANNOVAR: functional annotation of genetic variants from high-throughput sequencing data. Nucleic Acids Res. 2010;38:e164.
9. Richards S, Aziz N, Bale S, et al. Standards and guidelines for the interpretation of sequence variants: a joint consensus recommendation of the American College of Medical Genetics and Genomics and the Association for Molecular Pathology. Genet Med. 2015;17:405–24.
10. Cerami E, Gao J, Dogrusoz U, et al. The cBio cancer genomics portal: an open platform for exploring multidimensional cancer genomics data. Cancer Discov. 2012;2:401–4.
11. Gao J, Aksoy BA, Dogrusoz U, et al. Integrative analysis of complex cancer genomics and clinical profiles using the cBioPortal. Sci Signal. 2013;6:l1.
12. Chalmers ZR, Connelly CF, Fabrizio D, et al. Analysis of 100,000 human cancer genomes reveals the landscape of tumor mutational burden. Genome Med. 2017;9:34.
13. Kanehisa M, Goto S, Sato Y, et al. Data, information, knowledge and principle: back to metabolism in KEGG. Nucleic Acids Res. 2014;42:D199–205.
14. Sato Y, Yoshizato T, Shiraishi Y, et al. Integrated molecular analysis of clear-cell renal cell carcinoma. Nat Genet. 2013;45:860–7.
15. Caswell-Jin JL, Gupta T, Hall E, et al. Racial/ethnic differences in multiple-gene sequencing results for hereditary cancer risk. Genet Med. 2018;20:234–9.
16. Guo G, Gui Y, Gao S, et al. Frequent mutations of genes encoding ubiquitin-mediated proteolysis pathway components in clear cell renal cell carcinoma. Nat Genet. 2011;44:17–9.
17. Choueiri TK, Fay AP, Gagnon R, et al. The role of aberrant VHL/HIF pathway elements in predicting clinical outcome to pazopanib therapy in patients with metastatic clear-cell renal cell carcinoma. Clin Cancer Res. 2013;19:5218–26.
18. Shenoy N, Pagliaro L. Sequential pathogenesis of metastatic VHL mutant clear cell renal cell carcinoma: putting it together with a translational perspective. Ann Oncol. 2016;27:1685–95.
19. Hirsch MS, Signoretti S, Dal Cin P. Adult renal cell carcinoma: a review of established entities from morphology to molecular genetics. Surg Pathol Clin. 2015;8:587–621.
20. Nargund AM, Pham CG, Dong Y, et al. The SWI/SNF protein PBRM1 restrains VHL-loss-driven clear cell renal cell carcinoma. Cell Rep. 2017;18:2893–906.

21. Harlander S, Schonenberger D, Toussaint NC, et al. Combined mutation in Vhl, Trp53 and Rb1 causes clear cell renal cell carcinoma in mice. Nat Med. 2017;23:869–77.

22. Reisman D, Glaros S, Thompson EA. The SWI/SNF complex and cancer. Oncogene. 2009;28:1653–68.

23. Varela I, Tarpey P, Raine K, et al. Exome sequencing identifies frequent mutation of the SWI/SNF complex gene PBRM1 in renal carcinoma. Nature. 2011;469:539–42.

24. Nargund AM, Pham CG, Dong Y, et al. The SWI/SNF protein PBRM1 restrains VHL-loss-driven clear cell renal cell carcinoma. Cell Rep. 2017;18:2893–906.

25. Hogner A, Krause H, Jandrig B, et al. PBRM1 and VHL expression correlate in human clear cell renal cell carcinoma with differential association with patient's overall survival. Urol Oncol. 2018;36(94):e1–14.

26. Hakimi AA, Ostrovnaya I, Reva B, et al. Adverse outcomes in clear cell renal cell carcinoma with mutations of 3p21 epigenetic regulators BAP1 and SETD2: a report by MSKCC and the KIRC TCGA research network. Clin Cancer Res. 2013;19:3259–67.

27. Miura Y, Inoshita N, Ikeda M, et al. Loss of BAP1 protein expression in the first metastatic site predicts prognosis in patients with clear cell renal cell carcinoma. Urol Oncol. 2017;35:386–91.

28. Casuscelli J, Weinhold N, Gundem G, et al. Genomic landscape and evolution of metastatic chromophobe renal cell carcinoma. JCI Insight. 2017;2:92688.

29. Ersahin T, Tuncbag N, Cetin-Atalay R. The PI3K/AKT/mTOR interactive pathway. Mol BioSyst. 2015;11:1946–54.

30. Ribback S, Cigliano A, Kroeger N, et al. PI3K/AKT/mTOR pathway plays a major pathogenetic role in glycogen accumulation and tumor development in renal distal tubules of rats and men. Oncotarget. 2015;6:13036–48.

31. Bodnar L, Stec R, Cierniak S, et al. Clinical usefulness of PI3K/Akt/mTOR genotyping in companion with other clinical variables in metastatic renal cell carcinoma patients treated with everolimus in the second and subsequent lines. Ann Oncol. 2015;26:1385–9.

32. Abbas M, Steffens S, Bellut M, et al. Intratumoral expression of programmed death ligand 1 (PD-L1) in patients with clear cell renal cell carcinoma (ccRCC). Med Oncol. 2016;33:80.

# 11

# LncRNA DLX6-AS1 promoted cancer cell proliferation and invasion by attenuating the endogenous function of miR-181b in pancreatic cancer

Yong An[†], Xue-min Chen[†], Yong Yang, Feng Mo, Yong Jiang, Dong-lin Sun and Hui-hua Cai[*] ⓘ

## Abstract

**Background:** Pancreatic cancer, one of the most aggressive malignancies, ranks the fourth cause of cancer-related death worldwide. Aberrantly expressed long non-coding RNAs (lncRNAs) functioned as oncogenes or tumor suppressors in pancreatic cancer. This study aimed to determine the expression of lncRNA DLX6 antisense RNA 1 (DLX6-AS1) in pancreatic cancer tissues and to explore the DLX6-AS1-related pathway in pancreatic cancer.

**Materials and methods:** The gene expression levels were determined by quantitative real-time PCR, and protein expression levels were determined by western blot assay. CCK-8 assay, colony formation assay and Transwell migration and invasion assays were used to examine cell proliferation, migration and invasion. Luciferase reporter assay was used to confirm the binding between DLX6-AS1and its potential targets. In vivo study used the mouse xenograft model to test the anti-tumor effect of DLX6-AS1 knockdown.

**Results:** The high expression of DLX6-AS1 was observed in pancreatic cancer tissues, and high expression of DLX6-AS1 was positively correlated with larger tumor size, advanced TNM stage and lymph node metastasis. Knockdown of DLX6-AS1 dramatically impaired cancer cell proliferation, migration and invasion. MiR-181b was the downstream target of DLX6-AS1. Knockdown of miR-181b reversed the suppression of cell viability, migration and invasion abilities caused by DLX6-AS1 knockdown. MiR-181b was found to target Zinc finger E-box-binding homeobox 2 and to modulate epithelial-mesenchymal transition. Furthermore, DLX6-AS1 knockdown inhibited tumor growth and tumor metastasis in vivo.

**Conclusion:** Collectively, our data suggested that DLX6-AS1 promotes cancer cell proliferation and invasion by attenuating the endogenous function of miR-181b in pancreatic cancer.

**Keywords:** Pancreatic cancer, lncRNA DLX6-AS1, Proliferation, Migration and invasion, miR-181b, Zinc finger E-box-binding homeobox 2

*Correspondence: chh1168@163.com
[†]Yong An and Xue-min Chen contributed equally to this work
Department of Hepatobiliary Surgery, The First People's Hospital
of Changzhou, The Third Affiliated Hospital of Soochow University, 185
Juqian Street, Changzhou 213000, Jiangsu, China

## Background

Pancreatic cancer, one of the most aggressive malignancies, ranks the fourth cause of cancer-related death. Currently, there is lack of sensitive screening for early stage tumors. Up to date, surgery is the effective treatment for pancreatic cancer, however, the 5-year survival rate of the patients with pancreatic cancer is lower than 10% [1]. Unfortunately, 80% of the patients are not suitable for surgery and the recurrence rate in those who subjected to resection is very high [2]. Chemotherapy remains the primary treatment and the combination therapy including FOLFIRINOX, paclitaxel and gemcitabine is the first-line drug, but the outcome is not satisfactory [3, 4]. In terms of targeted drugs, the tyrosine-kinase inhibitor of epidermal growth factor receptor, Eroltinib, combined with gemcitabine, just made modest progress in survival benefit [5]. Consequently, the mechanisms underlying pancreatic cancer should be further investigated.

Recently, emerging evidence indicated the crucial roles of non-coding RNAs in various human diseases, and non-coding RNAs can be sub-grouped to small non-coding RNAs (< 200 nucleotides) and long non-coding RNAs (lncRNAs; > 200 nucleotides) [6]. LncRNAs take part in various physiological and pathological processes, including proliferation, differentiation, invasion, or chromosome inactivation [7]. Studies showed that lncRNA H19 was overexpressed in human pancreatic ductal adenocarcinoma and induced cancer cell proliferation by modulating cell cycle through E2F1 pathway [8]. LncRNA HOXA-AS2 was also up-regulated in pancreatic cancer tissues. Mechanistically, it promoted pancreatic cancer cell proliferation by interacting with enhancer of zeste homolog 2 and lysine specific demethylase 1 [9]. In addition, the microRNAs belongs to a class of small non-coding RNA with 18–22 nucleotides in length [10, 11]. Up to date, hundreds of identified miRNAs have been shown to function as key regulators in tumor development including pancreatic cancer. For example, miR-1271 served as a potent tumor suppressor by reducing AKT/mTOR signaling and promoting apoptosis [12]. Overexpression of miR-126 and miR-34a had superior anti-tumor effect in pancreatic cancer [13]. The lncRNA DLX6 antisense RNA 1 (DLX6-AS1) is a developmentally-regulated long non-coding RNA. According to GTEx Analysis, it is overexpressed in brain tissues in normal. High DLX6-AS1 expression was noticed in lung adenocarcinoma and associated with histological differentiation and TNM stage [14]. DLX6-AS1 was also up-regulated in hepatocellular carcinoma tissue and correlated with clinical prognosis [15]. However, how DLX6-AS1 regulates pancreatic cancer tumorigenesis and its underlying molecular mechanisms regarding pancreatic cancer development remain unknown.

In the present study, we detected the expression of DLX6-AS1 in pancreatic cancer tissues and cells and predicted its potentially targeted miRNA. We demonstrated that DLX6-AS1 up-regulated the expression of Zinc finger E-box-binding homeobox 2 (ZEB2) by sponging miR-181b, therefore promoting cell proliferation, invasion as well as epithelial-mesenchymal transition in pancreatic cancer cells.

## Materials and methods
### Human specimens
Eighty-four pairs of cancerous and adjacent normal tissues were collected from patients diagnosed with pancreatic cancer from 2015 to 2017 at the First People's Hospital of Changzhou. All the specimens were frozen in liquid nitrogen and stored at $-80$ °C for further use. The study was approved by the Ethics Committee of the First People's Hospital of Changzhou and written informed consent was signed and returned by each patient before using the tissues and clinical data.

### Cell culture
Human pancreatic duct epithelial cell Line (HPDE6-C7), and human pancreatic cancer cell lines CAPAN-1, BxPC-3, SW 1990 and PANC-1were purchased from ATCC (Manassas, USA). CAPAN-1 and BxPC-3 cells were cultured in RPMI-1640 medium (Gibco, Thermo Fisher Scientific, Waltham, USA) supplemented with 10% fetal bovine serum (FBS, Gibco, Thermo Fisher Scientific). PANC-1cells were cultured in Dulbecco's modified Eagle's medium (Gibco, Thermo Fisher Scientific) supplemented with 10% FBS (Gibco Thermo Fisher Scientific). SW 1990 cells were cultured in Leibovitz's L-15 medium and HPDE6-C7 was maintained in Keratinocyte Serum Free Medium supplemented with 25 mg/500 ml Bovine Pituitary Extract and 2.5 µg/500 ml Epidermal Growth Factor (Gibco, Thermo Fisher Scientific). They were all kept at 37 °C in a humidified atmosphere containing 5% $CO_2$.

### Oligonucleotides and transfection
The small interfering RNAs (siRNAs) for DLX6-AS1 [siDLX6-AS1 and siDLX6-AS1(a)] and the respective negative control siRNA, miR-181b mimics (5′-AACAUUCAUUGCUGUCGGUGGGU-3′), miR-181b inhibitors (5′-ACCCACCGACAGCAAUGAAUGUU-3′) and the respective negative control miRNAs were purchased from RiboBio (Guangzhou, China). Cell transfections (final concentration for siRNA transfection: 100 nM, final concentration for miRNAs transfection: 50 nM) were performed using Lipofectamine 2000 (Invitrogen, Carlsbad, USA) according to the manufacturer's protocol and the transfection efficiency was confirmed using

quantitative real-time PCR (qRT-PCR). All the experiments were performed in triplicate.

## RNA isolation and qRT-PCR

Total RNA was extracted from tissue or cells through TRIzol reagent (Invitrogen, Carlsbad, USA). The extracted RNA was then reversely transcribed into cDNA using PrimeScript™ 1st strand cDNA Synthesis Kit (Takara, Dalian, China). Real-time PCR was performed with SYBR Premix Ex Taq (Takara, Dalian, China) in the ABI7500 system. GAPDH or U6 was used as internal control for data analysis. All the experiments were performed in triplicate.

## CCK-8 assay

For proliferation assay, the transfected cells were seeded in 96-well plates at the density of 5000 cells/well overnight. At 0, 24, 48 and 72 h after transfection, the cells were incubated with 10 µl CCK-8 reagent for 2 h at 37 °C in the dark, and the OD value at 450 nm was read using a microplate reader (Bio-Rad Laboratories, Hercules, CA, USA) to determine the viability. All the experiments were performed in triplicate.

## Colony formation assay

The transfected cells were seeded in a 6-well plate at the density of 1000 cells/well and incubated in full culture medium at 37 °C. At 14 day, the cells were washed with PBS, fixed with methanol and stained with 1% crystal violet. The number of colonies was counted under a microscope. All the experiments were performed in triplicate.

## Transwell migration and invasion assays

Transwell migration and invasion assays were measured by Transwell chamber (8 µm pore size, Corning) without Matrigel for migration assay and with Matrigel for invasion assay. At 48 h after transfection, $1 \times 10^5$ cells were cultured in the upper chamber with serum-free median. The lower chamber was filled with median containing 10% FBS as the chemoattractant. After incubation for 48 h, cells in the upper membrane were removed with cotton swab while those that migrated or invaded were fixed in methanol, stained with 0.1% crystal violet and quantified under a microscope. All the experiments were performed in triplicate.

## Luciferase reporter assays

DLX6-AS1 fragments with the wild type (WT) or mutant (MUT) miR-181b binding sites were cloned to generate the plasmids pmirGLO-DLX6-AS1-WT or pmir-GLO- DLX6-AS1-MUT (Promega, Madison, USA). The 3′UTR of ZEB2 containing the wild type or mutant miR-181b binding sites were used to generate the plasmids

pmirGLO-ZEB2-WT and pmirGLO-ZEB2-MUT (Promega). HEK293T cells were co-transfected with luciferase plasmids and miR-181b mimics, or mimics NC by using Lipofectamine 2000 reagent according to the manufacture's instruction (Invitrogen). At 48 h after transfection, firefly and Renilla luciferase activities were measured by a Dual-Luciferase Reporter Assay System (Promega) and the experiments were performed in triplicate.

## Western blot

The tissue or cells were collected and total proteins were extracted and quantified. Equal amount of proteins was subjected to 10% SDS-PAGE and then transferred onto PVDF membranes (Millipore, Bedford, USA). After blocking with 5% fat-free milk, the membranes were probed with primary anti-ZEB2, anti-E-cadherin, anti-vimentin or anti-N-cadherin antibodies (Abcam, Cambridge, USA) at 4 °C overnight. Then membranes were incubated with horseradish peroxidase-conjugated IgG secondary antibody (Santa Cruz Biotechnology, Santa Cruz, USA) at 37 °C for 2 h. Enhanced chemiluminescence kit (Pierce, Waltham, China) with imaging system (Bio-Rad, Hercules, USA) were used to analyze the protein signals and β-actin was used as the internal control.

## Tumor growth and tumor metastasis assay in nude mice

Lentivirus expressing shDLX6-AS1 or shRNA control were designed and packaged by Genechem (Shanghai, China), and stable cell lines were established by infecting lentivirus into SW1990 cells and selected by puromycin (Sigma, St. Louis, USA). All the animal experiments were approved by the Animal Experimentation Ethics Committee of the First People's Hospital of Changzhou Hospital. For the tumor growth assay, twelve female BABL/c athymic nude mice (4–5 weeks old) were subjected to flank subcutaneous injection of SW1990 cells stably expressing shDLX6-AS1 or shNC. Tumor volume was measured every 5 day from the 10 day to the 35 day after inoculation. The volume was calculated as: volume $=$ (length $\times$ width$^2$)/2. At 35 day, the mice were sacrificed and the tumors were removed, weighed and snap-frozen for RNA extraction. For the tumor metastasis assay, twelve female BABL/c athymic nude mice (4–5 weeks old) were subjected to tail vein injection of SW1990 cells stably expressing shDLX6-AS1 or shNC. At 35 day, all the mice were sacrificed and the lung were excised, and the number of metastatic nodules in the lung was counted.

## Statistical analysis

Data were presented as mean $\pm$ standard deviation. The data analysis was performed by using GraphPad Prism software (Version 5.0, GraphPad, San Diego, USA). The significant differences in the clinical parameters between low expression and high expression of DLX6-AS1 groups were analyzed by Chi square test. Significant differences for the mean values between groups were determined by the Student's *t* test or one-way ANOVA, as appropriate. P value < 0.05 was considered statistically significant.

## Results

### Up-regulation of lncRNA DLX6-AS1 in pancreatic cancer tissues

The expression levels of lncRNA DLX6-AS1 in 84 pancreatic cancerous tissues and adjacent normal tissues were firstly evaluated by qRT-PCR. Expression level of DLX6-AS1 was up-regulated in cancerous tissues comparing with the adjacent normal counterparts (Fig. 1a). The expression of DLX6-AS1 in pancreatic cancer tissues was further divided into low expression group and high expression group based on the median values. High expression of DLX6-AS1 was positively correlated with

larger tumor size, advanced TNM stage and lymph node metastasis (Table 1). Meanwhile, we have sub-grouped pancreatic cancerous tissues as lymph node metastasis negative and positive groups, low TNM stages (I-II) and high TNM stages (III-IV) groups, as well as well/moderate and poor differentiated groups. As shown in Fig. 1b–d, the expression level of DLX6-AS1 in the lymph node metastasis negative group, low TNM stages group or well/moderate group was lower than that in the lymph node metastasis positive, high TNM stages or poor differentiated groups.

### Knockdown of lncRNA DLX6-AS1 suppressed pancreatic cancer cell proliferation, migration and invasion

The expression of DLX6-AS1 in human pancreatic cancer cell lines (CAPAN-1, BxPC-3, SW1990 and PANC-1) and human pancreatic duct epithelial cell line (HPDE6-C7) was determined by qRT-PCR. Elevated expression of DLX6-AS1 was observed in pancreatic cancer cell lines compared with HPDE6-C7

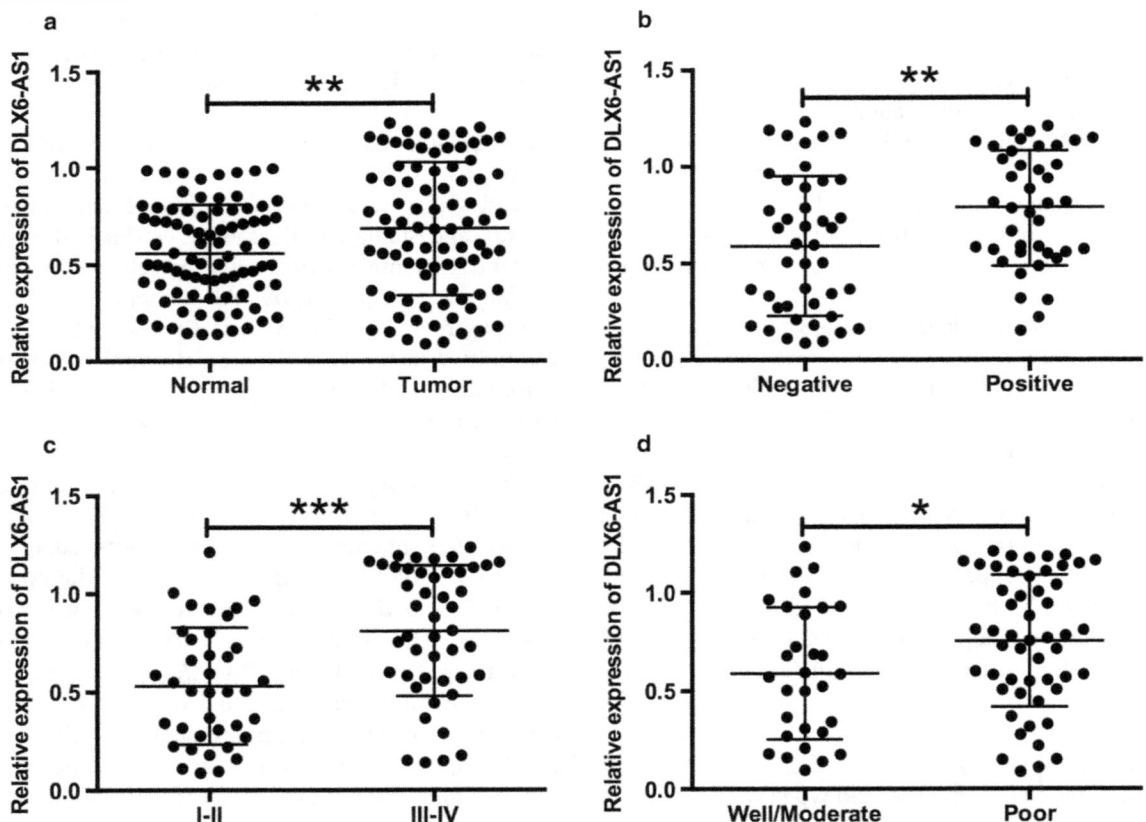

**Fig. 1** Up-regulation of lncRNA DLX6-AS1 in pancreatic cancer tissues. **a** The expression of DLX6-AS1 in pancreatic cancer tissues (n = 84) and normal adjacent pancreatic tissues (n = 84) was determined by qRT-PCR. **b** The expression of DLX6-AS1 in pancreatic cancer tissues from patients without lymph node metastasis (n = 43) and with lymph node metastasis (n = 41). **c** The expression of DLX6-AS1 in pancreatic cancer tissues from patients with TNM stages (I–II, n = 38; III-IV, n = 46). **d** The expression of DLX6-AS1 in well/moderate (n = 33) and poor differentiated (n = 51) pancreatic cancer tissues. *P < 0.05, **P < 0.01 and ***P < 0.001

**Table 1** Correlation between lncRNA DLX6-AS1 expression and clinicopathological parameters of patients with pancreatic cancer

| Clinical parameters | DLX6-AS1 expression | | P value |
|---|---|---|---|
| | Low (n = 41) | High (n = 43) | |
| Gender | | | |
| Male | 22 | 20 | 0.6627 |
| Female | 19 | 23 | |
| Age (years) | | | |
| < 60 | 15 | 17 | 0.825 |
| ≥ 60 | 26 | 26 | |
| Tumor size (cm) | | | |
| < 2 | 27 | 17 | 0.0181 |
| ≥ 2 | 14 | 26 | |
| TNM stage | | | |
| I–II | 25 | 13 | 0.0081 |
| III–IV | 16 | 30 | |
| Tumor differentiation | | | |
| Well/Moderate | 21 | 12 | 0.0438 |
| Poor | 20 | 31 | |
| Lymph node metastasis | | | |
| Negative | 28 | 15 | 0.0026 |
| Positive | 13 | 28 | |
| Distant metastasis | | | |
| Negative | 22 | 18 | 0.3822 |
| Positive | 19 | 25 | |

cells (Fig. 2a). To investigate the biological function of DLX6-AS1 in pancreatic cancer cells, CCK-8 assay, colony formation assay and Transwell migration/invasion assay were performed to measure the cell proliferation, migration and invasion in SW1990 and PANC-1 cells transfected with DLX6-AS1 siRNAs or scrambled siRNA. The knockdown efficiency of DLX6-AS1 siR-NAs [si-DLX6-AS1 and DLX6-AS1(a)] was firstly confirmed in both cell lines (Fig. 2b). CCK-8 assay results showed that both siDLX6-AS1 and siDLX6-AS1(a) suppressed cell viability of pancreatic cancer cells in a time-dependent number (Fig. 2c, d). As both siRNAs were effective in suppressing DLX6-AS1 expression and cell viability, siDLX6-AS1 was used for further

experimentation. Colony formation assay results demonstrated that DLX6-AS1 knockdown reduced the number of colonies compared to siNC group (Fig. 2e). Additionally, migration/invasion assay results showed that siDLX6-AS1 transfection suppressed cell migration and invasion abilities of SW1990 and PANC-1cells (Fig. 2f, g).

### DLX6-AS1 targeted miR-181b in pancreatic cancer cells

We used the DIANA tools to predict the potential targets of DLX6-AS1 and found that miR-181b contain the complementary binding site of DLX6-AS1. To confirm this, luciferase reporter vectors containing the wild type or mutated binding sites were constructed. They were co-transfected with miR-181b mimics or mimic NC into HEK293T cells. The results showed that miR-181b reduced the luciferase activity of wild type DLX6-AS1, but had no effect on the mutant one (Fig. 3a, b). Furthermore, SW1990 and PANC-1cells were transfected with siDLX6-AS1or siNC. The qRT-PCR results revealed that silencing DLX6-AS1 increased the expression level of miR-181b in both cell lines (Fig. 3c). Meanwhile, the miR-181b expression level in pancreatic cancer tissues was lower than that in the adjacent normal tissues (Fig. 3d). Furthermore, a negative correlation between DLX6-AS1 and miR-181b expression in the pancreatic cancer tissues was observed (Fig. 3e).

### DLX6-AS1 regulated cell viability and invasion through miR-181b

Firstly, we have checked the expression of miR-181b in four human pancreatic cancer cell lines and one normal pancreatic duct epithelial cell line (HPDE6-C7). Decreased expression of miR-181b was observed in cancer cell lines compared with HPDE6-C7 cells and miR-181b inhibitor transfection reduced the expression of miR-181b in both SW1990 and PANC-1 cells (Fig. 4a, b). Previously, we have shown that knockdown of DLX6-AS1 suppressed pancreatic cancer cell proliferation, migration and invasion. To explore whether DLX6-AS1 exerted biological effects through miR-181b, the cells were treated with siDLX6-AS1, together with miR-181b inhibitor or inhibitor NC. CCK-8 assay showed that miR-181b inhibitor reversed the reduction of cell viability as

(See figure on next page.)

**Fig. 2** Knockdown of lncRNA DLX6-AS1 suppressed pancreatic cancer cell proliferation, migration and invasion. **a** The expression of DLX6-AS1 in human pancreatic cancer cell lines and human pancreatic duct epithelial cell line (HPDE6-C7) was determined by qRT-PCR. **b** DLX6-AS1 siRNAs [siDLX6-AS1 and siDLX6-AS1(a)] transfection suppressed the expression of DLX6-AS1 in SW1990 cell sand PANC-1 cells. The cell proliferation of **c** SW1990 cells and **d** PANC-1 cells transfected with siNC, siDLX6-AS1 or siDLX6-AS1(a) was determined by CCK-8 assay. **e** Colony formation assay was performed to analyze the cell growth of SW1990 and PANC-1 cells transfected with siNC or siDLX6-AS1. **f** Cell migration and **g** cell invasion of SW1990 and PANC-1 cells transfected with siNC or siDLX6-AS1 were determined by Transwell migration assay and Transwell invasion assay, respectively. *P < 0.05, **P < 0.01 and ***P < 0.001

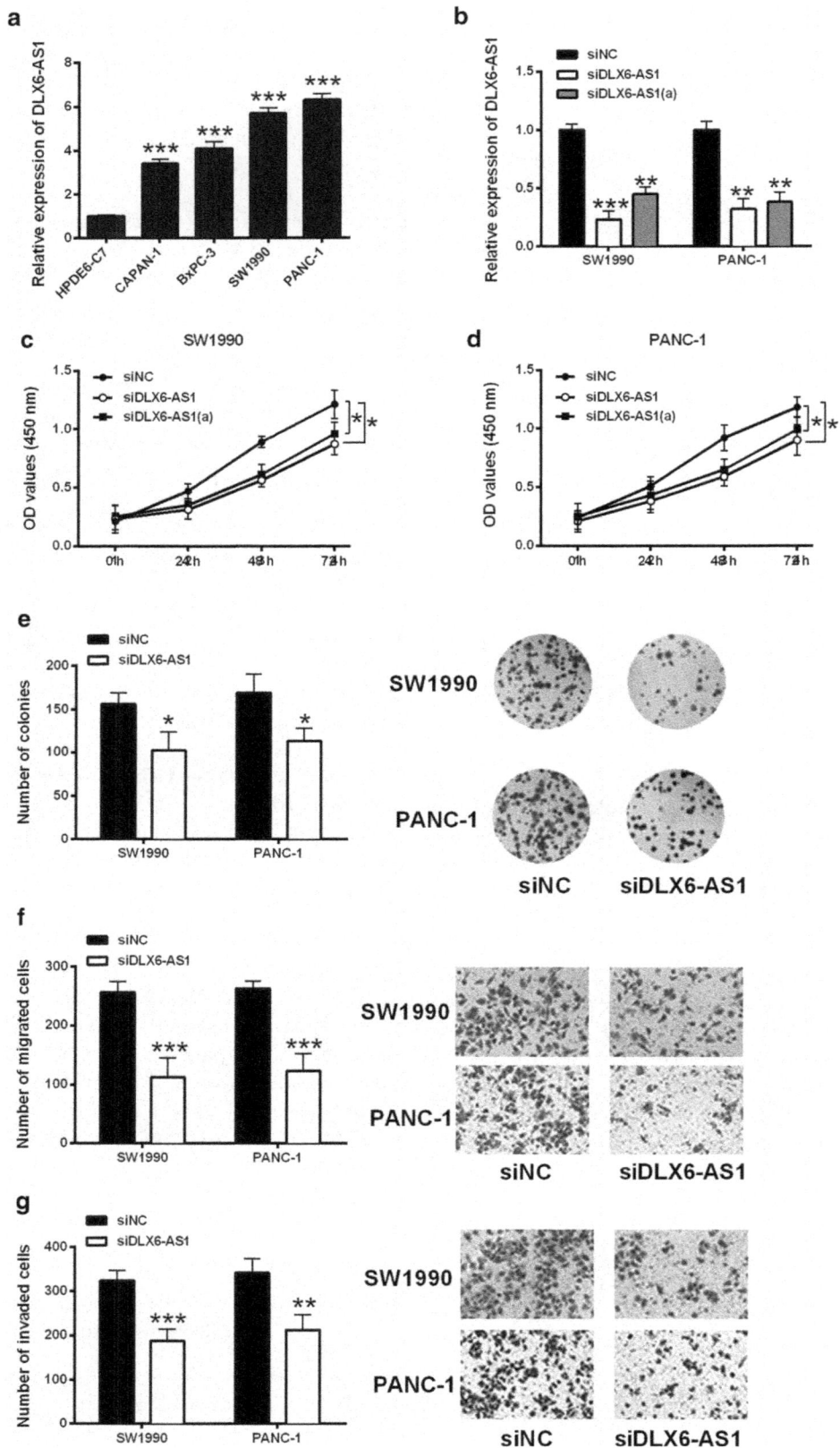

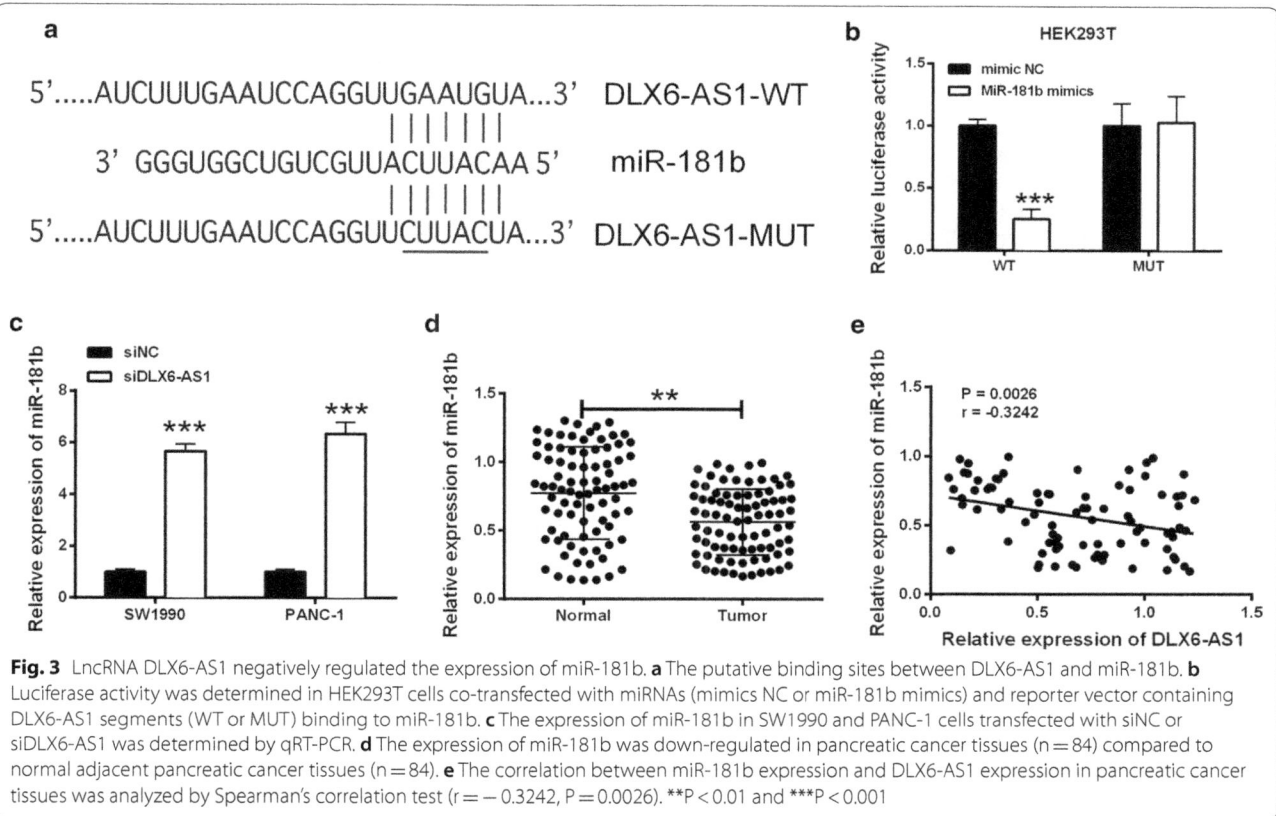

**Fig. 3** LncRNA DLX6-AS1 negatively regulated the expression of miR-181b. **a** The putative binding sites between DLX6-AS1 and miR-181b. **b** Luciferase activity was determined in HEK293T cells co-transfected with miRNAs (mimics NC or miR-181b mimics) and reporter vector containing DLX6-AS1 segments (WT or MUT) binding to miR-181b. **c** The expression of miR-181b in SW1990 and PANC-1 cells transfected with siNC or siDLX6-AS1 was determined by qRT-PCR. **d** The expression of miR-181b was down-regulated in pancreatic cancer tissues (n = 84) compared to normal adjacent pancreatic cancer tissues (n = 84). **e** The correlation between miR-181b expression and DLX6-AS1 expression in pancreatic cancer tissues was analyzed by Spearman's correlation test (r = − 0.3242, P = 0.0026). **P < 0.01 and ***P < 0.001

well as colony formation ability caused by DLX6-AS1 knockdown in SW1990 and PANC-1 cells (Fig. 4c–e). In addition, cell migration and invasion assay showed that miR-181b inhibitor abrogated the inhibitory effect of DLX6-AS1 knockdown on cell migration and invasion in SW1990 and PANC-1 cells (Fig. 4f, g).

### miR-181b targeted ZEB2 and regulated epithelial-mesenchymal transition (EMT) in pancreatic cancer cells

Similarly, we used the TargetScan to predict the potential targets of miR-181b and found that ZEB2 was one of the targets of miR-181b. Luciferase reporter assay showed miR-181b mimics reduced the luciferase activity of wild type ZEB2 3′UTR, but had no effect on the mutant one (Fig. 5a, b). Next, the mRNA expression level of ZEB2 was measured in cell lines and patient tissues. ZEB2 expression was reduced by miR-181b mimics transfection in SW1990 and PANC-1 cells (Fig. 5c) and the mRNA expression level of ZEB2 was higher in pancreatic tumor tissues than that in the paired adjacent ones (Fig. 5d). In addition, a negative correlation between miR-181b and ZEB2 mRNA expression in pancreatic cancer tissues was observed (Fig. 5c–e). Furthermore, the mRNA and protein levels of ZEB2 and EMT markers including

E-cadherin, vimentin and N-cadherin were examined. DLX6-AS1 knockdown decreased the mRNA and protein expression levels of ZEB2, vimentin and N-cadherin, and increased the mRNA and protein expression levels of E-cadherin, which was abrogated by miR-181b inhibitor transfection (Fig. 5f, g).

### DLX6-AS1 knock-down inhibited tumor growth in vivo

SW1990 cells stably transfected with shDLX6-AS1 or shNC were injected into the nude mice. As shown in Fig. 6a, DLX6-AS1 knockdown inhibited tumor growth comparing with shNC group. The tumor volume at 25, 30 and 35 d following injection was significantly lower in shDLX6-AS1 group than that in shNC group. The weight of dissected tumors in shDLX6-AS1 group was also lower than that in shNC group (Fig. 6a, b). The number of metastatic nodules in the lung from the shDLX6-AS1 group was significantly reduced compared to shNC group (Fig. 6c). Moreover, in consistent with the in vitro results, the expression of DLX6-AS1 was decreased and the expression of miR-181b was increased in shDLX6-AS1 group (Fig. 6d, e). In addition, the mRNA and protein levels of ZEB2, vimentin and N-cadherin was down-regulated while E-cadherin was up-regulated in shDLX6-AS1 (Fig. 6f, g).

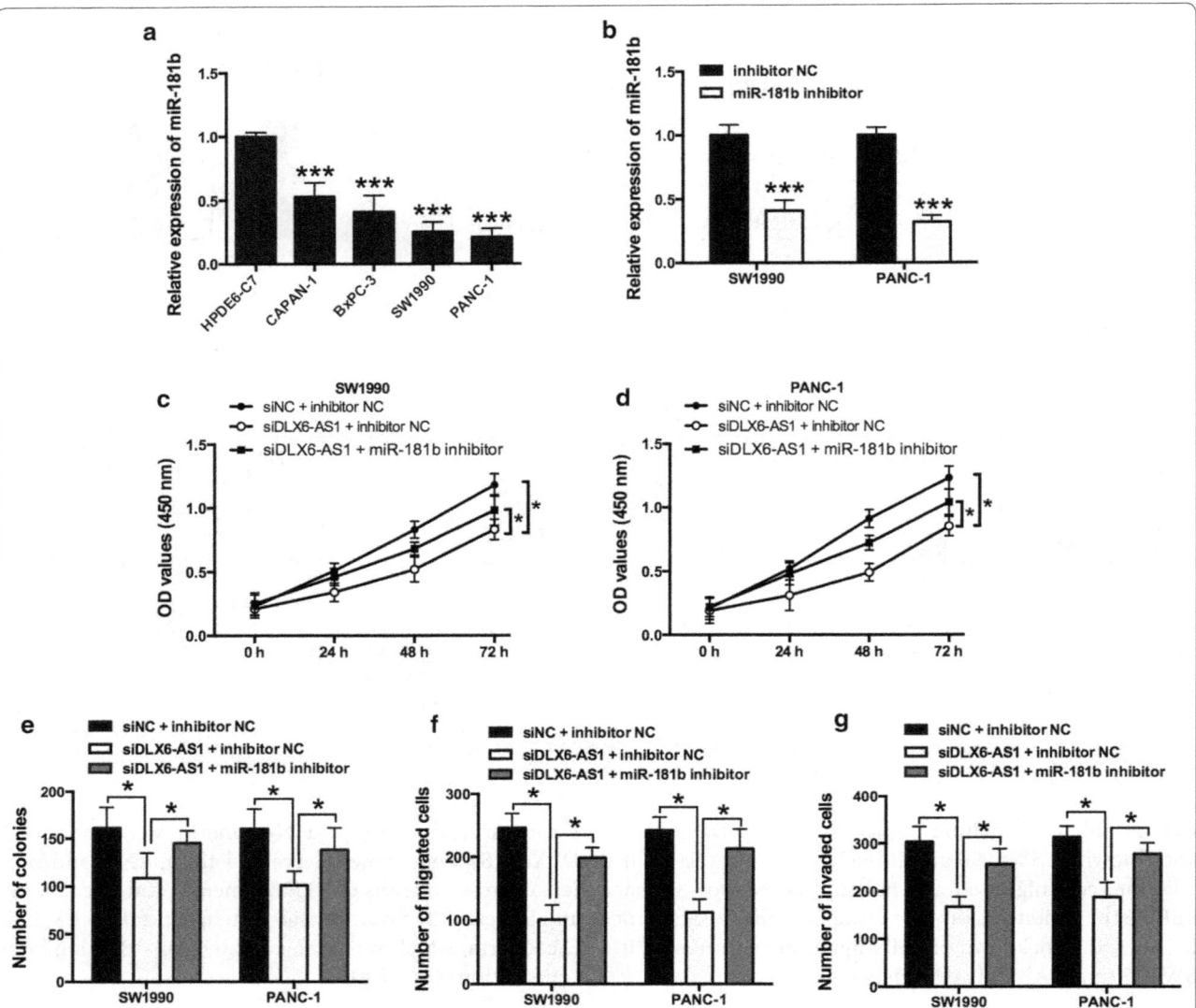

**Fig. 4** Knockdown of miR-181b attenuated DLX6-AS1-mediated effects on pancreatic cancer cell proliferation, migration and invasion. **a** The expression of miR-181b in human pancreatic cancer cell lines and human pancreatic duct epithelial cell line (HPDE6-C7) was determined by qRT-PCR. **b** The expression of miR-181b in SW1990 and PANC-1 cells transfected inhibitor NC or miR-181b inhibitor was determined by qRT-PCR. The cell proliferation of **c** SW1990 and **d** PANC-1 cells co-transfected with siNC + inhibitor NC, siDLX6-AS1 + inhibitor NC, or siDLX6-AS1 + miR-181b inhibitor was determined by CCK-8 assay. **e** Cell growth, **f** cell migration and **g** cell invasion of SW1990 and PANC-1 cells co-transfected with siNC + inhibitor NC, siDLX6-AS1 + inhibitor NC, or siDLX6-AS1 + miR-181b inhibitor were determined by colony formation assay, Transwell migration assay and Transwell invasion assay, respectively. *P < 0.05 and ***P < 0.001

## Discussion

In the early stage of pancreatic cancer, there are almost no symptoms. When patients have typical symptoms, they have already reached an advanced stage and showed tumor metastasis [16]. As a result, the prognosis for pancreatic cancer is poor and the 5-year overall survival is very low with median survival of only 6 months [17, 18]. These make us to seek more effective

therapies and advanced strategies for the treatment of pancreatic cancer.

Accumulating evidence has demonstrated the critical roles of lncRNAs in regulating pathological processes of pancreatic cancer. For instance, ectopic expression of AB209630 suppressed cell proliferation ability in pancreatic ductal adenocarcinoma cells resistant to gemcitabine through blocking the PI3K/AKT signaling pathway [19].

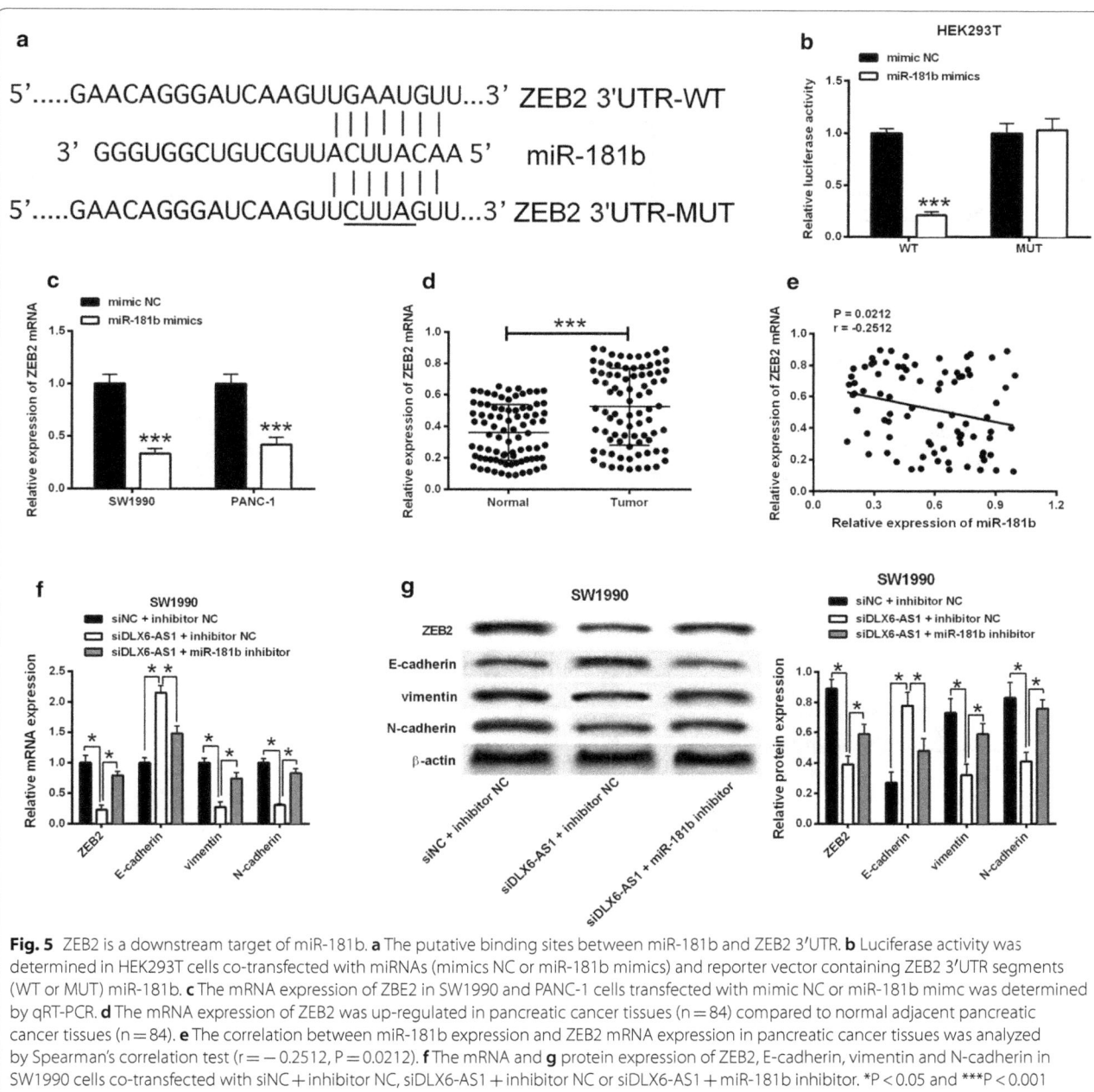

**Fig. 5** ZEB2 is a downstream target of miR-181b. **a** The putative binding sites between miR-181b and ZEB2 3′UTR. **b** Luciferase activity was determined in HEK293T cells co-transfected with miRNAs (mimics NC or miR-181b mimics) and reporter vector containing ZEB2 3′UTR segments (WT or MUT) miR-181b. **c** The mRNA expression of ZBE2 in SW1990 and PANC-1 cells transfected with mimic NC or miR-181b mimc was determined by qRT-PCR. **d** The mRNA expression of ZEB2 was up-regulated in pancreatic cancer tissues (n = 84) compared to normal adjacent pancreatic cancer tissues (n = 84). **e** The correlation between miR-181b expression and ZEB2 mRNA expression in pancreatic cancer tissues was analyzed by Spearman's correlation test (r = − 0.2512, P = 0.0212). **f** The mRNA and **g** protein expression of ZEB2, E-cadherin, vimentin and N-cadherin in SW1990 cells co-transfected with siNC + inhibitor NC, siDLX6-AS1 + inhibitor NC or siDLX6-AS1 + miR-181b inhibitor. *P < 0.05 and ***P < 0.001

UCA1 was up-regulated in pancreatic cancer tissues and correlated with poor clinical outcome, and promoted cell migration and invasion by the Hippo signaling pathway [20]. XLOC_000647 served as a tumor suppressor, impairing cell proliferation, invasion, and epithelial-mesenchymal transition abilities through NLRP3 inhibition in pancreatic cancer [21]. In this study, we identified the upregulation of DLX6-AS1 in pancreatic cancer. Besides, knockdown of DLX6-AS1 dramatically impaired pancreatic cancer cell proliferation, migration and invasion.

Recently, lncRNAs was found to function as competing endogenous RNAs to regulate the expression level of miRNA, thus playing crucial role in the development of cancer. For better understanding the mechanisms of DLX6-AS1 in pancreatic cancer, we found that miR-181b was of the downstream targets, and miR-181b has been reported as tumor suppressor in various cancers. In glioblastoma, lower level of miR-181b was correlated with more advanced grade patients. MiR-181b can modulate vascular cell adhesion molecule 1 expression

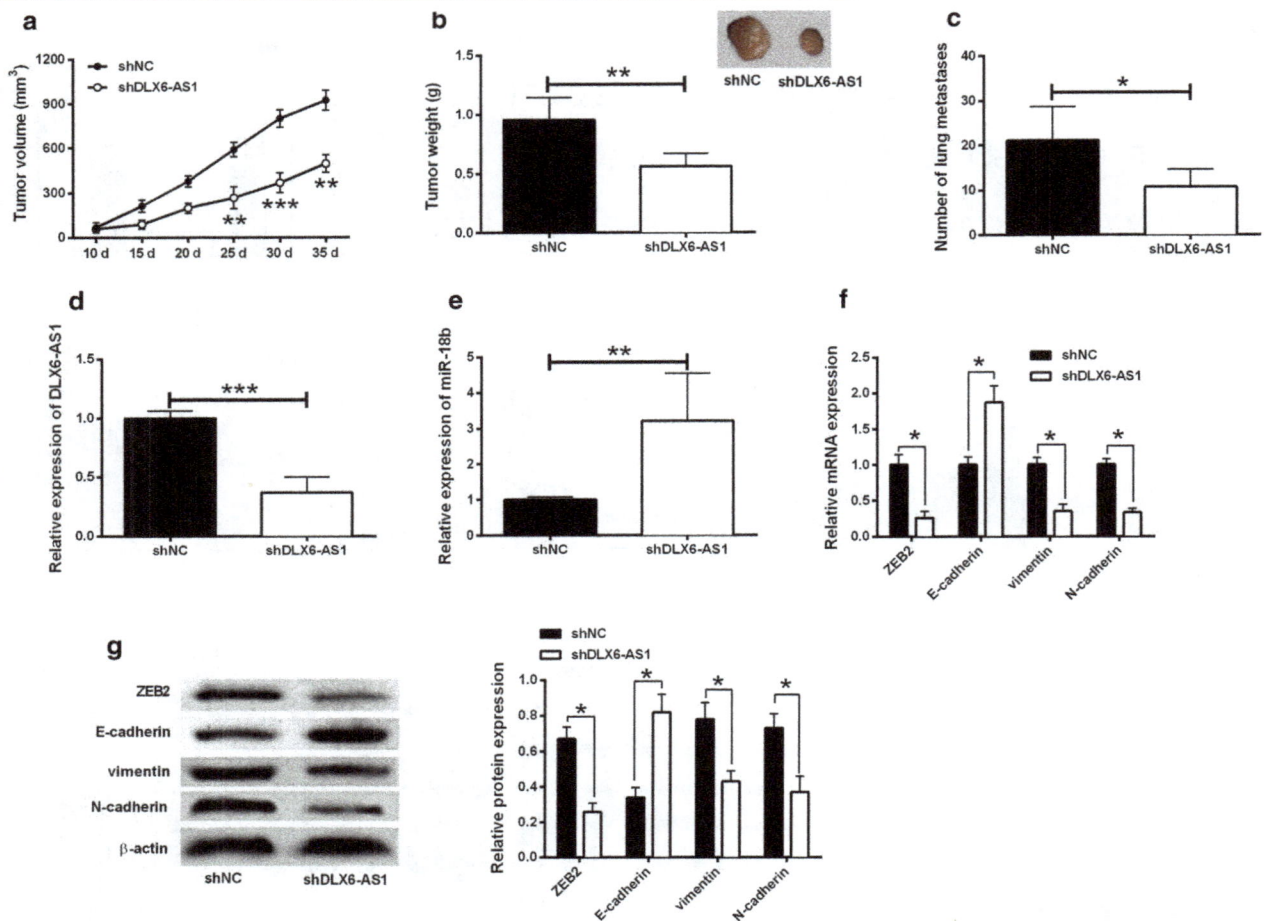

**Fig. 6** Knockdown of DLX6-AS1 inhibited in vivo tumor growth in nude mice. **a** The tumor volume at 25, 30 and 35 days following tumor cells injection was significantly lower in shDLX6-AS1 group than that in shNC group. **b** The weight of dissected tumors in shDLX6-AS1 group was lower than that in shNC group. **c** The number of metastatic nodules in the lung from shDLX6-AS1 group was reduced compared to that in shNC group. The expression of **d** DLX6-AS1 and **e** miR-181b in dissected tumor tissues from shNC group and shDLX6-AS1 group were determined qRT-PCR. **f** The mRNA and **g** protein expression of ZEB2, E-cadherin, vimentin and N-cadherin in the dissected tissues were determined by qRT-PCR and western blot, respectively. *P < 0.05, **P < 0.01 and ***P < 0.001

and monocyte adhesion in an epidermal growth factor receptor-dependent pathway [22]. MiR-181b suppressed cell cycle, cell viability and proliferation through down-regulation of FAMLF in burkitt lymphoma cells [23]. In breast cancer, ectopic expression of miR-181b inhibited the increase of NF-κB level induced by chemokine ligand 18 in cancer cells, thus suppressing cell survival rate and migration [24]. Consistent with the above reports, our results showed that miR-181b functioned as a tumor suppressor in pancreatic cancer. Its inhibition reversed the reduction of cell viability, migration and invasion abilities caused by DLX6-AS1 knockdown.

Furthermore, we investigated the molecular basis of miR-181b through TargetScan and found that ZEB2 was the downstream target of miR-181b. Here we found that

the expression level of ZEB2 in pancreatic cancer tissues was higher than that in the paired adjacent ones. ZEB2 belongs to the ZEB proteins family, and was reported to interact with SMAD protein, involving TGF-β-induced EMT. During EMT, epithelial cells obtain the motile and invasive abilities typical of mesenchymal cells, which is an important process for cancer metastasis and associated with poor prognosis [25, 26]. In terms of molecular level, this process is indicated by the expression changes of some markers, including loss of epithelial markers and the gain of mesenchymal markers. ZEB2 is reported to be a repressor of E-cadherin and the cadherin switching, like decrease in E-cadherin and increase in N-cadherin is a feature of EMT in malignant tumors [27, 28]. In the present study, in vitro data showed that DLX6-AS1 knockdown decreased ZEB2 expression level, followed by the increase of E-cadherin and decrease of vimentin and N-cadherin, which was abrogated by miR-181b inhibitors. In the mouse xenograft models, the mRNA level of ZEB2, vimentin and N-cadherin was downregulated while E-cadherin was up-regulated in the DLX6-AS1 knock-down group with reduced tumor size and suppressed tumor metastasis. Taken together, the effect of DLX6-AS1 on EMT depends on the regulation of ZEB2 through targeting miR-181b. In addition, our results showed that the effects of DLX6-AS1 knockdown on survival were marginal, and the effects of DLX6-AS1 knockdown and the rescue experiments have a greater effect on cell migration and EMT-related markers expression, indicating that dysregulation of DLX6-AS1 may be more important for pancreatic cancer metastasis rather than tumor maintenance.

## Conclusion

In conclusion, we investigated the uncharacterized role of DLX6-AS1 in pancreatic cancer and demonstrated that DLX6-AS1 promoted cancer cell proliferation and invasion by attenuating the endogenous function of miR-181b.

**Authors' contributions**
HC designed and conceived the whole study. YA and XC wrote the main manuscript. YA, XC and FM performed the experiments. YY, FM, YJ and DS performed data analysis. All authors contributed to manuscript revisions. All authors read and approved the final manuscript.

**Acknowledgements**
None.

**Competing interests**
The authors declare that they have no competing interests.

**Funding**
This study was supported by Natural Science Foundation of Jiangsu Province (No. BK20150254), Applied Basic Research of Changzhou Technology Bureau (No. CJ20140023) and National Natural Science Foundation of China (No. 81502002).

## References

1. Kamisawa T, Wood LD, Itoi T, Takaori K. Pancreatic cancer. Lancet. 2016;388(10039):73–85.

2. Di Marco M, Grassi E, Durante S, Vecchiarelli S, Palloni A, Macchini M, Casadei R, Ricci C, Panzacchi R, Santini D, et al. State of the art biological therapies in pancreatic cancer. World J Gastrointest Oncol. 2016;8(1):55–66.

3. Kipps E, Young K, Starling N. Liposomal irinotecan in gemcitabine-refractory metastatic pancreatic cancer: efficacy, safety and place in therapy. Ther Adv Med Oncol. 2017;9(3):159–70.

4. Rajabpour A, Afgar A, Mahmoodzadeh H, Radfar JE, Rajaei F, Teimoori-Toolabi L. MiR-608 regulating the expression of ribonucleotide reductase M1 and cytidine deaminase is repressed through induced gemcitabine chemoresistance in pancreatic cancer cells. Cancer Chemother Pharmacol. 2017;80(4):765–75.

5. Kim E, Kim K, Kyu Chie E, Oh DY, Tae Kim Y. Chemoradiotherapy after gemcitabine plus erlotinib in patients with locally advanced pancreatic cancer. J BUON. 2017;22(4):1046–52.

6. Djebali S, Davis CA, Merkel A, Dobin A, Lassmann T, Mortazavi A, Tanzer A, Lagarde J, Lin W, Schlesinger F, et al. Landscape of transcription in human cells. Nature. 2012;489(7414):101–8.

7. Gutschner T, Diederichs S. The hallmarks of cancer: a long non-coding RNA point of view. RNA Biol. 2012;9(6):703–19.

8. Ma L, Tian X, Guo H, Zhang Z, Du C, Wang F, Xie X, Gao H, Zhuang Y, Kornmann M, et al. Long noncoding RNA H19 derived miR-675 regulates cell proliferation by down-regulating E2F-1 in human pancreatic ductal adenocarcinoma. J Cancer. 2018;9(2):389–99.

9. Lian Y, Li Z, Fan Y, Huang Q, Chen J, Liu W, Xiao C, Xu H. The lncRNA-HOXA-AS2/EZH2/LSD1 oncogene complex promotes cell proliferation in pancreatic cancer. Am J Transl Res. 2017;9(12):5496–506.

10. Hayes J, Peruzzi PP, Lawler S. MicroRNAs in cancer: biomarkers, functions and therapy. Trends Mol Med. 2014;20(8):460–9.

11. Shah MY, Ferrajoli A, Sood AK, Lopez-Berestein G, Calin GA. microRNA therapeutics in cancer—an emerging concept. EBioMedicine. 2016;12:34–42.

12. Xie F, Huang Q, Liu CH, Lin XS, Liu Z, Liu LL, Huang DW, Zhou HC. MiR-1271 negatively regulates AKT/MTOR signaling and promotes apoptosis via targeting PDK1 in pancreatic cancer. Eur Rev Med Pharmacol Sci. 2018;22(3):678–86.

13. Feng SD, Mao Z, Liu C, Nie YS, Sun B, Guo M, Su C. Simultaneous overexpression of miR-126 and miR-34a induces a superior antitumor efficacy in pancreatic adenocarcinoma. OncoTargets Ther. 2017;10:5591–604.

14. Li J, Li P, Zhao W, Yang R, Chen S, Bai Y, Dun S, Chen X, Du Y, Wang Y, et al. Expression of long non-coding RNA DLX6-AS1 in lung adenocarcinoma. Cancer Cell Int. 2015;15:48.

15. Li L, Hou A, Gao X, Zhang J, Zhang L, Wang J, Li H, Song Y. Lentivirus-mediated miR-23a overexpression induces trophoblast cell apoptosis through inhibiting X-linked inhibitor of apoptosis. Biomed Pharmacother. 2017;94:412–7.

16. Ryan DP, Hong TS, Bardeesy N. Pancreatic adenocarcinoma. N Engl J Med. 2014;371(11):1039–49.

17. Hidalgo M. Pancreatic cancer. N Engl J Med. 2010;362(17):1605–17.

18. Vincent A, Herman J, Schulick R, Hruban RH, Goggins M. Pancreatic cancer. Lancet. 2011;378(9791):607–20.

19. Wang L, Wang F, Na L, Yu J, Huang L, Meng ZQ, Chen Z, Chen H, Ming LL, Hua YQ. LncRNA AB209630 inhibits gemcitabine resistance cell proliferation by regulating PI3K/AKT signaling in pancreatic ductal adenocarcinoma. Cancer Biomark. 2018;22(1):169–74.

20. Zhang M, Zhao Y, Zhang Y, Wang D, Gu S, Feng W, Peng W, Gong A, Xu M. LncRNA UCA1 promotes migration and invasion in pancreatic cancer cells via the Hippo pathway. Biochimica et biophysica acta. 2018;1864(5 Pt A):1770–82.

21. Hu H, Wang Y, Ding X, He Y, Lu Z, Wu P, Tian L, Yuan H, Liu D, Shi G, et al. Long non-coding RNA XLOC_000647 suppresses progression of pancreatic cancer and decreases epithelial-mesenchymal transition-induced cell invasion by down-regulating NLRP3. Mol Cancer. 2018;17(1):18.

22. Liu YS, Lin HY, Lai SW, Huang CY, Huang BR, Chen PY, Wei KC, Lu DY. MiR-181b modulates EGFR-dependent VCAM-1 expression and monocyte adhesion in glioblastoma. Oncogene. 2017;36(35):5006–22.

23. Li JG, Ding Y, Huang YM, Chen WL, Pan LL, Li Y, Chen XL, Chen Y, Wang SY, Wu XN. FAMLF is a target of miR-181b in Burkitt lymphoma. Braz J Med Biol Res. 2017;50(6):e5661.

24. Wang L, Wang YX, Chen LP, Ji ML. Upregulation of microRNA-181b inhibits CCL18-induced breast cancer cell metastasis and invasion via the NF-kappaB signaling pathway. Oncol Lett. 2016;12(6):4411–8.

25. Lim J, Thiery JP. Epithelial-mesenchymal transitions: insights from development. Development. 2012;139(19):3471–86.

26. Tam WL, Weinberg RA. The epigenetics of epithelial-mesenchymal plasticity in cancer. Nat Med. 2013;19(11):1438–49.

27. Zhu GJ, Song PP, Zhou H, Shen XH, Wang JG, Ma XF, Gu YJ, Liu DD, Feng AN, Qian XY, et al. Role of epithelial-mesenchymal transition markers E-cadherin, N-cadherin, beta-catenin and ZEB2 in laryngeal squamous cell carcinoma. Oncol Lett. 2018;15(3):3472–81.

28. Wang T, Chen X, Qiao W, Kong L, Sun D, Li Z. Transcription factor E2F1 promotes EMT by regulating ZEB2 in small cell lung cancer. BMC Cancer. 2017;17(1):719.

# miR-144/451 cluster plays an oncogenic role in esophageal cancer by inhibiting cell invasion

Zhikui Gao[1] (ID), Peng Zhang[2], Ming Xie[3], Han Gao[1], Lihong Yin[1] and Ran Liu[1*]

## Abstract

**Background:** miRNA clusters are widely expressed across species, accumulating evidence has illustrated that miRNA cluster functioned more efficiently than single miRNA in cancer oncogenesis. It is likely that miRNA clusters are more stable and reliable than individual miRNA to be biomarkers for diagnosis and therapy. We previously found low expression of miR-144/451 was closely related with the risk for esophageal cancer. Researches on miR-144/451 cluster were mostly focused on individual miRNA but not the whole cluster, the regulatory mechanism of miRNA cluster were largely unknown.

**Methods:** In present study, we firstly analysed biological functions of individual miRNAs of miR-144/451 in ECa9706 transfected with miRNA mimics. We further analysed the biological function of the whole cluster in stable trans-genic cell overexpressing miR-144/451. We then performed genome-wide mRNA microarray to detect differentially expressed gene profiles in stable transgenic cells.

**Results:** Overexpression of miR-144-3p promoted early apoptosis of ECa9706 and inhibited cell migration, cell inva-sion and cell proliferation. miR-144-5p and miR-451a inhibited cell proliferation, at the same time, miR-451a inhibited cell migration. Overexpression of miR-144/451 leads to the arrest cell cycle from S to G2 and G2 to M,while the inva-sion ability was obviously inhibited. We further observed c-Myc, p-ERK were downregulated in cells overexpressing miR-144/451, while p53 was up-regulated. The downstream effectors of c-Myc, MMP9 and p-cdc2 were downregu-lated in miR-144/451 stable transgenic cell. miR-144/451 may or partly inhibited cell cycles and invasion of ECa9706 through inhibiting ERK/c-Myc signaling pathway.

**Conclusion:** Collectively, we analysed the function of miR-144/451 cluster from individual to overall level. miR-144/451 cluster played proto oncogene role in esophageal cancer by inhibiting cell invasion.

**Keywords:** Esophageal cancer, miRNA cluster, miR-144-3p, miR-144-5p, miR-451a

## Background

Esophageal cancer is a common digestive system cancer with high incidence and mortality. According to statistics of WHO, esophageal cancer ranks as the fourth high-est cause of cancer-related mortality in the world, there are 456,000 new cases and 400,000 deaths in 2012, more than half of the new cases occurs in China [1]. It is worth mentioning the incidence is still growing. Although endoscopic resection is effective for esophageal cancer patients at early stage, the overall 5-year survival rate is still no more than 20% [2, 3]. There are no effective treat-ment for advanced esophageal cancer, so the key point for raising the survival rate of esophageal cancer is detect-ing and treating at early stage [4]. However, no obvious clinical symptom for esophageal cancer can be observed, searching for sensitive and specific biomarkers for early esophageal cancer becomes especially important.

Growing evidence showed that miRNAs played impor-tant roles in post transcriptional regulation by binding to

*Correspondence: ranliu@seu.edu.cn
[1] Key Laboratory of Environmental Medicine Engineering, Ministry of Education, School of Public Health, Southeast University, Nanjing 210009, China
Full list of author information is available at the end of the article

the 3′UTR region of mRNAs, directing the repression of protein expression [5]. Abnormal miRNA-mediated regulation can affect oncellular functions which were closely related to the occurrence of tumor, miRNAs seem to be important molecular markers in the diagnosis of tumor [6, 7]. Usually, miRNA genes were transcribed under the regulation of promoter and operon, in particular some were closely aligned on chromosome formed as a cluster. These clusters are suspected to transcribe together, though not exclusively, mediate synergistic or antagonistic regulatory effects. miRNA cluster is likely to be more stable and reliable than individual miRNA to be biomarkers for diagnosis [8, 9]. However, most of the studies on miRNA clusters focused on individual miRNAs but not the cluster, regulatory mechanisms of miRNA cluster were largely unknown.

miR-144/451 cluster is highly conversed in different species, miRbase database (http://www.mirba se.org/) shows miR-144/451 cluster is constituted by miR-144-3p, miR-144-5p, miR-451a, miR-4732-3p and miR-4732-5p (Table 1). In previous study, we discovered the low-expression of miR-144/451 was closely related with the risk for esophageal cancer [10]. miR-144-3p was reported to be related with gastric carcinoma, lung cancer, hepatoma and colorectal cancer [11–14], miR-144-5p was reported to be related with bladder cancer and colorectal cancer [15, 16], miR-451a was reported to be related with lung cancer, gastric carcinoma, colorectal cancer, liver cancer, breast cancer and osteosarcoma [17–22]. However, few is known about the function and mechanism of miR-144/451 in esophageal cancer. Most of the researches about miR-144/451 is focused only on single miRNAs but not on the cluster.

In present study, we analysed functions of individual miRNA of miR-144/451 in ECa9706, we established stable transgenic cells overexpressing miR-144/451 and analysed the function of the cluster. To better understand the potential mechanism of the cluster, genome-wide mRNA microarray and Western blot were performed. Results

of the present study may advance our understanding of the expression pattern and functional role of the miR-144/451 cluster in esophageal carcinoma.

## Materials and methods

### Cell line

ECa9706, ECa109, H5E46, Het-1A and HEK-293T cells were provided by Key Laboratory of Environmental Medicine Engineering, Ministry of Education, School of Public Health, Southeast University. Cells were grown in RPMI-1640 containing 10% fetal bovine serum (Gibico), 100 U/mL penicillin–streptomycin solution (Gibico) at 37 °C in incubator containing 5% $CO_2$ humidified atmosphere. Transient transfected Cells over-expressing miRNAs were obtained using micrON™ miRNA mimic (RiboBio). Lipofectamine® RNAiMAX Reagent (Invitrogen) were used for transfection according to manufacturer's instructions. Stable expression cell strain over-expressing miR-144/451 cluster were obtained using lentiviral transfection.

### Plasmids construction, virus production, and infection of target cells

To obtain pri-miR-144/451 cluster plasmid, a synthetic sequence within the range of upstream 200 bp to downstream 200 bp of pri-miR-144/451 was cloned into PCDH-CMV-MCS-EF1-Puro lentivirus plasmid. Plasmids of pMDLg/pRRE, pRSV-Rev, pMD2G and PCDH-CMV-MCS-EF1-Puro were transfected into HEK-293T for packaging lentivirus.

### Antibodies and reagents

PTEN (138G6) Rabbit Monoclonal antibody, Phospho-cdc2 (Tyr15) antibody, Phospho-p44/42 MAPK (ERK1/2) (Thr202/Tyr204) Rabbit Monoclonal antibody, p44/42 MAPK (Erk1/2) Rabbit Monoclonal antibody, Phospho-β-Catenin (Ser33/37/Thr41) antibody, Total-β-Catenin antibody, Phospho-c-Myc (Ser62) Rabbit Monoclonal antibody, p53 Rabbit Monoclonal antibody, Non-phospho (Active) β-Catenin (Ser33/37/Thr41) Rabbit Monoclonal antibody were obtained from Cell Signaling Technology (CST). Mouse anti-human C-myc monoclonal antibody, anti-MMP-9 antibody were obtained from Millipore.

### Apoptosis and cell cycle

For cells transfected with mimics, cell apoptosis were detected using Annexin V-APC/7-AAD Apoptosis Detection Kit (KGA1026, KeyGEN BioTECH) according to the manufacture's protocol, for cells stably transfected with Lentiviral vectors, cell apoptosis was detected using (KGA1026, KeyGEN BioTECH). Flow cytometry (PI staining) were used for detecting cell cycle using PI

**Table 1  Location and sequences of miR-144/451 cluster**

| miRNA | Sequence | Location (GRCh38) |
|-------|----------|-------------------|
| miR-144-3p | UACAGUAUAGAUGAUGUA CU | chr17: 28861584–28861603 |
| miR-144-5p | GGAUAUCAUCAUAUACUG UAAG | chr17: 28861547–28861568 |
| miR-451a | AAACCGUUACCAUUACUG AGUU | chr17: 28861385–28861406 |
| miR-4732-3p | GCCCUGACCUGUCCUGUU CUG | chr17: 28861663–28861685 |
| miR-4732-5p | UGUAGAGCAGGGAGCAGG AAGCU | chr17: 28861697–28861717 |

cell cycle Detection Kit (KGA107, KeyGEN BioTECH) according to the manufacture's protocol, experiments were done in triplicates.

## Cell proliferation assay

Cell proliferation were detected using 5-ethynyl-2′-deoxyuridine (EdU) labeling/detection kit (Ribobio). Firstly, cells with a density of $1 \times 104$ cells/well were planted on 96-well plates, after 24 h, 50 mM EdU were added into the plate for an additional 2 h. Then the cells were fixed with 4% formaldehyde in PBS for 30 min and incubate with glycine for 5 min. After washing with PBS and 0.5% TritonX-100 in PBS, cells were incubated with $1 \times$ Apollo dye at room temperature in dankness for 30 min. At last, wash cells with 0.5% TritonX-100 in PBS and methanol, incubate cells with $1 \times$ Hoechst 33342 dye at room temperature in dankness for 30 min. Preserve labeled cells in PBS. Observe and photograph using fluorescence microscopy, select five images randomly for cell counting, Assays were performed with five parallels.

## Invasion and migration

Cell invasion and migration were detected using 8.0 μm Transwell chamber (Corning). For cell migration, $5 \times 10^4$ cells were seeded into the upper chamber in serum-free media, the lower chamber were filled with RPMI-1640 containing 10% fetal bovine serum, culture for 24 h, color and count migrated cell. For cell invasion, $5 \times 10^5$ cells were seeded into the upper chamber using serum-free media, the lower chamber were filled with RPMI-1640 containing 50% fetal bovine serum, culture for 24 h, color and count invasive cells, experiments were done in triplicates.

## RNA extraction and genome-wide mRNA microarray

Total RNA were isolated using Trizol reagent (Invitrogen). RNA concentration were measured using Nanodrop 2000 (Thermo Fisher) and Agilent 2100 Bioanalyzer (Agilent). aRNA were obtained using GeneChip 3′IVT PLUS Kit (Affymetrix). mRNA profiles were detected using Affymetrix GeneChip primeview human Expression Array (100 format) in miR-144/451 overexpressing and negative control cells, experiments were done in triplicates.

## Bioinformatics analysis of microarray and target prediction

Ingenuity Pathway Analysis (IPA) were performed for analysing mRNA profiles detected by genome-wide mRNA microarray.

## Western blot analysis

Cellular protein were extracted with cold RIPA buffer (Beyotime) containing protease and phosphatase inhibitors (Millipore). Lysates were cleared by centrifugation at 14,000 rpm at 4 °C for 15 min. Protein concentration were detected using bicinchoninic acid (BCA) assay (Thermo Fisher). Aliquots of protein (20 μg) were separated by 10% SDS-PAGE and the separated proteins were transferred onto 0.45 μm PVDF membrane (Millipore). Membranes were blocked with 5% (w/v) non-fat milk in Tris–HCl buffered saline (pH 7.4) with Tween-20 and incubated with the primary antibody overnight at 4 °C. Subsequently, membranes were washed with Tris–HCl buffered saline and incubated with secondary antibody conjugated to horseradish peroxidase respectively diluted in 1:1000, at room temperature for 1 h. Membranes were washed in Tris–HCl buffered saline and bounds were detected with SuperSignal West Femto/Pico Kit (Thermo Fisher). Blots were visualized and quantified using Tanon-5200 Imaging System (Tanon).

## RT-QPCR

All primers (Bulge-Loop™ miRNA RT-QPCR Primer kits) for miRNA were purchased from Guangzhou Ribo-Bio Co., Ltd. All primers for mRNA were synthetized in GenScript Corporation, U6 was selected as internal reference for miRNAs. The Sequence for forward primer of pri-miRNA was ACAGTGCTTTTCAAGCCATGC, for reverse primer, the sequence was GGGTGCCCGGAC TAGTACAT. β-actin was selected as internal reference for detecting pri-miRNA, sequence for forward primer was: ATCCGCAAAGACCTGT, and for reverse primer the sequence was: GGGTGTAACGCAACTAAG.

Total RNA (~ 2 μg) were extracted using Trizol regent (Invitrogen). cDNA was synthesized using Moloney Murine Leukemia Virus (MMLV) reverse transcriptase (Promega) and ribonuclease inhibitor (Thermo Fisher). SYBR Green mastermix were purchased from Toyobo Technologies. QPCR reactions were performed using StepOnePlus system (Applied Biosystems). Data for miRNA and mRNA were normalized using U6 and β-actin respectively. Expression of miRNA and mRNA were presented as relative RNA expression using $\Delta\Delta C_T$ formula (the fold change in target gene expression was equal to $2^{-\Delta\Delta CT}$). All results were presented as mean of triplicates ± SD of three independent experiments.

## Statistical analysis

Statistical analysis was performed using SPSS 17.0. Group differences were explored by Student's t-test and analysis of variance (ANOVA). $P$ value < 0.05 was considered to be statistically significant.

## Results

### Expression of miR-144/451 in different cells

We detected the expression of miR-144/451 in ECa9706, ECa109, H5E46 and Het-1A. miR-144-3p, miR-144-5p, miR-451a and miR-4732-3p were low expressed (Fig. 1a), Eca9706 were selected for further experiment.

### Transfection efficiency of miRNA mimics

In ECa9706, miRNA mimics significantly up-regulated expression of miR-144-3p, miR-144-5p, miR-451a, miR-4732-3p and miR-4732-5p. Fold changes for all these five miRNAs were more than 1000.

### Effects of individual miRNAs on biological function

miR-144-3p decreased the proportion of cells in G2 phase, but in cells over-expressing miR-451a, the proportion of cells in G2 increased. In cells overexpressing miR-144-3p and miR-451a there are $(14.62 \pm 1.41)\%$ and $(22.84 \pm 0.97)\%$ cells in G2 phase respectively, while in control the proportion is $(18.20 \pm 1.12)\%$ (Fig. 1b). miR-144-3p significantly promoted cell apoptosis with the early apoptosis rate of $(18.70 \pm 2.11)\%$, while in control, the early apoptosis rate was $(9.00 \pm 1.15)\%$ (Fig. 1c). Proliferation rate of cells overexpressing miR-144-3p, miR-144-5p, miR-451a and miR-4732-3p were $(34.18 \pm 5.83)\%$, $(33.56 \pm 3.94)\%$, $(34.15 \pm 2.94)\%$ and $(31.50 \pm 2.01)\%$ respectively, in control the proliferation rate was $(41.16 \pm 2.13)\%$ (Fig. 1d). For cell migration, compared with the number of migrated cells of $36.67 \pm 3.58$ in control, miR-144-3p, miR-451a, miR-4732-3p and miR-4732-5p inhibited cell migration, the number of cells passed through the membrane were $15.63 \pm 1.00$, $21.27 \pm 1.70$, $26.97 \pm 3.47$ and $24.87 \pm 1.36$ respectively. No difference were observed between cells over-expressing miR-144-5p and the control (Fig. 1e). For cell invasion, miR-144-3p obviously inhibited invasive ability, only $12.07 \pm 1.10$ cells passed through reconstituted basement membrane in cells overexpressing miR-133-3p, while the number was $25.90 \pm 2.26$ in control. For cell proliferation, miR-144-3p, miR-144-5p, miR-451a and miR-4732-3p significantly inhibited proliferation of ECa9706 (Fig. 1e).

### Expression of miR-144/451 cluster in stable cell line

In cells overexpressing pri-miR-144/451, miR-144-3p, miR-144-5p and miR-451a were significantly up-regulated, the fold change were 152.22, 699.41 and 600.49 respectively. No significant difference of the expression of miR-4732-3p and miR-4732-5p were found between pri-miR-144/451 and the control. miR-4732-3p and miR-4732-5p seems not to be the member of miR-144/451 cluster (Table 2).

### Effects of miR-144/451 on biological function

Overexpression of miR-144/451 increased the proportion of cells in phase of G2 and S, thus cells in G1 apparently reduced (Fig. 2a). No difference of apoptosis rate between cell over-expressing miR-144/451 and the control cell were observed (Fig. 2b). Overexpression of miR-144/451 have no effect on cell proliferation and migration (Fig. 2c, d). Transwell assay showed overexpression of miR-144/451 obviously inhibited cell invasion, the inhibition rate reached 50% (Fig. 2d).

### Effects of miR-144/451 on gene expression

According to the standard of |Fold change| $\geq 1.3$ and $P$-value $< 0.05$, there are 17 up-regulated and 57 down-regulated genes in cells overexpressing miR-144/451 were detected (Fig. 3a, b), detailed data were shown in Additional file 1: Table S1.

### Possible upstream regulators of the differently expressed mRNAs

IPA were used for analysing the possible upstream regulators, TGFB1, TNF, MAPK1, ERK, TP53, P38 MAPK, SMAD3, TCF/LEF, MMP1, EGFR, MMP2, WNT5A were predicted to be possible upstream regulators, detailed data were shown in Additional file 2: Table S2. According to the predicted interaction of moleculars, we predicted possible networks, the most enriched network were given as Fig. 3c.

### Effect of miR-144-451 gene cluster on key protein

Stable transgenic and miRNA mimic transfected cells were collected individually. Protein expression of selected cells were detected using Western Blot. The expression of protein was evaluated by integrated option density (IOD), Relative expression were evaluated using the ratio of target protein and internal reference protein (Additional file 3: Table S3). Overexpression of miR-144/451 and individual miRNA have no effect on expression of total and unphosphorylated β-catenin. miR-144-3p, miR-144-5p, miR-451a, miR-4732-3p and miR-4732-5p slightly increased the expression of phosphorylated

---

(See figure on next page.)

**Fig. 1** Effects of overexpression of single miRNA on cell functions. **a** Effects of overexpression of sigle miRNA on cell cycle. **b** Effects of overexpression of single miRNA on cell apoptosis. **c** Effects of overexpression of single miRNA on cell proliferation. **d** Effects of overexpression of single miRNA on cell migration and invasion

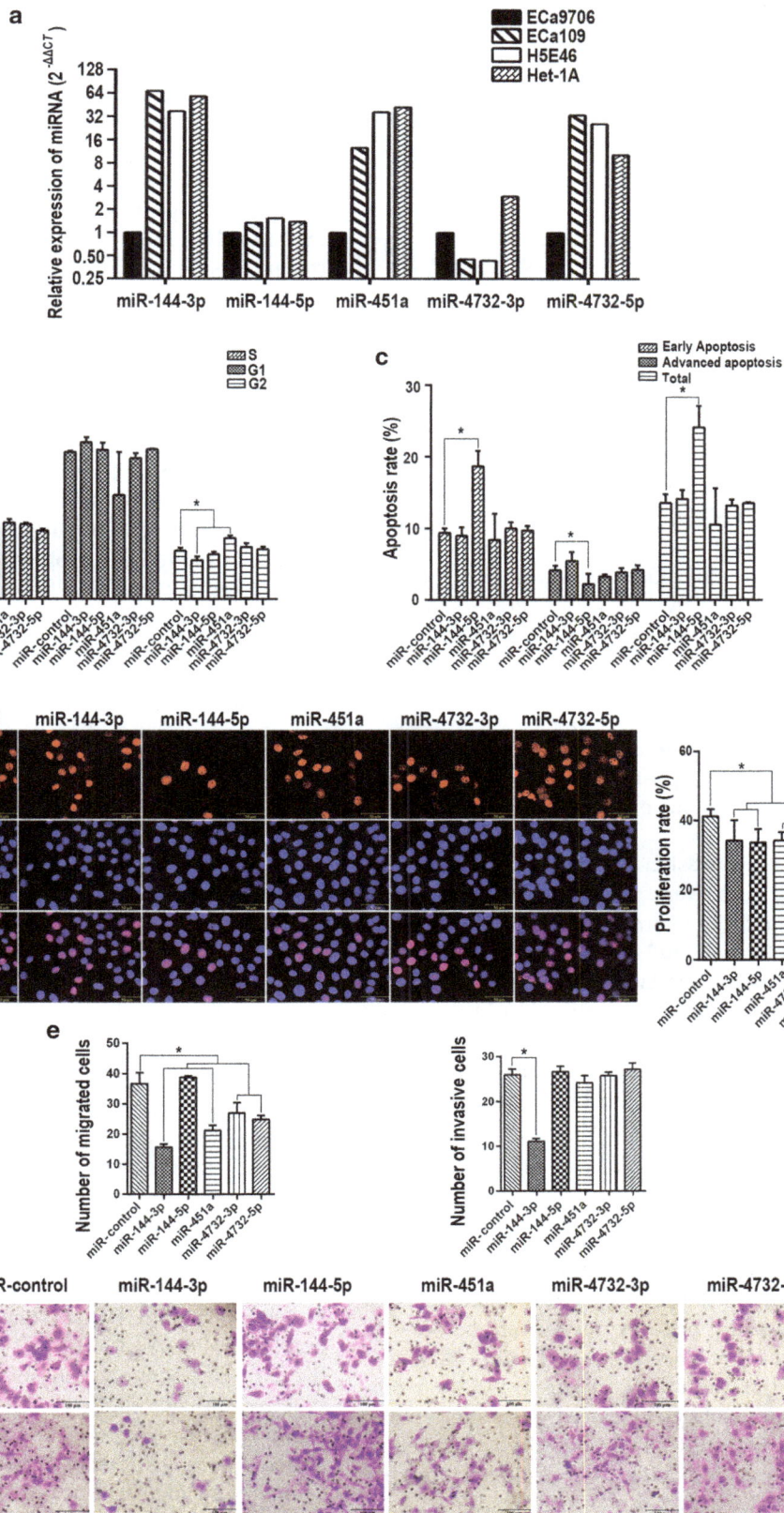

**Table 2 Expression of miR-144/451 in cells over-expressing pri-miR-144/451**

| miRNA | $\Delta C_T$ | | $\Delta\Delta C_T$ | $2^{-\Delta\Delta CT}$ | P value |
|---|---|---|---|---|---|
| | Mimic | Control | | | |
| miR-144-3p | 19.65±0.46 | 26.90±0.58 | − 7.25±0.46 | 152.22 | < 0.001 |
| miR-144-5p | 16.85±0.40 | 26.30±0.77 | − 9.45±0.50 | 699.41 | < 0.001 |
| miR-451a | 13.66±0.36 | 22.89±0.51 | − 9.23±0.36 | 600.49 | < 0.001 |
| miR-4732-3p | 16.69±0.15 | 17.13±0.36 | − 0.45±0.23 | 1.37 | 0.157 |
| miR-4732-5p | 19.50±0.46 | 20.87±0.05 | − 1.37±0.27 | 2.58 | 0.025 |
| pri-miRNA | 10.50±0.14 | 15.71±1.26 | − 5.21±0.73 | 37.01 | 0.002 |

β-catenin with the IOD of 1.01, 1.00, 1.00, 0.99 and 0.99 respectively, while the IOD for control was 0.92. In consistent, in cells over-expressing pri-miR-144/451, the expression of phosphorylated β-catenin was up-regulated (0.73 vs 0.53) (Fig. 4a).

miR-144-3p and miR-451 decreased the expression of total cMyc, but in miR-451a overexpressed cell total cMyc was down-regulated. miR-144-3p decreased the expression of phosphorylated c-Myc, but the cluster increased the expression of phosphorylated c-Myc (Fig. 4b).

Expression of p53 was increased in cells over-expressing miR-4732-5p and pri-miR-144/451, miR-144-3p decreased the expression of non-activated Caspase3 (Fig. 4c).

No difference of expression of PTEN and ERK1/2 were observed among cells overexpressing miRNA and miR-144/451 cluster and the control cells. miR-144-3p, miR-451a, miR-4732-3p and miR-144/451 cluster decreased the expression of phosphorylated ERK1/2 (Fig. 4d).

miR-144-3p, miR-4732-5p and miR-144/451 decreased the expression of MMP9 (Fig. 4e). The expression of phosphorylated cdc2 was decreased in cells over-expressing miR-144-3p and miR-144-5p but increased in cells overexpressing miR-144/451 (Fig. 4b).

## Discussion

miRNA cluster refers to miRNAs encoded closely on chromosome, these miRNAs commonly share the same promoter, and exhibit the similar expression pattern and function of regulating gene expression at the level of posttranscription. It has been reported miR-144-3p and miR-451a played as the tumor suppressor in lung cancer, gastric cancer, colorectal cancer, liver cancer and many other cancers, miR-144-5p has been reported to be tumor suppressor in bladder cancer [11–22]. In consistent, in present study, we discovered miR-144-3p,

miR-144-5p, miR-451a played a tumor suppressor role in esophageal cancer.

Considering the complexity the regulation of moleculars, the function of individual miRNA may not exactly reflect real function of the cluster. The maturity of miRNA needs undergo pri-miRNA transcripts, pre-miRNA and mature miRNA in turn [23], so we established cells over-expressing miR-144/451 by over-expressing pri-miR-144/451. In cells overexpressing pri-miR-144/451, the expression of miR-4732-3p and miR-4732-5p almost unchanged, considering the biological function of this two miRNAs are not remarkable as the other three, we infered that miR-4732-3p and miR-4732-5p were not the real member of miR-144/451 cluster.

The function of miR-144/451 cluster were not the summation of the individual miRNA, which were not entirely consistent with the individual miRNA. miR-144-3p, miR-451a, miR-4732-3p and miR-4732-5p inhibited cell migration, miR-144-3p, miR-144-5p, miR-451a and miR-4732-3p inhibited cell proliferation, however, no change of cell migration and proliferation were observed in cells over-expressing miR-144/451. The fold change in mimic transfected cell is larger than that in stable transfected cell, the complex interaction among these miRNAs may be responsible for this result.

To better understand the possible regulatory mechanism of miR-144/451, genome expression array were performed to detect the changed mRNA profiles between cells overexpressing miR-144/451 and control. The fold change of expression of mRNAs was not large in general, biological analysis suggested miR-144/451 is closely related with phosphorylation, miR-144/451 seemed mainly regulated post transcription. According to the result and the result of cell function, we selected the corresponding key proteins for verification.

Wnt signaling pathway regulates cell differentiation, proliferation, migration and many other functions, some components of Wnt signaling pathway were also implicated in other signaling pathways [24–26]. As a key component of Wnt signaling pathway, β-catenin regulates the activation of TCF/LEF, which plays important roles in transcription regulation [27]. Phosphorylated β-catenin was unstable and could be degraded by 26S protease, non-phosphorylated β-catenin was not easy to be degraded which leads to the accumulation of β-catenin, thereby phosphorylation state regulates transcription regulation. Phosphorylation of Thr41, Ser37 and Ser33 is the main degradation pathway [28, 29]. In present study, miR-144-3p, miR-144-5p and miR-451a increased the expression of phosphorylated β-catenin, these miRNAs played a synergistic effect on the inhibition of Wnt/β-catenin signaling pathway.

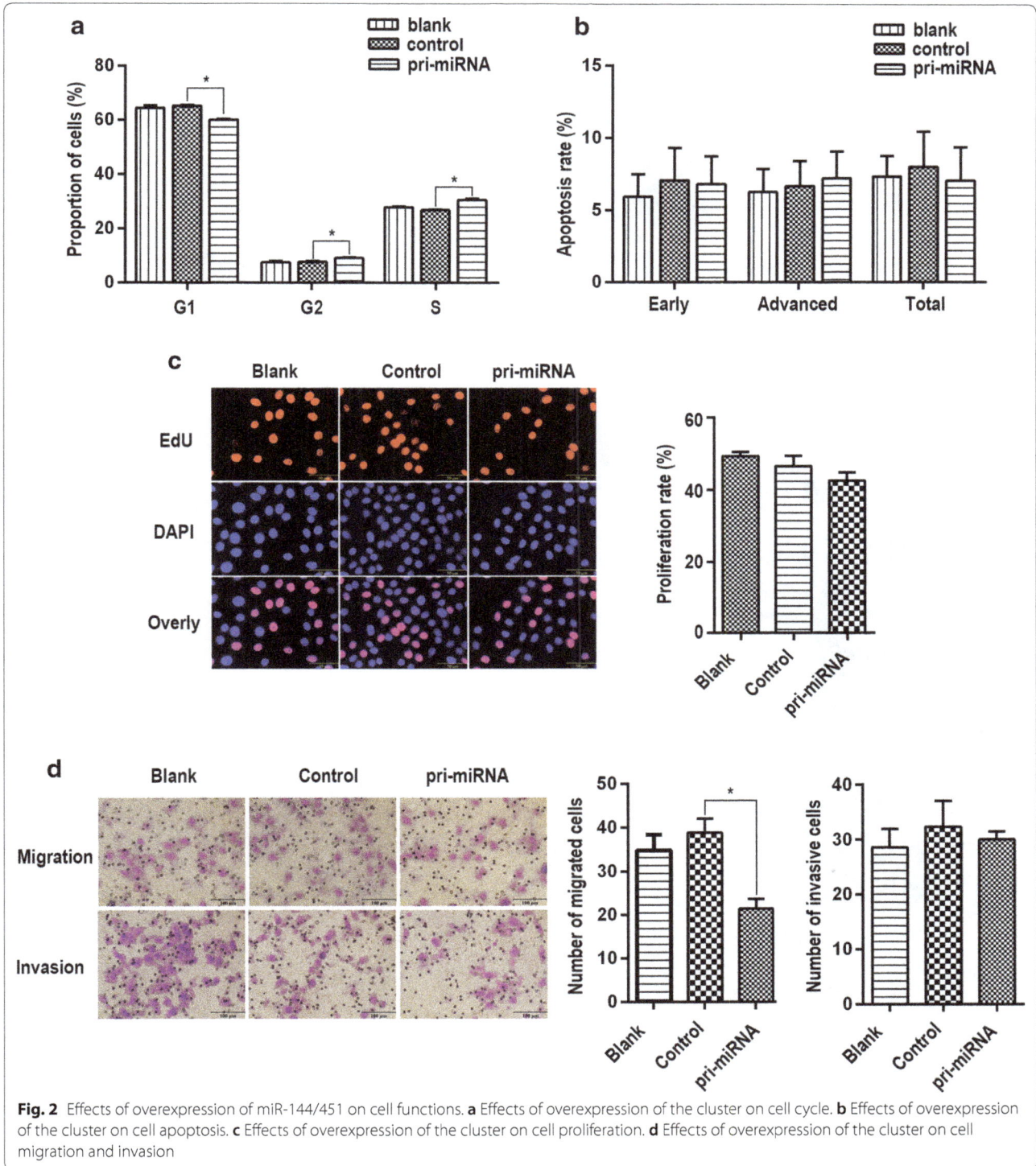

**Fig. 2** Effects of overexpression of miR-144/451 on cell functions. **a** Effects of overexpression of the cluster on cell cycle. **b** Effects of overexpression of the cluster on cell apoptosis. **c** Effects of overexpression of the cluster on cell proliferation. **d** Effects of overexpression of the cluster on cell migration and invasion

As transcription factor, c-Myc was reported to inhibit cell apoptosis and promote cell proliferation by activating key protein implicated in apoptosis and proliferation, such as RAS, RAF, BCL-2 and c-ABL [29–34]. Phosphorylation of the Ser62 Strengthened stability of c-Myc, therefore prolonged the half-life of c-Myc [35]. In this study, miR-144-3p decreased the expression of c-Myc, miR-144-5p and miR-451a increased the

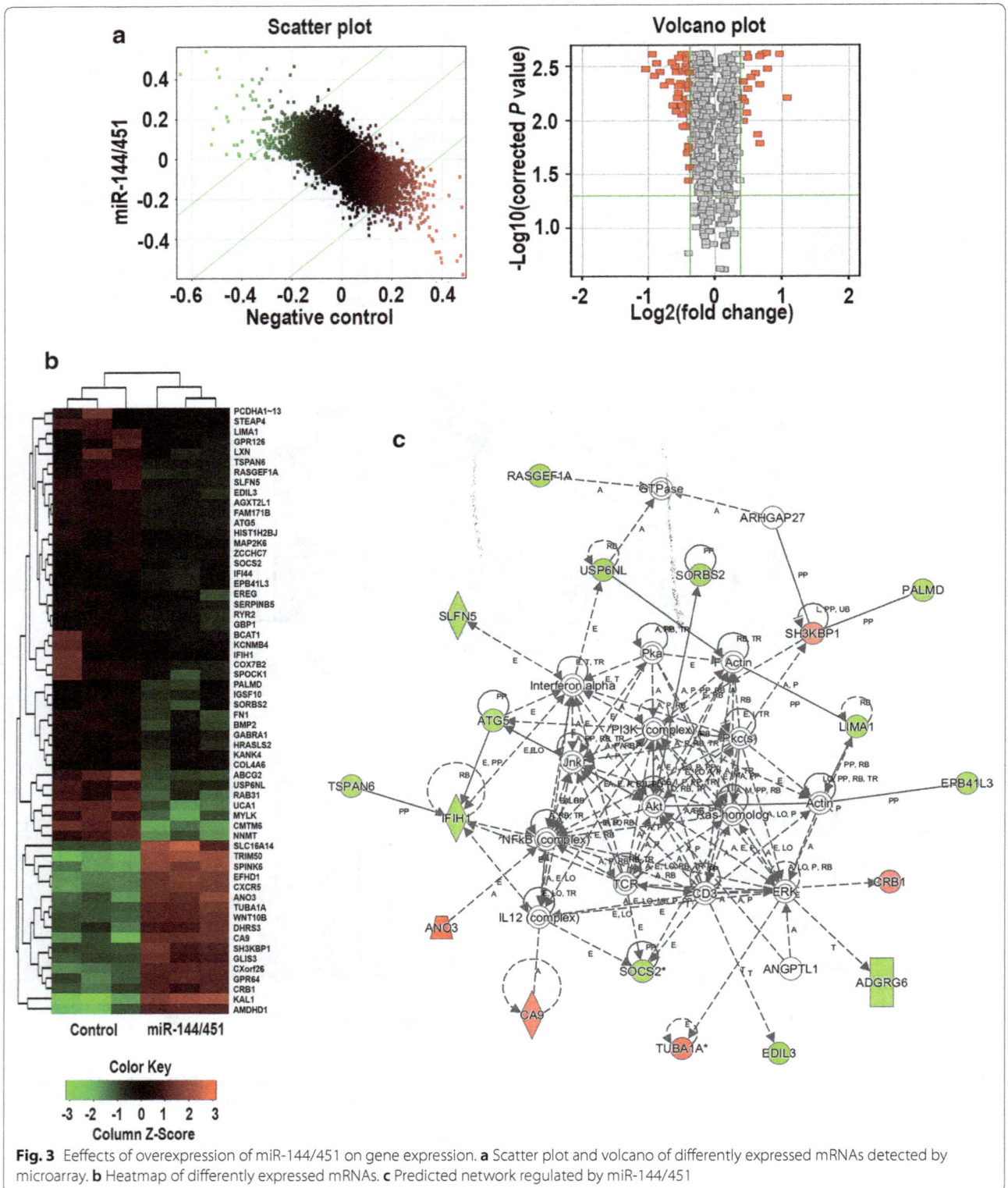

**Fig. 3** Eeffects of overexpression of miR-144/451 on gene expression. **a** Scatter plot and volcano of differently expressed mRNAs detected by microarray. **b** Heatmap of differently expressed mRNAs. **c** Predicted network regulated by miR-144/451

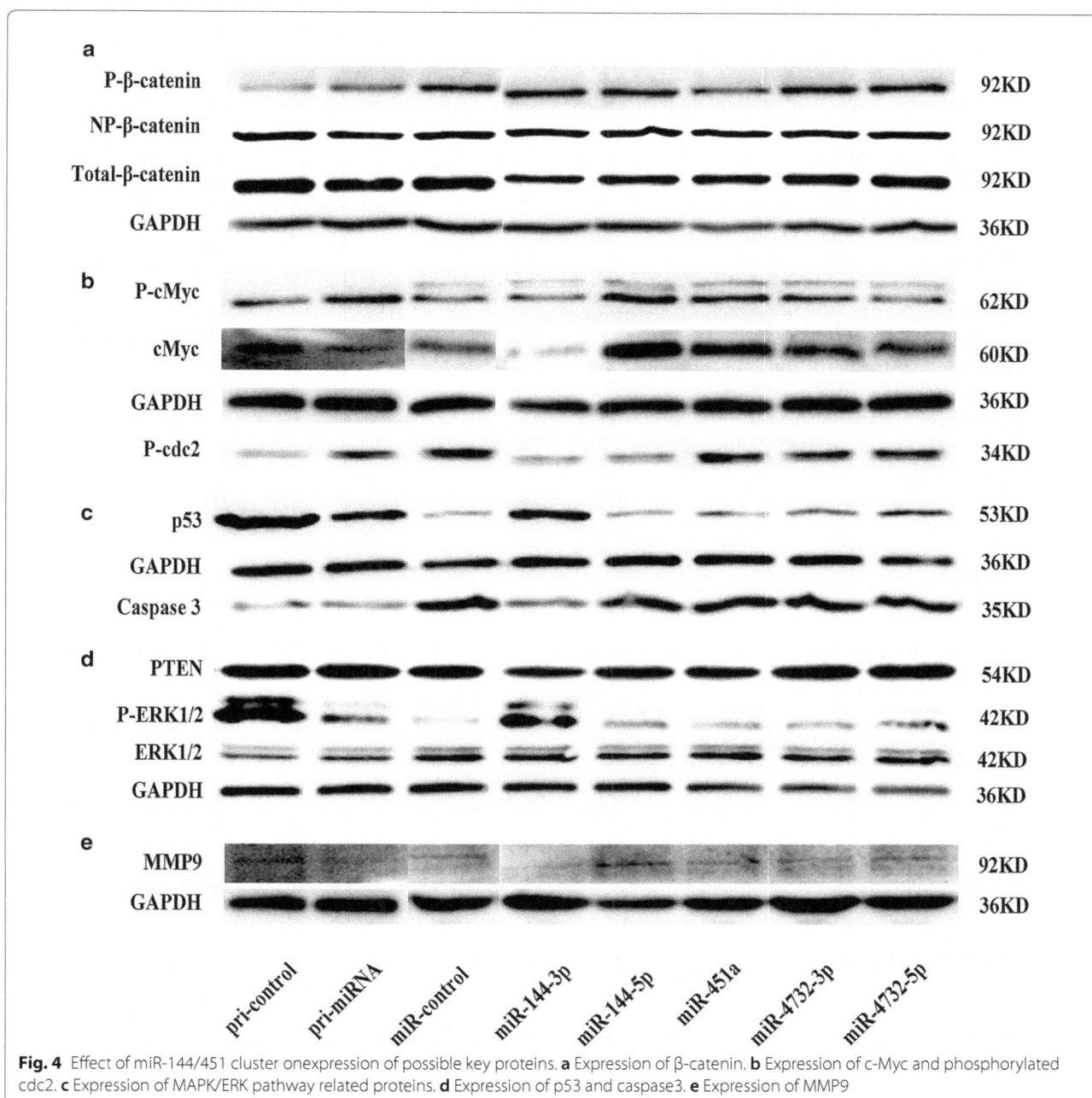

**Fig. 4** Effect of miR-144/451 cluster onexpression of possible key proteins. **a** Expression of β-catenin. **b** Expression of c-Myc and phosphorylated cdc2. **c** Expression of MAPK/ERK pathway related proteins. **d** Expression of p53 and caspase3. **e** Expression of MMP9

expression of c-Myc, miR-144/451 decreased the expression of c-Myc, however the expression of phosphorylated c-Myc was down-regulated, suggesting that the low expression of c-Myc may be mainly due to the inhibition of transcriptional translation but not degradation.

MAPK/ERK signaling pathway played important roles in a variety of tumors, by regulating cyclinD1, ERK regulates the transformation of cell cycle from G1 to S phase. The signaling pathway is reported to be closely related with matrix metalloproteinase (MMPs) which is essential for cell invasion [36, 37]. As the upstream regulatory protein of MAPK/ERK signaling pathway, in this study miR-144/451 have no effect on expression of PTEN [38], while the expression of phosphorylated ERK1/2 was decreased by over-expressing of miR-144/451 cluster, no change of the expression of Non- phosphorylated ERK1/2 were observed. The inhibition of MAPK/ERK signaling pathway may mainly caused by posttranscriptional modification of ERK1/2, miR-144-3p and miR-451a played a synergistic role in the inhibition of MAPK/ERK signaling pathway.

cdc2 plays important roles on regulating cell cycle. In advanced G2 phase, cdc2 combined with cyclinB to promote cell entry into M phase [39, 40]. Dephosphorylation of Tyr15 is essential to the activation of cdc2. miR-144/451 increased the expression of p-cdc2, which was consistent with the change of cell cycle.

In this study, over-expression of miR-144/451 up-regulated the expression of p53, interestingly, in miR-144-3p, miR-144-5p and miR-451a over-expressing cells no up-regulation of p53 were observed. miR-144/451 cluster is not a simple functional superposition of individual miRNAs. As key protein regulating cell apoptosis, Caspase3 exists in normal cells in the form of inactive zymogen, at early stage of apoptosis, Caspase3 can be activated and split into 12KD and 17KD products [41, 42]. In this study, miR-144-3p decreased the expression of 34KD Caspase3, no change in the expression of Caspase3 were observed in stable cell over-expressing miR-144/451, which were consistent with results of cell apoptosis.

## Conclusion

miR-144-451 inhibited invasion and cell cycle of EC9706. miR-144-3p promoted the apoptosis of EC9706, miR-451a can lead to the arrest of G2 phase, miR-144-3, miR-451a,miR-4732-3p inhibited the migration of cell, miR-144-3p inhibited the invasion of cell, the proliferation can be inhibited by miR-144-3p, miR-144-5p, miR-451a and miR-4732-3p. Wnt and MAPK/ERK/c-Myc signaling pathways were inhibited by miR-144-451 cluster, at while, miR-144/451 cluster downregulated the expression of MMP9 and upregulated the expression of p-cdc2 which may participated in the process of cell cycle arrest and invasion inhibition.

## Additional files

**Additional file 1: Table S1.** Abnormally expressed mRNAs in miR-144/451 overexpressing.

**Additional file 2: Table S2.** Upstream regulators of mRNAs abnormally expressed.

**Additional file 3: Table S3.** Relative expression of proteins.

## Abbreviations

EdU: 5-ethynyl-2′-deoxyuridine; IPA: Ingenuity Pathway Analysis; BCA: bicinchoninic acid; MMLV: Moloney Murine Leukemia Virus; IOD: integrated option density.

## Authors' contributions

ZG, RL and LY conceived and designed the experiments. ZG and HG performed the in vitro experiments, PZ and MX collected esophageal carcinoma tissues, ZG analyzed the data and wrote the paper. All authors read and approved the final manuscript.

## Author details

[1] Key Laboratory of Environmental Medicine Engineering, Ministry of Education, School of Public Health, Southeast University, Nanjing 210009, China. [2] Huzhou Center for Disease Control and Prevention, Huzhou 313000, China. [3] North China Petroleum Bureau General Hospital, Renqiu 062552, China.

## Acknowledgements

Not applicable.

## Competing interests

The authors declare that they have no competing interests.

## Funding

This work was supported by National Natural Science Foundation of China Grants (81872579, 81573108, 81573191), New Century Excellent Talents in University from Ministry of Education (NCET-13-0124) and Postgraduate Research & Practice Innovation Program of Jiangsu Province (KYCX17_0188), and Zhejiang Province Public Technology Application Research Project (No. 2016C33218).

## References

1. McGuire S. World cancer report 2014. Geneva: World Health Organization, International Agency for Research on Cancer, WHO Press; 2015.
2. Torre LA, et al. Global cancer statistics, 2012. CA Cancer J Clin. 2015;65(2):87–108.
3. Hammad H, Kaltenbach T, Soetikno R. Endoscopic submucosal dissection for malignant esophageal lesions. Curr Gastroenterol Rep. 2014;16(5):386.
4. Ikebe M, et al. Neoadjuvant therapy for advanced esophageal cancer: the impact on surgical management. Gen Thorac Cardiovasc Surg. 2016;64(7):386–94.
5. Bartel DP. MicroRNAs: target recognition and regulatory functions. Cell. 2009;136(2):215–33.
6. Ambros V. The functions of animal microRNAs. Nature. 2004;431(7006):350–5.
7. Esquela-Kerscher A, Slack FJ. Oncomirs—microRNAs with a role in cancer. Nat Rev Cancer. 2006;6(4):259–69.
8. Yu J, et al. Human microRNA clusters: genomic organization and expression profile in leukemia cell lines. Biochem Biophys Res Commun. 2006;349(1):59–68.
9. Wystub K, et al. miR-1/133a clusters cooperatively specify the cardiomyogenic lineage by adjustment of myocardin levels during embryonic heart development. PLoS Genetics. 2013;9(9):e1003793.
10. Gao Z, et al. Possible tumor suppressive role of the miR-144/451 cluster in esophageal carcinoma as determined by principal component regression analysis. Mol Med Rep. 2016;14(4):3805–13.
11. Zha W, et al. Roles of mir-144-ZFX pathway in growth regulation of non-small-cell lung cancer. PLoS ONE. 2013;8(9):e74175.
12. Liu J, et al. MicroRNA-144 inhibits the metastasis of gastric cancer by targeting MET expression. J Exp Clin Cancer Res. 2015;34:9.
13. Xiao R, Li C, Chai B. miRNA-144 suppresses proliferation and migration of colorectal cancer cells through GSPT1. Biomed Pharmacother. 2015;74:138–44.
14. Ma Y, et al. MicroRNA-144 suppresses tumorigenesis of hepatocellular carcinoma by targeting AKT3. Mol Med Rep. 2015;11(2):1378–83.
15. Matsushita R, et al. Tumour-suppressive microRNA-144-5p directly targets CCNE1/2 as potential prognostic markers in bladder cancer. Br J Cancer. 2015;113(2):282–9.
16. Turczynska KM, et al. Stretch-sensitive down-regulation of the mir-144/451 cluster in vascular smooth muscle and its role in AMP-activated protein kinase signaling. PLoS ONE. 2013;8(5):e65135.

17. Wang R, et al. MicroRNA-451 functions as a tumor suppressor in human non-small cell lung cancer by targeting ras-related protein 14 (RAB14). Oncogene. 2011;30(23):2644–58.

18. Babapoor S, et al. A novel miR-451a isomiR, associated with amelanotypic phenotype, acts as a tumor suppressor in melanoma by retarding cell migration and invasion. PLoS ONE. 2014;9(9):e107502.

19. Liu ZR, et al. miR-451a inhibited cell proliferation and enhanced tamoxifen sensitive in breast cancer via macrophage migration inhibitory factor. Biomed Res Int. 2015;2015:12.

20. Li H-P, et al. miR-451 inhibits cell proliferation in human hepatocellular carcinoma through direct suppression of IKK-beta. Carcinogenesis. 2013;34(11):2443–51.

21. Bergamaschi A, Katzenellenbogen BS. Tamoxifen downregulation of miR-451 increases 14-3-3 zeta and promotes breast cancer cell survival and endocrine resistance. Oncogene. 2012;31(1):39–47.

22. Yuan J, et al. The expression and function of miRNA-451 in osteosarcoma. Med Oncol. 2015;32(1):324.

23. Lee Y, et al. MicroRNA genes are transcribed by RNA polymerase II. EMBO J. 2004;23(20):4051–60.

24. Angbohang A, et al. Downregulation of the canonical WNT signaling pathway by TGF beta 1 inhibits photoreceptor differentiation of adult human Muller glia with stem cell characteristics. Stem Cells Dev. 2016;25(1):1–12.

25. Hamada F. Wnt signaling and cancer. Kaibogaku zasshi J Anat. 2009;84(4):111–2.

26. Clevers H. Wnt/beta-catenin signaling in development and disease. Cell. 2006;127(3):469–80.

27. Kikuchi A, Kishida S, Yamamoto H. Regulation of Wnt signaling by protein-protein interaction and post-translational modifications. Exp Mol Med. 2006;38(1):1–10.

28. Liu CM, et al. Control of beta-catenin phosphorylation/degradation by a dual-kinase mechanism. Cell. 2002;108(6):837–47.

29. Provost E, et al. Functional correlates of mutations in beta-catenin exon 3 phosphorylation sites. J Biol Chem. 2003;278(34):31781–9.

30. Xu JH, et al. Catenin regulates c-Myc and CDKN1A expression in breast cancer cells. Mol Carcinog. 2016;55(5):431–9.

31. Ponzielli R, et al. Cancer therapeutics: targeting the dark side of Myc. Eur J Cancer. 2005;41(16):2485–501.

32. Oster SK, et al. The myc oncogene: MarvelouslY Complex. Adv Cancer Res. 2002;84:81–154.

33. Nilsson JA, Cleveland JL. Myc pathways provoking cell suicide and cancer. Oncogene. 2003;22(56):9007–21.

34. Pelengaris S, Khan M, Evan GI. Suppression of Myc-induced apoptosis in beta cells exposes multiple oncogenic properties of Myc and triggers carcinogenic progression. Cell. 2002;109(3):321–34.

35. Wang W, et al. SCP1 regulates c-Myc stability and functions through dephosphorylating c-Myc Ser62. Oncogene. 2016;35(4):491–500.

36. Yang C-Q, et al. MCP-1 stimulates MMP-9 expression via ERK 1/2 and p38 MAPK signaling pathways in human aortic smooth muscle cells. Cell Physiol Biochem. 2014;34(2):266–76.

37. Chang MC, et al. Mesothelin enhances invasion of ovarian cancer by inducing MMP-7 through MAPK/ERK and JNK pathways. Biochem J. 2012;442:293–302.

38. Chetram MA, Hinton CV. PTEN regulation of ERK1/2 signaling in cancer. J Recept Signal Transduct Res. 2012;32(4):190–5.

39. Aleem E, Kiyokawa H, Kaldis P. Cdc2-cyclin E complexes regulate the G1/S phase transition. Nat Cell Biol. 2005;7(8):831-U93.

40. Sun W-J, et al. Romidepsin induces G2/M phase arrest via Erk/cdc25C/cdc2/cyclinB pathway and apoptosis induction through JNK/c-Jun/caspase3 pathway in hepatocellular carcinoma cells. Biochem Pharmacol. 2017;127:90–100.

41. Zheng TS, et al. Caspase-3 controls both cytoplasmic and nuclear events associated with Fas-mediated apoptosis in vivo. Proc Natl Acad Sci USA. 1998;95(23):13618–23.

42. Olie RA, et al. A novel antisense oligonucleotide targeting survivin expression induces apoptosis and sensitizes lung cancer cells to chemotherapy. Can Res. 2000;60(11):2805–9.

# Excessive mitochondrial fragmentation triggered by erlotinib promotes pancreatic cancer PANC-1 cell apoptosis via activating the mROS-HtrA2/Omi pathways

Jun Wan[1], Jie Cui[1], Lei Wang[2], Kunpeng Wu[1], Xiaoping Hong[1], Yulin Zou[1], Shuang Zhao[1] and Hong Ke[3*]

## Abstract

**Background:** Mitochondrial fragmentation drastically regulates the viability of pancreatic cancer through a poorly understood mechanism. The present study used erlotinib to activate mitochondrial fragmentation and then investigated the downstream events that occurred in response to mitochondrial fragmentation.

**Methods:** Cell viability and apoptosis were determined via MTT assay, TUNEL staining and ELISA. Mitochondrial fragmentation was measured via an immunofluorescence assay and qPCR. siRNA transfection and pathway blockers were used to perform the loss-of-function assays.

**Results:** The results of our study demonstrated that erlotinib treatment mediated cell apoptosis in the PANC-1 pancreatic cancer cell line via evoking mitochondrial fragmentation. Mechanistically, erlotinib application increased mitochondrial fission and reduced mitochondrial fusion, triggering mitochondrial fragmentation. Subsequently, mitochondrial fragmentation caused the overproduction of mitochondrial ROS (mROS). Interestingly, excessive mROS induced cardiolipin oxidation and mPTP opening, finally facilitating HtrA2/Omi liberation from the mitochondria into the cytoplasm, where HtrA2/Omi activated caspase-9-dependent cell apoptosis. Notably, neutralization of mROS or knockdown of HtrA2/Omi attenuated erlotinib-mediated mitochondrial fragmentation and favored cancer cell survival.

**Conclusions:** Together, our results identified the mROS-HtrA2/Omi axis as a novel signaling pathway that is activated by mitochondrial fragmentation and that promotes PANC-1 pancreatic cancer cell mitochondrial apoptosis in the presence of erlotinib.

**Keywords:** Erlotinib, Mitochondrial fragmentation, Mitochondrial apoptosis, mROS, HtrA2/Omi

## Background

Pancreatic cancer is the fourth leading cause of cancer-related death worldwide [1]. Although the incidence of pancreatic cancer is relatively low, approximately 3.2% of all new cancer cases in the United States, the 5-year survival rate is 8.5% in patients diagnosed with pancreatic cancer. In addition, the detection rate of early pancreatic cancer remains low due to the lack of specific symptoms. Accordingly, most patients (52%) are diagnosed with distant metastasis [2], and, unfortunately, the 5-year relative survival of patients with metastatic pancreatic cancer is less than 2% [3]. Although smoking and health history can affect the risk of pancreatic cancer, the pathogenesis of pancreatic cancer development is not completely understood. Therefore, exploring the molecular features of pancreatic cancer growth and death is vital to control the disease progression and bring more clinical benefits to patients with pancreatic cancer.

*Correspondence: Herojun2016@126.com
[3] Department of Oncology, Third Clinical Medical College, Three Gorges University, Gezhouba Group Central Hospital, No. 60 Qiaohu Lake Road, Xiling District, Yichang 443002, Hubei, China
Full list of author information is available at the end of the article

The biological behavior of cancer is closely regulated by mitochondria [4, 5]. Sufficient ATP supply, intracellular calcium homeostasis, metabolic signaling transduction, and cell apoptosis management are affected by mitochondria [6–8]. In addition, mitochondria are also the key target of several chemotherapeutics and radiotherapies [9]. A recent study has reported that pancreatic cancer death, proliferation and metastasis are modulated by mitochondrial homeostasis, especially mitochondrial fission [10]. Excessive mitochondrial fission induces cancer cell oxidative injury and subsequently mediates mitochondrial ATP depletion; this effect impairs PANC-1 cell proliferation and evokes mitochondrial apoptosis [10]. Notably, this conclusion is also supported by other studies. In colorectal cancer, the activation of mitochondrial fission is associated with SW837 cell apoptosis and migration inhibition [11]. In gastric cancer, abnormal mitochondrial fission contributes to cancer cell oxidative stress and energy undersupply [12]. In breast cancer, Drp1-mediated mitochondrial fission suppresses breast cancer cell invasion [13]. This information indicates that mitochondrial fission has a well-characterized role in the regulation of cancer viability. However, the downstream molecular events of mitochondrial fission activation remain to be discovered.

Based on a previous study in a mouse model of cardiac ischemia reperfusion injury, the activation of mitochondrial fission promotes the formation of mitochondrial fragmentation, and these mitochondrial debris contain a decreased mitochondrial potential [14]. In addition, mitochondrial fragmentation can activate cell death via two mechanisms [15]; one mechanism is driven via HK2/VDAC1 disassociation-mediated mPTP opening, and the other involves mROS-induced cardiolipin oxidation. Notably, mitochondrial ROS (mROS) overloading, as a primary result of mitochondrial fragmentation [16], has been noted in different disease models such as those of gastric cancer [17], breast cancer [18], and leukemia [19]. Subsequently, excessive mitochondrial oxidative injury can activate the HtrA2/Omi-related apoptotic pathway in a manner that is dependent on caspase-9 activity [11]. This evidence indicates that the downstream effectors of mitochondrial fragmentation include mROS overproduction, HtrA2/Omi upregulation, caspase-9 activation and mitochondrial apoptosis augmentation. Given these factors, we want to know whether mitochondrial fragmentation regulates pancreatic cancer viability via mROS-HtrA2/Omi-caspase-9 pathways.

To this end, erlotinib is the first-line anti-tumor drug for the treatment of pancreatic cancer in the clinic [20]. Several human studies have verified the efficacy of erlotinib in improving the 5-year survival rate of patients with pancreatic cancer [21, 22]. Molecular investigations

report that several biological processes are modulated by erlotinib, including mTOR inhibition [23], epidermal growth factor receptor downregulation [24], and epidermal interstitial transformation (EMT) suppression [25]. However, no study that explores the role of erlotinib in triggering mitochondrial stress has been conducted. In the present study, erlotinib was applied to activate mitochondrial fragmentation in a human PANC-1 pancreatic cancer cell line. Then, we explored the regulatory mechanism of mitochondrial fragmentation on cell viability in the presence of erlotinib.

## Methods and materials

### Pancreatic carcinoma cell lines

The PANC-1 (ATCC® CRL-1469™) and MIA PaCa-2 (ATCC® CRL-1420™) pancreatic cell lines were used in the present study. These cells were cultured in Dulbecco's modified Eagle's medium (DMEM) (Thermo Fisher Scientific, Waltham, MA) supplemented with 10% fetal bovine serum (FBS) (Thermo Fisher Scientific, Waltham, MA) at 37 °C in a 5% $CO_2$ atmosphere. Different doses of erlotinib (ERL, Sigma. Cat. No. SML2156) were incubated with the cancer cells for 24 h, and these concentrations of ERL were chosen according to a previous study [26]. FCCP (5 μm, Selleck Chemicals, Houston, TX, USA) and mitochondrial division inhibitor 1 (Mdivi1; 10 mM; Sigma-Aldrich; Merck KGaA) were used to activate and inhibit mitochondrial fragmentation, respectively, according to a previous study. To repress mROS overproduction, mitochondrial-targeted antioxidant MitoQ (2 μM, MedKoo Biosciences, Inc.; CAT#: 317102) was used.

### Western blotting and antibodies

Cells were scraped in RIPA lysis buffer (Beyotime, Shenzhen, Guangdong, China). The lysates (50–70 μg) were separated by 10% SDS-polyacrylamide gel (10–15%) electrophoresis (SDS-PAGE). Proteins were electrotransferred onto the Pure Nitrocellulose Blotting membrane (Life Sciences) (Millipore, Bedford, MA, USA) and then blocked with 5% nonfat milk for 2 h at room temperature [27]. After washing with TBST three times, the membranes were incubated at 4 °C overnight with the following primary antibodies: HrtA2/Omi (:1000; Abcam; #ab32092), caspase9 (1:1000, Cell Signaling Technology, #9504), Bax (1:1000, Cell Signaling Technology, #2772), Opa1 (1:1000, Abcam, #ab42364), Mfn2 (1:1000, Abcam, #ab56889), Tom20 (1:1000, Abcam, #ab186735), CDK4 (1:1000, Abcam, #ab137675), Cyclin D1 (1:1000, Abcam, #ab134175), Bcl2 (1:1000, Cell Signaling Technology, #3498), Bad (:1000; Abcam; #ab90435), survivin (1:1000, Cell Signaling Technology, #2808), cyt-c (1:1000; Abcam; #ab90529), complex III subunit core (CIII-core2, 1:1000,

Invitrogen, #459220), complex II (CII-30, 1:1000, Abcam, #ab110410), complex IV subunit II (CIV-II, 1:1000, Abcam, #ab110268). Next, the membranes were visualized using an enhanced chemiluminescence system (ECL; Pierce Company, USA) [28].

### MTT assay, caspase activity detection and LDH release assay

MTT was used to analyze the cellular viability [29]. Cells ($1 \times 10^6$ cells/well) were cultured on a 96-well plate at 37 °C with 5% $CO_2$. Then, 40 µl of MTT solution (2 mg/ml; Sigma-Aldrich) was added to the medium for 4 h at 37 °C with 5% $CO_2$. Subsequently, the cell medium was discarded, and 80 µl of DMSO was added to the wells for 1 h at 37 °C with 5% $CO_2$ in the dark. The OD of each well was observed at A490 nm via a spectrophotometer (Epoch 2; BioTek Instruments, Inc., Winooski, VT, USA). To analyze changes in caspase-9, caspase-9 activity kits (Beyotime Institute of Biotechnology, China; Catalog No. C1158) were used according to the manufacturer's protocol [30]. In brief, to measure caspase-9 activity, 5 µl of LEHD-p-NA substrate (4 mM, 200 µM final concentration) was added to the samples for 1 h at 37 °C. Then, the absorbance at 400 nm was recorded via a microplate reader to reflect the caspase-3 and caspase-9 activities. To analyze caspase-3 activity, 5 µl of DEVD-p-NA substrate (4 mM, 200 µM final concentration) was added to the samples for 2 h at 37 °C [31].

### ELISA

Glutathione (GSH, Thermo Fisher Scientific Inc., Waltham, MA, USA; Catalog No. T10095), glutathione peroxidase GPX, (Beyotime Institute of Biotechnology, China; Catalog No. S0056) and SOD (Thermo Fisher Scientific Inc., Waltham, MA, USA; Catalog No. BMS222TEN) were measured according to the manufacturer's instructions using a microplate reader (Epoch 2; BioTek Instruments, Inc.) [32]. Cellular ATP generation was measured to reflect mitochondrial function. Firstly, cells were washed three times with cold PBS at room temperature. Subsequently, a luciferase-based ATP assay kit (CellTiter-Glo® Luminescent Cell Viability Assay; cat. no. G7570; Promega Corporation, Madison, WI, USA) was used to analyze ATP content, according to the manufacturer's protocols. ATP production was measured using a microplate reader at the wavelength of 570 nm (Epoch 2; BioTek Instruments, Inc., Winooski, VT, USA) [33].

### Immunostaining

Cells were washed twice with PBS, permeabilized in 0.1% Triton X-100 overnight at 4 °C. After the fixation procedure, the sections were cryoprotected in a PBS solution supplemented with 0.9 mol/l of sucrose overnight at 4 °C [34]. The primary antibodies used in the present study were as follows: caspase9 (1:1000, Cell Signaling Technology, #9504), Mff (1:1000, Cell Signaling Technology, #86668), Tom20 (1:1000, Abcam, #ab186735), HrtA2/Omi (1:1000; Abcam; #ab32092).

### Small interfering RNA transfection

To inhibit HtrA2/Omi expression, two independent siRNAs against HtrA2/Omi were transfected into PANC-1 cells according to a previous study [27]. Briefly, the cells were seeded onto 6-well plates and then incubated with Opti-Minimal Essential Medium (Invitrogen; Thermo Fisher Scientific, Inc.) for 24 h. Then, Lipofectamine® 2000 transfection reagent (Thermo Fisher Scientific, Inc.) was added into the medium of PANC-1 cells and supplemented with 5 nmol/l siRNA solution. Transfection was performed for 48 h, and then the cells were collected. Western blotting was used to verify the transfection efficiency.

### Detection of mitochondrial membrane potential and mPTP opening

To observe the mitochondrial potential, JC-1 staining (Thermo Fisher Scientific Inc., Waltham, MA, USA; Catalog No. M34152) was used. Then, 10 mg/ml JC-1 was added to the medium for 10 min at 37 °C in the dark to label the mitochondria. Normal mitochondrial potential showed red fluorescence, and damaged mitochondrial potential showed green fluorescence [35]. The mPTP opening rate was detected using calcein-AM (Sigma, Cat. No. 17783) as described previously [36]. Briefly, cells were incubated with calcein-AM for 30 min at 37 °C in the dark. Next, PBS was used to wash the cells three times. Finally, the optical density (OD) at an absorbance of 579 nm was recorded using a multifunction microplate reader (Epoch 2; BioTek Instruments, Inc., Winooski, VT, USA). The mPTP opening rate was calculated as a ratio to that of the control group [14]. The relative mPTP opening was measured as a ratio to that of the control group.

### TUNEL assay and cardiolipin staining

Apoptotic cells were detected with an In Situ Cell Death Detection Kit (Thermo Fisher Scientific Inc., Waltham, MA, USA; Catalog No. C1024) according to the manufacturer's protocol. Briefly, cells were fixed with 4% paraformaldehyde at 37 °C for 15 min. Blocking buffer (3% $H_2O_2$ in $CH_3OH$) was added to the wells, and then cells were permeabilized with 0.1% Triton X-100 in 0.1% sodium citrate for 2 min on ice. The cells were incubated with TUNEL reaction mixture for 1 h at 37 °C.

DAPI (Sigma-Aldrich, St. Louis, MO, USA) was used to counterstain the nuclei, and the numbers of TUNEL-positive cells were recorded [37]. Cardiolipin oxidation was stained with 10-*N*-nonylacridine orange (NAO; 2 mmol/l; Molecular Probes, Eugene, OR, USA). Under normal conditions, NAO interacts with nonoxidized cardiolipin and generates a characteristic green fluorescence. However, upon cardiolipin oxidation, NAO cannot interact with cardiolipin, and this result is accompanied by a drop in green fluorescence. Accordingly, the green fluorescence intensity of NAO was used to quantify the cardiolipin oxidation with the help of Image-Pro Plus 6.0; Media Cybernetics, Rockville, MD, USA) [16].

### RNA extraction and qPCR analysis

For mRNA expression analysis, total RNA was isolated using Trizol (Invitrogen, Carlsbad, California, USA) according to a previous study. Then, cDNA was synthesized using 1 mg RNA and the First-Strand Synthesis Kit (Fermentas, Flamborough, Ontario, Canada) according to a previous study [38]. The cycling conditions were as follows: 92 °C for 7 min, 40 cycles of 95 °C for 20 s and 70 °C for 45 s. β-actin was amplified as an internal standard. All the primer sequences are listed below: Drp1 (forward prime 5′-CATGGACGAGCTGGCCTTC-3′, reverse prime 5′-ATCCTGTAGTGATGTATCAGG-3′), Mff (forward prime 5′-TGTCCAGTCCGTAACTGA C-3′, reverse prime 5′-TTCGATACCTGACTTAC-3′), Mfn2 (forward prime 5′-CCTCTTGATCCTGATCTT AACGT-3′, reverse prime 5′-GGACTACCTGATTGT CATTC-3′), OPA1 (forward prime 5′-GCTACTTGT GAGGTCGATTC-3′, reverse prime 5′-GCCGTATAC CGTGGTATGTCTG-3′) [14].

### EdU staining

EdU staining was performed to analyze the cell proliferation according to a previous study [39]. The EdU incorporation assay was performed using the EdU kit (cat. no. A10044; Thermo Fisher Scientific Inc.). Briefly, EdU (2 nM/well) was diluted in complete culture medium, and the cells were incubated with the dilution for 2 h at 37 °C. Subsequently, the cells were fixed with 4% paraformaldehyde for 15 min at 37 °C and were incubated with Apollo Staining reaction liquid for 30 min. DAPI was used to counterstain the nuclei for 15 min at room temperature under a digital microscope system (IX81; Olympus Corporation).

### Flow cytometry assay

Flow cytometry was applied as a quantitative method for evaluating mitochondrial ROS levels according to a previous study [4]. In brief, PANC-1 cells were seeded onto 6-well plates and then treated with erlotinib. Subsequently, the cells were isolated using 0.25% trypsin and then incubated with MitoSOX red mitochondrial superoxide indicator (Molecular Probes, USA) for 30 min in the dark at 37 °C. Subsequently, PBS was used to wash cell two times, and then the cells were analyzed with a FACS Calibur Flow cytometer. Data were analyzed by FACS Diva software. The experiment was repeated three times to improve the accuracy [39]. The number of apoptotic cells was analyzed quantitatively using the Annexin V–FITC/PI Apoptosis Detection Kit (BD Biosciences, USA). After treatment, the cells were harvested, resuspended in 200 µl of binding buffer, and then incubated with 5 µl of Annexin V–FITC/binding buffer mixture (30 min, 37 °C) in the dark. Subsequently, the cells were incubated with 10 µl of propidium iodide for 5 min and immediately analyzed by bivariate flow cytometry using a BD FACSCalibur cytometer [36].

### Statistical analysis

Data are expressed as the mean $\pm$ SE of triplicate samples. Statistical analysis for multiple comparisons was analyzed by a one-way analysis of variance (ANOVA) followed by Bonferroni's multiple comparison test. p values below 0.05 were considered statistically significant.

### Results

#### Erlotinib dose-dependently promotes PANC-1 pancreatic cancer cell apoptosis

First, erlotinib was incubated with PANC-1 pancreatic cancer cells. Then, cell viability was observed using the MTT assay and LDH-cytotoxicity assay. Compared to the control group, erlotinib treatment reduced the viability of PANC-1 cells (Fig. 1a, b), and this effect was achieved in a dose-dependent manner. This finding was also found in erlotinib-treated PaCa-2 pancreatic cancer cells (Fig. 1c, d). To explore whether the reduction in cell viability was attributable to excessive cell apoptosis, the TUNEL assay was used. The number of TUNEL-positive cells was

(See figure on next page.)

**Fig. 1** Erlotinib promotes PANC-1 apoptosis in a concentration-dependent fashion. **a** The MTT assay for PANC-1 viability. Different doses of erlotinib were added to the medium of PANC-1 cells. **b** LDH release was used to evaluate the cell death in PANC-1 cells in the presence of erlotinib. **c** The MTT assay for PaCa-2 cells in the presence of erlotinib treatment. **d** LDH release was used to evaluate the cell death in PaCa-2 cells in the presence of erlotinib. **e** TUNEL staining for apoptotic PANC-1 cells and PaCa-2 cells. The number of TUNEL-positive cells was recorded. **f** Quantification of the TUNEL assay in PANC-1 cells. **g** The TUNEL assay for PaCa-2 cells in response to erlotinib treatment. The percentage of TUNEL-positive PaCa-2 cells was recorded. **h, i** Caspase-3 activity was determined using an ELISA in PANC-1 cells and PaCa-2 cells. #$p < 0.05$ vs. control group

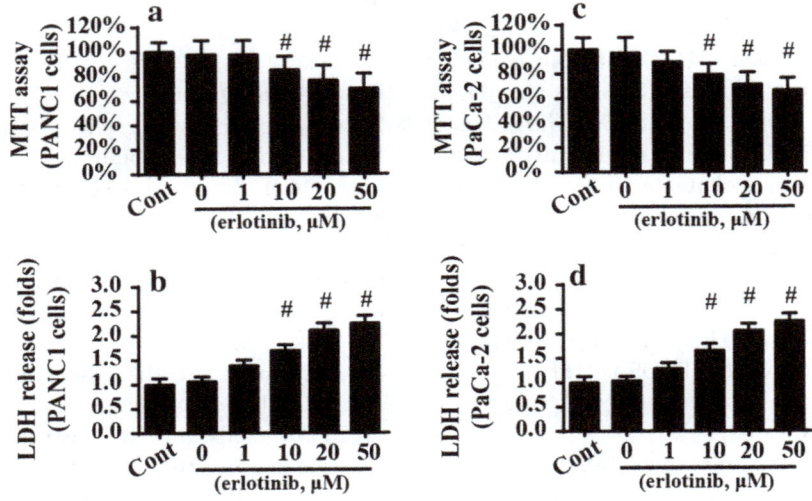

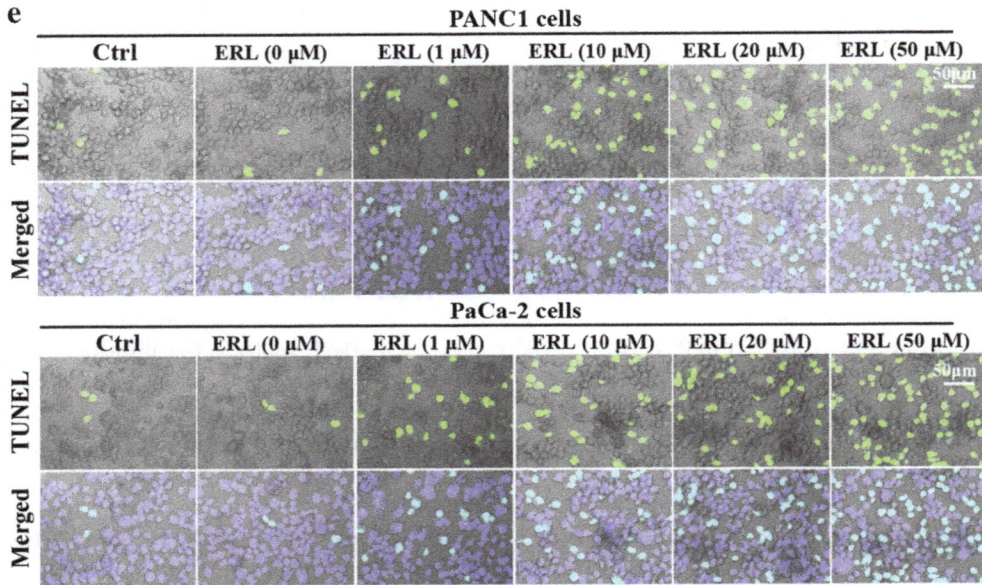

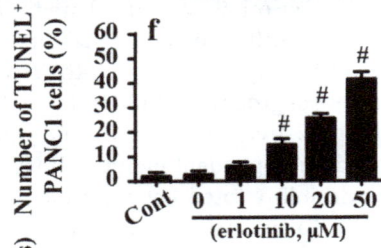

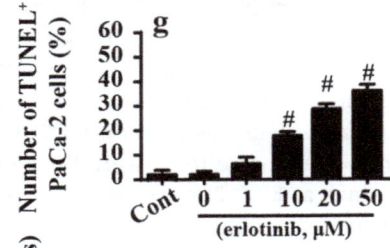

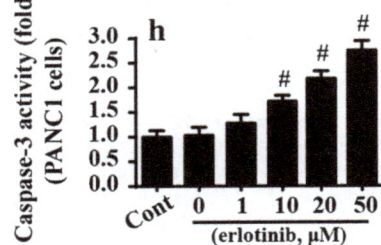

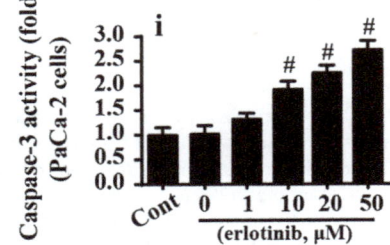

counted as the apoptotic index. As shown in Fig. 1e, f, erlotinib dose-dependently increased the apoptotic index in PANC-1 cells. Similarly, the number of TUNEL-positive cells was also elevated in PaCa-2 cells upon exposure to erlotinib (Fig. 1e, g). Furthermore, since cell apoptosis is primarily executed via caspase-3 activation, caspase-3 activity was determined via ELISA. Compared to the control group, caspase-3 activity was relatively increased in response to erlotinib treatment (Fig. 1h), which is suggestive of caspase-3 activation by erlotinib. This alteration was also noted in PaCa-2 cells (Fig. 1I). These data were further supported via quantitative analysis of cell apoptosis with the help of flow cytometry (Additional file 1: Figure S1). Together, our results indicated that erlotinib dose-dependently promoted PANC-1 and PaCa-2 cell apoptosis. Notably, no phenotypic difference was noted in erlotinib-mediated apoptosis in PANC-1 cells or PaCa2 cells, and thus PANC-1 cells were used in the following study. In addition, we have found that the minimum concentration of erlotinib that induces cell death was 10 μM, and thus, 10 μM erlotinib was used to conduct the molecular investigations.

### Erlotinib induces mitochondrial fragmentation in PANC-1 pancreatic cancer cells via elevating mitochondrial fission and repressing mitochondrial fusion

Subsequently, the mitochondrial morphology was observed via an immunofluorescence assay using a Tom-20 antibody [40]. Compared to the control group, we found that erlotinib treatment mediated the formation of mitochondrial fragmentation (Fig. 2a). Then, the average length of the mitochondria was measured after erlotinib treatment and was used to quantify mitochondrial fragmentation. As shown in Fig. 2b, the mean length of the mitochondria was ~9.1 μm at baseline. However, after treatment with erlotinib, the mean length of mitochondria was reduced to ~2.3 μm (Fig. 2b). In addition, the fluorescence intensity of Mff, an activator of mitochondrial fragmentation, was obviously increased in response to erlotinib treatment compared to that in control group (Fig. 2c). Subsequently, to further confirm the promotive effect of erlotinib on mitochondrial fragmentation,

Mdivi-1, an antagonist of mitochondrial fragmentation, was added into the medium of erlotinib-treated cells. Meanwhile, FCCP, an agonist of mitochondrial fragmentation, was used to incubate with normal cells, which was used as the positive control group. Then, mitochondrial fission, mitochondrial length and Mff expression were evaluated again. Compared to the control group, FCCP triggered mitochondrial fragmentation and upregulated Mff expression, similar to the results obtained via supplementation with erlotinib (Fig. 2a–c). However, Mdivi-1 treatment abrogated the promotive effect of erlotinib on mitochondrial fragmentation.

Notably, the fragmented mitochondria could be the result of increased mitochondrial fission and decreased mitochondrial fusion. To verify the alterations of mitochondrial fission/fusion, qPCR was performed to analyze the transcription factors that are related to mitochondrial fission/fusion. In response to erlotinib treatment, the transcription of pro-fission factors such as Drp1 and Mff were significantly upregulated (Fig. 2d–g), indicative of mitochondrial fission activation by erlotinib. In contrast, the transcription and expression of pro-fusion factors, such as Mfn2 and Opa1 were obviously downregulated in response to erlotinib treatment (Fig. 2d–j), suggesting that mitochondrial fusion was repressed by erlotinib. Together, our results confirmed that erlotinib promoted mitochondrial fragmentation in PANC-1 cells.

### Mitochondrial fragmentation induces oxidative stress via mitochondrial ROS (mROS)

Additional experiments were performed to explore the downstream events of mitochondrial fragmentation. Based on a previous study, mitochondrial fragmentation was associated with cellular oxidative stress via mROS overloading [41]. To confirm this, a mROS probe and flow cytometry were used to quantify mROS levels after erlotinib treatment. As shown in Fig. 3a, b, the level of mROS was significantly elevated in response to erlotinib treatment. To validate whether mitochondrial fragmentation was required for mROS overloading, Mdivi-1 and FCCP were used. FCCP treatment elevated the ROS production in control group, similar to the results obtained

(See figure on next page.)
**Fig. 2** Erlotinib activates mitochondrial fragmentation in PANC-1 cells. **a** Mitochondrial fragmentation was determined using an immunofluorescence assay. Tom-20 was used to stain the mitochondria, and the average length of the mitochondria was calculated to quantify mitochondrial fragmentation. Mff antibody was used to lable the Mff, an mitochondrial fragmentation activator. FCCP and Mdivi-1 were used to activate or inhibit mitochondrial fragmentation, respectively. **b** Quantification of the mitochondrial length. **c** The relative Mff fluorescence intensity was evaluated in the presence of erlotinib treatment. FCCP and Mdivi-1 was used to activate or inhibit mitochondrial fragmentation, respectively. Mdivi-1, an antagonist of mitochondrial fragmentation, was added into the medium of erlotinib-treated cells. Meanwhile, FCCP, an agonist of mitochondrial fragmentation, was used to incubate with normal cells, which was used as the positive control group. **d–g** The alterations of mitochondrial fission/fusion-related factors were measured using qPCR. Drp1 and Mff were pro-fission proteins, and their expressions were significantly increased in response to erlotinib treatment. In contrast, Mfn2 and Opa1 were pro-fusion factors, and their levels were downregulated by erlotinib application. **h–j** Western blotting for Mfn2 and Opa1 in response to erlotinib treatment. *$p < 0.05$

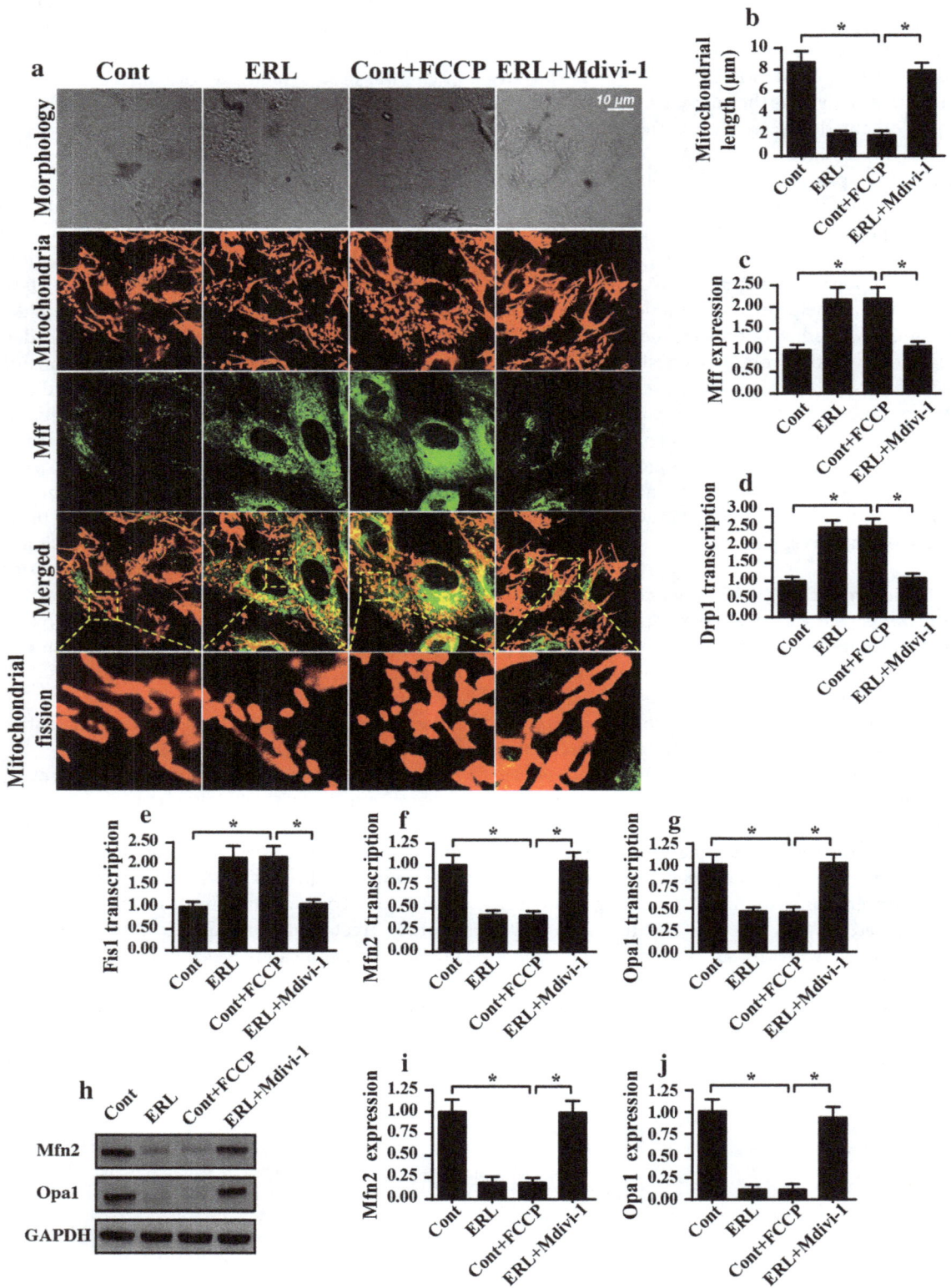

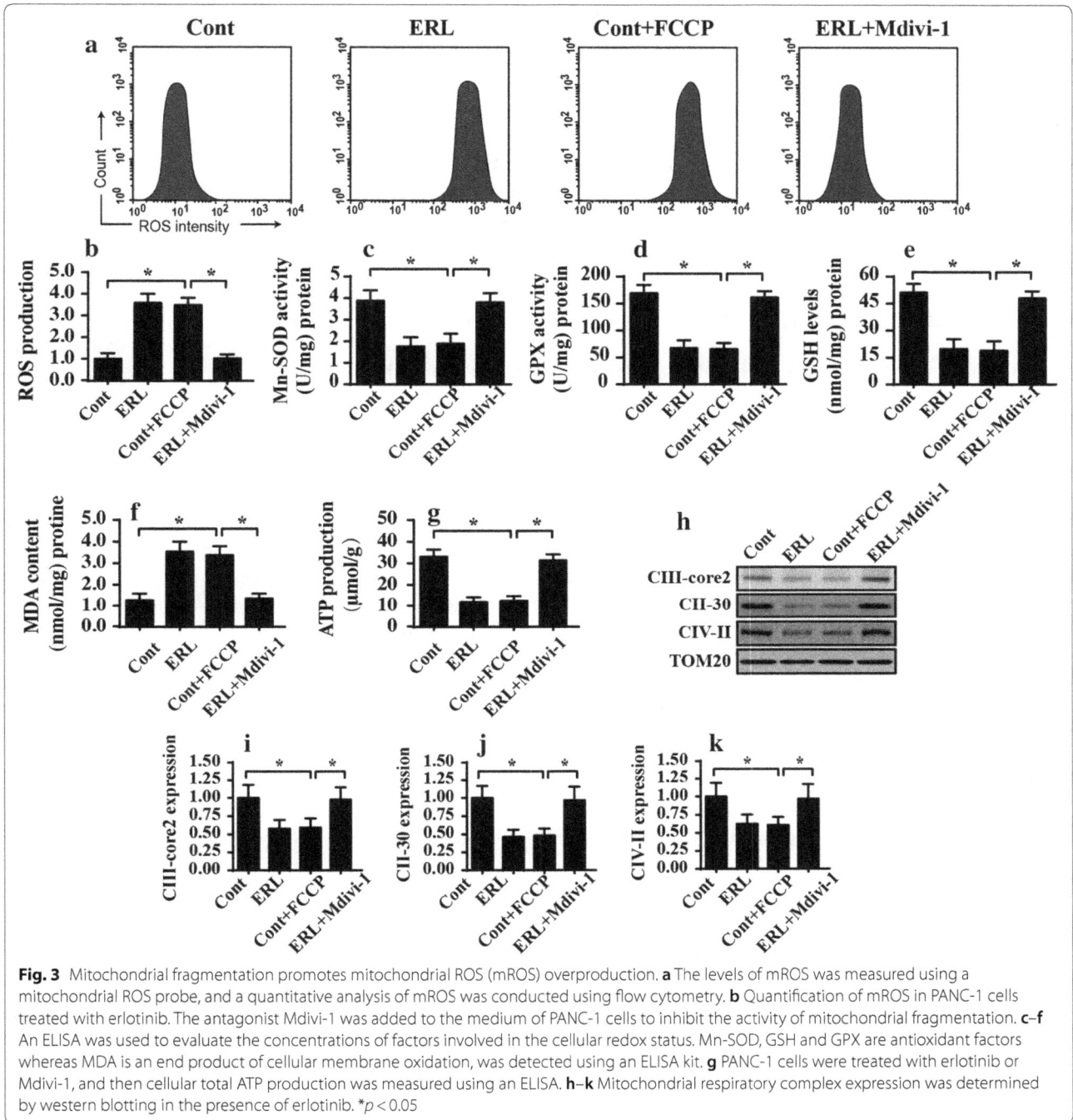

**Fig. 3** Mitochondrial fragmentation promotes mitochondrial ROS (mROS) overproduction. **a** The levels of mROS was measured using a mitochondrial ROS probe, and a quantitative analysis of mROS was conducted using flow cytometry. **b** Quantification of mROS in PANC-1 cells treated with erlotinib. The antagonist Mdivi-1 was added to the medium of PANC-1 cells to inhibit the activity of mitochondrial fragmentation. **c–f** An ELISA was used to evaluate the concentrations of factors involved in the cellular redox status. Mn-SOD, GSH and GPX are antioxidant factors whereas MDA is an end product of cellular membrane oxidation, was detected using an ELISA kit. **g** PANC-1 cells were treated with erlotinib or Mdivi-1, and then cellular total ATP production was measured using an ELISA. **h–k** Mitochondrial respiratory complex expression was determined by western blotting in the presence of erlotinib. *$p < 0.05$

vis supplementation of erlotinib, However, Mdivi-1 application attenuated erlotinib-mediated mROS overloading (Fig. 3a, b), indicating the necessary role that is played by mitochondrial fragmentation in mROS generation. Excessive mROS production would induce cellular oxidative injury. To confirm this, an ELISA assay was used to observe alterations in the levels of cellular antioxidants.

Compared to the control group, the concentration of Mn-SOD, GSH and GPX were markedly reduced after erlotinib treatment (Fig. 3c–e). In contrast, the level of MDA, an end product of the peroxidation of lipids in the cell membrane, was increased in response to erlotinib treatment (Fig. 3f). Interestingly, blockade of mitochondrial fragmentation via Mdivi-1 could decrease the level of antioxidants and suppress the production of MDA (Fig. 3c–f). Excessive oxidative injury can also disrupt cellular energy metabolism. Accordingly, total ATP production was measured using ELISA. Compared to the control group, erlotinib treatment significantly reduced the ATP production in PANC-1 cells (Fig. 3g), and this effect could be reversed by Mdivi-1. Furthermore, we also found that the expression of proteins related to mitochondrial ATP synthesis were notably downregulated in response to erlotinib (Fig. 3h–k); this effect was abrogated by Mdivi-1. Accordingly, our data indicated that mitochondrial fragmentation evoked mitochondrial ROS overloading and oxidative stress in PANC-1 cells.

### Mitochondrial fragmentation-mediated mROS promotes HtrA2/Omi liberation

Next, experiments were performed to observe the consequence of mROS-mediated cell oxidative stress. Based on a previous report [42], excessive mROS could cause mitochondrial membrane permeabilization, which facilitates the translocation of mitochondrial proapoptotic factors to the nucleus/cytoplasm [43]. In the present study, an immunofluorescence analysis demonstrated that erlotinib increased the migration of HtrA2/Omi to nucleus when compared to the control group (Fig. 4a, b). Interestingly, this effect of erlotinib could be abolished via Mdivi-1 (Fig. 4a, b). Subsequently, western blotting was performed to quantify HtrA2/Omi liberation. As shown in Fig. 4c–e, compared to the control group, erlotinib treatment increaased the levels of cytoplasmic HtrA2/Omi (cyto-Htra2/Omi) and reduced the expression of mitochondrial HtrA2/Omi (mito-HtrA2/Omi). Similar results were also observed in cytochrome c (cyt c) liberation from mitochondria into cytoplasm (Fig. 4c–f). However, Mdivi-1 treatment repressed the erlotinib-mediated HtrA2/Omi and cyt c translocation from mitochondria into the cytoplasm. These results indicated that mitochondrial fragmentation accounted for HtrA2/Omi liberation.

At the molecular level, HtrA2/Omi is primarily expressed in the inner membrane of mitochondria. Based on a recent study, the liberation of HtrA2/Omi from mitochondria into the cytoplasm is dependent on

cardiolipin oxidation and mPTP opening [15, 44]. First, the oxidation of cardiolipin lowers the affinity of HtrA2/Omi to the mitochondria. Second, the opening of mPTP provides a channel for HtrA2/Omi leakage [45]. Given the role of mitochondrial fragmentation in cellular oxidative stress via mROS overproduction, we asked whether mROS was required for the mitochondrial fragmentation-mediated HtrA2/Omi liberation via modulating cardiolipin oxidation and mPTP opening. To support our hypothesis, cardiolipin oxidation was determined via staining with NAO, which is a cardiolipin probe. Under physiological conditions, NAO could interact with cardiolipin to display a green fluorescence. In response to cardiolipin oxidation, NAO cannot bind to oxidized cardiolipin, and thus the green fluorescence is reduced. As shown in Fig. 4g, h, the fluorescence of cardiolipin was significantly downregulated in response to erlotinib, and this effect was reversed by Mdivi-1. To verify whether mROS was responsible for cardiolipin oxidation, mitoQ was used to neutralize the mitochondrial fragmentation-produced mROS. Interestingly, mitoQ treatment also reversed the green fluorescence intensity of cardiolipin (Fig. 4g, h), similar to the results obtained via supplementation with Mdivi-1. These results verified the role played by mROS in cardiolipin oxidation. In addition, we also found that the mPTP opening rate was significantly increased in response to erlotinib (Fig. 4i), and this effect was inhibited by Mdivi-1 or mitoQ (Fig. 4i). Together, our data demonstrated that the mitochondrial fragmentation-mediated mROS regulated HtrA2/Omi liberation via inducing cardiolipin oxidation and mPTP opening.

### Released HtrA2/Omi induces caspase-9-dependent apoptosis

After it is released into the cytoplasm, HtrA2/Omi can interact with and activate mitochondrial apoptosis in a manner that is dependent on caspase-9 activity [11]. Notably, an early feature of caspase-9-related apoptosis is the reduction of mitochondrial potential. In the present study, a JC-1 kit was used to stain for the mitochondrial potential. The results indicated that erlotinib treatment significantly reduced the mitochondrial potential (Fig. 5a, b), and this effect was inhibited by Mdivi-1. To confirm

(See figure on next page.)

**Fig. 4** Mitochondrial fragmentation-mediated mROS induces HtrA2/Omi liberation. **a, b** Immunofluorescence measurements of HtrA2/Omi in response to erlotinib treatment. Mdivi-1 was used to inhibit mitochondrial fragmentation. **c–f** Cytoplasmic HtrA2/Omi (cyto-HrA2/Omi), cytoplasmic cyt c (cyto-cyt c), mitochondrial HtrA2/Omi (mito-HtrA2/Omi) and mitochondrial cyt c (mito-cyt c) were determined using western blotting analysis. **g, h** Cardiolipin oxidation was observed using an NAO probe. In response to cardiolipin oxidation, NAO could not bind to oxidized cardiolipin, and thus the green fluorescence was reduced. Accordingly, the relative fluorescence intensity was recorded to quantify cardiolipin oxidation. MitoQ was added to the medium of PANC-1 cells to neutralize the mROS that were produced by mitochondrial fragmentation. **i** mPTP opening was determined using tetramethylrhodamine ethyl ester. The relative mPTP opening rate was quantified as a ratio to that of control group. $*p < 0.05$

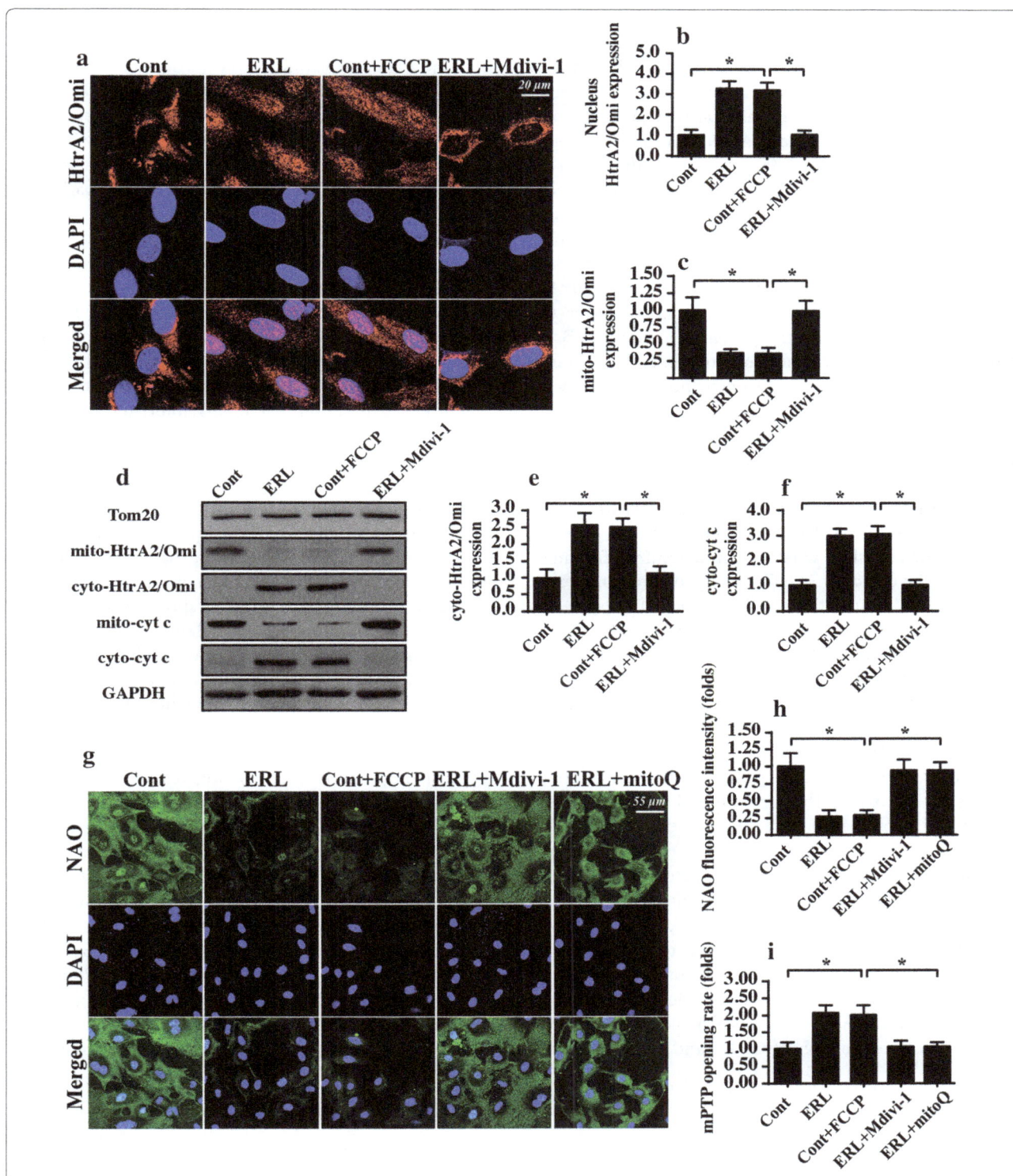

whether HtrA2/Omi accounted for the mitochondrial potential collapse, two independent siRNAs were used. After knockdown of HtrA2/Omi, the mitochondrial potential was analyzed again. Compared to the erlotinib-treated group, the loss of HtrA2/Omi stabilized the mitochondrial potential (Fig. 5a, b), an effect that was similar to the results obtained via treatment with Mdivi-1. Furthermore, the last characteristic of caspase-9-related apoptosis is the activation of caspase-9, an effect that is accompanied by an increase in proapoptotic proteins. In the present study, the protein activity (Fig. 5c) and expression (Fig. 5d, e) of caspase-9 were both upregulated in answer to erlotinib stress and these effects could be repressed by Mdivi-1 or HtrA2/Omi siRNA. As a consequence of caspase-9 activation, the levels of proapoptotic factors such as Bad and Bax were significantly increased in response to erlotinib treatment, and this effect was negated by Mdivi-1 treatment or HtrA2/Omi siRNA transfection (Fig. 5f–j). By comparison, the expression of antiapoptotic proteins, including Bcl-2 and survivin, were obviously downregulated by erlotinib (Fig. 5f–j) and were reversed to near-normal levels with Mdivi-1 treatment or HtrA2/Omi knockdown. Together, our results indicated that mitochondrial fragmentation activated caspase-9-dependent apoptosis via HtrA2/Omi.

### Mitochondrial fragmentation also modulated PANC-1 cell proliferation via mROS-HtrA2/Omi pathways

To this end, we asked whether mitochondrial fragmentation was involved in PANC-1 cell proliferation via the mROS-HtrA2/Omi pathways. First, the EdU assay was conducted to observe cellular proliferation. As shown in Fig. 6a, b, compared to the control group, erlotinib treatment significantly reduced the ratio of EdU-positive cells; this effect was repressed by Mdivi-1 (Fig. 6a, b). In addition, the neutralization of mROS via mitoQ and knockdown of HtrA2/Omi via siRNA transfection also reversed the number of EdU-positive cells after erlotinib treatment (Fig. 6a, b). These results indicated that mitochondrial fragmentation affected the cell proliferation in PANC-1 cell via the mROS-HtrA2/Omi axis. Further, the cell proliferation is primarily regulated by CDK4 and Cyclin D1. Cyclin D1 and cyclin E interact with each other and generate cyclin-dependent kinase (Cdk)4/6-cyclin D and/or Cdk2-cyclin E complexes, which accelerate transition from the G0/G1 to S stage, according to the previous study [46]. We have provided the references for this. With the help of a western blotting assay, we found that the expression of CDK4 and Cyclin D1 were

both reduced in response to erlotinib treatment, and this effect was negated by Mdivi-1 (Fig. 6c–e). Interestingly, the neutralization of mROS via mitoQ and knockdown of HtrA2/Omi via siRNA transfection also reversed the levels of CDK4 and Cyclin D1. Together, our results confirmed that PANC-1 cell proliferation was modulated by erlotinib via mitochondrial fragmentation in a manner that was dependent on the mROS-HtrA2/Omi pathways.

## Discussion

According to the previous findings, mitochondrial fission has been acknowledged as a potential target to reduce the proliferation, migration and survival of PANC-1 pancreatic cancer cells [10]. Excessive mitochondrial fission promotes mitochondrial fragmentation [15]. Fragmented mitochondria induce damage to mitochondrial structure and function, eventually interrupting the cellular ATP supply and activating the apoptosis response [47, 48]. However, the detailed molecular mechanism by which mitochondrial fragmentation triggers mitochondrial damage and cellular apoptosis remains unclear. Our study provides an answer to this question. We used different doses of ERL to screen its proapoptotic effect in two types of cancer cell lines. Then, we used the minimal lethal dose of ERL to investigate its apoptotic mechanism, with a focus on mitochondrial damage. We observed the minimal lethal dose of ERL has an ability to induce the mitochondrial fragmentation and this finding may explain one of the mechanisms by which ERL mediated cancer cell apoptosis. Notably, whether higher dose of ERL could activate other signaling pathway to induce cell apoptosis requires further investigation. Our data illustrated that erlotinib treatment promoted mitochondrial fragmentation that occurred via increased mitochondrial fission and decreased mitochondrial fusion. Subsequently, excessive mitochondrial fragmentation triggered mROS overloading, leading to cellular oxidative stress and disordered energy metabolism. In addition, mROS overproduction was closely associated with cardiolipin oxidation and mPTP opening, favoring HtrA2/Omi liberation from mitochondria into the cytoplasm. As a consequence of HtrA2/Omi leakage, reduction of the mitochondrial potential and caspase-9 activation were

(See figure on next page.)

**Fig. 5** Released HtrA2/Omi triggers an activation of caspase-9-related cellular apoptosis. **a, b** The mitochondrial potential was determined using a JC-1 kit in PANC-1 cells. Mdivi-1 was used to inhibit mitochondrial fragmentation. Furthermore, two independent siRNAs against HtrA2/Omi were transfected into PANC-1 cells to suppress HtrA2/Omi expression. The red-to-green ratio was recorded to quantify the mitochondrial potential. **c** The activation of caspase-9 was measured using an ELISA to evaluate the activity of caspase-9. Mdivi-1 was used to inhibit mitochondrial fragmentation. Furthermore, two independent siRNAs against HtrA2/Omi were transfected into PANC-1 cells to suppress HtrA2/Omi expression. **d, e** Expression of caspase-9 was determined via immunofluorescence. **f–j** Western blotting was performed to detect alterations in proapoptotic proteins and antiapoptotic factors. Mdivi-1 was used to inhibit mitochondrial fragmentation. Additionally, two siRNAs against HtrA2/Omi were transfected into PANC-1 cells to suppress HtrA2/Omi expression. *$p < 0.05$

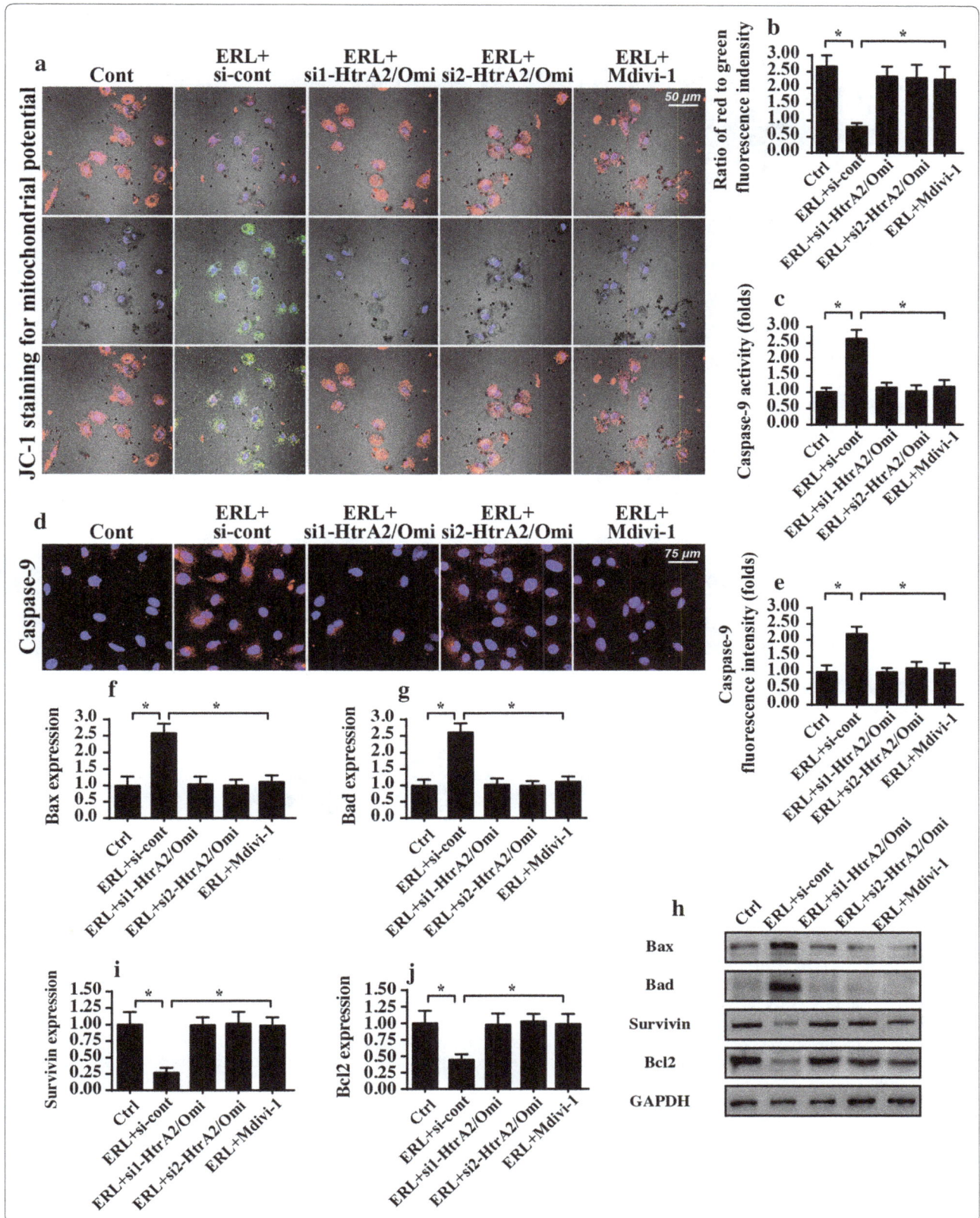

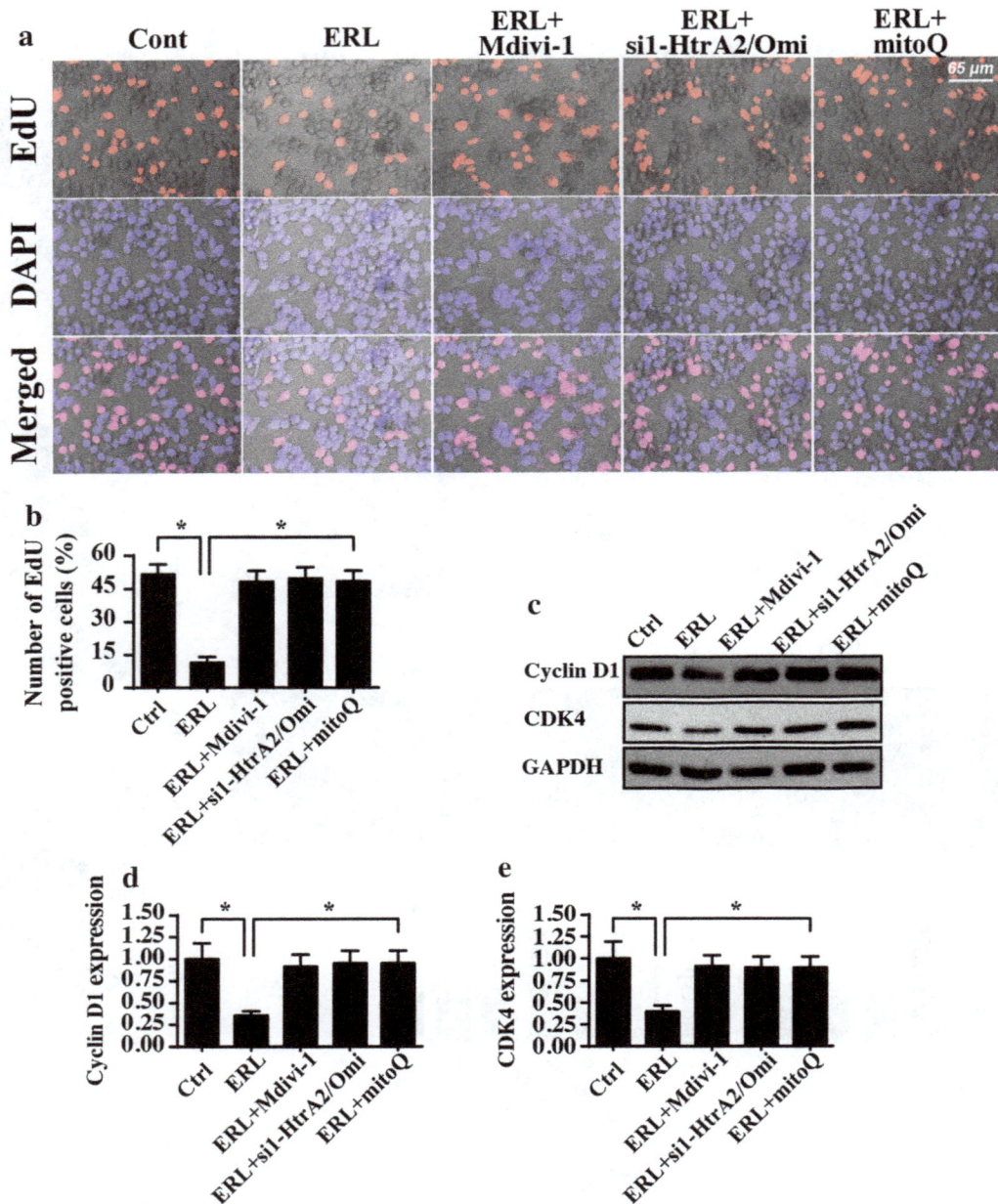

**Fig. 6** Mitochondrial fragmentation regulates the proliferation of PANC-1 cells via the mROS-HtrA2/Omi pathways. **a** The EdU assay was used to observe the cellular proliferation in response to erlotinib treatment. Mdivi-1 was used to inhibit mitochondrial fragmentation. Furthermore, two siRNAs against HtrA2/Omi were transfected into PANC-1 cells to suppress HtrA2/Omi expression. Additionally, mitoQ was added into the medium of PANC-1 cells to attenuate the production of mROS. **b** The quantification of EdU-positive cells. **c–e** CDK4 and Cyclin D1 expression were evaluated via western blotting. Mdivi-1 was used to inhibit mitochondrial fragmentation. In addition, two siRNAs against HtrA2/Omi were transfected into PANC-1 cells to suppress HtrA2/Omi expression. Furthermore, mitoQ was added to the medium of PANC-1 cells to attenuate the production of mROS. *$p < 0.05$

noted, and these alterations were accompanied by an upregulation of proapoptotic proteins and a downregulation of antiapoptotic factors. Overall, we demonstrated for the first time that erlotinib-activated mitochondrial fragmentation mediated PANC-1 apoptosis via the mROS-HtrA2/Omi pathways. This finding fills the knowledge gap regarding how mitochondrial fragmentation induces mitochondrial damage and triggers the apoptotic pathway.

Mitochondrial fission and fusion are a part of mitochondrial dynamics. Under physiological conditions, the mitochondrial network undergoes moderate fission and fusion to fill the requirements for cellular metabolism [49, 50]. Mild levels of mitochondrial fission help the mitochondria in generating daughter mitochondria, whereas moderate levels of mitochondrial fusion provides the energy for communication between the mitochondrial network [51, 52]. Interestingly, uncontrolled mitochondrial fission generates massive amounts of fragmented mitochondria and disrupts mitochondrial homeostasis. Previous studies have identified mitochondrial fragmentation, which is produced by mitochondrial fission, as the apoptotic trigger in various disease models. For instance, in fatty liver disease, mitochondrial fragmentation promotes the apoptosis of hepatocytes and the progression of liver fibrosis by decreasing mitophagy [53]. In neurodegenerative illness such as Alzheimer's disease, excessive mitochondrial fragmentation disturbs mitochondrial energy metabolism and causes neuronal oxidative injury [54]. In addition, in rectal cancer, activated mitochondrial fragmentation limits tumor proliferation and augments cancer apoptosis [11]. In accordance with these findings, our data also illustrated the necessary role played by mitochondrial fragmentation in initiating pancreatic cancer PANC-1 cell death. Thus, mitochondrial fragmentation would be considered as a tumor-suppressor, and strategies to promote mitochondrial fragmentation are of significant importance in the design of anti-cancer drugs.

Although the proapoptotic effect of mitochondrial fragmentation has been well-documented, the detailed mechanisms by which mitochondrial fragmentation induces mitochondrial damage and activates cellular apoptosis are incompletely understood. In the present study, we found that mitochondrial fragmentation modulated mitochondrial homeostasis and cell viability through two mechanisms. One mechanism was driven by the promotion of mROS-mediated cell oxidative injury, and the other involved the HtrA2/Omi liberation-induced caspase-9 activation. First, mitochondrial fragmentation generated superfluous amounts of mROS, and the excess mROS induced cardiolipin oxidation and mPTP opening [55]. Subsequently, oxidized cardiolipin and increased mPTP opening worked together to augment the liberation of HtrA2/Omi from mitochondria into the cytoplasm, where Htra2/Omi reduced the mitochondrial potential and induced caspase-9 activation. This information was also consistent with previous studies. In cardiac ischemia–reperfusion injury, excessive mitochondrial fragmentation-induced mitochondrial DNA damage evokes mROS overproduction and cardiolipin oxidation [14, 15]. Additionally, in oral cancer, mitochondrial fragmentation-related cardiolipin oxidation and mPTP opening eventually contribute to caspase-involved cellular apoptosis [56].

In the present study, we used erlotinib to activate mitochondrial fragmentation and found that erlotinib-mediated PANC-1 cellular apoptosis could be inhibited by Mdivi-1, which is an antagonist of mitochondrial fragmentation. To the best of our knowledge, this is the first study to investigate the role of erlotinib in mitochondrial stress. Although erlotinib has been tested in several human clinical studies [57, 58], its pharmacological mechanism has not been adequately explored. Our study proposed that the anti-cancer property of erlotinib relied on the activation of mitochondrial fragmentation by upregulating mitochondrial fission and downregulating mitochondrial fusion. Notably, the dose selection of ERL was according to a previous study [26] and this selection may be also relied on the types of cancer cell lines. In clinical practice, different doses of ERL have been used according to the tumor staging and pathologic grading. Further insight is required to figure out the appropriate concentration of ERL on different types of pancreatic cancer. Besides, there are several limitations in the present study. Although we used two pancreatic cancer cell lines to screen the role of erlotinib, an animal study is necessary to further support our finding. In addition, human evidence is also required to validate the tumor-suppressive effects of mitochondrial fragmentation in response to erlotinib treatment.

## Conclusion

Collectively, our results reported that mitochondrial fragmentation, which was activated by erlotinib, regulated the viability of the PANC-1 pancreatic cancer cell line via the mROS-HtrA2/Omi pathways. This conclusion provides a potential target to modify pancreatic cancer viability via augmenting mitochondrial fragmentation and activating the mROS-HtrA2/Omi pathways.

## Additional file

**Additional file 1: Figure S1.** The proapoptotic effect of erlotinib on PANC1 cells using Annexin V/PI staining. Early apoptosis (Annexin V+/PI- cells) and late apoptosis (Annexin V+/PI+ cells) were counted. #p<0.05 vs. control group.

**Authors' contributions**
JW, JC, and LW were involved in the conception and design, performance of experiments, data analysis and interpretation, and manuscript writing. KPW, XPH, YLZ, HK and SZ were involved in data analysis and interpretation. All authors read and approved the final manuscript.

## Author details
[1] Department of Pharmacy, Third Clinical Medical College, Three Gorges University, Gezhouba Group Central Hospital, Yichang 443002, Hubei, China. [2] Department of Pathogenic Biology, School of Medicine, China Three Gorges University, Yichang 443002, Hubei, China. [3] Department of Oncology, Third Clinical Medical College, Three Gorges University, Gezhouba Group Central Hospital, No. 60 Qiaohu Lake Road, Xiling District, Yichang 443002, Hubei, China.

## Acknowledgements
Not applicable.

## Competing interests
The authors declare that they have no competing interests.

## Funding
This study was supported by grants from the Hubei Province Health and Family Planning Scientific Research Project (WJ2017F085) and the Youth Project of China Three Gorges University (KJ2016A018).

## References
1. Zhou H, Yue Y, Wang J, Ma Q, Chen Y. Melatonin therapy for diabetic cardiomyopathy: A mechanism involving Syk-mitochondrial complex I-SERCA pathway. Cell Signal. 2018;47:88–100.
2. Rossi ML, Rehman AA, Gondi CS. Therapeutic options for the management of pancreatic cancer. World J Gastroenterol. 2014;20(32):11142–59.
3. Zhu H, Jin Q, Li Y, Ma Q, Wang J, Li D, Zhou H, Chen Y. Melatonin protected cardiac microvascular endothelial cells against oxidative stress injury via suppression of IP3R-[Ca(2+)]c/VDAC-[Ca(2+)]m axis by activation of MAPK/ERK signaling pathway. Cell Stress Chaperones. 2018;23(1):101–13.
4. Shi C, Cai Y, Li Y, Li Y, Hu N, Ma S, Hu S, Zhu P, Wang W, Zhou H. Yap promotes hepatocellular carcinoma metastasis and mobilization via governing cofilin/F-actin/lamellipodium axis by regulation of JNK/Bnip3/SERCA/CaMKII pathways. Redox Biol. 2018;14:59–71.
5. Viale A, Pettazzoni P, Lyssiotis CA, Ying H, Sanchez N, Marchesini M, Carugo A, Green T, Seth S, Giuliani V, et al. Oncogene ablation-resistant pancreatic cancer cells depend on mitochondrial function. Nature. 2014;514(7524):628–32.
6. Li G, Gan Y, Fan Y, Wu Y, Lin H, Song Y, Cai X, Yu X, Pan W, Yao M, et al. Enriched environment inhibits mouse pancreatic cancer growth and down-regulates the expression of mitochondria-related genes in cancer cells. Sci Rep. 2015;5:7856.
7. Zhou H, Li D, Zhu P, Hu S, Hu N, Ma S, Zhang Y, Han T, Ren J, Cao F, et al. Melatonin suppresses platelet activation and function against cardiac ischemia/reperfusion injury via PPARgamma/FUNDC1/mitophagy pathways. J Pineal Res. 2017;63(4):e12438.
8. Zhu P, Hu S, Jin Q, Li D, Tian F, Toan S, Li Y, Zhou H, Chen Y. Ripk3 promotes ER stress-induced necroptosis in cardiac IR injury: A mechanism involving calcium overload/XO/ROS/mPTP pathway. Redox Biol. 2018;16:157–68.
9. Xia J, Inagaki Y, Gao J, Qi F, Song P, Han G, Sawakami T, Gao B, Luo C, Kokudo N, et al. Combination of cinobufacini and doxorubicin increases apoptosis of hepatocellular carcinoma cells through the Fas- and mitochondria-mediated pathways. Am J Chin Med. 2017;45(7):1537–56.
10. Pan L, Zhou L, Yin W, Bai J, Liu R. miR-125a induces apoptosis, metabolism disorder and migration impairment in pancreatic cancer cells by targeting Mfn2-related mitochondrial fission. Int J Oncol. 2018;53(1):124–36.
11. Li H, He F, Zhao X, Zhang Y, Chu X, Hua C, Qu Y, Duan Y, Ming L. YAP inhibits the apoptosis and migration of human rectal cancer cells via suppression of JNK-Drp1-mitochondrial Fission-HtrA2/Omi pathways. Cell Physiol Biochem. 2017;44(5):2073–89.
12. Yan H, Xiao F, Zou J, Qiu C, Sun W, Gu M, Zhang L. NR4A1-induced increase in the sensitivity of a human gastric cancer line to TNFalpha-mediated apoptosis is associated with the inhibition of JNK/Parkin-dependent mitophagy. Int J Oncol. 2018;52(2):367–78.
13. Zhang J, Zhang Y, Wu W, Wang F, Liu X, Shui G, Nie C. Guanylate-binding protein 2 regulates Drp1-mediated mitochondrial fission to suppress breast cancer cell invasion. Cell Death Dis. 2017;8(10):e3151.
14. Zhou H, Wang J, Zhu P, Zhu H, Toan S, Hu S, Ren J, Chen Y. NR4A1 aggravates the cardiac microvascular ischemia reperfusion injury through suppressing FUNDC1-mediated mitophagy and promoting Mff-required mitochondrial fission by CK2alpha. Basic Res Cardiol. 2018;113(4):23.
15. Zhou H, Hu S, Jin Q, Shi C, Zhang Y, Zhu P, Ma Q, Tian F, Chen Y. Mff-dependent mitochondrial fission contributes to the pathogenesis of cardiac microvasculature ischemia/reperfusion injury via induction of mROS-mediated cardiolipin oxidation and HK2/VDAC1 disassociation-involved mPTP opening. J Am Heart Assoc. 2017. https://doi.org/10.1161/JAHA.116.005328.
16. Zhou H, Shi C, Hu S, Zhu H, Ren J, Chen Y. BI1 is associated with microvascular protection in cardiac ischemia reperfusion injury via repressing Syk-Nox2-Drp1-mitochondrial fission pathways. Angiogenesis. 2018;21(3):599–615.
17. Yuan X, Zhou Y, Wang W, Li J, Xie G, Zhao Y, Xu D, Shen L. Activation of TLR4 signaling promotes gastric cancer progression by inducing mitochondrial ROS production. Cell Death Dis. 2013;4:e794.
18. Hong H, Tao T, Chen S, Liang C, Qiu Y, Zhou Y, Zhang R. MicroRNA-143 promotes cardiac ischemia-mediated mitochondrial impairment by the inhibition of protein kinase Cepsilon. Basic Res Cardiol. 2017;112(6):60.
19. Dall'Acqua S, Linardi MA, Bortolozzi R, Clauser M, Marzocchini S, Maggi F, Nicoletti M, Innocenti G, Basso G, Viola G. Natural daucane esters induces apoptosis in leukaemic cells through ROS production. Phytochemistry. 2014;108:147–56.
20. Salminen A, Kaarniranta K, Kauppinen A. Integrated stress response stimulates FGF21 expression: Systemic enhancer of longevity. Cell Signal. 2017;40:10–21.
21. Zhou H, Zhang Y, Hu S, Shi C, Zhu P, Ma Q, Jin Q, Cao F, Tian F, Chen Y. Melatonin protects cardiac microvasculature against ischemia/reperfusion injury via suppression of mitochondrial fission-VDAC1-HK2-mPTP-mitophagy axis. J Pineal Res. 2017;63(1):e12413.
22. Xie CG, Sun SL, Wei SM, Xu XM, Shao LM, Chen JM, Cai JT. Downregulation of GEP100 improved the growth inhibition effect of erlotinib through modulating mesenchymal epithelial transition process in pancreatic cancer. Pancreas. 2018;47(6):732–7.
23. Nunez-Gomez E, Pericacho M, Ollauri-Ibanez C, Bernabeu C, Lopez-Novoa JM. The role of endoglin in post-ischemic revascularization. Angiogenesis. 2017;20(1):1–24.
24. Kadera BE, Toste PA, Wu N, Li L, Nguyen AH, Dawson DW, Donahue TR. Low expression of the E3 ubiquitin ligase CBL confers chemoresistance in human pancreatic cancer and is targeted by epidermal growth factor receptor inhibition. Clin Cancer Res. 2015;21(1):157–65.
25. Zhou H, Ma Q, Zhu P, Ren J, Reiter RJ, Chen Y. Protective role of melatonin in cardiac ischemia-reperfusion injury: From pathogenesis to targeted therapy. J Pineal Res. 2018;64(3):e12471.
26. Shan F, Shao Z, Jiang S, Cheng Z. Erlotinib induces the human non-small-cell lung cancer cells apoptosis via activating ROS-dependent JNK pathways. Cancer Med. 2016;5(11):3166–75.
27. Couto JA, Ayturk UM, Konczyk DJ, Goss JA, Huang AY, Hann S, Reeve JL, Liang MG, Bischoff J, Warman ML, et al. A somatic GNA11 mutation is associated with extremity capillary malformation and overgrowth. Angiogenesis. 2017;20(3):303–6.
28. Zhou H, Li D, Zhu P, Ma Q, Toan S, Wang J, Hu S, Chen Y, Zhang Y. Inhibitory effect of melatonin on necroptosis via repressing the Ripk3-PGAM5-CypD-mPTP pathway attenuates cardiac microvascular ischemia-reperfusion injury. J Pineal Res. 2018;65:e12503.
29. Kingery JR, Hamid T, Lewis RK, Ismahil MA, Bansal SS, Rokosh G, Townes TM, Ildstad ST, Jones SP, Prabhu SD. Leukocyte iNOS is required for inflammation and pathological remodeling in ischemic heart failure. Basic Res Cardiol. 2017;112(2):19.
30. Feng D, Wang B, Wang L, Abraham N, Tao K, Huang L, Shi W, Dong Y, Qu Y. Pre-ischemia melatonin treatment alleviated acute neuronal injury after ischemic stroke by inhibiting endoplasmic reticulum stress-dependent autophagy via PERK and IRE1 signalings. J Pineal Res. 2017. https://doi.org/10.1111/jpi.12395.
31. Brasacchio D, Alsop AE, Noori T, Lufti M, Iyer S, Simpson KJ, Bird PI, Kluck RM, Johnstone RW, Trapani JA. Epigenetic control of mitochondrial cell death through PACS1-mediated regulation of BAX/BAK oligomerization. Cell Death Differ. 2017;24(6):961–70.
32. Li R, Xin T, Li D, Wang C, Zhu H, Zhou H. Therapeutic effect of Sirtuin 3 on ameliorating nonalcoholic fatty liver disease: the role of the ERK-CREB pathway and Bnip3-mediated mitophagy. Redox Biol. 2018;18:229–43.

Excessive mitochondrial fragmentation triggered by erlotinib promotes pancreatic cancer PANC-1 cell...

167

33. Ligeza J, Marona P, Gach N, Lipert B, Miekus K, Wilk W, Jaszczynski J, Stelmach A, Loboda A, Dulak J, et al. MCPIP1 contributes to clear cell renal cell carcinomas development. Angiogenesis. 2017;20(3):325–40.

34. Yang X, Xu Y, Wang T, Shu D, Guo P, Miskimins K, Qian SY. Inhibition of cancer migration and invasion by knocking down delta-5-desaturase in COX-2 overexpressed cancer cells. Redox Biol. 2017;11:653–62.

35. Lin S, Hoffmann K, Gao C, Petrulionis M, Herr I, Schemmer P. Melatonin promotes sorafenib-induced apoptosis through synergistic activation of JNK/c-jun pathway in human hepatocellular carcinoma. J Pineal Res. 2017. https://doi.org/10.1111/jpi.12398.

36. Zhou H, Zhu P, Wang J, Zhu H, Ren J, Chen Y. Pathogenesis of cardiac ischemia reperfusion injury is associated with CK2alpha-disturbed mitochondrial homeostasis via suppression of FUNDC1-related mitophagy. Cell Death Differ. 2018;25(6):1080–93.

37. Zhou H, Wang J, Zhu P, Hu S, Ren J. Ripk3 regulates cardiac microvascular reperfusion injury: the role of IP3R-dependent calcium overload, XO-mediated oxidative stress and F-action/filopodia-based cellular migration. Cell Signal. 2018;45:12–22.

38. Sarkar C, Ganju RK, Pompili VJ, Chakroborty D. Enhanced peripheral dopamine impairs post-ischemic healing by suppressing angiotensin receptor type 1 expression in endothelial cells and inhibiting angiogenesis. Angiogenesis. 2017;20(1):97–107.

39. Iggena D, Winter Y, Steiner B. Melatonin restores hippocampal neural precursor cell proliferation and prevents cognitive deficits induced by jet lag simulation in adult mice. J Pineal Res. 2017. https://doi.org/10.1111/jpi.12397.

40. Garcia-Nino WR, Correa F, Rodriguez-Barrena JI, Leon-Contreras JC, Buelna-Chontal M, Soria-Castro E, Hernandez-Pando R, Pedraza-Chaverri J, Zazueta C. Cardioprotective kinase signaling to subsarcolemmal and interfibrillar mitochondria is mediated by caveolar structures. Basic Res Cardiol. 2017;112(2):15.

41. Gadicherla AK, Wang N, Bulic M, Agullo-Pascual E, Lissoni A, De Smet M, Delmar M, Bultynck G, Krysko DV, Camara A, et al. Mitochondrial Cx43 hemichannels contribute to mitochondrial calcium entry and cell death in the heart. Basic Res Cardiol. 2017;112(3):27.

42. Rossello X, Riquelme JA, He Z, Taferner S, Vanhaesebroeck B, Davidson SM, Yellon DM. The role of PI3 Kalpha isoform in cardioprotection. Basic Res Cardiol. 2017;112(6):66.

43. Rossello X, Yellon DM. The RISK pathway and beyond. Basic Res Cardiol. 2017;113(1):2.

44. Das N, Mandala A, Naaz S, Giri S, Jain M, Bandyopadhyay D, Reiter RJ, Roy SS. Melatonin protects against lipid-induced mitochondrial dysfunction in hepatocytes and inhibits stellate cell activation during hepatic fibrosis in mice. J Pineal Res. 2017. https://doi.org/10.1111/jpi.12404.

45. Liu Z, Gan L, Xu Y, Luo D, Ren Q, Wu S, Sun C. Melatonin alleviates inflammasome-induced pyroptosis through inhibiting NF-kappaB/GSDMD signal in mice adipose tissue. J Pineal Res. 2017. https://doi.org/10.1111/jpi.12414.

46. Zhou H, Li D, Shi C, Xin T, Yang J, Zhou Y, Hu S, Tian F, Wang J, Chen Y. Effects of Exendin-4 on bone marrow mesenchymal stem cell proliferation, migration and apoptosis in vitro. Sci Rep. 2015;5:12898.

47. Zhou H, Wang S, Zhu P, Hu S, Chen Y, Ren J. Empagliflozin rescues diabetic myocardial microvascular injury via AMPK-mediated inhibition of mitochondrial fission. Redox Biol. 2018;15:335–46.

48. Hu Z, Cheng J, Xu J, Ruf W, Lockwood CJ. Tissue factor is an angiogenic-specific receptor for factor VII-targeted immunotherapy and photodynamic therapy. Angiogenesis. 2017;20(1):85–96.

49. Zhou H, Wang S, Hu S, Chen Y, Ren J. ER-mitochondria microdomains in cardiac ischemia-reperfusion injury: a fresh perspective. Front Physiol. 2018;9:755.

50. Fuhrmann DC, Brune B. Mitochondrial composition and function under the control of hypoxia. Redox Biol. 2017;12:208–15.

51. Kozlov AV, Lancaster JR Jr, Meszaros AT, Weidinger A. Mitochondria-meditated pathways of organ failure upon inflammation. Redox Biol. 2017;13:170–81.

52. Jin Q, Li R, Hu N, Xin T, Zhu P, Hu S, Ma S, Zhu H, Ren J, Zhou H. DUSP1 alleviates cardiac ischemia/reperfusion injury by suppressing the Mff-required mitochondrial fission and Bnip3-related mitophagy via the JNK pathways. Redox Biol. 2018;14:576–87.

53. Zhou H, Du W, Li Y, Shi C, Hu N, Ma S, Wang W, Ren J. Effects of melatonin on fatty liver disease: the role of NR4A1/DNA-PKcs/p53 pathway, mitochondrial fission, and mitophagy. J Pineal Res. 2018. https://doi.org/10.1111/jpi.12450.

54. Lei Q, Tan J, Yi S, Wu N, Wang Y, Wu H. Mitochonic acid 5 activates the MAPK-ERK-yap signaling pathways to protect mouse microglial BV-2 cells against TNFalpha-induced apoptosis via increased Bnip3-related mitophagy. Cell Mol Biol Lett. 2018;23:14.

55. Zhou H, Zhu P, Guo J, Hu N, Wang S, Li D, Hu S, Ren J, Cao F, Chen Y. Ripk3 induces mitochondrial apoptosis via inhibition of FUNDC1 mitophagy in cardiac IR injury. Redox Biol. 2017;13:498–507.

56. Lee K, Back K. Overexpression of rice serotonin N-acetyltransferase 1 in transgenic rice plants confers resistance to cadmium and senescence and increases grain yield. J Pineal Res. 2017;62(3):e12392.

57. Abravan A, Eide HA, Knudtsen IS, Londalen AM, Helland A, Malinen E. Assessment of pulmonary (18)F-FDG-PET uptake and cytokine profiles in non-small cell lung cancer patients treated with radiotherapy and erlotinib. Clin Transl Radiat Oncol. 2017;4:57–63.

58. Liu D, Zeng X, Li X, Mehta JL, Wang X. Role of NLRP3 inflammasome in the pathogenesis of cardiovascular diseases. Basic Res Cardiol. 2017;113(1):5.

# Prognostic value of microvessel density in cervical cancer

Xiaoli Hu, Hailing Liu, Miaomiao Ye and Xueqiong Zhu*⬤

## Abstract

**Background:** Several epidemiological researches have indicated that microvessel density (MVD), reflecting angiogenesis, was a negatively prognostic factor of cervical cancer. However, the results were inconsistent. Therefore, we performed a meta-analysis to evaluate the association between microvessel density and the survival probability of patients with cervical cancer.

**Method:** There was a comprehensive search of the PubMed, EMBASE and Cochrane databases up to August 31, 2017. Based on a fixed-effects or random-effects model, the hazard ratio (HR) and 95% confidence intervals (CIs) were calculated from researches on overall survival (OS) and disease-free survival (DFS).

**Result:** Totally, we included 13 observational researches, involving 1097 patients with cervical cancer. The results showed that high level of microvessel density was negatively correlated with OS (HR = 1.79, 95% CIs 1.31–2.44, $I^2 = 60.7\%$, $P = 0.003$) and DFS (HR = 1.47, 95% CIs 1.13–1.80, $I^2 = 0\%$, $P = 0.423$) of cervical cancer patients. In subgroup analysis, high counts of MVD were significantly associated with a poor survival (including OS and DFS) of the patients detected by anti-factor VIII antibodies or in European origin.

**Conclusion:** The present meta-analysis indicated that survival with high level of MVD was significant poorer than with low MVD in cervical cancer patient. Standardization of MVD assessment is needed.

**Keywords:** Microvessel density, Survival, Cervical neoplasia, Meta-analysis

## Background

Cervical cancer is the third most frequent gynecological neoplasms worldwide and one of the leading causes of cancer-related death among women in developing countries [1]. This disease is responsible for approximately 265,000 deaths annually in the world, 87% occurring in low-income countries [2]. Although independent prognostic factors such as lymph node status, tumor size, pathologic grading of tumor and International Federation of Gynecology and Obstetrics (FIGO) stage contribute to a better comprehension of the disease progression [3, 4]. However, such factors couldn't predict individual clinical outcome absolutely in cervical cancer. Thus, there need more prognostic markers to further improve predictive accuracy.

*Correspondence: zjwzzxq@163.com
Department of Obstetrics and Gynecology, The Second Affiliated Hospital of Wenzhou Medical University, Wenzhou 325000, Zhejiang, China

Angiogenesis have been reported to play a crucial role in the growth, metastasis and progression of various types of cancers like breast cancer and renal cell carcinoma [5, 6]. When a tumor exceeds the size of 1 mm, its further growth needs angiogenesis, which can form new blood vessels and further lead to tumor metastasis. There are a variety of biomarkers to quantify intratumoral angiogenesis, including vascular endothelial growth factor (VEGF), basic fibroblast growth factor (bFGF) and microvessel density (MVD).

At present, MVD assessment is the most common method to evaluate intratumor angiogenesis in cancer. In early 1990s, MVD was firstly introduced as an indicator by Weidner et al. [7] to assess the microvessels density in patients with invasive breast cancer. Additionally, the most commonly used antibodies for microvessel staining are CD31, CD34, CD105 (Endoglin) and anti-factor VIII (Von Willebrand Factor). Over the past two decades, some studies had reported MVD as a prognosis factor in various tumors such as gastric carcinoma [8].

However, the value of microvessel density as a prognostic indicator of cervical cancer was controversial. Several researches demonstrated that the expression of MVD significantly associated with poor overall survival (OS) or progression free survival (PFS) for cervical cancer [9, 10]. But some studies were unable to indicate a significant relationship between MVD and poor survival in cervical cancer patients [11, 12].

Therefore, we conducted a meta-analysis in order to evaluate the prognostic value of microvessel density in patients with cervical carcinoma. Meanwhile, this study may help to provide a valuable prognostic indicator and guide the management of the cervical cancer patients in the future.

## Methods
### Search strategy
Two investigators conducted a comprehensive search in electronic databases of PubMed, EMBASE and Cochrane library for relevant researches up to 31 August 2017. The following Medical Subject Heading terms and keywords were used: ("cervical cancer" or "cervical tumor" or "cervical tumour" or "cervical malignance" or "cervical carcinoma" or "uterine cervical neoplasms" or "cervical neoplasm") and ("microvessel density" or "MVD" or "angiogenesis" or "neovascularization") and ("prognosis" or "outcome" or "survival" or "prognostic") with no restrictions. Meanwhile, we also performed a manual search of references cited in the retrieved studies and published reviews.

### Selection criteria
To be eligible, researches must be consistent with the following inclusion criteria: (1) All included patients with cervical carcinoma diagnosed by the pathological results; (2) reported the association between MVD and survival outcomes, such as overall survival (OS) and disease free survival (DFS); (3) papers were restricted to human studies published as full-length articles in English. Exclusion criteria were (1) reviews, letters, case reports, or editorial comments; (2) duplicate publications; (3) full text unavailable; (4) insufficient data for calculating the hazard ratios (HRs) and 95% confidence intervals (CIs).

The candidate studies were identified by two independent reviewers according to the titles and abstracts to exclude irrelevant studies. Then full texts of the remaining researches were scanned carefully to decide whether to include the studies, and any different opinion was resolved through discussion. Multivariate data were the priority choice when both multivariate and univariate data were offered. However, we also accepted univariate data when no multivariate results were provided.

### Data extraction and quality assessment
The following information were extracted carefully from all including studies by two authors by means of a standardized data table which included following items: the first author; the year of publication; the location of study; the number of included patients; the age range of participants; FIGO stage; the antibody to assess MVD; the duration of follow up; the cutoff value of MVD (usually with median MVD as cutoff); the types of survival analyses; HRs and 95% CI for overall survival/disease-free survival; the result of the study. The result for every single study was marked "positive" when higher MVD predicted poorer survival and "negative" when higher MVD did not indicate lower survival rate or even once supported a better survival.

Quality assessment of the including studies was evaluated by two investigators independently using the 9-star Newcastle–Ottawa Scale (NOS) [13]. According to the scoring system, we defined the research quality as high with scores which were equal to or greater than 7.

### Statistical analysis
The prognostic efficiency of MVD on cervical carcinoma was calculated by using the HRs and 95% CIs. When the effect values couldn't be provided directly by the study, we calculated HR value and 95% corresponding CIs in the Kaplan–Meier curve at particular time points using the methods introduced by Parmar et al. [14]. An observed HR > 1 indicated a bad prognosis in cervical cancer patient with the high MVD. Statistical heterogeneity from all the publications was tested by Cochran's Q test and Higgins I-squared statistics [15]. Meanwhile, a fixed-effects model was adopted to assess the pooled value when $I^2 < 50\%$ and $P > 0.10$ which indicated that no obvious heterogeneity was found. Otherwise, a random-effects model was applied. All statistical analyses were performed with STATA 11.0 (STATA Corp, College Station, Texas).

In addition, Subgroup analyses were conducted to calculate the potential source of heterogeneity according to geographical regions and antibodies for detecting MVD. A sensitivity analysis evaluating the consistency of the combined outcomes was adopted. The possible publication bias was assessed by Begg's tests [16]. All P-value were two-tailed and statistical significance was obvious as $P < 0.05$.

## Results

### Literature search

At the beginning, there were a total of 580 articles identified from three databases (262 from PubMed, 298 from EMBASE, 18 from Cochrane databases) according to the inclusion criteria. After screening the title, abstract and key words, 427 articles were deleted when met duplication. Followed by excluded researches which were obvious irrelevant, or didn't meet the inclusion criteria, we adopted a number of 13 independent and observational studies involving 1097 patients [9–11, 17–26]. The flow chart presented in Fig. 1 showed the study selection process in detail.

### Study characteristics

Table 1 presented the main characteristics of the 13 studies included in the meta-analysis. These researches were published between 1995 and 2014, and the sample sizes ranged from 30 to 173. As for the region, three studies were conducted from America [9, 21, 24], seven in Europe [10, 17, 18, 22, 23, 25, 26] and three in Asian country [11, 19, 20]. In addition, there were four different antibodies enrolled in the included studies to assess the microvessel density. Anti-factor VIII antibody was used in six studies [10, 18–20, 22, 26], CD 31 was conducted in four studies [17, 21, 23, 24], CD 34 was in two articles [9, 11], CD 105 was applied in two studies [21, 23], respectively. And all of the protein-levels of antibody were detected by immunohistochemistry (IHC). Among

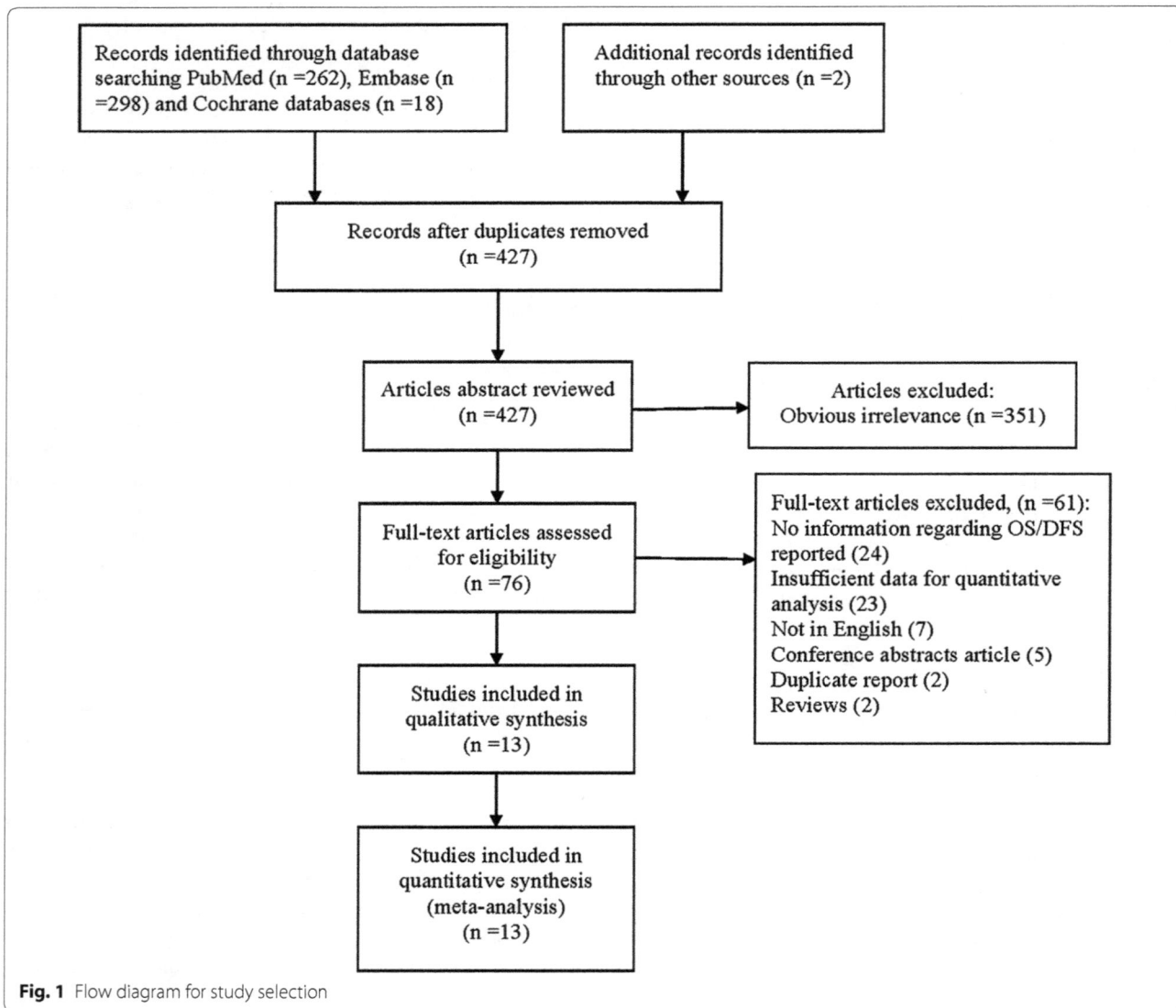

**Fig. 1** Flow diagram for study selection

**Table 1 Main characteristics of included studies**

| Study (year, population) | Age | FIGO stage | Sample size | Antibody | Follow-up (month) | Method for MVD | Cutoff of MVD | HR (95% CIs) | Survival analysis | Results | NOS |
|---|---|---|---|---|---|---|---|---|---|---|---|
| Cantu et al. (2003, Mexico) [9] | 48 (28–70) | II–III | 118 | CD34 | 60 (median) | Hot spot | 20 | DFS: 1.63 (1.71–2.65) | DFS | Positive | 7 |
| Cooper et al. (1998, England) [10] | 50 (29–81) | I–III | 111 | Anti-factor VIII | 55 (28–117) (median) | Hot spot | 10 | OS: 1.68 (1.03–2.74); DFS: 2.2 (1.09–4.44) | OS, DFS | Positive | 8 |
| Dellas et al. (1997, Switzerland) [17] | NR | IB | 58 | CD31 | 67 (median) | Hot spot | NR | OS: 1.5 (1.04–2.16) | OS | Positive | 7 |
| Hockel et al. (2001, Germany) [18] | NR | IB1–VIB | 52 | Anti-factor VIII | 26 (4–96) (median) | Hot spot | 40 | OS: 3.17 (1.32–7.63); DFS: 2.08 (1.22–3.54) | OS, DFS | Positive | 8 |
| Kaku et al. (1998, Japan) [19] | 46 (25–67) | I–II | 56 | Anti-factor VIII | 99 (61–175) (median) | Hot spot | 75 | OS: 3.31 (1.21–9.07) | OS | Positive | 8 |
| Lee et al. (2006, Korea) [11] | 48 (31–69) | IB–IIB | 85 | CD34 | 60 | IHC | 30.5 | OS: 1.11 (0.63–1.98); DFS: 1.04 (0.59–1.85) | OS, DFS | No significance | 9 |
| Moriyama et al. (2009, Japan) [20] | 55.9 (33–72) | IB–IIB | 57 | Anti-factor VIII | 10.5–174.3 | Hot spot | 0.8% | OS: 2.92 (1.11–7.69) | OS | Positive | 8 |
| Randall et al. (2009, America) [21] | 39.1 | IA2, IB, IIA | 173 | CD31, CD105 | 105.9 (2.7–184.8) (median) | Hot spot | 110 in CD31, 28 in CD105 | CD31-OS: 0.36 (0.17–0.79); CD105-OS: 1.76 (0.89–3.48) | OS | Positive in CD31 | 8 |
| Schlenger et al. (1995, Germany) [22] | 53 (26–80) | IB–IVA | 39 | Anti-factor VIII | 18 (4–41) (median) | IHC | 83 | DFS: 1.46 (1.05–2.03) | DFS | Positive | 8 |
| Tjalma et al. (1998, Belgium) [25] | 54 (24–91) | IA–IVB | 114 | CD31 | 39 (1–203) | Hot spot | 261 | OS: 2.17 (1.15–4.1) | OS | Positive | 7 |
| Van et al. (2006, America) [24] | 42±11 (26–79) | IB–IVA | 38 | CD31 | 17±17 (1–71) (mean) | IHC | NR | OS: 2.54 (1.11–5.82) | OS | Positive | 7 |
| Zijlmans et al. (2009, Netherlands) [23] | 45 (29–72) | IB–VIB | 30 | CD105 | NR | Hot Spot | NR | OS: 3.81 (0.46–31.42); DFS: 3.23 (1.38–7.57) | OS, DFS | Positive | 8 |
| Obermair et al. (1998, Austria) [26] | 43 (23–70) | IB | 166 | Anti-factor VIII | 85 (5–170) (median) | Hot Spot | 20 | OS: 2.56 (1.59–4.11) | OS | Positive | 7 |

*HR* hazard ratio, *CIs* confidence intervals, *NA* not available, *OS* overall survival, *DFS/PFS/MFS/RFS* disease-free survival/progress-free survival/metastasis-free survival/recurrence-free survival

them, MVD count in ten studies was performed by hotspot method which was introduced by Weidner et al. [7], while the hotspot method was not mentioned in other three articles. Thus, 14 researches (from 13 articles) involving 1097 patients were available for this meta-analysis. We included 11 studies which gave a description of the association between OS and MVD, and six researches involved other outcomes such as DFS. Otherwise, we defined the study as '− 1' and '− 2' if more than one outcome or antibody were applied in the same study [27, 28]. Meanwhile, the quality of included researches were assessed by using the Newcastle–Ottawa Scale and found to range from 7 stars to 9 stars, showing that the studies were in high quality.

### Association of MVD and OS of cervical cancer

The pooled HR for the 11 studies assessing the association between MVD and cervical cancer with OS was 1.7 (95% CIs 1.31–2.44, random-effects, Fig. 2), suggesting that high MVD level was associated with a poor prognosis of overall survival in cervical cancer patients. Since the heterogeneity among studies was significant

($I^2 = 60.7\%$, $P = 0.003$), random-effects model was applied for statistical analysis. Meanwhile, subgroup meta-analysis according types of antibodies and population was conducted to evaluate the possible source of heterogeneity among these studies (Figs. 3 and 4).

In the subgroup analysis by different antibodies, the prognostic value of MVD for OS was significant in the "anti-factor VIII" subgroup (HR = 2.34, 95% CIs 1.75–3.12, $I^2 = 0\%$, n = 5), while there was not statistically significant association in "CD31" subgroup (HR = 1.33, 95% CIs 0.65–2.72, $I^2 = 81.2\%$, n = 4), "CD34" subgroup (HR = 1.11, 95% CIs 0.63–1.97, n = 1) and "CD105" subgroup (HR = 1.89, 95% CIs 0.99–3.62, $I^2 = 0\%$, n = 2).

There was another subgroup about source regions of included studies, a pooled HR was 1.93 (95% CIs 1.53–2.44, $I^2 = 4.8\%$, n = 6) in Europe population, indicating a significantly poorer survival in cervical cancer patients with higher MVD in European countries. However, MVD level was not significantly associated with OS in Asia (HR = 2.01, 95% CIs 0.94–4.31, $I^2 = 60.1\%$, n = 3) and American locations (HR = 1.17, 95% CIs 0.37–3.69, $I^2 = 85.5\%$, n = 3).

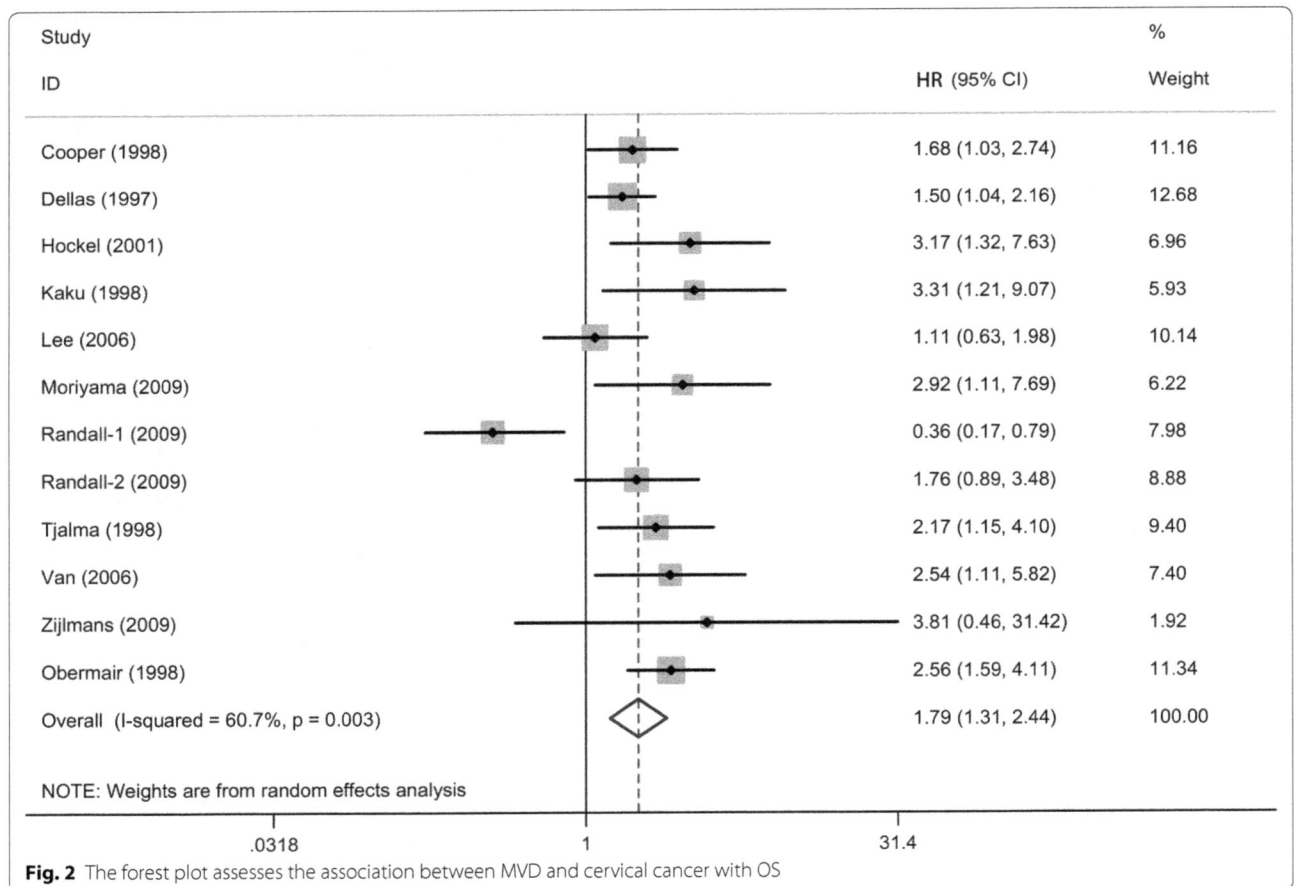

| Study ID | HR (95% CI) | % Weight |
|---|---|---|
| Cooper (1998) | 1.68 (1.03, 2.74) | 11.16 |
| Dellas (1997) | 1.50 (1.04, 2.16) | 12.68 |
| Hockel (2001) | 3.17 (1.32, 7.63) | 6.96 |
| Kaku (1998) | 3.31 (1.21, 9.07) | 5.93 |
| Lee (2006) | 1.11 (0.63, 1.98) | 10.14 |
| Moriyama (2009) | 2.92 (1.11, 7.69) | 6.22 |
| Randall-1 (2009) | 0.36 (0.17, 0.79) | 7.98 |
| Randall-2 (2009) | 1.76 (0.89, 3.48) | 8.88 |
| Tjalma (1998) | 2.17 (1.15, 4.10) | 9.40 |
| Van (2006) | 2.54 (1.11, 5.82) | 7.40 |
| Zijlmans (2009) | 3.81 (0.46, 31.42) | 1.92 |
| Obermair (1998) | 2.56 (1.59, 4.11) | 11.34 |
| Overall (I-squared = 60.7%, p = 0.003) | 1.79 (1.31, 2.44) | 100.00 |

NOTE: Weights are from random effects analysis

.0318    1    31.4

**Fig. 2** The forest plot assesses the association between MVD and cervical cancer with OS

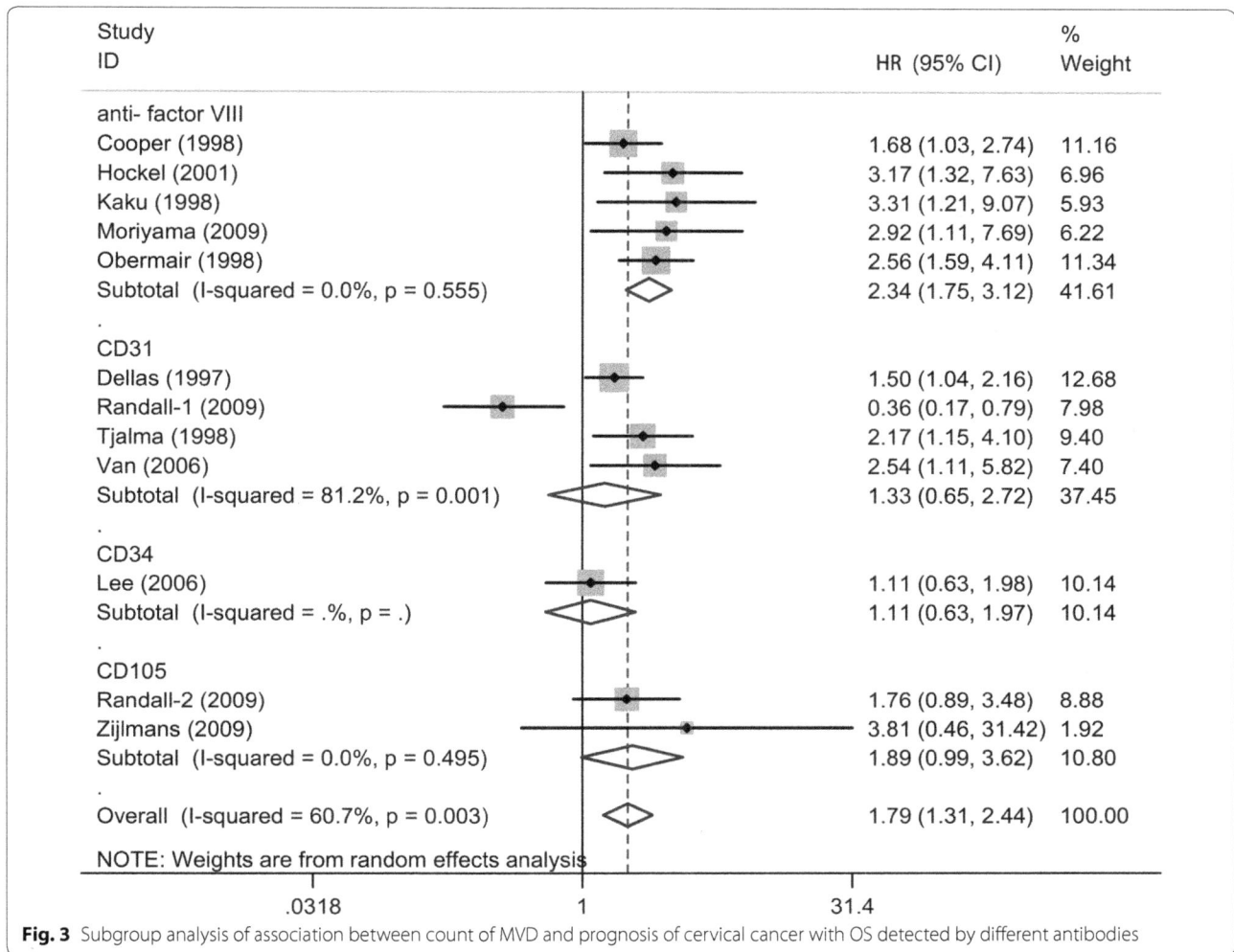

| Study ID | | HR (95% CI) | % Weight |
|---|---|---|---|
| anti- factor VIII | | | |
| Cooper (1998) | | 1.68 (1.03, 2.74) | 11.16 |
| Hockel (2001) | | 3.17 (1.32, 7.63) | 6.96 |
| Kaku (1998) | | 3.31 (1.21, 9.07) | 5.93 |
| Moriyama (2009) | | 2.92 (1.11, 7.69) | 6.22 |
| Obermair (1998) | | 2.56 (1.59, 4.11) | 11.34 |
| Subtotal (I-squared = 0.0%, p = 0.555) | | 2.34 (1.75, 3.12) | 41.61 |
| | | | |
| CD31 | | | |
| Dellas (1997) | | 1.50 (1.04, 2.16) | 12.68 |
| Randall-1 (2009) | | 0.36 (0.17, 0.79) | 7.98 |
| Tjalma (1998) | | 2.17 (1.15, 4.10) | 9.40 |
| Van (2006) | | 2.54 (1.11, 5.82) | 7.40 |
| Subtotal (I-squared = 81.2%, p = 0.001) | | 1.33 (0.65, 2.72) | 37.45 |
| | | | |
| CD34 | | | |
| Lee (2006) | | 1.11 (0.63, 1.98) | 10.14 |
| Subtotal (I-squared = .%, p = .) | | 1.11 (0.63, 1.97) | 10.14 |
| | | | |
| CD105 | | | |
| Randall-2 (2009) | | 1.76 (0.89, 3.48) | 8.88 |
| Zijlmans (2009) | | 3.81 (0.46, 31.42) | 1.92 |
| Subtotal (I-squared = 0.0%, p = 0.495) | | 1.89 (0.99, 3.62) | 10.80 |
| | | | |
| Overall (I-squared = 60.7%, p = 0.003) | | 1.79 (1.31, 2.44) | 100.00 |

NOTE: Weights are from random effects analysis

.0318                    1                    31.4

**Fig. 3** Subgroup analysis of association between count of MVD and prognosis of cervical cancer with OS detected by different antibodies

## Association of MVD and DFS of cervical cancer

We analyzed the relationship between the level of MVD and DFS among cervical cancer patients. There was no heterogeneity of data ($I^2 = 0\%$), in which a fixed-effect model was selected to assess the pooled outcome (Fig. 5). As a result, MVD level was associated with a worse DFS of cervical cancer patients (HR = 1.47, 95% CIs 1.13–1.80, n = 6).

Furthermore, subgroup analyses based on antibody and region were used to explore the influencing factors which may impacted the overall outcomes (Figs. 6 and 7). Divided by different immunohistochemical biomarkers among the subgroups, "anti-factor VIII" antibody (HR = 1.60, 95% CIs 1.16–2.03, $I^2 = 0$, n = 3) showed the significantly negative association between MVD and DFS among cervical cancer patients, but not in "CD34" subgroup (HR = 1.23, 95% CIs 0.71–1.75, $I^2 = 8.4\%$, n = 2).

In addition, the included studies were stratified into the three regional distribution of patients (Europe, Asia and America). Negative effected of MVD on DFS in European countries were found in patients with cervical cancer (HR = 1.63, 95% CIs 1.20–2.06, $I^2 = 0\%$, n = 4), but not in Asia location (HR = 1.47, 95% CIs 1.13–1.80, $I^2 = 0\%$, n = 2).

### Sensitivity analysis

In sensitivity analysis, the leave-one-out method was applied to assess the stability of the pooled outcomes. Eligible studies were sequentially removed one by one to evaluate the influence of each included study on the overall HR. After leaving out any single study, statistical significance of the OS or DFS did not change, suggesting no individual study had excessive influence of the association of MVD and cervical cancer (Fig. 8a, b).

### Publication bias

The presence of publication bias for the overall relationship between MVD level and the prognosis of cervical

| Study ID | | HR (95% CI) | % Weight |
|---|---|---|---|
| **Europe** | | | |
| Cooper (1998) | | 1.68 (1.03, 2.74) | 11.16 |
| Dellas (1997) | | 1.50 (1.04, 2.16) | 12.68 |
| Hockel (2001) | | 3.17 (1.32, 7.63) | 6.96 |
| Tjalma (1998) | | 2.17 (1.15, 4.10) | 9.40 |
| Zijlmans (2009) | | 3.81 (0.46, 31.42) | 1.92 |
| Obermair (1998) | | 2.56 (1.59, 4.11) | 11.34 |
| Subtotal (I-squared = 4.8%, p = 0.386) | | 1.93 (1.53, 2.44) | 53.46 |
| **Asia** | | | |
| Kaku (1998) | | 3.31 (1.21, 9.07) | 5.93 |
| Lee (2006) | | 1.11 (0.63, 1.98) | 10.14 |
| Moriyama (2009) | | 2.92 (1.11, 7.69) | 6.22 |
| Subtotal (I-squared = 60.1%, p = 0.082) | | 2.01 (0.94, 4.31) | 22.29 |
| **America** | | | |
| Randall-1 (2009) | | 0.36 (0.17, 0.79) | 7.98 |
| Randall-2 (2009) | | 1.76 (0.89, 3.48) | 8.88 |
| Van (2006) | | 2.54 (1.11, 5.82) | 7.40 |
| Subtotal (I-squared = 85.5%, p = 0.001) | | 1.17 (0.37, 3.69) | 24.25 |
| Overall (I-squared = 60.7%, p = 0.003) | | 1.79 (1.31, 2.44) | 100.00 |

NOTE: Weights are from random effects analysis

.0318                    1                    31.4

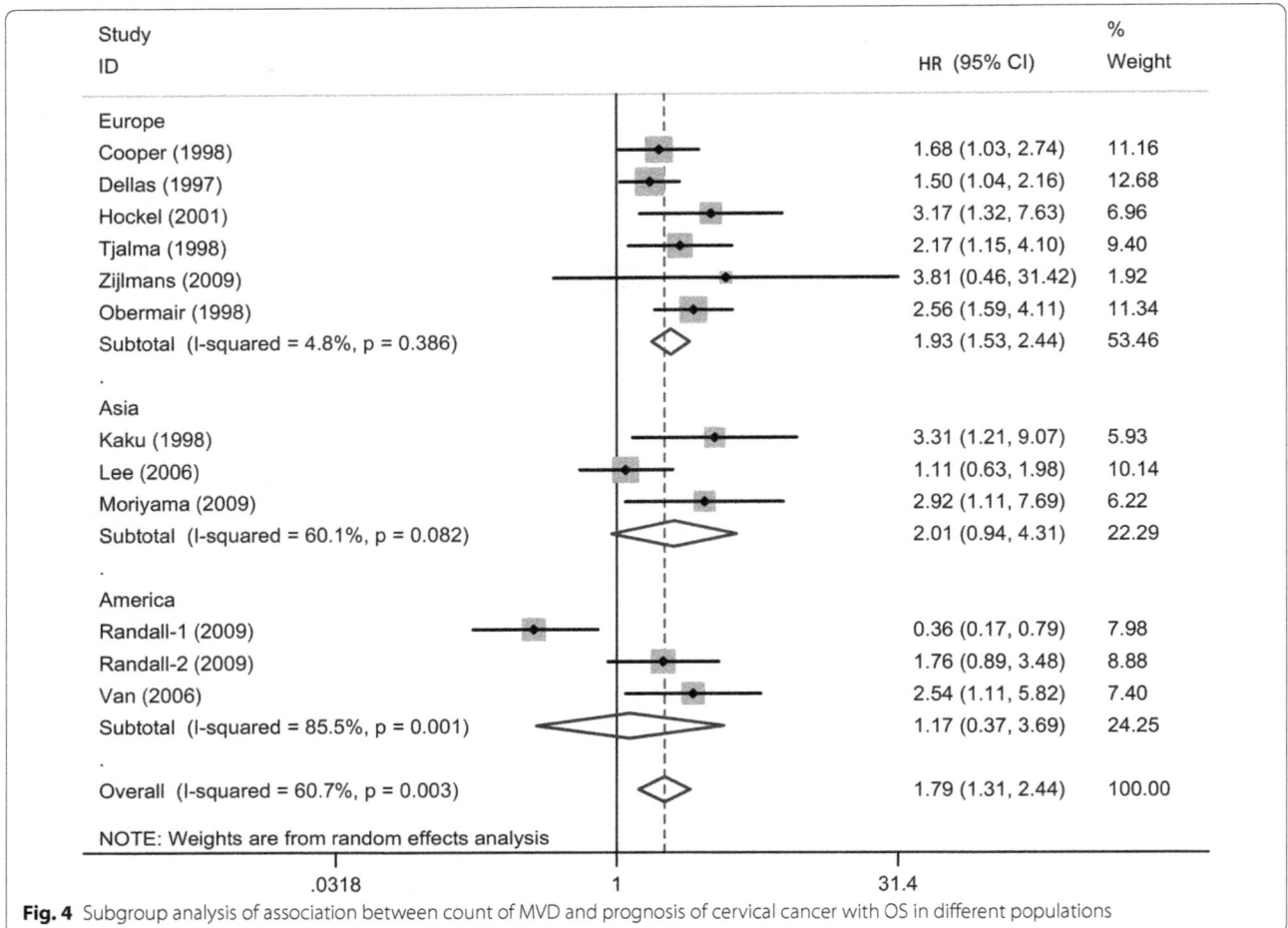

**Fig. 4** Subgroup analysis of association between count of MVD and prognosis of cervical cancer with OS in different populations

was calculated by using the Begg's rank correlation test ($P = 0.15$ for OS; $P = 0.238$ for DFS). Funnel plots were graphically symmetric, indicating that there was no significant publication bias among the included articles (Fig. 9a, b).

## Discussion

A number of studies have showed that MVD played the potential role as prognostic biomarker for many cancers. In our present meta-analysis, we confirmed that high counts of MVD, a marker of angiogenesis, was significantly associated with worse prognosis in patients with cervical cancer. Moreover, results were also conducted in subgroup analyses for patients detected by different antibodies or in various countries. Although some modest bias cannot be excluded, this was the first meta-analysis of published articles to assess the relationship between MVD count and prognosis in cervical cancer.

Between-study heterogeneity was significant in our meta-analysis for OS ($I^2 = 60.7\%$). However, there was no heterogeneity for DFS ($I^2 = 0\%$). We tried to reduce the variability by screening the researches using the same standard, which was to divide studies into different subgroups, such as the regional distributions and staining markers. However, the heterogeneity could not be eliminated in general. But the heterogeneity had decreased in some subgroups such as the Europe group ($I^2 = 4.8\%$ and 11.8%) and the group using anti-factor VIII as biomarkers on OS ($I^2 = 0\%$) for the MVD group. These results showed that all the different factors played important roles in the generation of heterogeneity which couldn't be eliminated at the same time.

Obviously, our study showed that the selection of antibody as a biomarker for MVD assessment played an important role for conclusion. There were eight studies in our meta-analysis using factor VIII as an endothelial biomarker, eight studies using other antibodies such as CD31, CD34 and CD105. We have established that the counts of MVD assessed by factor VIII were significantly related with the poor outcomes of cervical cancer, including OS and DFS. However, there was no statistical significance in the association between the levels of MVD

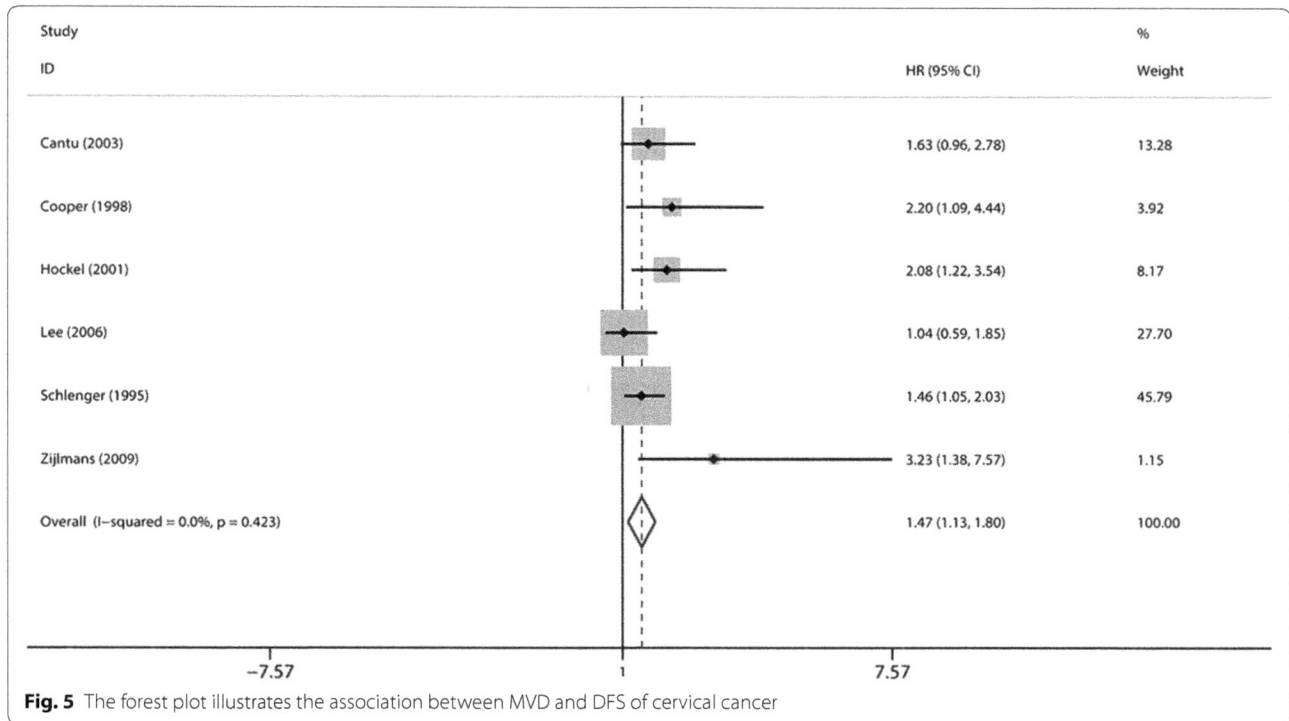

**Fig. 5** The forest plot illustrates the association between MVD and DFS of cervical cancer

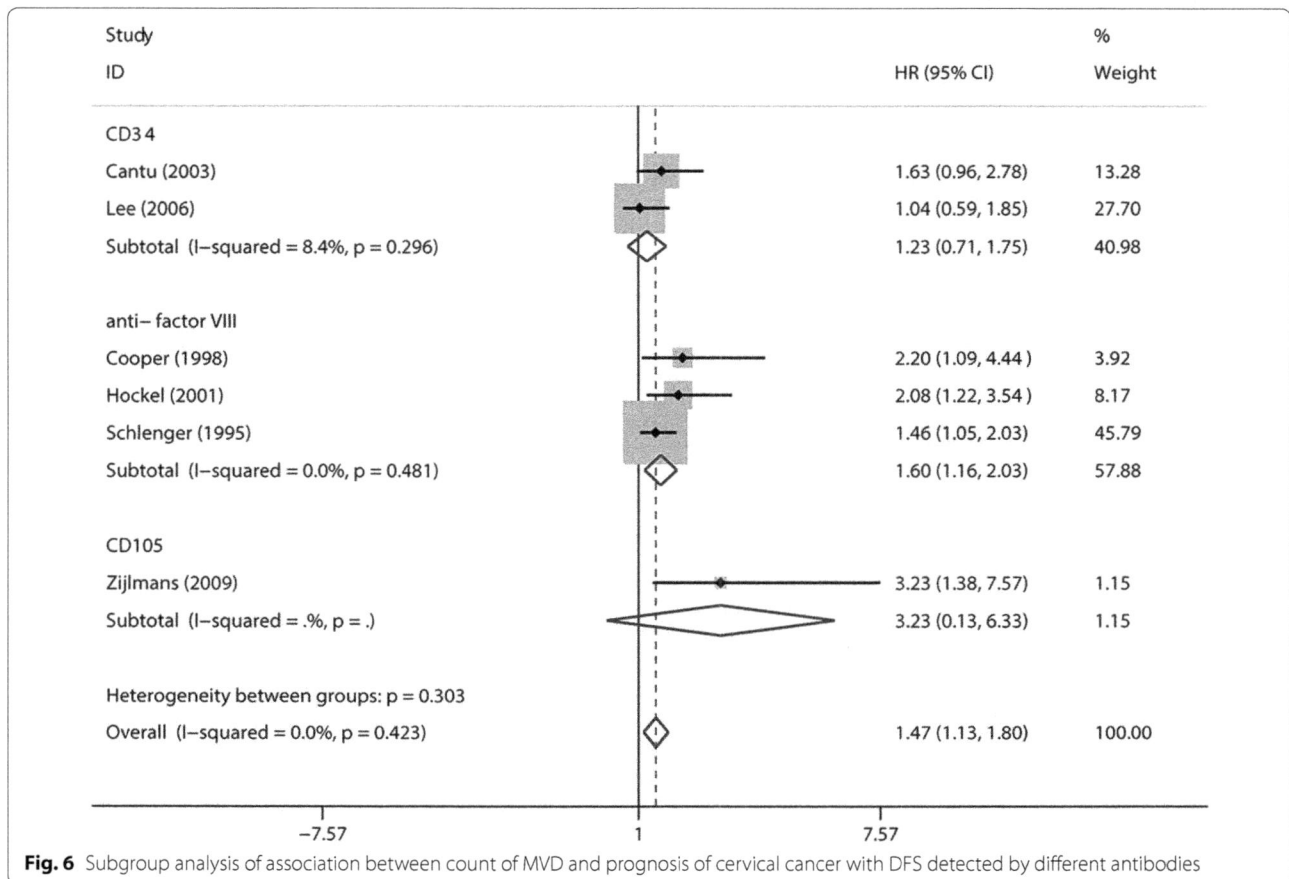

**Fig. 6** Subgroup analysis of association between count of MVD and prognosis of cervical cancer with DFS detected by different antibodies

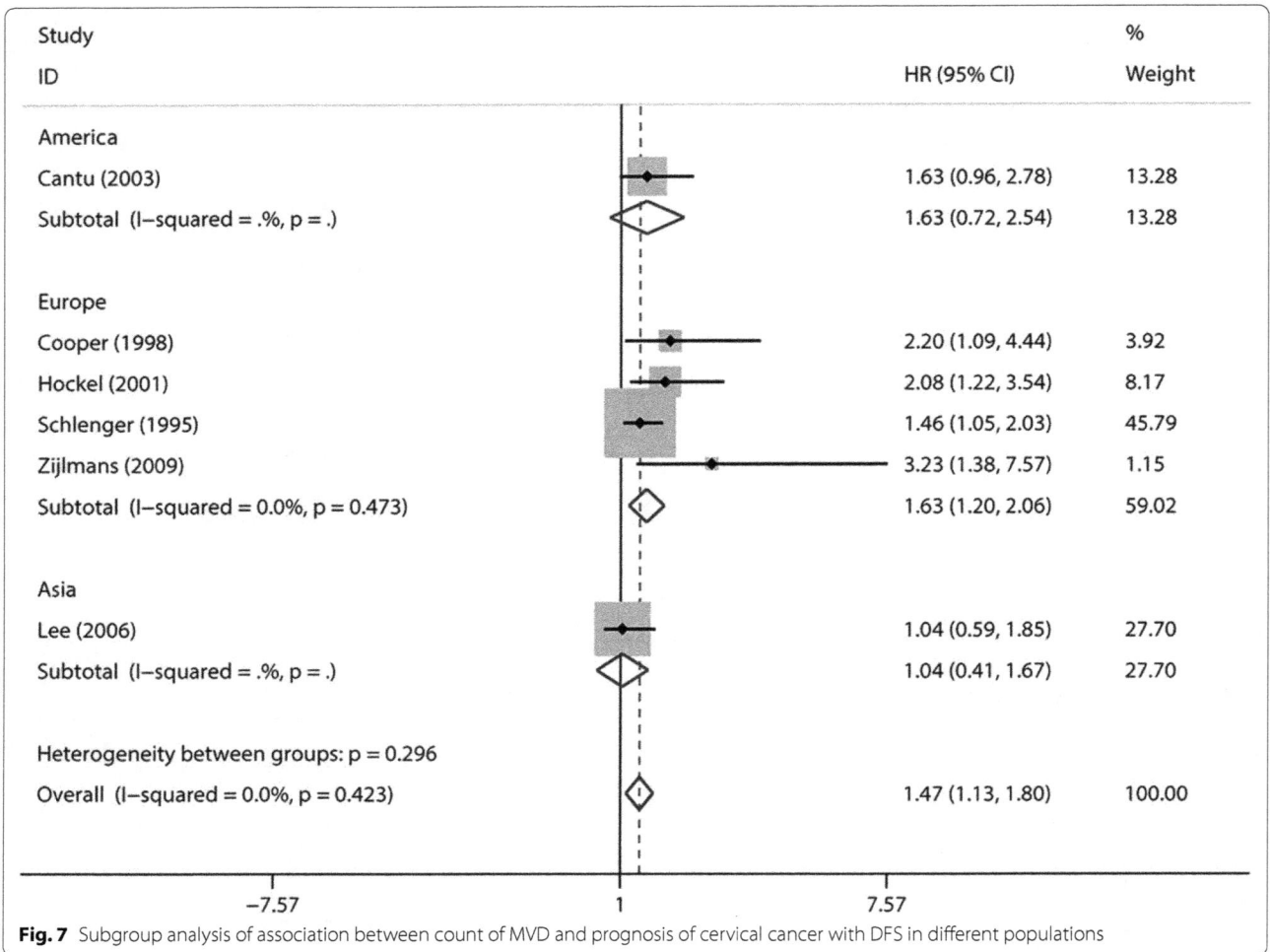

**Fig. 7** Subgroup analysis of association between count of MVD and prognosis of cervical cancer with DFS in different populations

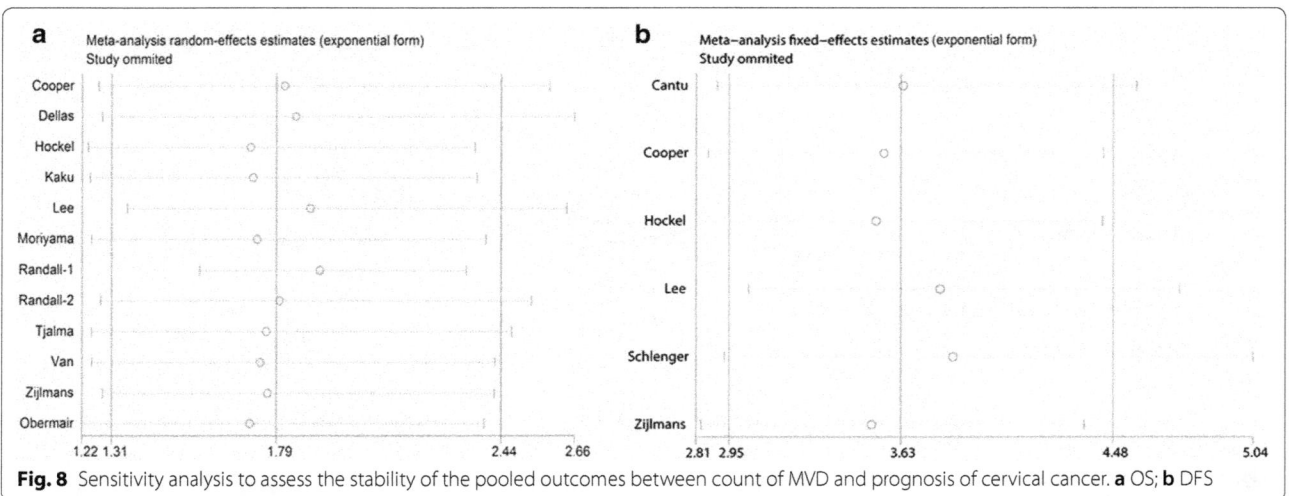

**Fig. 8** Sensitivity analysis to assess the stability of the pooled outcomes between count of MVD and prognosis of cervical cancer. **a** OS; **b** DFS

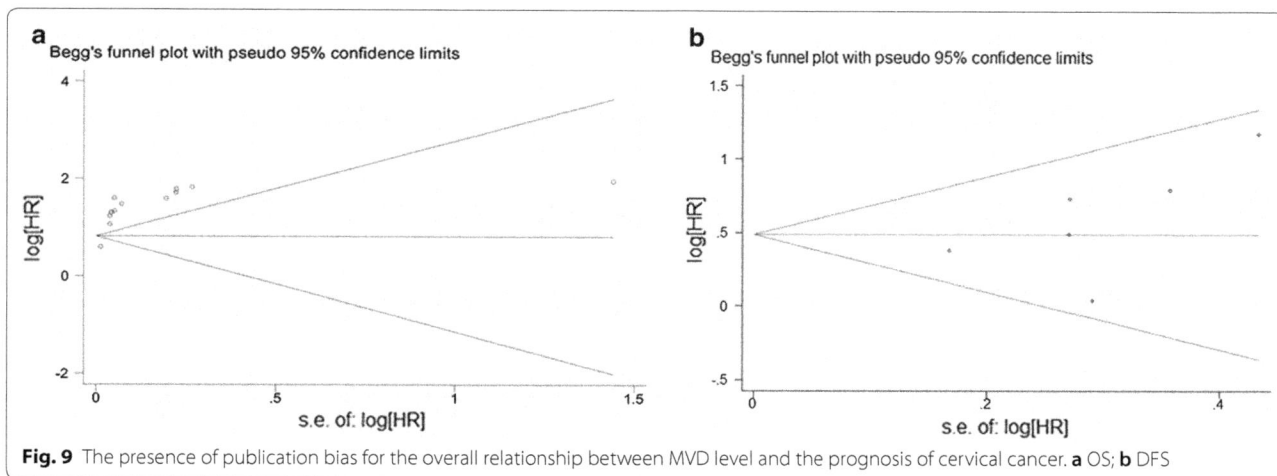

**Fig. 9** The presence of publication bias for the overall relationship between MVD level and the prognosis of cervical cancer. **a** OS; **b** DFS

assessed by anti-CD31, CD34 or CD105 with the prognosis of cervical cancer patients for OS or DFS. Weider et al. [7] chose an antibody against factor VIII-related antigen to mark mainly the endothelia of mature vessels. This biomarker was still the most commonly used in the related studies about microvessel density, however factor VIII did not express in all endothelial cells. And factor VIII also expressed in lymphatic endothelium and platelets, which would result in cross-reactivity with non-endothelium [29]. At present, for these antibodies expressed in lymphatic endothelium and platelets leading to appropriate marker for MVD in tumor has not been established. Recently, other antibodies were used to assess the counts of MVD in cervical cancer [30, 31], such as CD31 (also known as platelet endothelial cell adhesion molecule), CD34 and CD105 (also known as Endoglin). It indicated that CD34 had an improved sensitivity and specificity than factor VIII for endothelial cells activated by regional tumor angiogenesis [32]. Uzzan et al. [27] found that the microvessel counting evaluated by anti-CD31 or anti-CD34 were approximately 30% higher than factor VIII. Therefore, we considered that no statistical significance of relationship between counts of MVD assessed by other biomarkers including CD31, CD34 and CD105, and prognosis of cervical cancer patients was limited by a few number of related studies. Thus, more high-quality studies concerning the MVD detecting and MVD count should be acquired in future. Meanwhile, we found that there were more researches about the relation between MVD and prognosis of cervical cancer patients in Europe group than in Asia and America. When stratified by geographical area, our subgroup analysis indicated that patients with cervical cancer who had a higher level of MVD would had the poorer survival in Europe

countries, while the results could not be verified in Asia and America. It was probably because of the insufficient quantity in above-mentioned two regions.

In addition, several limitations of this meta-analysis should also be discussed. First of all, the choice of cutoff values for high MVD varied among the studies, some included articles mainly used median level, while others applied mean or even an inaccurate bound. These differences were responsible for the difficulty in determining a standard cut off value in clinical practice. Therefore, future researches should aim to standardize MVD assessment method. Secondly, for HRs couldn't be provided directly or calculated from the data in some studies, we need to extract the data from survival curve graphs. Furthermore, it is inevitable that the patient's baseline status in included studies were different, such as age, menopausal status, tumor type, tumor size, lymph node status, the immunohistochemical marker for MVD detecting and duration of follow-up. Finally, all the included studies in our meta-analysis were retrospective observational researches, more prone to bias than randomized controlled trails.

## Conclusions

To conclude, despite above-mentioned limitations, our meta-analysis strongly showed a poor survival of high counts of MVD in patients with cervical cancer, including OS and DFS, respectively. Moreover, these MVD-related biomarkers could be further used in the prognosis prediction of cervical cancer in clinical practice. However, future basic researches and randomized controlled studies with large samples are needed to conduct the prognostic value of MVD for patients with cervical cancer.

## Abbreviations

MVD: microvessel density; HR: hazard ratio; CIs: confidence intervals; OS: overall survival; DFS: disease-free survival; FIGO: International Federation of Gynecology and Obstetrics; VEGF: vascular endothelial growth factor; bFGF: basic fibroblast growth factor; NOS: the 9-star Newcastle–Ottawa Scale; IHC: immunohistochemistry; NA: not available.

## Authors' contributions

XLH and XQZ designed the study; XLH and HL searched and selected the articles, conducted the data extraction and did the statistical analysis; XLH and MMY wrote the manuscript. All authors read and approved the final manuscript.

## Acknowledgements

Not applicable.

## Competing interests

The authors declare that they have no competing interests.

## Funding

This work was supported by grants from Center for Uterine Cancer Diagnosis & Therapy Research of Zhejiang Province and Key Lab of Wenzhou City-Gynecological Oncology (No. ZD201603).

## References

1. Siegel RL, Miller KD, Jemal A. Cancer statistics, 2018. CA Cancer J Clin. 2018;68(1):7–30.

2. Kress CM, Sharling L, Owen-Smith AA, Desalegn D, Blumberg HM, Goedken J. Knowledge, attitudes, and practices regarding cervical cancer and screening among Ethiopian health care workers. Int J Womens Health. 2015;7:765–72.

3. Intaraphet S, Kasatpibal N, Siriaunkgul S, Sogaard M, Patumanond J, Khunamornpong S, Chandacham A, Suprasert P. Prognostic impact of histology in patients with cervical squamous cell carcinoma, adenocarcinoma and small cell neuroendocrine carcinoma. Asian Pac J Cancer Prev. 2013;14(9):5355–60.

4. Horn LC, Bilek K, Fischer U, Einenkel J, Hentschel B. A cut-off value of 2 cm in tumor size is of prognostic value in surgically treated FIGO stage IB cervical cancer. Gynecol Oncol. 2014;134(1):42–6.

5. Leek RD. The prognostic role of angiogenesis in breast cancer. Anticancer Res. 2001;21(6B):4325–31.

6. Jilaveanu LB, Puligandla M, Weiss SA, Wang XV, Zito C, Flaherty KT, Boeke M, Neumeister V, Camp RL, Adeniran A, et al. Tumor microvessel density as a prognostic marker in high-risk renal cell carcinoma patients treated on ECOG-ACRIN E2805. Clin Cancer Res. 2018;24(1):217–23.

7. Weidner N, Semple JP, Welch WR, Folkman J. Tumor angiogenesis and metastasis—correlation in invasive breast carcinoma. N Engl J Med. 1991;324(1):1–8.

8. Cao F, Hu YW, Li P, Liu Y, Wang K, Ma L, Li PF, Ni CR, Ding HZ. Lymphangiogenic and angiogenic microvessel density in chinese patients with gastric carcinoma: correlation with clinicopathologic parameters and prognosis. Asian Pac J Cancer Prev. 2013;14(8):4549–52.

9. Cantu De Leon D, Lopez-Graniel C, Frias Mendivil M, Chanona Vilchis G, Gomez C, De La Garza Salazar J. Significance of microvascular density (MVD) in cervical cancer recurrence. Int J Gynecol Cancer. 2003;13(6):856–62.

10. Cooper RA, Wilks DP, Logue JP, Davidson SE, Hunter RD, Roberts SA, West CM. High tumor angiogenesis is associated with poorer survival in carcinoma of the cervix treated with radiotherapy. Clin Cancer Res. 1998;4(11):2795–800.

11. Lee JS, Choi YD, Lee JH, Nam JH, Choi C, Lee MC, Park CS, Kim HS, Min KW. Expression of PTEN in the progression of cervical neoplasia and its relation to tumor behavior and angiogenesis in invasive squamous cell carcinoma. J Surg Oncol. 2006;93(3):233–40.

12. Petsuksiri J, Chuangsuwanich T, Pattaranutaporn P, Kanngurn S. Angiogenesis in stage IIIB squamous cell carcinoma of uterine cervix: reproducibility of measurement and preliminary outcome as a prognostic factor. J Med Assoc Thai. 2004;87(7):794–9.

13. Dai C, Wang M, Lu J, Dai Z, Lin S, Yang P, Tian T, Liu X, Min W, Dai Z. Prognostic and predictive values of PD-L1 expression in patients with digestive system cancer: a meta-analysis. OncoTargets Ther. 2017;10:3625–34.

14. Parmar MK, Torri V, Stewart L. Extracting summary statistics to perform meta-analyses of the published literature for survival endpoints. Stat Med. 1998;17(24):2815–34.

15. Higgins JP, Thompson SG, Deeks JJ, Altman DG. Measuring inconsistency in meta-analyses. BMJ. 2003;327(7414):557–60.

16. Sterne JA, Egger M, Smith GD. Systematic reviews in health care: investigating and dealing with publication and other biases in meta-analysis. BMJ. 2001;323(7304):101–5.

17. Dellas A, Moch H, Schultheiss E, Feichter G, Almendral A, Gudat F, Torhorst J. Association of tumor induced vascularization with clinicopathological parameters in cervical neoplasm. Int J Oncol. 1997;11(1):105–9.

18. Hockel S, Schlenger K, Vaupel P, Hockel M. Association between host tissue vascularity and the prognostically relevant tumor vascularity in human cervical cancer. Int J Oncol. 2001;19(4):827–32.

19. Kaku T, Hirakawa T, Kamura T, Amada S, Kinukawa N, Kobayashi H, Sakai K, Ariyoshi K, Sonoda K, Nakano H. Angiogenesis in adenocarcinoma of the uterine cervix. Cancer. 1998;83(7):1384–90.

20. Moriyama S, Kotera K, Khan KN, Sato F, So Y, Fujishita A, Matsuda K, Nakajima H, Ishimaru TEA. Prognostic significance of tumor volume and microvessel density in squamous cell carcinoma of uterine cervix. Acta Med Nagasakiensia. 2009;53(4):77–84.

21. Randall LM, Monk BJ, Darcy KM, Tian C, Burger RA, Liao SY, Peters WA, Stock RJ, Fruehauf JP. Markers of angiogenesis in high-risk, early-stage cervical cancer: a Gynecologic Oncology Group study. Gynecol Oncol. 2009;112(3):583–9.

22. Schlenger K, Hockel M, Mitze M, Schaffer U, Weikel W, Knapstein PG, Lambert A. Tumor vascularity—a novel prognostic factor in advanced cervical carcinoma. Gynecol Oncol. 1995;59(1):57–66.

23. Zijlmans HJ, Fleuren GJ, Hazelbag S, Sier CF, Dreef EJ, Kenter GG, Gorter A. Expression of endoglin (CD105) in cervical cancer. Br J Cancer. 2009;100(10):1617–26.

24. van der Veldt AA, Hooft L, van Diest PJ, Berkhof J, Buist MR, Comans EF, Hoekstra OS, Molthoff CF. Microvessel density and p53 in detecting cervical cancer by FDG PET in cases of suspected recurrence. Eur J Nucl Med Mol Imaging. 2006;33(12):1408–16.

25. Tjalma W, Van Marck E, Weyler J, Dirix L, Van Daele A, Goovaerts G, Albertyn G, van Dam P. Quantification and prognostic relevance of angiogenic parameters in invasive cervical cancer. Br J Cancer. 1998;78(2):170–4.

26. Obermair A, Wanner C, Bilgi S, Speiser P, Kaider A, Reinthaller A, Leodolter S, Gitsch G. Tumor angiogenesis in stage IB cervical cancer: correlation of microvessel density with survival. Am J Obstet Gynecol. 1998;178(2):314–9.

27. Uzzan B, Nicolas P, Cucherat M, Perret GY. Microvessel density as a prognostic factor in women with breast cancer: a systematic review of the literature and meta-analysis. Cancer Res. 2004;64(9):2941–55.

28. Yu M, Liu L, Liang C, Li P, Ma X, Zhang Q, Wei Y. Intratumoral vessel density as prognostic factors in head and neck squamous cell carcinoma: a meta-analysis of literature. Head Neck. 2014;36(4):596–602.

29. Nowak A, Grzegrzolka J, Paprocka M, Piotrowska A, Rys J, Matkowski R, Dziegiel P. Nestin-positive microvessel density is an independent prognostic factor in breast cancer. Int J Oncol. 2017;51(2):668–76.
30. Barbu I, Craitoiu S, Simionescu CE, Dragnei AM, Margaritescu C. CD105 microvessels density, VEGF, EGFR-1 and c-erbB-2 and their prognostic correlation in different subtypes of cervical adenocarcinoma. Rom J Morphol Embryol. 2013;54(3):519–30.
31. Vieira SC, Silva BB, Pinto GA, Vassallo J, Moraes NG, Santana JO, Santos LG, Carvasan GA, Zeferino LC. CD34 as a marker for evaluating angiogenesis in cervical cancer. Pathol Res Pract. 2005;201(4):313–8.
32. Tanigawa N, Amaya H, Matsumura M, Shimomatsuya T, Horiuchi T, Muraoka R, Iki M. Extent of tumor vascularization correlates with prognosis and hematogenous metastasis in gastric carcinomas. Cancer Res. 1996;56(11):2671–6.

# IL-2 augments the sorafenib-induced apoptosis in liver cancer by promoting mitochondrial fission and activating the JNK/TAZ pathway

Xiaoyan Ding, Wei Sun and Jinglong Chen[*]

## Abstract

**Background:** Sorafenib is the standard targeted drug used to treat hepatocellular carcinoma (HCC), but the therapeutic response between individuals varies markedly. Recently, cytokine-based immunotherapy has been a topic of intense discussion in the fight against cancer. The aim of this study was to explore whether cytokine IL-2 could augment the anti-tumour effects of sorafenib on HCC.

**Methods:** HepG2 and Huh7 cells were co-treated with sorafenib and IL-2 in vitro, and cellular viability and death were analysed through the MTT assay, TUNEL staining, LDH release assay, and western blotting. Mitochondrial function was measured via ELISA, immunofluorescence, and western blotting. Pathway blockers were used to establish the role of the JNK-TAZ pathways in regulating cancer cell phenotypes.

**Results:** Our data demonstrated that sorafenib treatment increased the HCC apoptotic rate, repressed cell proliferation, and inhibited migratory responses, and these effects were enhanced by IL-2 supplementation. Mechanistically, the combination of IL-2 and sorafenib interrupted mitochondrial energy metabolism by downregulating mitochondrial respiratory proteins. In addition, IL-2 and sorafenib co-treatment promoted mitochondrial dysfunction, as evidenced by the decreased mitochondrial potential, elevated mitochondrial ROS production, increased leakage of mitochondrial pro-apoptotic factors, and activation of the mitochondrial death pathway. A molecular investigation revealed that mitochondrial fission was required for the IL-2/sorafenib-mediated mitochondrial dysfunction. Mitochondrial fission was triggered by sorafenib and was largely amplified by IL-2 supplementation. Finally, we found that IL-2/sorafenib regulated mitochondrial fission via the JNK-TAZ pathways; blockade of the JNK-TAZ pathways abrogated the inhibitory effects of L-2/sorafenib on cancer survival, growth and mobility.

**Conclusions:** Altogether, these data strongly suggest that additional supplementation with IL-2 enhances the anti-tumour activity of sorafenib by promoting the JNK-TAZ-mitochondrial fission axis. This finding will pave the way for new treatment modalities to control HCC progression by optimizing sorafenib-based therapy.

**Keywords:** IL-2, Sorafenib, Mitochondrial fission, Liver cancer, JNK-TAZ pathways

*Correspondence: chejl6412@163.com
Cancer Center, Beijing Ditan Hospital, Capital Medical University, No 8,
Jingshundong Street Chaoyang District, Beijing 100015, China

## Background

Hepatocellular carcinoma (HCC), the sixth most common cancer worldwide, accounts for ~5.7% of the overall incidence of cancer [1]. Several risk factors have been associated with the development of HCC, including (but not limited to) hepatitis B infection, alcohol consumption, diabetes mellitus and smoking [2]. Despite advancements in uncovering the molecular aetiology of HCC, treatments for HCC are still unsatisfactory; the 5-year survival rate remains approximately 26% in patients receiving standard chemotherapy and/or radiotherapy [3].

Targeted therapy has been tested in several clinical trials and has been proven to provide a survival advantage for patients with HCC. Sorafenib is the first approved targeted therapy drug and is also the first-line FDA-approved tyrosine kinase inhibitor, improving the median overall survival time from 7.9 to 10.7 months in patients with HCC [4]. At the molecular level, sorafenib represses Raf kinase, a key protein mediating cancer proliferation [5]. Sorafenib also suppresses angiogenesis by modulating the Ras/Raf/MEK/ERK signalling pathway and VEGFR [6]. Notably, the tolerance and efficacy of sorafenib in Child–Pugh B patients have not been determined, and several reports argue that sorafenib does not seem to be an option for these patients [7]. Furthermore, the clinical benefit of sorafenib treatment is limited to an overall increase in survival time of 3 months [8]. Thus, these data indicate the therapeutic potential of sorafenib against the progression of HCC but suggest that it is also clinically necessary to optimize sorafenib-based treatment by combining it with other therapeutic strategies, such as immunotherapy.

Immunotherapy has demonstrated great promise in specifically killing cancer cells by multiple mechanisms [9]. Cytokine-based immunotherapy is currently a topic of intense discussion in the fight against cancer [10]. For example, supplementation with IL-7 has been found to repress the progression of acute lymphoblastic leukaemia [11], and in pancreatic cancer, the inhibition of IL-6 suppresses the metastatic invasion and migration of tumours [12]. Moreover, the regulation of CXCL13 modifies breast cancer cell viability via the CXCR5/ERK pathway [13]. In animal studies and cell experiments on liver cancer, the cytokine IL-2 has been documented to be a potential therapeutic target to limit tumour growth [14, 15]. In a clinical trial with small sample sizes, administration of IL-2 was found to play a beneficial role in suppressing the development and progression of HCC [16]. This finding was also supported by a previous study in which an IL-2 vaccine mediated the regression of HCC in mice [15]. As there is strong evidence supporting the suppressive effects of IL-2-based therapy against HCC

progression, it is worthwhile to explore whether IL-2, in combination with sorafenib, can further reduce the proliferation of liver cancer cells.

Mitochondrial fission, which initiates the mitochondrial apoptosis pathway, is an early hallmark of cancer cell death [17, 18]. Excessive mitochondrial fission disrupts mitochondrial energy metabolism, evokes oxidative stress, causes cellular calcium overload, and promotes the activation of pro-apoptotic factors [19, 20]. Several attempts have been made to induce the activation of mitochondrial fission in various tumours such as those in pancreatic cancer [21], endometriosis [22], and breast cancer [23]. Based on the data gained from these studies, we wanted to determine whether IL-2 could augment sorafenib-mediated HCC apoptosis by activating mitochondrial fission. The JNK and TAZ pathways are the primary upstream regulators for mitochondrial fission in liver cancer and in breast cancer [24, 25]; however, whether IL-2 is capable of modifying mitochondrial fission via the JNK-TAZ axis has remained unknown. Thus, the aim of our study was to explore the efficacy of IL-2 in combination with sorafenib on inducing HCC apoptosis, with a focus on mitochondrial fission and the JNK-TAZ pathways.

## Materials and methods

### Cell culture and treatment

The HepG2 liver cancer cell line was purchased from the American Type Culture Collection (ATCC® HB-8065™). The Huh7 liver cancer cell line and L02 normal liver cell line were purchased from the Cell Bank of the Chinese Academy of Sciences. The HepG2 and Huh7 cells were cultured in DMEM medium (#12800-017, Gibco) with 10% FBS (#10437-028, Gibco) at 37 °C/5% $CO_2$. To induce damage, the cancer cells were treated with sorafenib (5 µM) for approximately 12 h. Another group of cells was treated with IL-2 (0–20 ng/ml) for 12 h according to a previous study [16]. To inhibit the activity of the JNK pathway, cells were treated with SP600125 (SP, 10 µM, Selleck Chemicals) 2 h before sorafenib/IL-2 treatment [26].

### Cellular viability and death evaluation

Cellular viability was measured with MTT and LDH release assays. The MTT assay was performed according to the methods used in a previous study [27]. Cells were plated onto a 96-well plate with the IL-2 and sorafenib treatment. MTT solution (Beyotime, China, Cat. No. C0009) was then added into the medium, and the cells were incubated for approximately 2 h at 37 °C/5% $CO_2$. The optical density (OD) of the MTT solution was recorded using a microplate reader (490 nm absorbance; Epoch 2; BioTek Instruments, Inc., Winooski, VT, USA).

An LDH release assay was conducted using a commercial kit (Beyotime, China, Cat. No. C0016) according to the manufacturer's instructions [28].

Cellular death was measured via a TUNEL assay and the measurement of caspase-3 activity. TUNEL staining was performed using a One Step TUNEL Apoptosis Assay Kit (Beyotime, China, Cat. No. C1086) according to the manufacturer's instructions. Caspase-3 activity was estimated using the Caspase 3 Activity Assay Kit (Beyotime, China, Cat. No. C1115), and the relative caspase-3 activity was measured compared to that of the control group using a microplate reader (430 nm absorbance; Epoch 2; BioTek Instruments, Inc., Winooski, VT, USA) [29].

## Oxidative stress measurement

Cellular oxidative stress was determined via ELISA as described in a previous study. Cells were washed with PBS and lysed using RIPA Lysis Buffer (Beyotime, China, Cat. No. P0013C). Then, the proteins were collected through high-speed centrifugation, and the concentrations of GSH (Beyotime, China, Cat. No. S0073), SOD (Beyotime, China, Cat. No. S0086) and GPX (Beyotime, China, Cat. No. S0058) were measured using commercial kits according to the manufacturers' instructions [30].

## EdU staining and transwell assay

To analyse the cellular proliferation, EdU staining was conducted using the BeyoClick™ EdU Cell Proliferation Kit with Alexa Fluor 594 (Beyotime, China, Cat. No. C00788L). Cells were first washed with PBS. Fresh DMEM was then added, and 10 μM EdU was added into the medium. The cells were incubated for 2 h at 37 °C/5% $CO_2$. After the incubation, the cells were again washed with PBS to remove the DMEM and the free EdU probe. The cells were then fixed in 4% paraformaldehyde at room temperature for 30 min before being stained with DAPI for 3 min. After an additional wash in PBS, the cells were observed under an inverted microscope [31].

A transwell assay was carried out to observe the cell migration response based on the methods of a previous study [32]. Cells at a density of $1 \times 10^3$ were added into the upper chamber. DMEM with 2% FBS was loaded into the lower chamber. Subsequently, the cells were cultured at 37 °C/5% $CO_2$ for 12 h. After the culture period, the non-migrated cells were removed, and the migrated cells were fixed with 3.7% paraformaldehyde for 30 min at room temperature. The migrated cells were then stained with 0.05% crystal violet for 15 min at room temperature in the dark. The number of migrated cells was recorded, and images were captured under an inverted microscope.

## Mitochondrial function detection

Mitochondrial function was measured by analysing the mitochondrial membrane potential, the mitochondrial permeability transition pore (mPTP) opening rate and the mitochondrial ROS generation. The mitochondrial membrane potential was determined by JC-1 staining [33]. Live cells were washed with PBS, and a JC-1 solution was then added to the medium. The cells were incubated at 37 °C/5% $CO_2$ for 30 min, washed with PBS, loaded with DAPI, and then observed under a fluorescence microscope. The mPTP opening rate was recorded as described by a previous study. Cells were first washed with PBS and incubated with calcein-AM/cobalt at 37 °C/5% $CO_2$ for 30 min. The cells were then washed with PBS again to remove the free probe. The optical density (OD) was recorded using a microplate reader (540 nm absorbance; Epoch 2; BioTek Instruments, Inc., Winooski, VT, USA). The mPTP opening rate was expressed relative to that of the control group [34]. Mitochondrial ROS production was measured via flow cytometry as described by a previous study. Cells were washed three times in PBS and incubated with MitoSOX Red Mitochondrial Superoxide Indicator (Molecular Probes, USA) for 30 min at 37 °C/5% $CO_2$ in the dark. After incubation, the cells were washed three times in PBS at room temperature, and the mitochondrial ROS production was measured via flow cytometry [35].

## Western blotting

Cells were lysed in RIPA Lysis Buffer (Beyotime, China, Cat. No. P0013C). After high-speed centrifugation, the proteins were collected and quantified with the Enhanced BCA Protein Assay Kit (Beyotime, China, Cat. No. P0009). Subsequently, 40–60 μg of protein was loaded onto 10% SDS-PAGE gels and transferred to PVDF membranes. The membranes were washed with TBST and then blocked with 5% non-fat milk for 45 min at room temperature [36]. The membranes were then incubated at 4 °C overnight with the primary antibodies [CXCR4 (1:1000, Abcam, #ab1670), CXCR7 (1:1000, Abcam, #ab38089), cyclin D1 (1:1000, Abcam, #ab134175), PCNA (1:1000, Abcam, #ab18197), CDK4 (1:1000, Abcam, #ab137675), cadherin (1:1000, Abcam, #ab133168), vimentin (1:1000, Abcam, #ab8978), TAZ (1:1000, Abcam, #ab224239), complex III subunit core (CIII-core2, 1:1000, Invitrogen, #459220), complex II (CII-30, 1:1000, Abcam, #ab110410), complex IV subunit II (CIV-II, 1:1000, Abcam, #ab110268), Drp1 (1:1000, Abcam, #ab56788), Fis1 (1:1000, Abcam, #ab71498), Opa1 (1:1000, Abcam, #ab42364), Mfn1 (1:1000, Abcam, #ab57602), Mff (1:1000, Cell Signaling Technology, #86668), Bcl2 (1:1000, Cell Signaling Technology, #3498), Bax (1:1000, Cell Signaling Technology, #2772), caspase-9 (1:1000, Cell Signaling

Technology, #9504), Bad (1:1000; Abcam; #ab90435), Tom20 (1:1000, Abcam, #ab186735), cyt-c (1:1000; Abcam; #ab90529), GAPDH (1:1000, Cell Signaling Technology, #5174), JNK (1:1000; Cell Signaling Technology, #4672), and p-JNK (1:1000; Cell Signaling Technology, #9251)]. After being washed with TBST, the membranes were incubated with the secondary antibodies for 45 min at room temperature. The bands were observed with an enhanced chemiluminescence (ECL) substrate kit (Beyotime, China, Cat. No. P0018F). The mean densities of the bands were represented as the optical density in units/mm$^2$ and normalized to that of loading control (Quantity One, version 4.6.2; Bio-Rad Laboratories, Inc.)

## Immunofluorescence

Cells were washed with PBS at room temperature to remove the DMEM. Then, the cells were fixed in 3.7% paraformaldehyde for 30 min at room temperature and permeabilized with 0.1% Triton X-100 for 10 min at 4 °C. The cells were then washed with PBS, and 10% goat serum albumin was used to block the samples for 45 min at room temperature. The samples were again washed with PBS, and the primary antibodies [p-JNK (1:500; Cell Signaling Technology, #9251), cyt-c (1:500; Abcam; #ab90529), Drp1 (1:500, Abcam, #ab56788), CDK4 (1:500, Abcam, #ab137675), cyclin D1 (1:500, Abcam, #ab134175), and Tom20 (1:500, Abcam, #ab186735)] were added. The samples were incubated overnight at 4 °C. After being washed with PBS three times to remove the primary antibodies, the cells were incubated with the secondary antibodies for 45 min at room temperature [37]. After the cells were again washed with PBS to remove the free second antibodies and were loaded with DAPI, they were observed under an inverted microscope. Mitochondrial fission was observed via immunofluorescence using the Tom20 antibody. Images were captured, and the average length of the mitochondria was used to quantify the mitochondrial fission [38].

## Statistical analysis

All statistical analyses in the present study were performed in SPSS software (version 19.0). Our data are expressed as the mean ± SEM. Results for more than two groups were evaluated by one-way analysis of variance followed by Bonferroni's multiple comparison test. A P value < 0.05 was considered significant.

## Results

### IL-2 promotes sorafenib-mediated apoptosis in HepG2 and Huh7 cells

First, sorafenib was added into the medium of liver cancer cell lines (HepG2 cells and Huh7 cells) to repress the cancer cell viability. Compared to the control group, the sorafenib treatment group displayed markedly reduced cell viability, as assessed via MTT assay (Fig. 1a, b), suggesting that sorafenib is cytotoxic to liver cancer cell lines. Similarly, the cell death rate, as evaluated by the LDH release assay, also increased in response to sorafenib treatment in both the HepG2 and the Huh7 cells (Fig. 1c, d). To explore whether the tumour-suppressive effect of sorafenib could be enhanced by combining sorafenib with IL-2-based therapy, different doses of IL-2 were added to the medium. As shown in Fig. 1a, b, the cell viability of both HepG2 cells and Huh7 cells progressively decreased with increasing IL-2 concentrations. IL-2 treatment also dose-dependently elevated the cell death index, as determined by the LDH release assay (Fig. 1c, d). Altogether, these results indicated that IL-2 supplementation augmented the anti-tumour effect of sorafenib in HepG2 and Huh7 cells. The minimum toxic concentration of IL-2 was 5 ng/ml; therefore, that dose was used in subsequent functional studies. To exclude the influence of IL-2/sorafenib co-treatment on normal hepatocytes, L02 normal liver cells were treated with IL-2 and sorafenib. As shown in Additional file 1: Figure S1, we found that neither IL-2 nor sorafenib treatment affected the viability of L02 cells, as assessed via MTT assay and LDH release assay. Subsequently, TUNEL staining was used to detect cell apoptosis after IL-2 and sorafenib co-treatment in HepG2 cells. As shown in Fig. 1e−g, the number of TUNEL-positive cells increased with sorafenib treatment and was further elevated in response to IL-2 administration in both HepG2 cells and Huh7 cells. Similarly, caspase-3 activity increased in response to sorafenib treatment, and this effect was enhanced by IL-2 treatment (Fig. 1h, i). In all, our data indicated that IL-2 supplementation augmented sorafenib-mediated cell apoptosis in both HepG2 cells and Huh7 cells.

### IL-2 further repressed cell migration and proliferation in the presence of sorafenib

Cancer proliferation was observed via EdU assay. The results shown in Fig. 2a−c revealed that sorafenib attenuated the percentage of EdU$^+$ cells regardless of whether they were HepG2 cells or Huh7 cells. Interestingly, the anti-proliferative capacity of sorafenib was strengthened by IL-2 treatment (Fig. 2a−c), suggesting that IL-2 in combination with sorafenib further disrupted cancer growth. Similar results were observed for the expression of proteins related to the cell cycle. Cyclin D1, PCNA and CDK4 were abundant in the control group and were reduced in response to sorafenib treatment (Fig. 2d−j). IL-2 administration caused a further decline in the expression of cyclin D1, PCNA and CDK4 in both HepG2 cells and Huh7 cells (Fig. 2d−j). Taken together, our data support a synergistic role for sorafenib and IL-2 in repressing the multiplication of cancer cells.

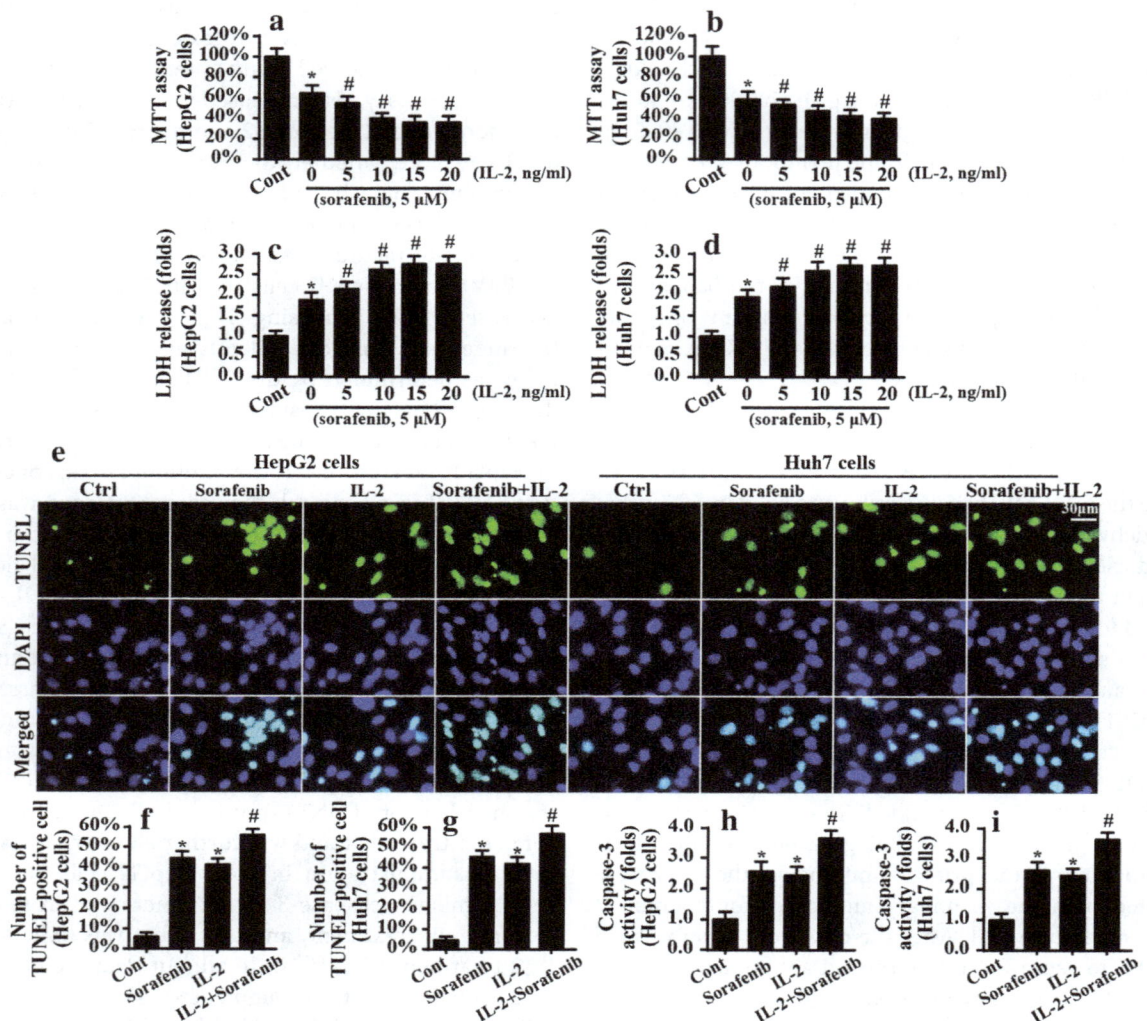

**Fig. 1** IL-2 treatment enhanced the pro-apoptotic effects of sorafenib. **a, b** Cell viability was measured via MTT assay in HepG2 cells and Huh7 cells. The different doses of IL-2 were added in the presence of 5 μM sorafenib. **c, d** Cell death was evaluated via LDH release assay in HepG2 cells and Huh7 cells. The different doses of IL-2 were added in the presence of 5 μM sorafenib. **e–g** A TUNEL assay was performed to observe the cell apoptotic rate. IL-2 (5 ng/ml) treatment was carried out in the presence of 5 μM sorafenib. **h, i** Caspase-3 activity was measured in HepG2 cells and Huh7 cells. IL-2 (5 ng/ml) treatment was carried out in the presence of 5 μM sorafenib. *$P < 0.05$ vs. control group; #$P < 0.05$ vs. sorafenib group. *Cont* control

To examine cell migration, a transwell assay was performed. The number of migrated cells was reduced by sorafenib treatment and was further depressed with IL-2 treatment (Fig. 2k–m). In addition, proteins related to cancer migration, such as cadherin and vimentin, were negatively regulated by sorafenib, and this effect was enhanced by IL-2 treatment in both HepG2 and Huh7 cells (Fig. 2n–r). In summary, the sorafenib-induced impairment of migration was strengthened by IL-2. Because no phenotypic differences were noted between

(See figure on next page.)
**Fig. 2** IL-2 further repressed cell migration and proliferation in the presence of sorafenib. **a–c** An EdU assay was used to observe the proliferative cells. The number of EdU-positive cells was recorded. **d–j** Western blotting analysis for the proteins related to cell proliferation. IL-2 (5 ng/ml) treatment was carried out in the presence of 5 μM sorafenib. **k–m** A transwell assay was conducted to determine the cell migration in response to IL-2 and sorafenib co-treatment. **n–r** The proteins related to cell migration were analysed via western blotting. IL-2 (5 ng/ml) treatment was carried out in the presence of 5 μM sorafenib. *$P < 0.05$ vs. control group; #$P < 0.05$ vs. sorafenib group. *Cont* control

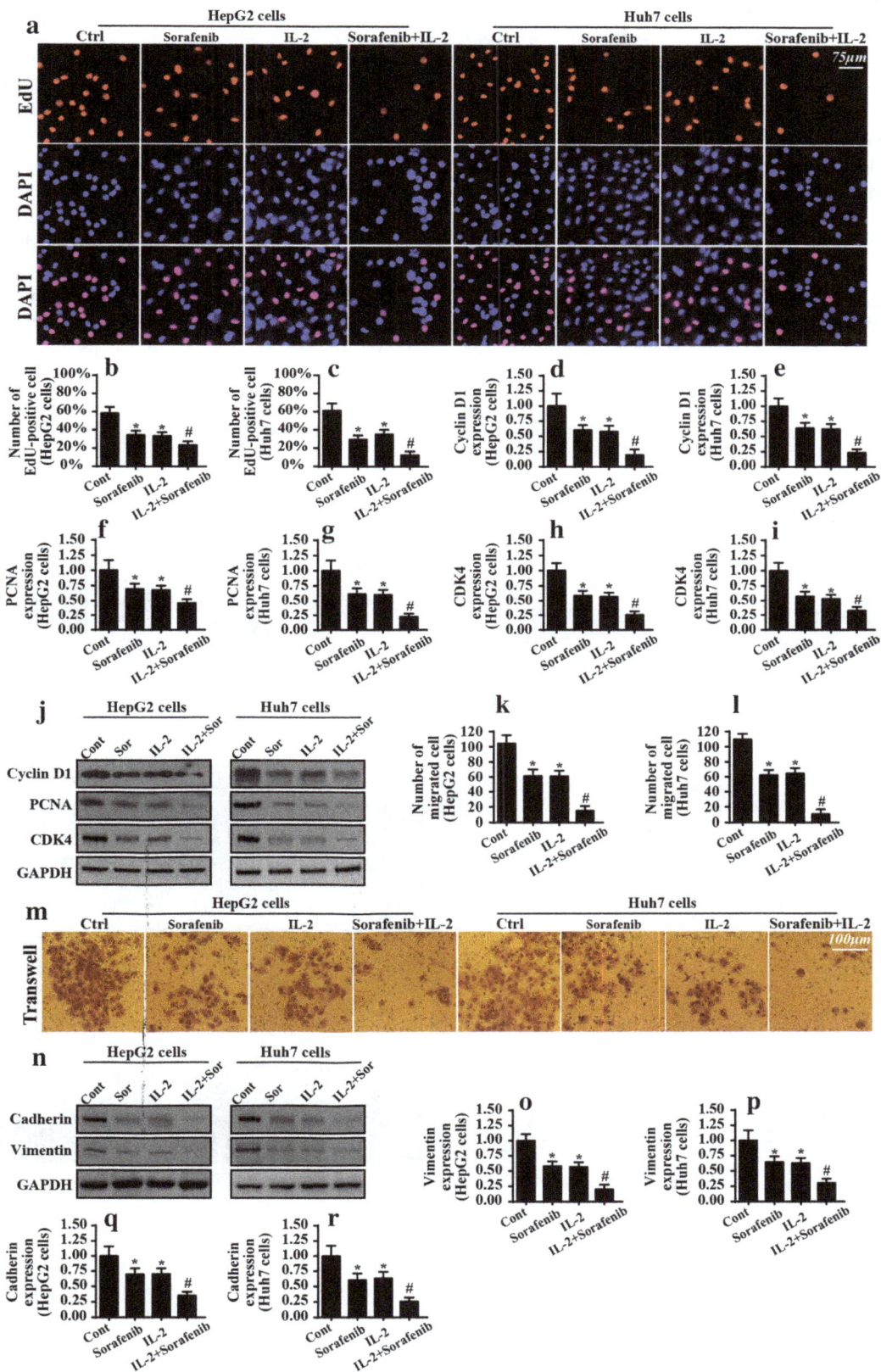

HepG2 and Huh7 cells with regards to apoptosis, proliferation or migration, the HepG2 cell line was used for subsequent molecular experiments.

## IL-2 in combination with sorafenib interrupts mitochondrial metabolism

Cellular proliferation, migration and survival are heavily dependent on the production of sufficient energy by the mitochondria; thus, mitochondrial metabolism was monitored. Cellular ATP production was repressed by sorafenib in HepG2 cells, and this effect was reinforced by IL-2 supplementation (Fig. 3a). Mitochondrial energy production primarily relies on the activity of mitochondrial respiratory enzymes [20, 39], which convert the mitochondrial membrane potential into the chemical ATP. Interestingly, the expression levels of the mitochondrial respiratory proteins were downregulated by

sorafenib (Fig. 3b–e); this tendency was exacerbated by IL-2 treatment. In addition, the mitochondrial potential, as assessed by JC-1 staining, was also negatively regulated by sorafenib (Fig. 3f–g). IL-2 treatment further repressed the mitochondrial potential, as evidenced by a lower ratio of red/green fluorescence intensity.

Finally, we measured the amount of glucose remaining in the medium to directly evaluate the cellular mitochondrial metabolism. Compared to the control group, the sorafenib treatment group showed reduced glucose uptake from the medium (Fig. 3h). Lactate production was also reduced in response to sorafenib treatment (Fig. 3j). IL-2 supplementation further repressed glucose absorption and lactate generation (Fig. 3h–j), indicating the cessation of glucose absorption, consumption and metabolism, possibly due to mitochondrial dysfunction. Altogether, our data highlight a

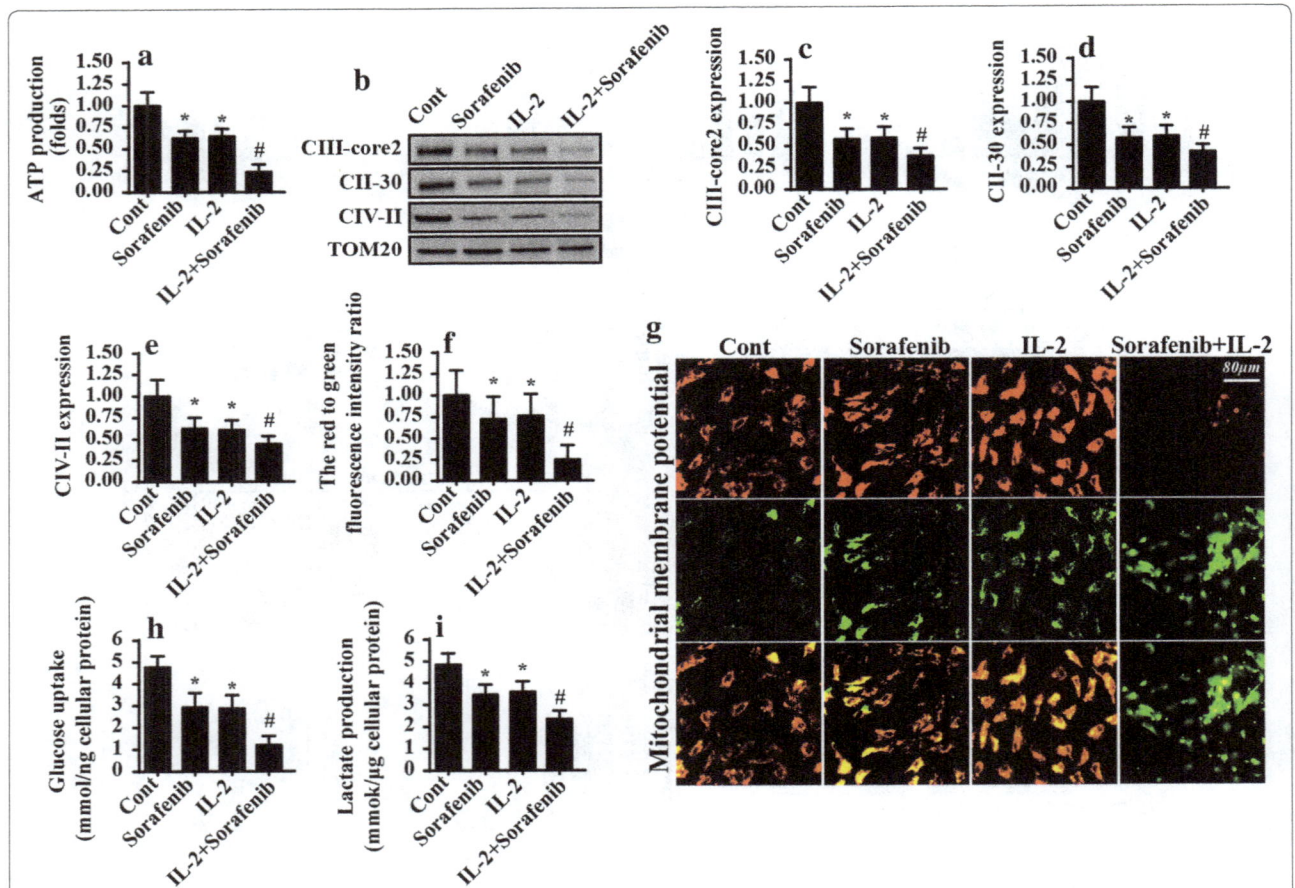

**Fig. 3** IL-2 and sorafenib co-treatment inhibited mitochondrial energy metabolism. **a** ATP production was measured in HepG2 cells subjected to IL-2 and sorafenib co-treatment. **b–e** Mitochondrial respiratory proteins were analysed via western blotting in HepG2 cells. IL-2 (5 ng/ml) treatment was carried out in the presence of 5 μM sorafenib. **f, g** Mitochondrial potential was detected through JC-1 staining. Red fluorescence, which indicated normal mitochondrial potential, was converted into green fluorescence after a reduction in mitochondrial potential. **h, i** The remaining glucose and the produced LDH in the medium were analysed for HepG2 cells. IL-2 (5 ng/ml) treatment was carried out in the presence of 5 μM sorafenib. *$P < 0.05$ vs. control group; #$P < 0.05$ vs. sorafenib group. *Cont* control

IL-2 augments the sorafenib-induced apoptosis in liver cancer by promoting mitochondrial fission...

187

causal relationship between IL-2 administration and mitochondrial dysfunction when sorafenib is present.

## IL-2 induces mitochondrial apoptosis in sorafenib-treated cells

Given the links between IL-2 and mitochondrial dysfunction, we tested whether IL-2 would amplify sorafenib-activated mitochondrial apoptosis in HepG2 cells. As shown in Fig. 4a, b, mitochondrial ROS production, an early molecular event in mitochondrial apoptosis, increased significantly in response to sorafenib treatment in HepG2 cells, and ROS generation was further evoked by IL-2 (Fig. 4a, b). The sorafenib-mediated ROS production was closely associated with a drop in the concentration of antioxidants such as GSH, SOD and GPX (Fig. 4c–e). IL-2 treatment contributed to a further loss of these antioxidants, suggesting a permissive role for IL-2 in cancer oxidative stress.

A late molecular feature of mitochondrial damage is the opening of the mitochondrial permeability transition pore (mPTP), a channel necessary to enable the transmission of mitochondrial pro-apoptotic factors into the cytoplasm/nucleus [40, 41]. Sorafenib-mediated mPTP opening was enhanced by IL-2 in HepG2 cells (Fig. 4f). We also found through immunofluorescence assay that cyt-c, a type of mitochondrial pro-apoptotic protein, was released into the nucleus upon sorafenib treatment due to the prolonged open state of the mPTP (Fig. 4g, h). IL-2 treatment facilitated the cyt-c translocation, as determined by analysis of the fluorescence intensity of cyt-c in the nucleus (Fig. 4g, h). This finding was also validated via western blotting. The level of mitochondrial cyt-c declined in sorafenib-treated cells; this decrease was accompanied by an increase in the expression of cytoplasmic cyt-c (Fig. 4i, j), an effect that was enhanced by IL-2. We also found that mitochondrial apoptotic proteins such as Bad, Bax and caspase-9 were all upregulated by sorafenib treatment (Fig. 4i–o). This upregulation was followed by a fall in the content of anti-apoptotic factors (Fig. 4i–o). The sorafenib-initiated mitochondrial apoptosis was amplified by IL-2 (Fig. 4i–o). Taken together, our data

illustrate that IL-2 can promote sorafenib-mediated mitochondrial apoptosis in HepG2 cells.

## Mitochondrial fission is augmented by IL-2 in the presence of sorafenib

To explain the additional action of IL-2 in activating mitochondrial apoptosis in the presence of sorafenib, we focused on mitochondrial fission, which is the upstream trigger of mitochondrial apoptosis through multiple biological processes [19, 20]. Mitochondrial fission was first examined by western blotting. Mitochondrial fission-related proteins such as Drp1, Fis1 and Mff [42] were slightly upregulated in sorafenib-treated cells (Fig. 5a–f) and were highly elevated in response to IL-2 supplementation. These data indicate that mitochondrial fission seems to be initiated by sorafenib and is further amplified by IL-2 supplementation. In addition, we examined the proteins related to mitochondrial fusion, the defensive system used to correct excessive mitochondrial division. Compared to those in the control group, the levels of mitochondrial fusion-related proteins, such as Mfn1 and Opa1, were marginally downregulated in the sorafenib-treated group (Fig. 5a–f), and this effect was exaggerated by IL-2. These data suggest that IL-2 helps sorafenib to hinder the mitochondrial fusion system, indirectly promoting mitochondrial fission.

Subsequently, an immunofluorescence assay for mitochondria was conducted to observe the mitochondrial fission. In sorafenib-treated cells, the mitochondrial network divided into several fragmented mitochondria in response to mitochondrial fission (Fig. 5g). This alteration was more prominent in IL-2-challenged cells. We further measured the average length of the mitochondria to quantify the mitochondrial fission. The average length of the mitochondria was reduced to some extent under sorafenib treatment (Fig. 5h), and this effect was augmented by IL-2. Overall, we confirmed that IL-2 promotes sorafenib-triggered mitochondrial fission in HepG2 cells.

## IL-2 regulates mitochondrial fission via the JNK-TAZ pathways

The mechanism by which IL-2 boosts mitochondrial fission in the presence of sorafenib was unclear. Since JNK and TAZ have been well documented as activators of

(See figure on next page.)

**Fig. 4** IL-2 activated the mitochondrial apoptotic pathway in the presence of sorafenib. **a, b** Mitochondrial ROS production was detected in HepG2 cells. IL-2 (5 ng/ml) treatment was carried out in the presence of 5 µM sorafenib. **c–e** The antioxidants in HepG2 cells under IL-2 and sorafenib co-treatment were measured via ELISA. **f** The mPTP opening rate was analysed to determine the mitochondrial damage. IL-2 (5 ng/ml) treatment was carried out in the presence of 5 µM sorafenib. **g, h** Cyt-c liberation was observed via immunofluorescence. **i–o** Mitochondrial apoptotic proteins were analysed by western blotting. The sorafenib-mediated upregulation of apoptotic proteins was further augmented by IL-2 treatment. $*P < 0.05$ vs. control group; $^{\#}P < 0.05$ vs. sorafenib group. *Cont* control

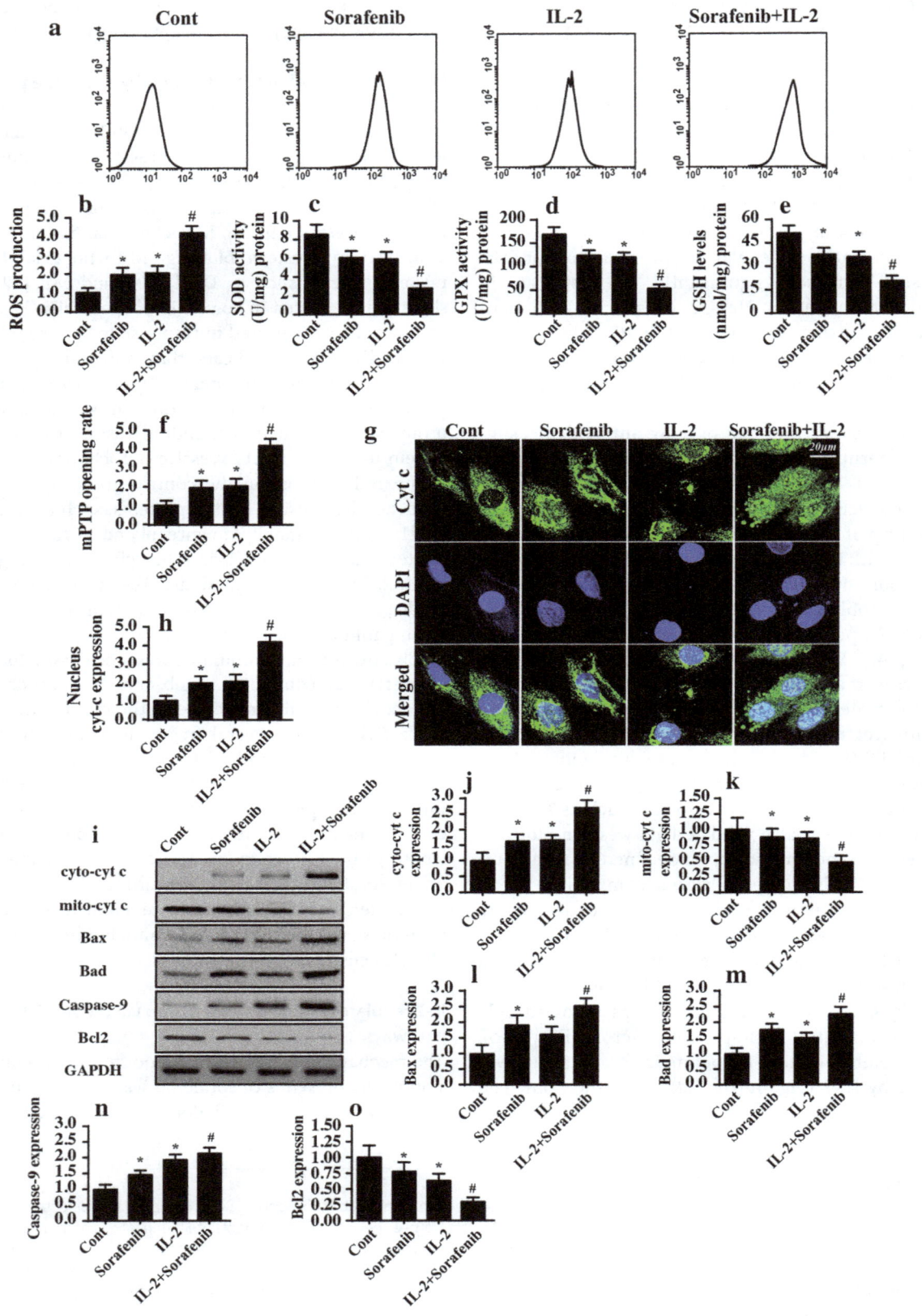

IL-2 augments the sorafenib-induced apoptosis in liver cancer by promoting mitochondrial fission...

189

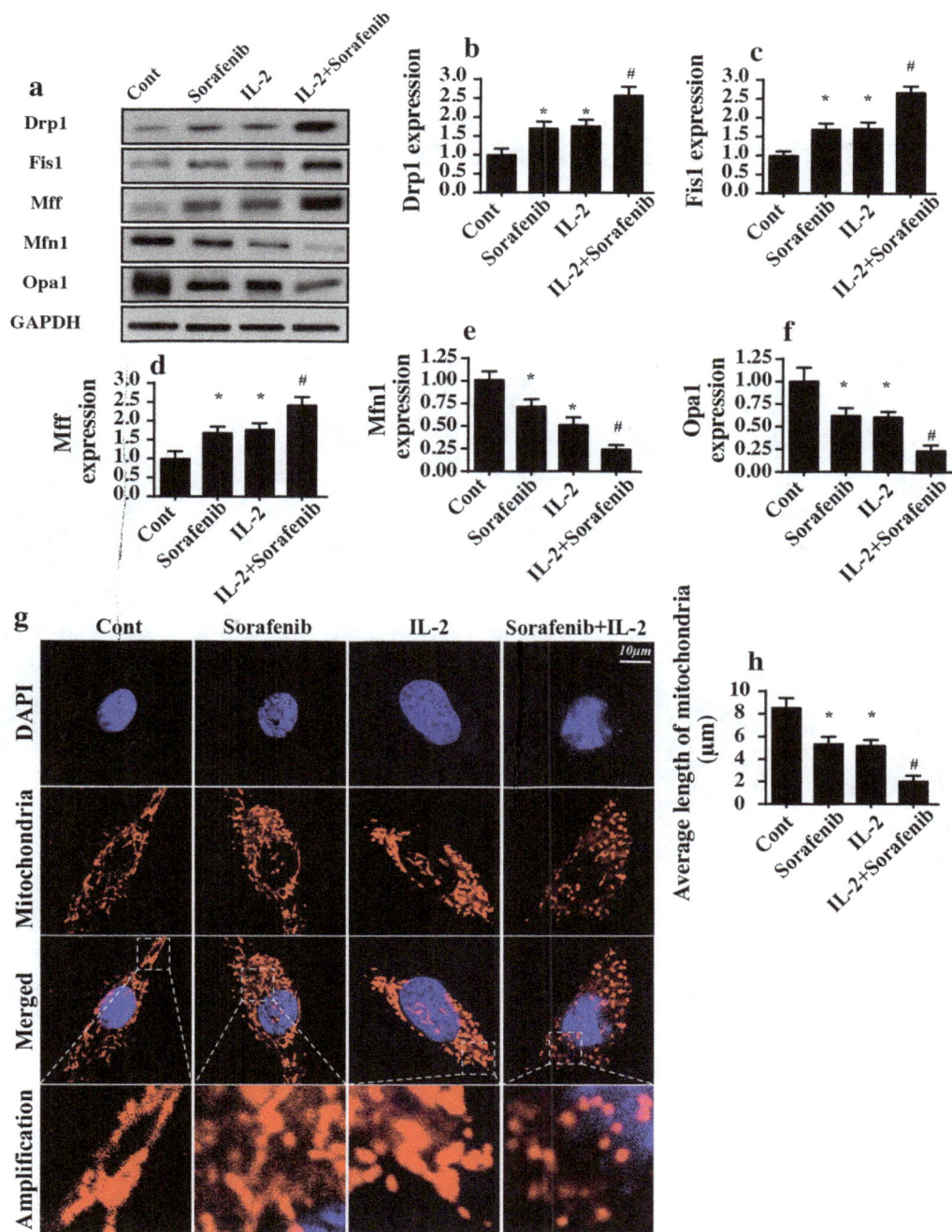

**Fig. 5** IL-2 enhanced sorafenib-initiated mitochondrial fission. **a–f** Western blotting was used to analyse the proteins related to mitochondrial fusion and mitochondrial fission. Drp1, Fis1 and Mff are factors involved in mitochondrial fission. In contrast, mitochondrial fusion is regulated by Mfn1 and Opa1. IL-2 and sorafenib co-treatment elevated the mitochondrial fission proteins and repressed the mitochondrial fusion factors. **g, h** Mitochondrial fission was observed via immunofluorescence using the Tom20 antibody. Then, the average length of mitochondria was measured in HepG2 cells. *$P < 0.05$ vs. control group; #$P < 0.05$ vs. sorafenib group. *Cont* control

mitochondrial fission, we wondered whether JNK-TAZ pathways were also involved in IL-2-exacerbated mitochondrial fission in the presence of sorafenib. Western blotting analysis revealed that both JNK phosphorylation and TAZ expression were slightly increased in response to sorafenib treatment (Fig. 6a–c) and were considerably

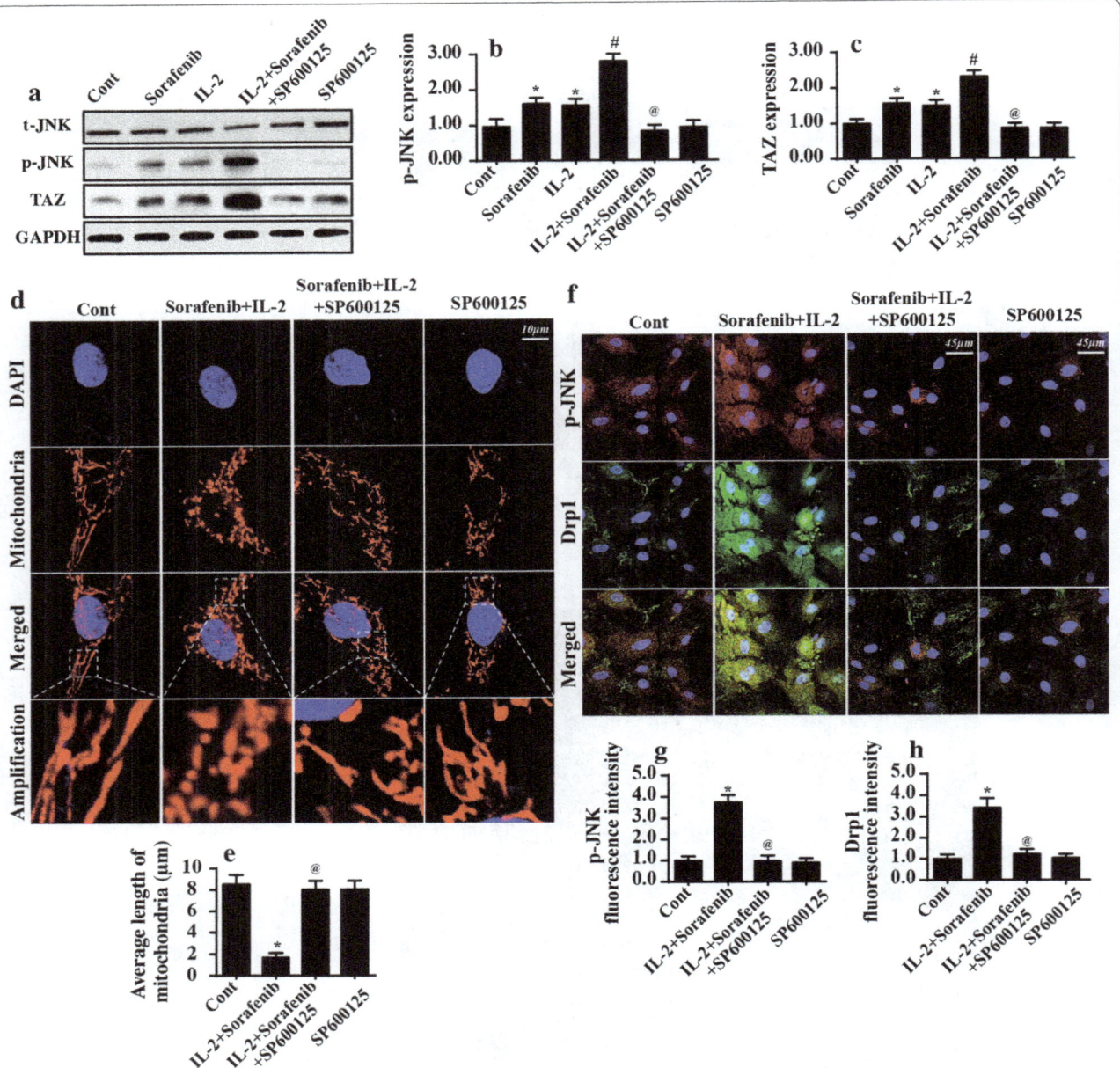

**Fig. 6** IL-2 and sorafenib co-treatment regulated mitochondrial fission via the JNK-TAZ pathways. **a–c** JNK phosphorylation and TAZ expression were measured via western blotting. SP600125, an inhibitor of JNK, was used to inhibit the activity of the JNK-TAZ pathways. **d, e** Mitochondrial fission was observed via immunofluorescence, and the average length of the mitochondria was recorded. **f–h** The regulatory effects of IL-2 and sorafenib co-treatment on the JNK-TAZ pathways and mitochondrial fission were monitored via immunofluorescence. IL-2 and sorafenib co-treatment promoted the upregulation of JNK phosphorylation, which was accompanied by an increase in Drp1, a factor for mitochondrial fission. *P < 0.05 vs. control group; @P < 0.05 vs. IL-2+ sorafenib group. *Cont* control

upregulated with IL-2 supplementation. These findings suggest that the JNK-TAZ pathways are regulated by IL-2 and sorafenib co-treatment.

To demonstrate whether the JNK-TAZ pathways were required to initiate mitochondrial fission, we inhibited JNK activity with a pathway blocker, SP600125. The

inhibitory efficiency was validated via western blotting as shown in Fig. 6a–c. After blockade of JNK, the mitochondrial fission was monitored by immunofluorescence as described previously. Compared to the fragmented mitochondria under IL-2 and sorafenib co-treatment, the mitochondria of SP600125-treated cells maintained an interconnected phenotype (Fig. 6d). Similarly, the average length of the mitochondria was increased after SP600125 treatment when compared to the average length after IL-2 and sorafenib co-treatment (Fig. 6e). We also measured the alteration of mitochondrial fission-related proteins, such as Drp1, through co-immunofluorescence. The fluorescence intensity of Drp1 closely paralleled the content of p-JNK upon IL-2 and sorafenib co-treatment (Fig. 6f–h); higher p-JNK expression was accompanied by increased Drp1 fluorescence intensity. However, inhibition of JNK abrogated the stimulatory effect of IL-2/sorafenib on Drp1 expression (Fig. 6f–h). Collectively, the above data verify the necessity of the JNK-TAZ pathways in IL-2/sorafenib-mediated mitochondrial fission.

### JNK-TAZ pathways are also involved in IL-2-mediated migration inhibition and proliferation arrest

Finally, we wanted to know whether the JNK-TAZ pathways also participate in the migration and proliferation of HepG2 cells. An immunofluorescence assay for cell cycle proteins confirmed that IL-2/sorafenib promoted the expression of CDK4 and cyclin D1 (Fig. 7a–c), and this effect was negated by blocking the JNK-TAZ pathways. In addition, the EdU assay also illustrated that IL-2/sorafenib co-treatment attenuated the ratio of EdU-positive cells by activating the JNK-TAZ pathways (Fig. 7d, e). These data indicate that IL-2/sorafenib-modulated cancer proliferation is dependent on the activity of the JNK-TAZ pathways.

With respect to cancer migration, molecular regulators, such as CXCR4 and CXCR7, were reduced by IL-2/sorafenib co-treatment and were reversed to near-normal levels after the inactivation of the JNK-TAZ pathways (Fig. 7f–h). These data illustrate the critical role played by the JNK-TAZ pathways in cancer migration.

### Discussion

Despite advances in the molecular understanding of HCC, few effective drugs are available in clinical practice to prevent its development. Sorafenib, a first-line targeted therapy drug, has shown a significant survival benefit for patients with HCC in global multiple-centre clinical trials [43, 44]. However, its efficacy is limited to a 3-month extension in survival time [45, 46]. Although several attempts have been made to elucidate the resistance mechanism of HCC against sorafenib, no solid conclusions have been drawn [47]. Several studies have suggested that the alteration of glucose metabolism and/or the downregulation of the Raf-1 kinase inhibitory protein could be possible resistance mechanisms in patients receiving sorafenib [48, 49]. In the present study, our data suggest an option to enhance the therapeutic efficacy of sorafenib in killing liver cancer cells. A combination of

sorafenib and IL-2 reduced the viability of liver cancer cell lines in vitro compared to the viability after sorafenib treatment alone. Moreover, cancer cell migration and proliferation were also repressed by sorafenib in conjunction with IL-2. At the molecular level, IL-2 supplementation assisted sorafenib in inducing mitochondrial injury by activating fatal mitochondrial fission. We also demonstrated that IL-2, in the presence of sorafenib, modified mitochondrial fission via the JNK-TAZ pathways. This is the first investigation to present a novel way to enhance the anti-tumour effect of sorafenib on liver cancer in vitro. Our findings will pave the way for new treatment modalities to control HCC progression by optimizing sorafenib-based therapy.

In the present study, we demonstrated that IL-2 facilitated the pro-apoptotic effects of sorafenib by augmenting mitochondrial fission. Mitochondrial fission is a physical process that modulates the quantity and quality of mitochondrial mass [50]. Moderate mitochondrial fission is necessary for cellular metabolism through the timely production of daughter mitochondria [51]. Moreover, mitochondrial fission helps mitochondria to remove damaged parts, thus enabling mitochondrial turnover and renewal [52]. However, excessive mitochondrial fission converts the mitochondrial network into discontinuous debris, leading to mitochondrial dysfunction. Previous studies on cardiac ischemia/reperfusion have demonstrated that mitochondrial fission activates mitochondrial apoptosis via the HK2-VDAC1-mPTP pathway and the mROS/cardiolipin/cyt-c axis [42]. More recent studies on pancreatic cancer have also found that cancer cell proliferation, migration and survival are closely regulated by mitochondrial fission [21]. Similar findings have been reported for colorectal cancer [53], endometriosis [22], and liver cancer [25]. Consistent with these reports, our data also identify mitochondrial fission as the critical upstream signal for mitochondrial homeostasis in liver cancer cells.

We also demonstrated in this study that mitochondrial fission is drastically activated by IL-2 in the presence of sorafenib, and this regulatory mechanism is dependent on the JNK-TAZ pathways. Notably, no studies investigating the detailed role of IL-2 in mitochondrial fission have yet been conducted. Thus, our investigation provides the first evidence that the tumour-suppressive effects of IL-2 on liver cancer may be attributable to the activation of mitochondrial fission. Notably, the apoptotic rate of HepG2 cells was progressively increased with a rise in the dose of IL-2. The minimum toxic concentration of IL-2 was 5 ng/ml, and therefore, this dose was used to explore whether IL-2 could augment the efficiency of sorafenib-based therapy. Subsequently, we demonstrated that IL-2 regulates mitochondrial fission via

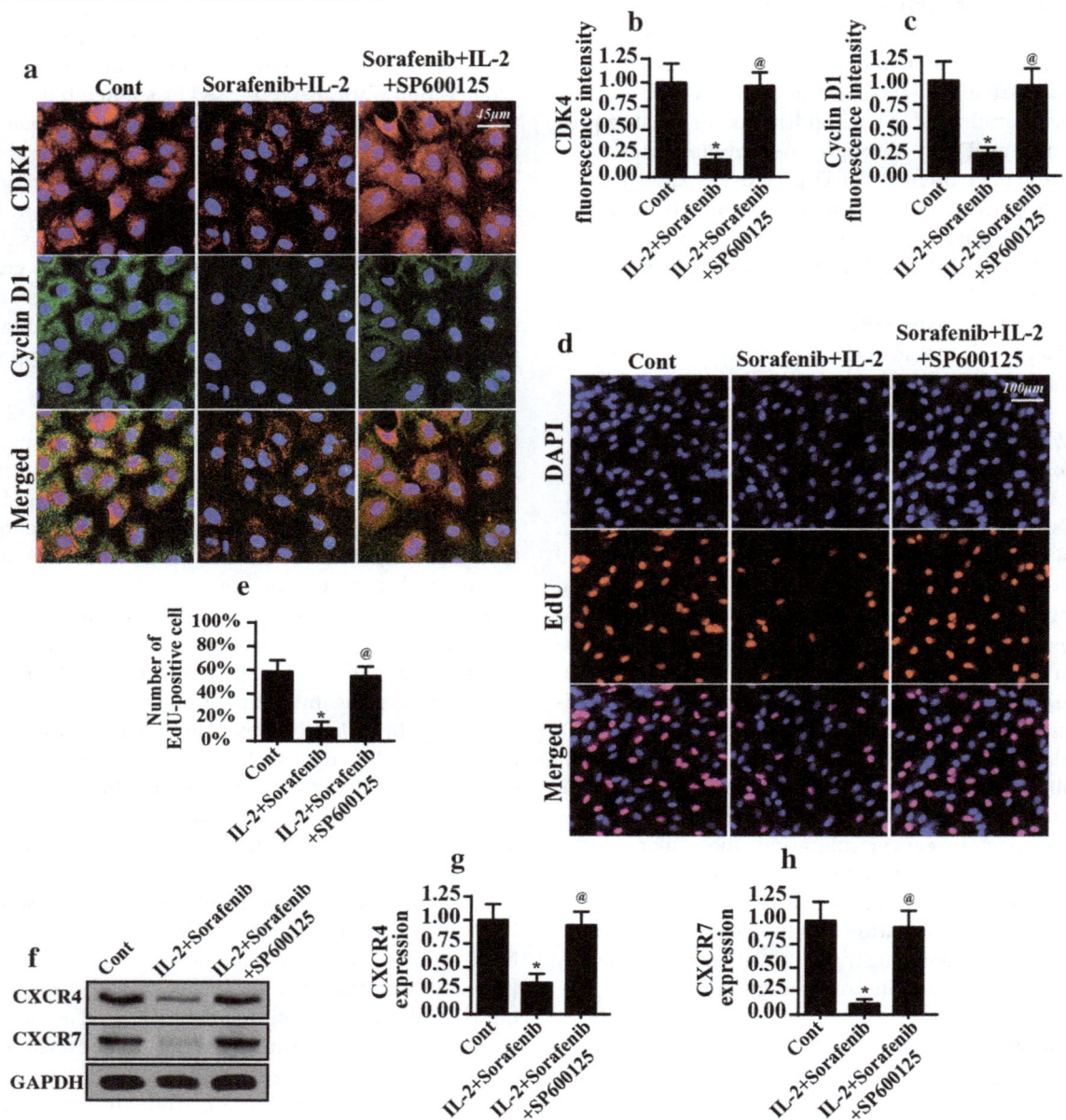

**Fig. 7** Cell migration and proliferation were also regulated by IL-2/sorafenib co-treatment through the JNK-TAZ pathways. **a–c** Immunofluorescence assay for cell proliferation-related factors. IL-2/sorafenib co-treatment elevated the expression of CDK4 and cyclin D1, which was repressed by SP600125, an inhibitor of the JNK-TAZ pathways. **d, e** An EdU assay was performed to quantify the cell proliferation. The number of EdU-positive cells was recorded. **f–h** Cell migration factors such as CXCR4 and CXCR7 were measured via western blotting. *$P < 0.05$ vs. control group; @$P < 0.05$ vs. IL-2+ sorafenib group. *Cont* control

the JNK-TAZ pathways. Previous studies have reported the critical role of JNK and TAZ in activating mitochondrial fission in several disease models. For example, in human rectal cancer cells, activation of the JNK pathway promotes mitochondrial fission, thereby reducing cancer cell survival and migration [53]. In primary hepatocytes, the inhibition of mitochondrial fission through the

modulation of JNK protects the cells against senecionine-induced mitochondrial apoptosis [54]. In breast cancer cells, disruption of the JNK pathway inhibits mitochondrial fission and represses cancer cell proliferation and survival [55]. The above information lays a foundation to help us understand the role of JNK in regulating mitochondrial fission. With respect to TAZ, an early study revealed that mitochondrial fission could be controlled by TAZ through the regulation of mitochondrial lipid synthesis [56]. Subsequent experiments verified that breast cancer migration is highly controlled by TAZ through mitochondrial fission [57]. Furthermore, TAZ has been found to promote mitochondrial fission and induce stem cell differentiation [58]. Such results describe the causal relationship between TAZ and mitochondrial fission. Similar to these findings, our study revealed that the JNK-TAZ pathways are activated by IL-2 in the presence of sorafenib and contribute to mitochondrial fission, ultimately repressing liver cancer cell survival, migration and proliferation. These findings inform us of the anti-tumour molecular mechanisms activated by IL-2 in combination with sorafenib and suggest that strategies targeting mitochondrial fission and the JNK-TAZ axis would yield additional clinical benefits for patients suffering from HCC. To the end, we also found that the survival rate and proliferative index of HepG2 cells were still high in response to IL-2/sorafenib co-treatment. Accordingly, more attempts are required to further enhance the sensitivity of HCC to sorafenib-based therapy. Although we observed the inhibitory effect of IL-2/sorafenib co-treatment on HepG2 cell migration, the IL-2/sorafenib-mediated cell apoptosis and proliferation arrest may also influence the HepG2 cell migration. Further investigation of the direct role of IL-2/sorafenib co-treatment in HCC migration is required.

## Conclusions

Taken together, our data indicate that additional supplementation with IL-2 can enhance the tumour-killing activity of sorafenib. IL-2 in combination with sorafenib repressed liver cancer cell proliferation, migration and survival by promoting mitochondrial dysfunction. The synergetic effects of IL-2 and sorafenib were primarily dependent on mitochondrial fission through the activation of the JNK-TAZ pathways. These findings provide new insights into the mechanisms of these drugs and suggest novel strategies to induce cancer cell death with sorafenib therapy.

## Additional file

**Additional file 1: Figure S1.** The influence of IL-2 and sorafenib treatment on the viability of L02 normal liver cells. A. MTT assay was used to evaluate the cell viability. B. LDH release assay was performed to detect the cell death in response to Il-2 and sorafenib treatment.

## Abbreviations

TAZ: transcriptional co-activator with PDZ-binding motif; Cyt-c: cytochrome c; mPTP: mitochondrial permeability transition pore; IL-2: interleukin-2; HCC: hepatocellular carcinoma.

**Authors' contributions**
XYD and WS conceived the research; XYD and JLC performed the experiments; all authors participated in discussing and revising the manuscript. All authors read and approved the final manuscript.

**Acknowledgements**
Not applicable.

**Competing interests**
The authors declare that they have no competing interests.

**Funding**
This study was supported by Foundation of Clinical Research Cooperation Capital Medical University (Project Number: 16JL77).

**References**
1. Zhou H, Li D, Zhu P, Hu S, Hu N, Ma S, et al. Melatonin suppresses platelet activation and function against cardiac ischemia/reperfusion injury via PPARgamma/FUNDC1/mitophagy pathways. J Pineal Res. 2017;63(4):e12438.
2. Li R, Xin T, Li D, Wang C, Zhu H, Zhou H. Therapeutic effect of Sirtuin 3 on ameliorating nonalcoholic fatty liver disease: the role of the ERK-CREB pathway and Bnip3-mediated mitophagy. Redox Biol. 2018;18:229–43.
3. Zhu H, Jin Q, Li Y, Ma Q, Wang J, Li D, et al. Melatonin protected cardiac microvascular endothelial cells against oxidative stress injury via suppression of IP3R-[Ca$^{2+}$]c/VDAC-[Ca$^{2+}$]m axis by activation of MAPK/ERK signaling pathway. Cell Stress Chaperones. 2018;23(1):101–13.
4. Llovet JM, Ricci S, Mazzaferro V, Hilgard P, Gane E, Blanc JF, de Oliveira AC, Santoro A, Raoul JL, Forner A, et al. Sorafenib in advanced hepatocellular carcinoma. N Engl J Med. 2008;359(4):378–90.
5. Kolch W, Kotwaliwale A, Vass K, Janosch P. The role of Raf kinases in malignant transformation. Expert Rev Mol Med. 2002;4(8):1–18.
6. Lee HJ, Jung YH, Choi GE, Ko SH, Lee SJ, Lee SH, et al. BNIP3 induction by hypoxia stimulates FASN-dependent free fatty acid production enhancing therapeutic potential of umbilical cord blood-derived human mesenchymal stem cells. Redox Biol. 2017;13:426–43.
7. Sun T, Liu H, Ming L. Multiple roles of autophagy in the sorafenib resistance of hepatocellular carcinoma. Cell Physiol Biochem. 2017;44(2):716–27.
8. Ray EM, Sanoff HK. Optimal therapy for patients with hepatocellular carcinoma and resistance or intolerance to sorafenib: challenges and solutions. J Hepatocell Carcinoma. 2017;4:131–8.
9. Xu F, Jin T, Zhu Y, Dai C. Immune checkpoint therapy in liver cancer. J Exp Clin Cancer Res. 2018;37(1):110.
10. Lee S, Loecher M, Iyer R. Immunomodulation in hepatocellular cancer. J Gastrointest Oncol. 2018;9(1):208–19.
11. Bingol B, Sheng M. Mechanisms of mitophagy: PINK1, Parkin, USP30 and beyond. Free Radic Biol Med. 2016;100:210–22.
12. Zhou H, Du W, Li Y, Shi C, Hu N, Ma S, et al. Effects of melatonin on fatty liver disease: the role of NR4A1/DNA-PKcs/p53 pathway, mitochondrial fission, and mitophagy. J Pineal Res. 2018;64(1):e12450.
13. Xu L, Liang Z, Li S, Ma J. Signaling via the CXCR5/ERK pathway is mediated by CXCL13 in mice with breast cancer. Oncol Lett. 2018;15(6):9293–8.
14. Pan C, Xiang L, Pan Z, Wang X, Li J, Zhuge L, Fang P, Xie Q, Hu X. MiR-544 promotes immune escape through downregulation of NCR1/NKp46 via targeting RUNX3 in liver cancer. Cancer Cell Int. 2018;18:52.
15. Rezzola S, Nawaz IM, Cancarini A, Ravelli C, Calza S, Semeraro F, et al. 3D endothelial cell spheroid/human vitreous humor assay for the charac-

15. terization of anti-angiogenic inhibitors for the treatment of proliferative diabetic retinopathy. Angiogenesis. 2017;20(4):629–40.

16. Karwi QG, Bice JS, Baxter GF. Pre- and postconditioning the heart with hydrogen sulfide (H2S) against ischemia/reperfusion injury in vivo: a systematic review and meta-analysis. Basic Res Cardiol. 2017;113(1):6.

17. Zhou H, Li D, Zhu P, Ma Q, Toan S, Wang J, Hu S, Chen Y, Zhang Y. Inhibitory effect of melatonin on necroptosis via repressing the Ripk3-PGAM5-CypD-mPTP pathway attenuates cardiac microvascular ischemia-reperfusion injury. J Pineal Res. 2018. https://doi.org/10.1111/jpi.12503.

18. Zhou H, Zhang Y, Hu S, Shi C, Zhu P, Ma Q, Jin Q, Cao F, Tian F, Chen Y. Melatonin protects cardiac microvasculature against ischemia/reperfusion injury via suppression of mitochondrial fission-VDAC1-HK2-mPTP-mitophagy axis. J Pineal Res. 2017. https://doi.org/10.1111/jpi.12413.

19. Zhou H, Shi C, Hu S, Zhu H, Ren J, Chen Y. BI1 is associated with microvascular protection in cardiac ischemia reperfusion injury via repressing Syk-Nox2-Drp1-mitochondrial fission pathways. Angiogenesis. 2018;21(3):599–615.

20. Zhou H, Wang J, Zhu P, Zhu H, Toan S, Hu S, Ren J, Chen Y. NR4A1 aggravates the cardiac microvascular ischemia reperfusion injury through suppressing FUNDC1-mediated mitophagy and promoting Mff-required mitochondrial fission by CK2alpha. Basic Res Cardiol. 2018;113(4):23.

21. Pan L, Zhou L, Yin W, Bai J, Liu R. miR-125a induces apoptosis, metabolism disorder and migrationimpairment in pancreatic cancer cells by targeting Mfn2-related mitochondrial fission. Int J Oncol. 2018;53(1):124–36.

22. Zhao Q, Ye M, Yang W, Wang M, Li M, Gu C, Zhao L, Zhang Z, Han W, Fan W, et al. Effect of Mst1 on endometriosis apoptosis and migration: role of Drp1-related mitochondrial fission and parkin-required mitophagy. Cell Physiol Biochem. 2018;45(3):1172–90.

23. Zhou H, Zhu P, Guo J, Hu N, Wang S, Li D, et al. Ripk3 induces mitochondrial apoptosis via inhibition of FUNDC1 mitophagy in cardiac IR injury. Redox Biol. 2017;13:498–507.

24. von Eyss B, Jaenicke LA, Kortlever RM, Royla N, Wiese KE, Letschert S, McDuffus LA, Sauer M, Rosenwald A, Evan GI, et al. A MYC-driven change in mitochondrial dynamics limits YAP/TAZ function in mammary epithelial cells and breast cancer. Cancer Cell. 2015;28(6):743–57.

25. Shi C, Cai Y, Li Y, Li Y, Hu N, Ma S, Hu S, Zhu P, Wang W, Zhou H. Yap promotes hepatocellular carcinoma metastasis and mobilization via governing cofilin/F-actin/lamellipodium axis by regulation of JNK/Bnip3/SERCA/CaMKII pathways. Redox Biol. 2018;14:59–71.

26. Ackermann M, Kim YO, Wagner WL, Schuppan D, Valenzuela CD, Mentzer SJ, Kreuz S, Stiller D, Wollin L, Konerding MA. Effects of nintedanib on the microvascular architecture in a lung fibrosis model. Angiogenesis. 2017;20(3):359–72.

27. Blackburn NJR, Vulesevic B, McNeill B, Cimenci CE, Ahmadi A, Gonzalez-Gomez M, Ostojic A, Zhong Z, Brownlee M, Beisswenger PJ, et al. Methylglyoxal-derived advanced glycation end products contribute to negative cardiac remodeling and dysfunction post-myocardial infarction. Basic Res Cardiol. 2017;112(5):57.

28. Brasacchio D, Alsop AE, Noori T, Lufti M, Iyer S, Simpson KJ, Bird PI, Kluck RM, Johnstone RW, Trapani JA. Epigenetic control of mitochondrial cell death through PACS1-mediated regulation of BAX/BAK oligomerization. Cell Death Differ. 2017;24(6):961–70.

29. Banerjee K, Keasey MP, Razskazovskiy V, Visavadiya NP, Jia C, Hagg T. Reduced FAK-STAT3 signaling contributes to ER stress-induced mitochondrial dysfunction and death in endothelial cells. Cell Signal. 2017;36:154–62.

30. Zhang Y, Zhou H, Wu W, Shi C, Hu S, Yin T, Ma Q, Han T, Zhang Y, Tian F, et al. Liraglutide protects cardiac microvascular endothelial cells against hypoxia/reoxygenation injury through the suppression of the SR-Ca(2+)-XO-ROS axis via activation of the GLP-1R/PI3K/Akt/survivin pathways. Free Radic Biol Med. 2016;95:278–92.

31. Hu SY, Zhang Y, Zhu PJ, Zhou H, Chen YD. Liraglutide directly protects cardiomyocytes against reperfusion injury possibly via modulation of intracellular calcium homeostasis. J Geriatr Cardiol. 2017;14(1):57–66.

32. Du GQ, Shao ZB, Wu J, Yin WJ, Li SH, Wu J, Weisel RD, Tian JW, Li RK. Targeted myocardial delivery of GDF11 gene rejuvenates the aged mouse heart and enhances myocardial regeneration after ischemia-reperfusion injury. Basic Res Cardiol. 2017;112(1):7.

33. Zhou H, Wang J, Zhu P, Hu S, Ren J. Ripk3 regulates cardiac microvascular reperfusion injury: the role of IP3R-dependent calcium overload, XO-mediated oxidative stress and F-action/filopodia-based cellular migration. Cell Signal. 2018;45:12–22.

34. Dufour F, Rattier T, Shirley S, Picarda G, Constantinescu AA, Morle A, Zakaria AB, Marcion G, Causse S, Szegezdi E, et al. N-glycosylation of mouse TRAIL-R and human TRAIL-R1 enhances TRAIL-induced death. Cell Death Differ. 2017;24(3):500–10.

35. Alghanem AF, Wilkinson EL, Emmett MS, Aljasir MA, Holmes K, Rothermel BA, Simms VA, Heath VL, Cross MJ. RCAN1.4 regulates VEGFR-2 internalisation, cell polarity and migration in human microvascular endothelial cells. Angiogenesis. 2017;20(3):341–58.

36. Gadicherla AK, Wang N, Bulic M, Agullo-Pascual E, Lissoni A, De Smet M, Delmar M, Bultynck G, Krysko DV, Camara A, et al. Mitochondrial Cx43 hemichannels contribute to mitochondrial calcium entry and cell death in the heart. Basic Res Cardiol. 2017;112(3):27.

37. Glab JA, Doerflinger M, Nedeva C, Jose I, Mbogo GW, Paton JC, Paton AW, Kueh AJ, Herold MJ, Huang DC, et al. DR5 and caspase-8 are dispensable in ER stress-induced apoptosis. Cell Death Differ. 2017;24(5):944–50.

38. Jin Q, Li R, Hu N, Xin T, Zhu P, Hu S, Ma S, Zhu H, Ren J, Zhou H. DUSP1 alleviates cardiac ischemia/reperfusion injury by suppressing the Mff-required mitochondrial fission and Bnip3-related mitophagy via the JNK pathways. Redox Biol. 2018;14:576–87.

39. Zhou H, Yue Y, Wang J, Ma Q, Chen Y. Melatonin therapy for diabetic cardiomyopathy: a mechanism involving Syk-mitochondrial complex I-SERCA pathway. Cell Signal. 2017;47:88–100.

40. Zhu P, Hu S, Jin Q, Li D, Tian F, Toan S, Li Y, Zhou H, Chen Y. Ripk3 promotes ER stress-induced necroptosis in cardiac IR injury: a mechanism involving calcium overload/XO/ROS/mPTP pathway. Redox Biol. 2018;16:157–68.

41. Zhou H, Zhu P, Wang J, Zhu H, Ren J, Chen Y. Pathogenesis of cardiac ischemia reperfusion injury is associated with CK2alpha-disturbed mitochondrial homeostasis via suppression of FUNDC1-related mitophagy. Cell Death Differ. 2018;25(6):1080–93.

42. Zhou H, Hu S, Jin Q, Shi C, Zhang Y, Zhu P, Ma Q, Tian F, Chen Y. Mff-dependent mitochondrial fission contributes to the pathogenesis of cardiac microvasculature ischemia/reperfusion injury via induction of mROS-mediated cardiolipin oxidation and HK2/VDAC1 disassociation-involved mPTP opening. J Am Heart Assoc. 2017;6(3):e005328.

43. Ziogas IA, Tsoulfas G. Evolving role of sorafenib in the management of hepatocellular carcinoma. World J Clin Oncol. 2017;8(3):203–13.

44. Jahandiez V, Cour M, Bochaton T, Abrial M, Loufouat J, Gharib A, Varennes A, Ovize M, Argaud L. Fast therapeutic hypothermia prevents post-cardiac arrest syndrome through cyclophilin D-mediated mitochondrial permeability transition inhibition. Basic Res Cardiol. 2017;112(4):35.

45. Kim DW, Talati C, Kim R. Hepatocellular carcinoma (HCC): beyond sorafenib-chemotherapy. J Gastrointest Oncol. 2017;8(2):256–65.

46. Sarkar C, Ganju RK, Pompili VJ, Chakroborty D. Enhanced peripheral dopamine impairs post-ischemic healing by suppressing angiotensin receptor type 1 expression in endothelial cells and inhibiting angiogenesis. Angiogenesis. 2017;20(1):97–107.

47. Zhou H, Wang S, Zhu P, Hu S, Chen Y, Ren J. Empagliflozin rescues diabetic myocardial microvascular injury via AMPK-mediated inhibition of mitochondrial fission. Redox Biol. 2018;15:335–46.

48. Kim JS, Choi GH, Jung Y, Kim KM, Jang SJ, Yu ES, Lee HC. Downregulation of Raf-1 kinase inhibitory protein as a sorafenib resistance mechanism in hepatocellular carcinoma cell lines. J Cancer Res Clin Oncol. 2018. https://doi.org/10.1007/s00432-018-2672-y.

49. Chiou JF, Tai CJ, Huang MT, Wei PL, Wang YH, An J, Wu CH, Liu TZ, Chang YJ. Glucose-regulated protein 78 is a novel contributor to acquisition of resistance to sorafenib in hepatocellular carcinoma. Ann Surg Oncol. 2010;17(2):603–12.

50. Fuhrmann DC, Brune B. Mitochondrial composition and function under the control of hypoxia. Redox Biol. 2017;12:208–15.

IL-2 augments the sorafenib-induced apoptosis in liver cancer by promoting mitochondrial fission...

195

51. Das N, Mandala A, Naaz S, Giri S, Jain M, Bandyopadhyay D, Reiter RJ, Roy SS. Melatonin protects against lipid-induced mitochondrial dysfunction in hepatocytes and inhibits stellate cell activation during hepatic fibrosis in mice. J Pineal Res. 2017. https://doi.org/10.1111/jpi.12404.

52. Sun Y, Li Q, Zhang J, Chen Z, He Q, Liu X, Zhao N, Yin A, Huang H, He M, et al. Autophagy regulatory molecule, TMEM74, interacts with BIK and inhibits BIK-induced apoptosis. Cell Signal. 2017;36:34–41.

53. Li H, He F, Zhao X, Zhang Y, Chu X, Hua C, Qu Y, Duan Y, Ming L. YAP inhibits the apoptosis and migration of human rectal cancer cells via suppression of JNK-Drp1-mitochondrial fission-HtrA2/Omi pathways. Cell Physiol Biochem. 2017;44(5):2073–89.

54. Yang X, Wang H, Ni HM, Xiong A, Wang Z, Sesaki H, Ding WX, Yang L. Inhibition of Drp1 protects against senecionine-induced mitochondria-mediated apoptosis in primary hepatocytes and in mice. Redox Biol. 2017;12:264–73.

55. Lee MS, Yin TC, Sung PH, Chiang JY, Sun CK, Yip HK. Melatonin enhances survival and preserves functional integrity of stem cells: a review. J Pineal Res. 2017. https://doi.org/10.1111/jpi.12372.

56. Mayr JA. Lipid metabolism in mitochondrial membranes. J Inherit Metab Dis. 2015;38(1):137–44.

57. Shin D, Kim EH, Lee J, Roh JL. RITA plus 3-MA overcomes chemoresistance of head and neck cancer cells via dual inhibition of autophagy and antioxidant systems. Redox Biol. 2017;13:219–27.

58. Noguchi M, Kasahara A. Mitochondrial dynamics coordinate cell differentiation. Biochem Biophys Res Commun. 2018;500(1):59–64.

# 16

# Prognostic value of Kindlin-2 expression in patients with solid tumors

Sheng Liu[†], Sheng Chen[†], Kaige Ma and Zengwu Shao[*] [iD]

## Abstract

**Background:** Kindlin-2 is one of the Kindlin family members which are evolutionarily conserved focal adhesion proteins with integrin β-binding affinity. Recently, accumulative studies have suggested that Kindlin-2 plays important roles in tumor biology. However, the prognostic significance of Kindlin-2 in patients with solid tumors remains controversial. Therefore, this study aimed to clarify the prognostic value of Kindlin-2 in solid tumors via meta-analysis.

**Methods:** A comprehensive search was performed in PubMed, Embase, Web of Science and EBSCO for all relevant studies reporting the prognostic significance of Kindlin-2 expression in solid cancer patients. The summary hazard ratio (HR) and corresponding 95% confidence interval (CI) were calculated to estimate the association between Kindlin-2 expression with survival of solid cancer patients.

**Results:** We included 14 eligible studies containing 1869 patients in our meta-analysis. The pooled results indicated that high Kindlin-2 expression was significantly associated with poor overall survival (OS) (pooled HR 1.66, 95% CI 1.44–1.92, $P < 0.0001$), disease-free survival (DFS)/recurrence-free survival (RFS)/progression-free survival (PFS) (pooled HR 1.73, 95% CI 1.16–2.57, $P = 0.0067$). For certain tumor types, high Kindlin-2 expression was significantly correlated with a poor outcome in patients with solid tumors, including pancreatic ductal adenocarcinoma (DFS/RFS/PFS), esophageal squamous cell carcinoma (OS, DFS/RFS/PFS), hepatocellular carcinoma (OS), clear cell renal cell carcinoma (OS), bladder cancer (OS, DFS/RFS/PFS), chondrosarcoma (OS), osteosarcoma (OS), gastric cancer (DFS/RFS/PFS), and glioma (OS).

**Conclusions:** Our meta-analysis demonstrated that high Kindlin-2 expression might indicate poor outcome in patients with solid tumors and could serve as a prognostic biomarker for solid cancer patients.

**Keywords:** Kindlin-2, Solid tumor, Cancer, Prognosis, Meta-analysis

## Background

Cancer is one of the leading contributors to heavy health care burden and disease-related mortality worldwide, with approximately 1,735,350 new cancer cases and 609,640 cancer-related deaths in the United States in 2018 [1, 2]. Although great advances in early detection and treatments have been made in recent years, the prognosis of cancer patients is still poor [3, 4]. Therefore, novel prognostic biomarkers are urgently needed for precisely predicting the outcome and providing therapeutic targets for cancer patients.

The Kindlin family is composed of three members of evolutionarily conserved focal adhesion proteins (Kindlin-1, -2 and -3) in mammal, which share the same 4.1-ezrin-radixin-moesin (FERM) domain, but have different expression distribution [5]. Kindlins can exert extensive biological functions in cell proliferation, migration, differentiation and cell death through binding with integrin β cytoplasmic tails and activating integrins, which have been linked to many hereditary disease and acquired disease of human [6]. Kindlin-1 (also known as FERMT1) is highly expressed in the skin and other tissues, whose deficiency and mutation can cause Kindler Syndrome [7, 8]. Kindlin-3 (also known as FERMT3) is

*Correspondence: szwpro@163.com
[†]Sheng Liu and Sheng Chen contributed equally to this work
Department of Orthopaedics, Union Hospital, Tongji Medical College, Huazhong University of Science and Technology, Wuhan 430022, China

generally expressed in the notochord, central nervous system, cement gland, and etc., mutations in which can contribute to leukocyte adhesion deficiency type III [8, 9].

Kindlin-2 (also known as FERMT2) was detected in various cell types, including fibroblast cells, smooth muscle cells and endothelial cells [10]. As a broadly distributed focal adhesion protein, Kindlin-2 has binding sites for various interaction partners, such as integrin, actin, the filamin-binding protein migfilin, integrin-linked kinase (ILK) [11, 12]. Previous studies demonstrated that Kindlin-2 could interact with integrin and these partners to activate Wnt signaling, transforming growth factor β (TGF-β) signaling,epidermal growth factor receptor (EGFR) signaling, Hedgehog and extracellular regulated protein kinases (ERK) signaling pathways, which play vital roles in tumor progression [13]. Recently, increasing evidences indicated the correlation between Kindlin-2 expression and prognosis in various types of solid tumors [14–28]. However, several studies demonstrated negative role or no significant association [14, 24, 28, 29]. Therefore, we performed this meta-analysis to explore the prognostic value of Kindlin-2 expression in patients with solid tumors.

## Materials and methods

### Study strategy

This meta-analysis study was based on the Preferred Reporting Items for Systematic Reviews and Meta-Analyses (PRISMA) guidelines [30]. Two authors (Sheng Liu and Sheng Chen) independently carried out the search. PubMed, Embase, Web of Science and EBSCO were searched for articles reporting the prognostic role of Kindlin-2 expression in patients with solid tumors. The search strategy based on MeSH words was "Kindlin-2 OR FEMRT2 OR pleckstrin homology domain-containing family C member 1 (PLEKHC1) OR uncoordinated protein 112 (UNC112) OR mitogen-inducible gene-2 (MIG-2) OR UNC112 related protein 2 short form (URP2SF)" AND "tumor OR neoplasm OR cancer OR carcinoma OR malignancy" AND "prognosis OR prognostic OR survival". The retrieval ended on 10 July, 2018. The references lists in identified articles were screened carefully lest relevant studies should be omitted.

### Inclusion and exclusion criteria

We included all articles meeting the criteria as follows: (1) cohort study; (2) Kindlin-2 expression in cancer tissue or relevant tissue; (3) the prognostic outcome of Kindlin-2 different expression group; (4) available data such as Kaplan–Meier (KM) plot, the hazard ratio (HR) and 95% confidence intervals (CI). Studies of non-human research, reviews, letters, case reports, laboratory articles, non-English articles and conference abstracts were excluded. Two authors (Sheng Liu and Sheng Chen) independently screened the titles and abstracts of identified articles, and excluded those considered irrelevant. Further evaluation was conducted by viewing the full text carefully. Disagreements were resolved by consulting with a third author (Zengwu Shao).

### Data extraction

Two researchers (Sheng Liu and Sheng Chen) independently extracted the relevant data from all eligible articles. The following data of each study was extracted: first author, publication year, original country, number of enrolled patients, tumor type, detected methods, cut-off value, high expression presentations, follow-up time, and HR and 95% CI of the high Kindlin-2 expression group versus the low one for various outcomes. The HR and 95% CI were extracted preferentially from multivariable analyses such as Cox proportional-hazards model. When the HRs were not provided, we extracted the survival information from the original study data (KM plot or the required data) using the software Engauge Digitizer 10.5 [31] and estimated the survival data by Tierney's method [32].

### Quality assessment

The quality of each study was assessed by two investigators (Sheng Liu and Sheng Chen) independently using the Newcastle–Ottawa Quality Assessment Scale (NOS). Any disagreement was resolved by discussing with another investigator (Kaige Ma). The scales allocate the total score for each study ranged from 0 to 9 for the quality of selection, comparability, exposure and outcomes of included studies. The studies with scores $\geq 6$ were considered as high-quality studies.

### Statistical analysis

The statistical analysis was performed using the software R 3.4.4 [33], meta package [34] and meta for package [35]. Pooled HRs and their corresponding 95% CIs were used to describe the prognostic value of Kindlin-2 expression. The heterogeneity was assessed using the Cochran Q-test and I-squared test. If $I^2 < 50\%$ or $P > 0.05$, it was indicated that no heterogeneity existed among studies, and a fixed-effects model was performed. Otherwise, it was considered as significant heterogeneity and the random-effects model was applied. Meta-regression and subgroup analysis were performed with the studies sorted into subgroups according to similar variables. Sensitivity analysis was applied to evaluate the stability of the results. Funnel plot and Egger's test were applied to assess the potential publication bias. Statistical significance was defined as $P$ value $< 0.05$.

## Results

### Eligible studies and their characteristics

According to the searching strategy above mentioned, 120 records were retrieved from the databases. After 72 duplicated records were removed, the remaining articles were screened. Then, 22 of 48 records were excluded because of several reasons: nine articles did not report Kindlin-2 expression as a prognostic variable; three did not involve a tumor; the remaining articles were six meeting articles, two patent articles and two review articles. When the further full-text review was finished, eleven basic research articles and one in non-English were excluded. Finally, the meta-analysis was performed for the remaining 14 articles (Fig. 1).

The included articles all had cohort study and published in the recent decade (2008–2017). In total, 1869 patients in the 16 cohorts were enrolled from China, Japan and Greece. They were diagnosed with pancreatic ductal adenocarcinoma (PDAC), esophageal squamous cell carcinoma (ESCC), bladder cancer (BC), chondrosarcoma (CHS), hepatocellular carcinoma (HCC), osteosarcoma (OSS), glioma, serous epithelial ovarian cancers (sEOC), gastric cancer (GC), or clear cell renal cell carcinoma (ccRCC). The expression of Kindlin-2 was detected by immunohistochemistry (IHC) or Western Blot (WB) in these studies, although the cut-off value varied in different studies. At least overall survival (OS) was used as the prognostic outcome in every study. HRs with their 95% CIs based on Cox proportional-hazards model (Cox) were reported in 11 studies directly. In the remaining three studies, the data were calculated from the KM plots or the P-value of log-rank test. Every study's NOS score was more than 6 points, which meant favorable methodology. The main characteristics of the eligible studies were summarized in Table 1. And the main clinicopathologic

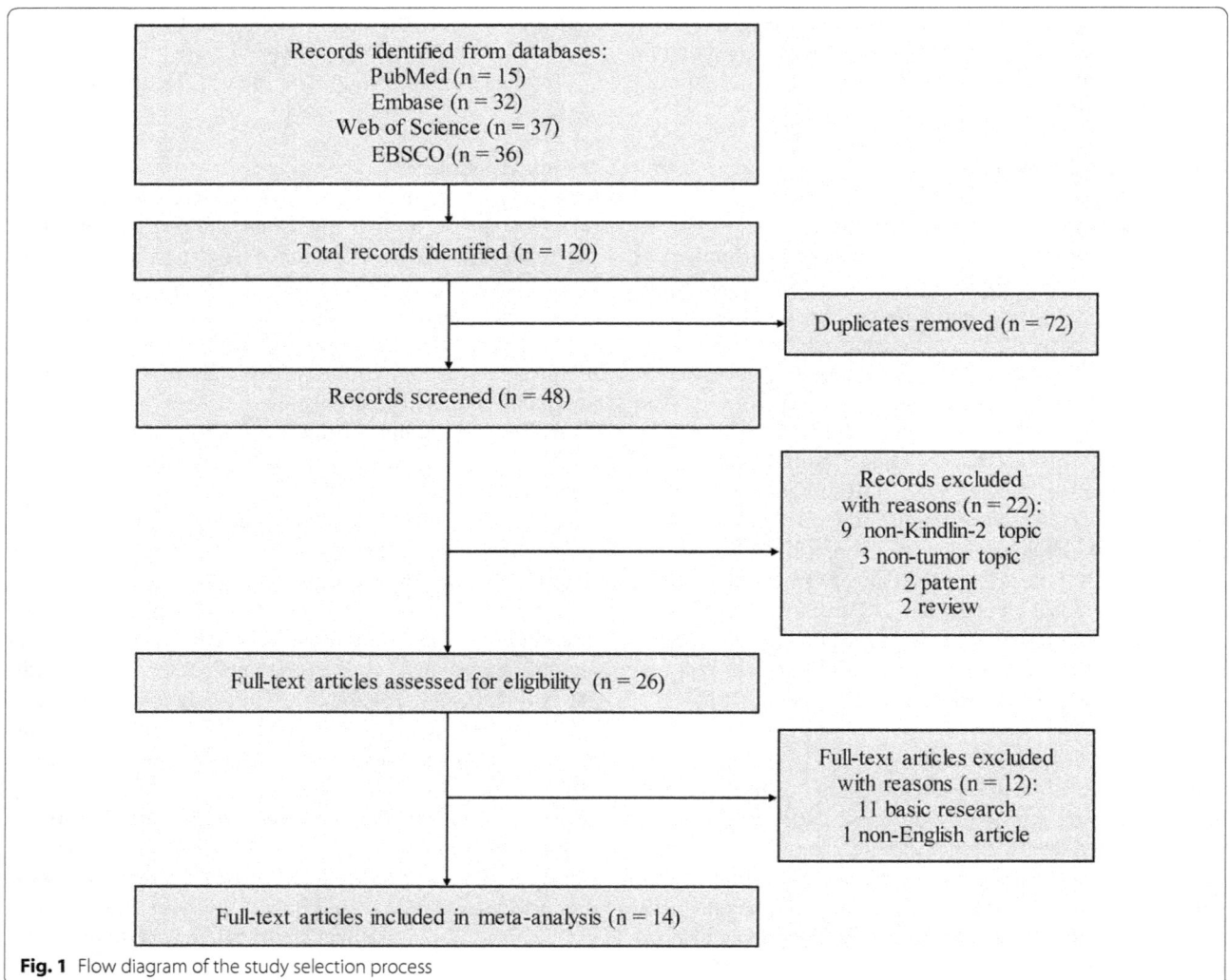

**Fig. 1** Flow diagram of the study selection process

features and their distribution of patients in these studies were shown on Table 2. Kindlin-2 expression was reported to have a significant association with several variables, including age, tumor size, stage, tumor category, lymphatic and vascular invasion, metastasis and response to chemotherapy ($P < 0.05$) (Table 2).

### Correlation between Kindlin-2 expression and survival outcomes of solid tumors

According to the protocol described above, the meta-analysis was performed and its main results were listed in Table 3. There were four survival outcomes evaluated in the included studies, including OS, disease-free survival (DFS), recurrence-free survival (RFS), progression-free survival (PFS). Given that they are similar in definition and number of studies evaluating RFS and PFS was limited (Table 1), we combined the latter three ones together as DFS/RFS/PFS. Thus, this meta-analysis was conducted with two groups: OS and DFS/RFS/PFS.

For the first group, there was no significant statistical heterogeneity ($I^2 = 36.3\%$, $P = 0.0729$). Then, we pooled the HRs and 95% CIs by the fixed-effects model. It was indicated that high Kindlin-2 expression in cancer patients was significantly associated with a poor outcome (for OS, HR 1.66, 95% CI 1.44–1.92, $P < 0.0001$) (Fig. 2 and Table 3).

For the second group, there was obvious heterogeneity ($I^2 = 76.9\%$, $P < 0.0001$). Hence, the random-effects model was performed, and the correlation between high Kindlin-2 expression and poor outcomes was still statistically significant (for DFS/RFS/PFS, HR 1.73, 95% CI 1.16–2.57, $P = 0.0067$) (Fig. 2 and Table 3).

### Subgroup analysis and meta-regression analysis

In order to identify factors that could explain the heterogeneity of the two above groups, subgroup analysis was performed focusing on six features able to analyze: number of patients in single study (less than 100 or not), tumor type (from digestive system or not), sample type (from cancer tissue or stroma tissue), maximum follow-up time (less than 60 months or not), HR extraction (from COX model or not), NOS score (less than 8 or not) (Fig. 3 and Table 3). However, other features were not analyzed due to the deficient report or inconsistent cut-off value. Through the subgroup analysis, we found that the correlation between high expression of Kindlin-2 and OS or DFS/RFS/PFS of solid tumor patients remained significant in all features above except for the subgroup of studies with the following features: patient quantity more than 100 (for OS, HR 1.39, 95% CI 0.88–2.22, $P = 0.1611$); tumor type not from digestive system (for OS, HR 1.31, 95% CI 0.55–3.09, $P = 0.5378$); HR not extracted from COX model (for OS, HR 1.60, 95% CI 0.75–3.43,

$P = 0.2185$; for DFS/RFS/PFS, HR 0.72, 95% CI 0.30–1.72, $P = 0.4542$); NOS score no less than 8 (for OS, HR 1.92, 95% CI 0.61–6.02, $P = 0.2624$) (Table 3). To explore the potential sources of heterogeneity, meta-regression analysis was performed according to the covariates including above features. The result illustrated that the above features might be not the source of heterogeneity as moderators except for maximum follow-up time (for DFS/RFS/PFS, $P = 0.0258$) and HR extraction (for DFS/RFS/PFS, $P = 0.0085$) (Table 3). Importantly, the pooled data from 11 cohorts and 1527 patients showed that Kindlin-2 could be an independent factor for prognosis of solid tumor patients (for OS, HR 1.70, 95% CI 1.46–1.98, $P < 0.0001$; for DFS/RFS/PFS, HR 2.23, 95% CI 1.51–3.28, $P < 0.0001$) (Table 3).

### Correlation between Kindlin-2 expression and survival outcomes of specific tumor types

The prognostic value of Kindlin-2 expression in different tumors was further investigated. We found that high expression of Kindlin-2 in PDAC patients showed an obvious correlation with poor OS (HR 1.60, 95% CI 1.10–2.34, $P = 0.015$) (Fig. 4), but showed no statistically significant association with poor DFS/RFS/PFS (HR 1.44, 95% CI 0.972–2.13, $P = 0.069$) (Fig. 4). Through meta-analysis, we also observed that high Kindlin-2 expression significantly correlated with poor OS in patients with ESCC (HR 1.71, 95% CI 1.19–2.47, $P = 0.004$), HCC (HR 2.33, 95% CI 1.38–3.93, $P = 0.002$), ccRCC (HR 1.75, 95% CI 1.22–2.52, $P = 0.003$) (Fig. 4). The pooled data also showed statistically association between high Kindlin-2 expression with poor RFS/DFS/PFS in ESCC (HR 1.59, 95% CI 1.10–2.28, $P = 0.0129$), HCC (HR 4.30, 95% CI 1.81–10.19), ccRCC (HR 1.47, 95% CI 1.05–2.06) (Fig. 4).

Consistent with their original article, the remaining HRs and their 95% CI showed that high Kindlin-2 expression had a significant relation with a worse prognosis in BC (for OS, HR 1.73, 95% CI 1.23–2.44; for DFS/RFS/PFS, HR 1.41, 95% CI 0.73–2.74), CHS (for OS, HR 3.56, 95% CI 1.22–10.36), GC (for OS, HR 2.83, 95% CI 0.63–12.73; for DFS/RFS/PFS, HR 5.17, 95% CI 3.06–8.72), glioma (for OS, HR 1.50, 95% CI 1.11–2.02), OS (for OS, HR 6.89, 95% CI 1.79–26.53; for DFS/RFS/PFS, HR 7.23, 95% CI 1.85–28.22), while it had a significant association with the better prognostic outcome of SEOC (for OS, HR 0.48, 95% CI 0.24–0.98; for DFS/RFS/PFS, HR 0.27, 95% CI 0.10–0.72) (Fig. 4).

### Publication bias assessment and sensitivity analysis

Funnel plot, Begger's test and Egger's test were applied to assess small-scale study effect for this meta-analysis. The plots seemed asymmetric (Fig. 5), although both Begger's and Egger's tests were not statistically

**Table 1** The main characteristics of the eligible studies

| Study (Author and year) | Country | size | Tumor type | Sample type | Method (antibody data) | Negative control | Expression location | Cut-off value: (intention) or (IPS=x*y) | High expression ratio: n/N (%) | Follow-up time: mean (min-max) (mon) | Survival outcome | Conclusion (UA/MA) | Multivariate analysis | HR extraction | NOS score |
|---|---|---|---|---|---|---|---|---|---|---|---|---|---|---|---|
| Yoshida et al. 2017 (I) [14] | Japan | 79 | PDAC | ac (Ca) Startle (St) | IHC (M, Merck Millipore) | NT + NP | NR | 50% | Ca: 54/79 (68%) St: 49/79 (62%) | NR | OS; RFS OS; RFS | NS; NS; NS; P | No | KM plot | 8 |
| Zhan et al. 2015 [15] | China | 31 | PDAC | ac | IHC (Millipore) | PBS | NR | 50% | 15/31 (48%) | 47 (3–73) | OS | P | No | P-value | 7 |
| Mahawith-itwong et al. 2013 [16] | Japan | 95 | PDAC | sf | IHC (R, Protein TechGroup, 1:100) | NR | NR | (4*3) 4/12 | 34/95 (64.2%) | 24 (3–136); 14 (0–136) | OS; DFS | P/NS; P/– | Yes | Cox P-value | 7 |
| Cao et al. 2015 (II) [17] | China | 110 | ESCC | scc | IHC (M, Origen,1:50) | NR | C + N | (3*4) NR | 34/65 (52%) | 36.5 (0–148.7) | OS; DFS | –/P; –/P | Yes | Cox | 6 |
| Cao et al. 2015 (II) [17] | China | 147 | ESCC | scc | IHC (M, Origen,1:50) | NR | C + N | (3*4) NR | 20/64 (31%) | 28.8 (27–72) | OS; DFS | P; P | Yes | Cox | 6 |
| Wu et al. 2017 [18] | China | 203 | BC | sf | IHC (M, Santa Cruz, 1:500) | PBS | NR | (3*4) 6/12 | 109/203 (54%) | 64 (49–78) | OS; CSS; DFS | P/P; P/–; P/– | Yes | Cox | 6 |
| Papachris-tou et al. 2008 [19] | Greece etc. | 60 | CHS | sf | IHC (M, home-made, 1/50) | TBS | C | 33% | 51/60 (85%) | 67.9 (40.9, 2–180) | OS | P | No | P-value | 8 |
| Ge et al. 2015 [20] | China | 72 | HCC | ac | IHC (R, ab152106, 1:100) | PBS | NR | (4*3) 4/12 | 43/72 (60%) | NR (17.96–43.11) | OS; DFS | P/P; P/P | Yes | Cox | 7 |
| Lin et al. 2017 [21] | China | 127 | HCC | ac | IHC (M, MAB2617, Billerica, 1:100) | NR | C | (3*4) 4/12 | 103/127 (81%) | 22 (1–94) | OS | P/P | Yes | Cox | 8 |
| Ning et al. 2017 [22] | China | 100 | OSS | Sarcoma | IHC (R, Milli-pore, 1:150) | PBS | N | (3*4) 4.56/12 | 51/100 (51%) | 29.82 (5.26–38.89) | OS; DFS | P/P; P/P | Yes | Cox | 7 |
| Ou et al. 2016 [23] | China | 188 | Glioma | Carci-noma | IHC (1:100) | NR | NR | 4/12 | 132/188 (70%) | NR (0–39) | OS | P/P | Yes | Cox | 8 |
| Ren et al. 2014 [24] | China | 113 | sEOC | scc | IHC (R, Dako, 1:2000) | PBS | NR | (4*4) 12/16 | 91/113 (80%) | NR | OS; PFS | N/NS; N/N | Yes | KM-plot | 6 |
| Shen et al. 2012 [25] | China | 40 | GC | ac | WB (R, ab74030, Abcam, 1:600) | actin | NR | Ratio: K2/actin > 2 | 22/40 (55%) | 37.1 (5–77) | OS; PFS | P/NS; P/P | Yes | Cox | 8 |
| Li et al 2017 [26] | China | 109 | ccRCC | ac | IHC (M, Mil-lipore) | NT | C | 50% | 70/109 (64%) | 69 (0.94–82) | OS | P/NS | Yes | Cox | 7 |

**Table 1** (continued)

| Study (Author and year) | Country | size | Tumor type | Sample type | Method (antibody data) | Negative control | Expression location | Cut-off value: (intention) or (IPS=x*y) | High expression ratio: n/N (%) | Follow-up time: mean (min–max) (mon) | Survival outcome | Conclusion (UA/MA) | Multivariate analysis | HR extraction | NOS score |
|---|---|---|---|---|---|---|---|---|---|---|---|---|---|---|---|
| Yan et al. 2016 [27] | China | 336 | ccRCC | ac | IHC (M, ab117962, Abcam, 1:100) | NR | NR | (3*3) 4/9 | 199/336 (59%) | NR (10–60) | OS; DFS | –/P; –/P | Yes | Cox | 7 |

(I) This article (Yoshida [14]) was listed two cohort study because the sample types contains cancer tissue and startle cell. (II) and (III) This article (Cao [17]) included patients from generation dataset (II) and validation dataset (III). Antibody data mainly contains the species (mouse, rabbit), code, manufacturer, and concentration ratio

n: number of patients; PDAC: pancreatic ductal adenocarcinoma; ESCC: esophageal squamous cell carcinoma; BC: bladder cancer; CHS: chondrosarcoma; HCC: hepatocellular carcinoma; OSS: osteosarcoma; sEOC: serous epithelial ovarian cancers; GC: gastric cancers; ccRCC: clear cell renal cell carcinoma; Ca: cancer tissue, St: startle cell; sf: stromal fibroblasts; scc: squamous cell carcinoma; IHC: immunohistochemistry; WB: Western Blot; NR: no report; NT: non-cancer tissue; NP: non-tumor patient; PBS: phosphate buffered solution; TBS: triethanolamine buffered solution; C: cytoplasm, N: cellular nucleus; IPS: immunohistochemical positive score; x: up-limit of the averaged staining intensity score; y: up-limit of the score standing for stained cells proportion; *: multiplication of the two score; Ratio: the ratio of gray value; UA: univariate analysis; MA: multivariate analysis; NS: not significant, P: positive for the conclusion that Kindlin-2 high expression is associated with poor prognostic outcome, N: negative for the conclusion; Cox: Cox proportional-hazards model; NOS: the Newcastle–Ottawa Quality Assessment Scale

**Table 2 The main clinicopathologic features of patients and their distribution in the eligible studies**

| Study (Author and year) | n | Age (years or numbers): [mean or median (range)] (cut-off: low/high) | Sex (M/F) | Histological differentiation (I/II/III) | Tumor size (cm) (cut-off) (low/high) | Tumor category (grade) | Lymphatic invasion (∓) | Vascular invasion (low/high) | Metastasis (∓) | Staging method | Stage (cut-off) | Other therapy (no/yes) |
|---|---|---|---|---|---|---|---|---|---|---|---|---|
| Yoshida et al. 2017 (I) [14] | 79 | 65 (mean) (41–85) (65):39/40 | 51/28 | 9/63/7 | NR | NR | 19/60 | 32/47 | NR | NR | NR | C: 9/70 R: 68/11 |
| Zhan et al. 2015 [15] | 31 | NR | NR | NR | NR | NR | NR | NR | NR | NR | NR | NR |
| Mahawithit-wong et al. 2013 [16] | 95 | 65 (mean) (36–86) (65): 52/43 | 58/37 | 10/33/52 | NR | (T1/2/3/4) 9/3/82/1 | 34/61* | 38/57 | NR | UICC | NR | C: 10/85 R: 78/17 |
| Cao et al. 2015 (II) [17] | 110 | (58): 55/55 | 80/30 | 33/67/10 | (3, 5) 32/45/11 | (T1, 2/3, 4) 7/103 | 57/53 | NR | NR | TNM | (IIB/IIIA) 59/51 | 99/12 |
| Cao et al. 2015 (III)[17] | 147 | (58): 79/68 | 113/34 | 23/109/15 | (3, 5) 38/71/36 | (T1, 2/3, 4) 20/127 | 64/83 | NR | NR | TNM | (IIB/IIIA) 70/77 | 104/43 |
| Wu et al. 2017 [18] | 203 | (65): 109/94 | 165/38 | (Low/high) 96/107* | (3) 140/63 | NR | NR | NR | NR | TNM | (I/II) 8/115* | NR |
| Papachristou et al. 2008 [19] | 60 | 54 (mean) (21–85) | 34/26 | 20/29/11* | (8) 23/37 | NR | NR | NR | NR | NR | NR | NR |
| Ge et al. 2015 [20] | 72 | (53): 35/37 | 60/12 | NR | (5) 29/43* | NR | NR | Cap: 44/28* Mic: 49/23* | NR | TNM | (II/III) 41/31 | NR |
| Lin et al. 2017 [21] | 127 | (60): 111/16 | 17/110 | NR | (3) 10/117 | NR | NR | Cap: 40/87 Mic: 66/61* | 9/115* | NR | (II/III) 11/116 | NR |
| Ning et al. 2017 [22] | 100 | (18): 40/60 | 68/32 | (Low/high) 15/85* | NR | NR | NR | NR | 60/40* | NR | NR | RC: 50/50* |
| Ou et al. 2016 [23] | 188 | 39 (mean) (39): 98/90* | 103/85 | NR | NR | NR | NR | NR | NR | NR | (II/III) 85/103* | NR |
| Ren et al. 2014 [24] | 113 | (50): 28/85* | –/113 | (Low/high) 26/87* | NR | NR | NR | NR | 49/34 | FIGO | (I/II/III/IV) 9/13/73/10 | RC: 21/68 |
| Shen et al. 2012 [25] | 40 | 67 (mean) (47–93) (60): 14/26 | 30/10 | 4/8/28 | NR | (T1, 2/3, 4) 8/32* | N1/2/3 21/10/9* | NR | 37/3 | Pathologic | (II/II) 8/32* | NR |
| Li et al. 2017 [26] | 109 | (60):62/47 | 67/42 | 36/41/32* | NR | (Tx/1/2/34) 4/68/20/17 | Nx/0/1 2/99/8* | NR | NR | AJCC | (II/III) 70/39 | NR |
| Yan et al. 2016 [27] | 336 | (65):177/159 | 240/96 | NR | (4) 176/160 | (T1, 2/3, 4) 167/169 | 202/134 | NR | 269/67* | TNM | (II/III) 124/212* | NR |

(I) This article (Yoshida [14]) was listed two cohort study because the sample types contains cancer tissue and startle cell. (II) and (III) This article (Cao [17]) included patients from generation dataset (II) and validation dataset (III)

n: number of patients; NR: no report; Cap: capillary invasion; Mic: microvascular invasion; C: chemotherapy; R: radiotherapy; RC: response for chemotherapy

*Means that Kindlin-2 expression was reported to have a significant relation with the variable in the study

**Table 3  The pooled HR and 95% CI for the prognostic value of Kindlin-2 expression**

| Outcome group | Subgroup | No. of studies | No. of patients | Model | Pooled HR (95% CI) | P value of pooled HR | Heterogeneity | | P value of meta-regression |
|---|---|---|---|---|---|---|---|---|---|
| | | | | | | | I² (%) | P value | |
| Overall | | | | | | | | | |
| OS | Overall | 16 | 1869 | Fixed | 1.6612 [1.4400; 1.9164] | <0.0001 | 36.3 | 0.0729 | – |
| DFS/RFS/PFS | | 11 | 1374 | Random | 1.7309 [1.1643; 2.5733] | 0.0067 | 76.9 | <0.0001 | |
| Sample size | | | | | | | | | |
| OS | ≥ 100 | 9 | 1433 | Random | 1.6074 [1.2435; 2.0777] | 0.0003 | 52.5 | 0.03 | 0.3455 |
| | < 100 | 7 | 436 | Fixed | 1.9081 [1.3873; 2.6245] | 0.0001 | 0.0 | 0.45 | |
| DFS/RFS/PFS | ≥ 100 | 6 | 1009 | Random | 1.3943 [0.8759; 2.2194] | 0.1611 | 70.7 | <0.01 | 0.2277 |
| | < 100 | 5 | 365 | Random | 2.2280 [1.1574; 4.2886] | 0.0165 | 78.0 | <0.01 | |
| Tumor type (from which system) | | | | | | | | | |
| OS | Digestive | 9 | 780 | Fixed | 1.7955 [1.4224; 2.2664] | <0.0001 | 0.0 | 0.79 | 0.5000 |
| | Non-digestive | 7 | 1089 | Random | 1.6305 [1.1236; 2.3662] | 0.0101 | 67.0 | <0.01 | |
| DFS/RFS/PFS | Digest | 7 | 622 | Random | 2.0137 [1.2856; 3.1542] | 0.0022 | 72.2 | <0.01 | 0.3149 |
| | Non-digestive | 4 | 752 | Random | 1.3101 [0.5547; 3.0945] | 0.5378 | 81.9 | <0.01 | |
| Sample type (from which tissue) | | | | | | | | | |
| OS | Cancer | 13 | 1492 | Random | 1.7897 [1.3855; 2.3118] | <0.0001 | 46.1 | 0.03 | 0.5741 |
| | Stroma | 3 | 377 | Fixed | 1.5830 [1.1958; 2.0957] | 0.0013 | 0.0 | 0.57 | |
| DFS/RFS/PFS | Cancer | 8 | 997 | Random | 1.8358 [1.0668; 3.1589] | 0.0283 | 83.4 | <0.01 | 0.6650 |
| | Stroma | 3 | 377 | Fixed | 1.5566 [1.0726; 2.2590] | 0.0199 | 0.0 | 0.74 | |
| Max follow-up time (months) | | | | | | | | | |
| OS | ≥ 60 | 13 | 1509 | Random | 1.6442 [1.3212; 2.0462] | 0.0207 | 31.7 | 0.13 | 0.4370 |
| | < 60 | 3 | 360 | Random | 2.4020 [1.1431; 5.0471] | <0.0001 | 66.3 | 0.05 | |
| DFS/RFS/PFS | ≥ 60 | 9 | 1202 | Random | 1.4740 [0.9864; 2.2028] | 0.0583 | 76.7 | <0.01 | 0.0258** |
| | < 60 | 2 | 172 | Fixed | 4.9891 [2.4072; 10.3405] | <0.0001 | 0.0 | 0.53 | |
| HR extraction | | | | | | | | | |
| OS | COX | 11 | 1527 | Fixed | 1.7024 [1.4600; 1.9851] | <0.0001 | 0.0 | 0.61 | 0.4737 |
| | Non-COX | 5 | 342 | Random | 1.6093 [0.7542; 3.4340] | 0.2185* | 72.7 | <0.01 | |
| DFS/RFS/PFS | COX | 8 | 1103 | Random | 2.2266 [1.5122; 3.2785] | <0.0001 | 72.1 | <0.01 | 0.0085** |
| | Non-COX | 3 | 271 | Random | 0.7158 [0.2982; 1.7182] | 0.4542* | 66.7 | 0.05 | |
| NOS score | | | | | | | | | |
| OS | ≥ 8 | 6 | 553 | Fixed | 1.6820 [1.3178; 2.1470] | <0.0001 | 0.0 | 0.64 | 0.6371 |
| | < 8 | 10 | 1316 | Random | 1.6701 [1.2539; 2.2243] | 0.0005 | 55.3 | 0.02 | |
| DFS/RFS/PFS | ≥ 8 | 3 | 198 | Random | 1.9211 [0.6133; 6.0179] | 0.2624* | 86.8 | <0.01 | 0.6479 |
| | < 8 | 8 | 1176 | Random | 1.6244 [1.0899; 2.4211] | 0.0172 | 69.8 | <0.01 | |

*Means that the P value of pooled HR is more than 0.05

**Means the P value from the test of moderators in the meta-regression is lower than 0.05

significant (Begger's $P=0.105$, Egger's $P=0.207$). Then, we introduced trim-and-filled model to neutralize the potential bias (Fig. 5), and statistical significance of the correlation still existed (for OS, HR 1.55, 95% CI 1.35–1.77, $P<0.0001$). Hence, no significant publication bias existed and exerted a strong impact on the pooled results in this meta-analysis.

To evaluate the effect of each study on the pooled results, we performed sensitivity analysis by omitting each single study sequentially. No study displayed an apparent influence on the overall results of OS and DFS/RFS/PFS (Fig. 6).

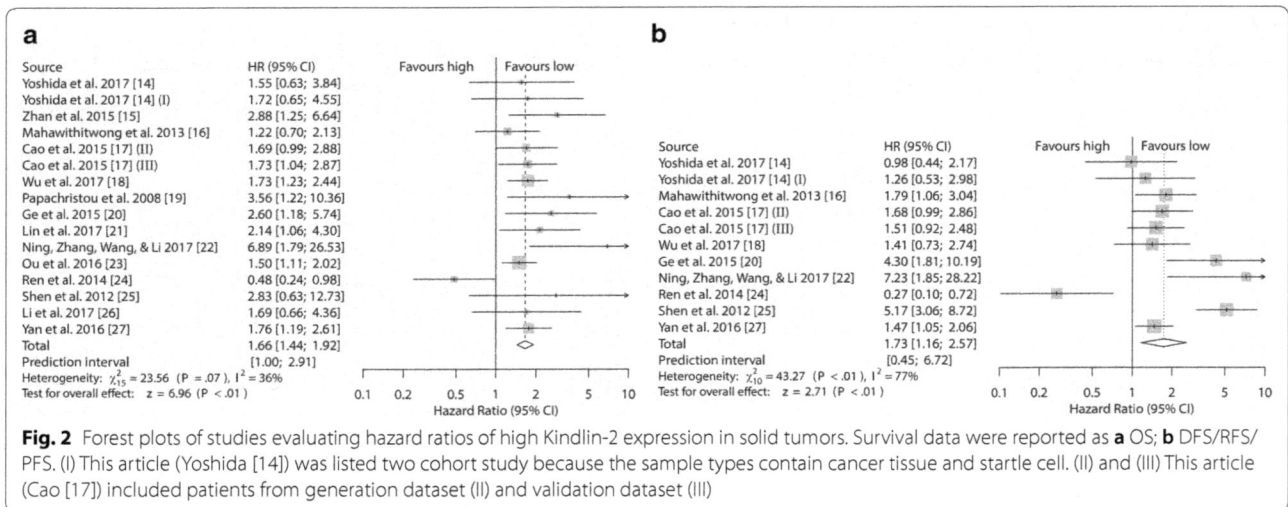

**Fig. 2** Forest plots of studies evaluating hazard ratios of high Kindlin-2 expression in solid tumors. Survival data were reported as **a** OS; **b** DFS/RFS/PFS. (I) This article (Yoshida [14]) was listed two cohort study because the sample types contain cancer tissue and startle cell. (II) and (III) This article (Cao [17]) included patients from generation dataset (II) and validation dataset (III)

## Discussion

The human Kindlin-2 gene, also known as mitogen inducible gene-2 (MIG-2), was originally identified in the human diploid fibroblast cell line WI-38 by differential cDNA library screening and is located on chromosome 14q22.1 [20, 36]. Recently, increasing evidences have suggested that Kindlin-2 expression levels significantly correlate with tumor invasion, lymph node metastasis and worse survival in different cancers, such as breast cancer, bladder cancer [5]. However, Ren et al. reported that Kindlin-2 inhibited the growth and migration of colorectal cancer cells [29], and Shi et al. found that Kindlin-2 could act as a suppressor of mesenchymal cancer cell invasion [37]. Owing to limited numbers of patients and conflicting conclusion in existing studies, the association between Kindlin-2 and prognosis of cancer patients remains controversial.

To our knowledge, there is no systemic review focusing on the correlation between Kindlin-2 expression and prognosis of cancer patients. Therefore, we performed this meta-analysis for critically assessing the prognostic significance of Kindlin-2 expression and to determine whether high Kindlin-2 expression is associated with poor prognosis of cancer patients or not. Our results showed that high Kindlin-2 expression was significantly associated with poor OS of patients with various solid tumors. Meanwhile, the correlation between high Kindlin-2 expression and poor DFS/RFS/PFS was not homogenous, but still significant. Then, we performed the

subgroup analysis for potential heterogeneity according to number of patients in single study, tumor type, sample type, maximum follow-up time, HR extraction, NOS score. We found that there remains an obvious relation between high Kindlin-2 expression and poor prognosis of tumor patients when concerning the above features except for the subgroups as follow: patient quantity more than 100; tumor type not from digestive system; HR not extracted from COX model; NOS score no less than 8. Given that the numbers of studies in these subgroups were limited, the correlating features may be not the source of the heterogeneity, which was consistent with the result of the following meta-regression. In the meta-regression analysis, we did found the lightly significant coefficient role in subgroup according to maximum follow-up time and HR extraction. It meant that the two potential moderators might partly account for the heterogeneity of the DFS/RFS/PFS group. Moreover, Kindlin-2 exerted a significant impact on worse prognosis of PDAC (DFS/RFS/PFS), ESCC (OS, DFS/RFS/PFS), HCC (OS), ccRCC (OS), BC (OS, DFS/RFS/PFS), CHS (OS), OSS (OS), GC (DFS/RFS/PFS) and glioma (OS), but not of PDAC (OS), GC (OS), sEOC (OS, DFS/RFS/PFS). The results revealed that Kindlin-2 expression had a varying correlation with prognostic outcomes of different tumor types. No significant publication bias existed in this meta-analysis and exerted a strong impact on the pooled result. Meanwhile, no study displayed an apparent influence on the overall results of OS and DFS/RFS/

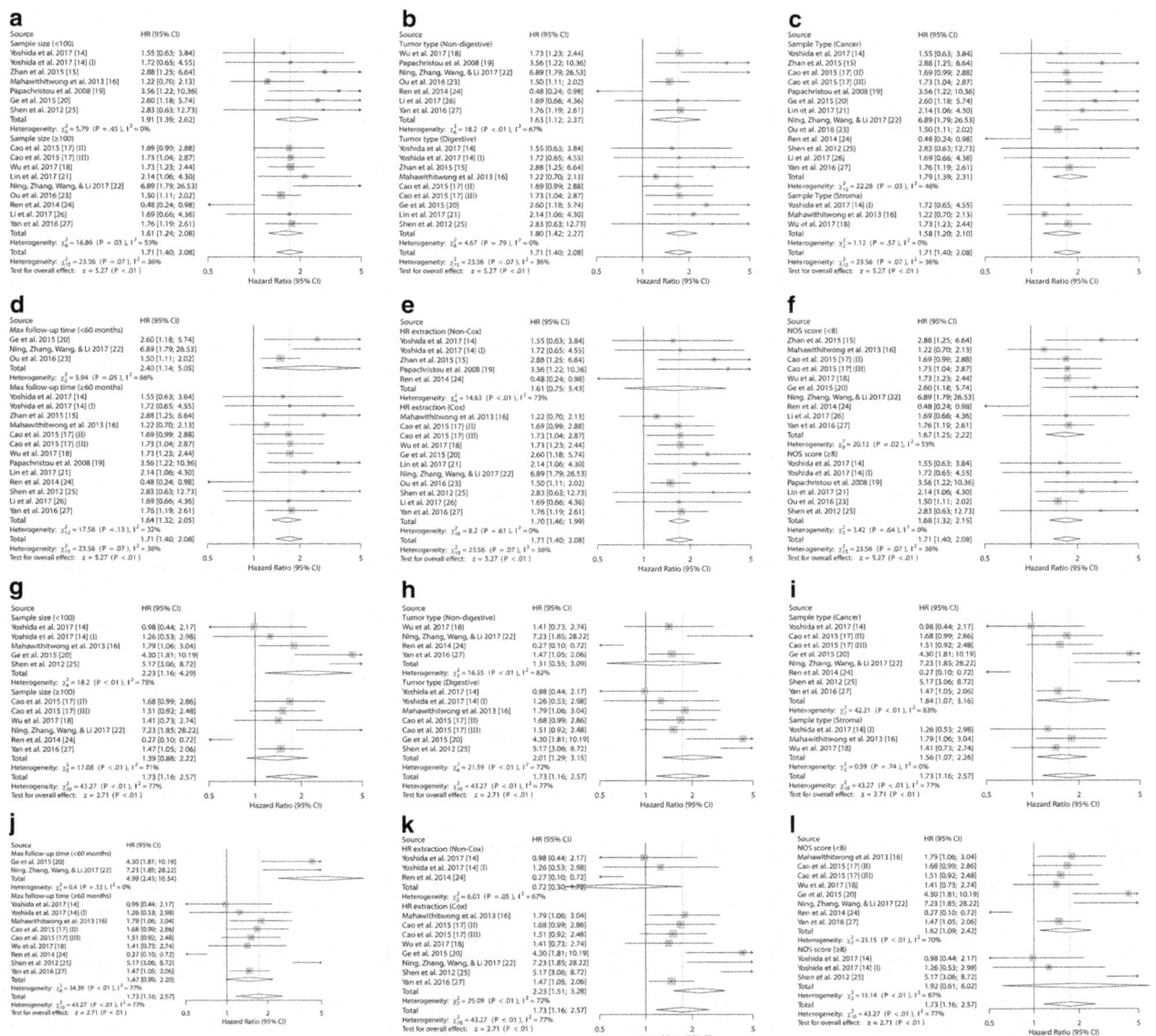

**Fig. 3** Forest plots of study subgroups according to the variables. Survival data were reported as (**a–f**) OS; **g–l** DFS/RFS/PFS. (I) This article (Yoshida [14]) was listed two cohort study because the sample types contain cancer tissue and startle cell. (II) and (III) This article (Cao [17]) included patients from generation dataset (II) and validation dataset (III)

PFS. Taken together, Kindlin-2 expression could serve as a prognostic biomarker, which might help clinicians to make the best choices for cancer patients.

However, the exact mechanism behind the varying correlation of Kindlin-2 and poor prognosis has been not fully investigated. It was reported in previous studies

that Kindlin-2 could be acted as an activator of integrin in the development of cancers [5]. And recent studies demonstrated that Kindlin-2 might exert a significant impact on poor prognosis by mainly modulating integrin signaling pathway and several other related signaling pathways, such as Wnt [21], TGF-β [15], EGFR [38]

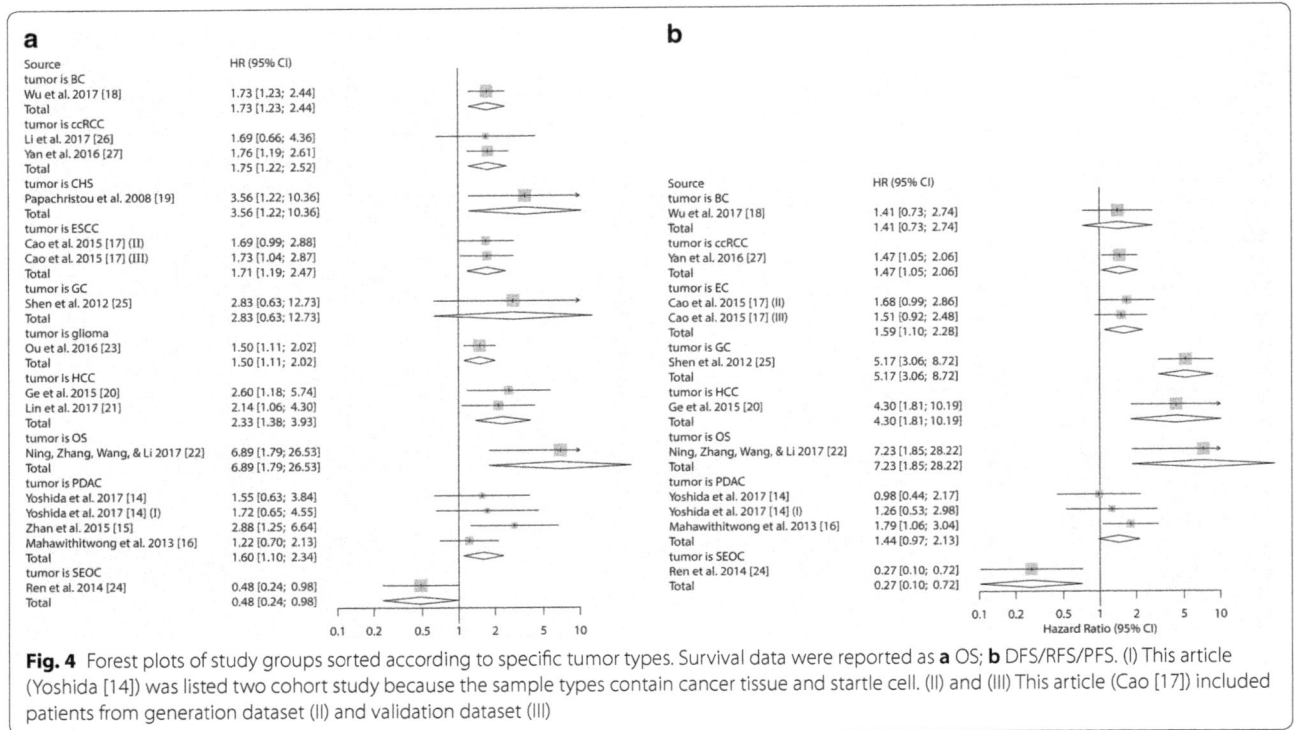

**Fig. 4** Forest plots of study groups sorted according to specific tumor types. Survival data were reported as **a** OS; **b** DFS/RFS/PFS. (I) This article (Yoshida [14]) was listed two cohort study because the sample types contain cancer tissue and startle cell. (II) and (III) This article (Cao [17]) included patients from generation dataset (II) and validation dataset (III)

and miR-200b [39]. These pathways were highly related with cell proliferation, migration, invasion [23, 38, 40], vascular function [41] and epithelial-to-mesenchymal transition (EMT) program [42], which might result in the poor prognosis of patients with solid tumor. Given that integrin regulates a variety of cell functions in cancer cell, e.g. PDAC [43], inhibition of integrin signaling might be more efficient than direct inhibition of integrin. Then Kindlin-2, an essential activator of integrin, might be a promising target, which is supported by our result and a previous study reporting that several hallmarks of PDAC cell in vitro were inhabited when Kindlin-2 was stably down-regulated [15]. Previous research also concluded that embryonic dermal origins could influence the expression level of Kindlin-2 in various organs [44]. It implied that varying prognostic value of Kindlin-2 might be dependent on tumors' embryonic dermal origins. In summary, high Kindlin-2 expression might indicate poor outcome in cancer patients and might be a promising therapeutic target for solid tumor.

Certainly, there were some limitations in our meta-analysis study. First, overall impact of Kindlin-2

expression on DFS/RFS/PFS was still inconclusive. Future study is needed to explore whether it is more accurate in predicting prognosis. Second, the number of studies for each specific tumor type there was limited. Third, the method we applied for extracting HR from KM plot was not as precise as the original study. Cut-off values of some key variables also differed among these studies. Potential heterogeneity might generate bias in the overall result. Hence, more studies with high quality are necessary for precisely illustrating the correlation between Kindlin-2 expression and prognosis of patients with various solid tumors.

## Conclusions

In conclusion, our results demonstrated that Kindlin-2 expression had a significant correlation with prognostic outcomes of patients with different solid tumors. Elevated expression level of Kindlin-2 was significantly associated with a poor prognosis in patients with PDAC (DFS/RFS/PFS), ESCC (OS, DFS/RFS/PFS), HCC (OS), ccRCC (OS), BC (OS, DFS/RFS/PFS), CHS (OS), OSS (OS), GC (DFS/RFS/PFS) and glioma (OS), but not

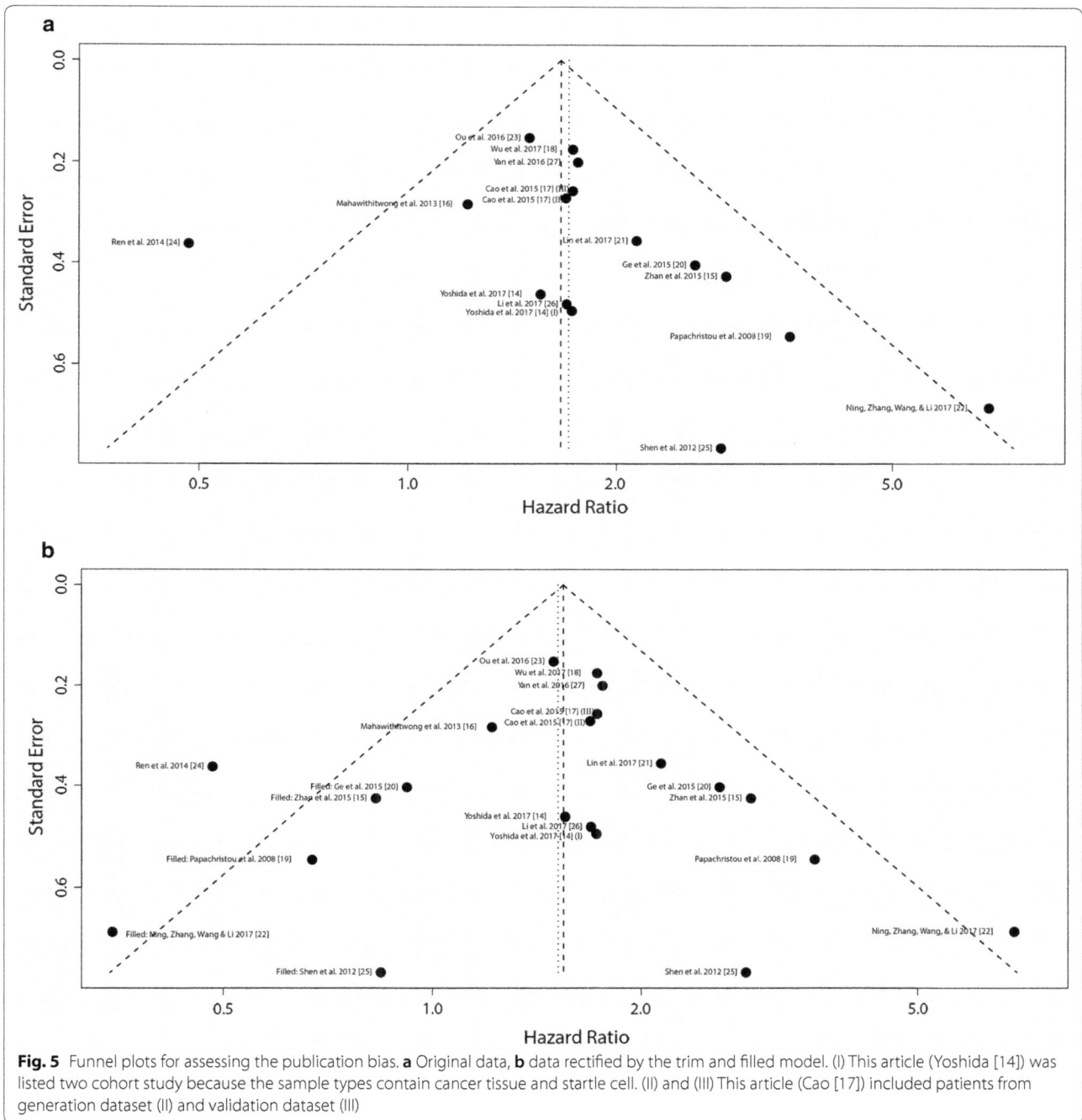

**Fig. 5** Funnel plots for assessing the publication bias. **a** Original data, **b** data rectified by the trim and filled model. (I) This article (Yoshida [14]) was listed two cohort study because the sample types contain cancer tissue and startle cell. (II) and (III) This article (Cao [17]) included patients from generation dataset (II) and validation dataset (III)

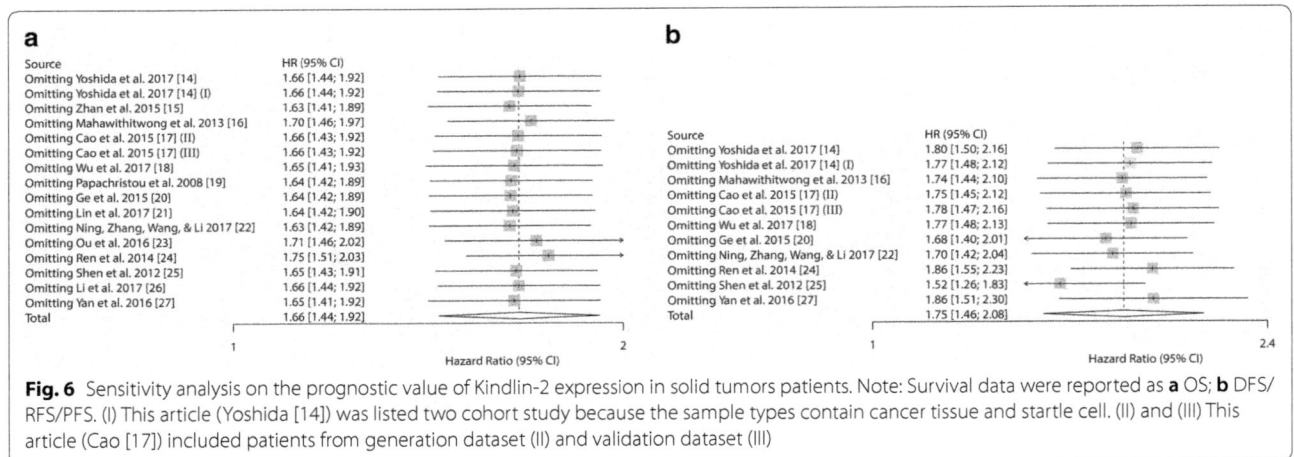

**Fig. 6** Sensitivity analysis on the prognostic value of Kindlin-2 expression in solid tumors patients. Note: Survival data were reported as **a** OS; **b** DFS/RFS/PFS. (I) This article (Yoshida [14]) was listed two cohort study because the sample types contain cancer tissue and startle cell. (II) and (III) This article (Cao [17]) included patients from generation dataset (II) and validation dataset (III)

PDAC (OS), GC (OS), sEOC (OS, DFS/RFS/PFS). More researches are warranted for accurately clarifying the association between Kindlin-2 expression and prognosis of solid cancer patients.

### Abbreviations

HR: hazard ratio; CI: confidence interval; OS: overall survival; DFS: disease-free survival; RFS: recurrence-free survival; PFS: progression-free survival; FERM: 4.1-ezrin-radixin-moesin; ILK: integrin-linked kinase; TGF-β: transforming growth factor β; EGFR: epidermal growth factor receptor; ERK: extracellular regulated protein kinases; KM: Kaplan–Meier; PDAC: pancreatic ductal adenocarcinoma; ESCC: esophageal squamous cell carcinoma; BC: bladder cancer; CHS: chondrosarcoma; HCC: hepatocellular carcinoma; OSS: osteosarcoma; sEOC: serous epithelial ovarian cancers; GC: gastric cancer; ccRCC: clear cell renal cell carcinoma; IHC: immunohistochemistry; WB: Western Blot; MIG-2: mitogen inducible gene-2; EMT: epithelial-to-mesenchymal transition.

### Authors' contributions

SL and SC collected, extracted and analyzed the data, wrote the paper; KGM and ZWS performed quality assessment and analyzed the data. ZWS conceived and designed this study. All authors reviewed the final manuscript. All authors read and approved the final manuscript.

### Acknowledgements

We would like to thank the researchers and study participants for their contributions.

### Competing interests

The authors declare that they have no competing interests.

### Funding

This study was supported by Grants 2016YFC1100100 from The National Key Research and Development Program of China, Grants 91649204 from Major Research Plan of National Natural Science Foundation of China.

### References

1. Torre LA, Bray F, Siegel RL, Ferlay J, Lortet-Tieulent J, Jemal A. Global cancer statistics, 2012. CA Cancer J Clin. 2015;65(2):87–108.

2. Siegel RL, Miller KD, Jemal A. Cancer statistics, 2018. CA Cancer J Clin. 2018;68(1):7–30.

3. Haberlin C, O'Dwyer T, Mockler D, Moran J, O'Donnell DM, Broderick J. The use of eHealth to promote physical activity in cancer survivors: a systematic review. Support Care Cancer. 2018;26:3323–36.

4. Hu B, Fan H, Lv X, Chen S, Shao Z. Prognostic significance of CXCL5 expression in cancer patients: a meta-analysis. Cancer Cell Int. 2018;18:68.

5. Rognoni E, Ruppert R, Fassler R. The kindlin family: functions, signaling properties and implications for human disease. J Cell Sci. 2016;129(1):17–27.

6. Meves A, Stremmel C, Gottschalk K, Fassler R. The Kindlin protein family: new members to the club of focal adhesion proteins. Trends Cell Biol. 2009;19(10):504–13.

7. Siegel DH, Ashton GH, Penagos HG, Lee JV, Feiler HS, Wilhelmsen KC, South AP, Smith FJ, Prescott AR, Wessagowit V, et al. Loss of kindlin-1, a human homolog of the Caenorhabditis elegans actin-extracellular-matrix linker protein UNC-112, causes Kindler syndrome. Am J Hum Genet. 2003;73(1):174–87.

8. Canning CA, Chan JS, Common JE, Lane EB, Jones CM. Developmental expression of the fermitin/kindlin gene family in Xenopus laevis embryos. Dev Dyn. 2011;240(8):1958–63.

9. Mory A, Feigelson SW, Yarali N, Kilic SS, Bayhan GI, Gershoni-Baruch R, Etzioni A, Alon R. Kindlin-3: a new gene involved in the pathogenesis of LAD-III. Blood. 2008;112(6):2591.

10. Ussar S, Wang HV, Linder S, Fassler R, Moser M. The Kindlins: subcellular localization and expression during murine development. Exp Cell Res. 2006;312(16):3142–51.

11. Harburger DS, Bouaouina M, Calderwood DA. Kindlin-1 and -2 directly bind the C-terminal region of beta integrin cytoplasmic tails and exert integrin-specific activation effects. J Biol Chem. 2009;284(17):11485–97.

12. Moser M, Legate KR, Zent R, Fassler R. The tail of integrins, talin, and kindlins. Science. 2009;324(5929):895–9.

13. Zhan J, Zhang H. Kindlins: roles in development and cancer progression. Int J Biochem Cell Biol. 2018;98:93–103.

14. Yoshida N, Masamune A, Hamada S, Kikuta K, Takikawa T, Motoi F, Unno M, Shimosegawa T. Kindlin-2 in pancreatic stellate cells promotes the progression of pancreatic cancer. Cancer Lett. 2017;390:103–14.

15. Zhan J, Song J, Wang P, Chi X, Wang Y, Guo Y, Fang W, Zhang H. Kindlin-2 induced by TGF-beta signaling promotes pancreatic ductal adenocarcinoma progression through downregulation of transcriptional factor HOXB9. Cancer Lett. 2015;361(1):75–85.

16. Mahawithitwong P, Ohuchida K, Ikenaga N, Fujita H, Zhao M, Kozono S, Shindo K, Ohtsuka T, Mizumoto K, Tanaka M. Kindlin-2 expression in peritumoral stroma is associated with poor prognosis in pancreatic ductal adenocarcinoma. Pancreas. 2013;42(4):663–9.

17. Cao HH, Zhang SY, Shen JH, Wu ZY, Wu JY, Wang SH, Li EM, Xu LY. A three-protein signature and clinical outcome in esophageal squamous cell carcinoma. Oncotarget. 2015;6(7):5435–48.

18. Wu J, Yu C, Cai L, Lu Y, Jiang L, Liu C, Li Y, Feng F, Gao Z, Zhu Z, et al. Effects of increased Kindlin-2 expression in bladder cancer stromal fibroblasts. Oncotarget. 2017;8(31):50692–703.

19. Papachristou DJ, Gkretsi V, Rao UN, Papachristou GI, Papaefthymiou OA, Basdra EK, Wu C, Papavassiliou AG. Expression of integrin-linked kinase and its binding partners in chondrosarcoma: association with prognostic significance. Eur J Cancer. 2008;44(16):2518–25.

20. Ge YS, Liu D, Jia WD, Li JS, Ma JL, Yu JH, Xu GL. Kindlin-2: a novel prognostic biomarker for patients with hepatocellular carcinoma. Pathol Res Pract. 2015;211(3):198–202.

21. Lin J, Lin W, Ye Y, Wang L, Chen X, Zang S, Huang A. Kindlin-2 promotes hepatocellular carcinoma invasion and metastasis by increasing Wnt/beta-catenin signaling. J Exp Clin Cancer Res. 2017;36(1):134.

22. Ning K, Zhang H, Wang Z, Li K. Prognostic implications of Kindlin proteins in human osteosarcoma. OncoTargets Ther. 2017;10:657–65.

23. Ou Y, Zhao Z, Zhang W, Wu Q, Wu C, Liu X, Fu M, Ji N, Wang D, Qiu J, et al. Kindlin-2 interacts with beta-catenin and YB-1 to enhance EGFR transcription during glioma progression. Oncotarget. 2016;7(46):74872–85.

24. Ren C, Du J, Xi C, Yu Y, Hu A, Zhan J, Guo H, Fang W, Liu C, Zhang H. Kindlin-2 inhibits serous epithelial ovarian cancer peritoneal dissemination and predicts patient outcomes. Biochem Biophys Res Commun. 2014;446(1):187–94.

25. Shen Z, Ye Y, Dong L, Vainionpaa S, Mustonen H, Puolakkainen P, Wang S. Kindlin-2: a novel adhesion protein related to tumor invasion, lymph node metastasis, and patient outcome in gastric cancer. Am J Surg. 2012;203(2):222–9.

26. Li M, Pei X, Wang G, Zhan J, Du J, Jiang H, Tang Y, Zhang H, He H. Kindlin 2 promotes clear cell renal cell carcinoma progression through the Wnt signaling pathway. Oncol Rep. 2017;38(3):1551–60.

27. Yan M, Zhang L, Wu Y, Gao L, Yang W, Li J, Chen Y, Jin X. Increased expression of kindlin-2 is correlated with hematogenous metastasis and poor prognosis in patients with clear cell renal cell carcinoma. FEBS Open Bio. 2016;6(7):660–5.

28. Lu F, Zhang YQ, Guo XJ, Qian XL, Li YQ, Fu L. Expression of integrin beta1 and Kindlin-2 in invasive micropapillary carcinoma of the breast. Chin J Cancer Prev Treat. 2015;22(12):929–35.

29. Ren Y, Jin H, Xue Z, Xu Q, Wang S, Zhao G, Huang J, Huang H. Kindlin-2 inhibited the growth and migration of colorectal cancer cells. Tumour Biol. 2015;36(6):4107–14.

30. Moher D, Liberati A, Tetzlaff J, Altman DG, Group P. Preferred reporting items for systematic reviews and meta-analyses: the PRISMA statement. Open Med. 2009;3(3):e123–30.

31. Mark Mitchell BM, Tobias Winchen, Zbigniew Jędrzejewski-Szmek, The Gitter Badger, & badshah400. markummitchell/engauge-digitizer: Version 10.4 Display and Export Enhancements (Version v10.4) Zenodo. 2017. https://doi.org/10.5281/zenodo.1006837.

32. Tierney JF, Stewart LA, Ghersi D, Burdett S, Sydes MR. Practical methods for incorporating summary time-to-event data into meta-analysis. Trials. 2007;8:16.

33. Team RC. R: a language and environment for statistical computing. R Foundation for Statistical Computing; 2018. https://www.R-project.org. Accessed 15 June 2018.

34. Schwarzer G. meta: an R package for meta-analysis. R News. 2007;7(3):40–5.

35. Viechtbauer W. Conducting meta-analyses in R with the metafor package. J Stat Softw. 2010;36(3):1–48.

36. Wick M, Burger C, Brusselbach S, Lucibello FC, Muller R. Identification of serum-inducible genes: different patterns of gene regulation during G0 → S and G1 → S progression. J Cell Sci. 1994;107(Pt 3):227–39 (preceding table of contents).

37. Shi X, Wu C. A suppressive role of mitogen inducible gene-2 in mesenchymal cancer cell invasion. Mol Cancer Res. 2008;6(5):715–24.

38. Guo B, Gao J, Zhan J, Zhang H. Kindlin-2 interacts with and stabilizes EGFR and is required for EGF-induced breast cancer cell migration. Cancer Lett. 2015;361(2):271–81.

39. Yu Y, Wu J, Guan L, Qi L, Tang Y, Ma B, Zhan J, Wang Y, Fang W, Zhang H. Kindlin 2 promotes breast cancer invasion via epigenetic silencing of the microRNA200 gene family. Int J Cancer. 2013;133(6):1368–79.

40. Wu X, Liu W, Jiang H, Chen J, Wang J, Zhu R, Li B. Kindlin-2 siRNA inhibits vascular smooth muscle cell proliferation, migration and intimal hyperplasia via Wnt signaling. Int J Mol Med. 2016;37(2):436–44.

41. Malinin NL, Pluskota E, Byzova TV. Integrin signaling in vascular function. Curr Opin Hematol. 2012;19(3):206–11.

42. Sossey-Alaoui K, Pluskota E, Szpak D, Schiemann WP, Plow EF. The Kindlin-2 regulation of epithelial-to-mesenchymal transition in breast cancer metastasis is mediated through miR-200b. Sci Rep. 2018;8(1):7360.

43. Grzesiak JJ, Ho JC, Moossa AR, Bouvet M. The integrin-extracellular matrix axis in pancreatic cancer. Pancreas. 2007;35(4):293–301.

44. Zhan J, Yang M, Chi X, Zhang J, Pei X, Ren C, Guo Y, Liu W, Zhang H. Kindlin-2 expression in adult tissues correlates with their embryonic origins. Sci China Life Sci. 2014;57(7):690–7.

# 17

# Identification of RPL5 and RPL10 as novel diagnostic biomarkers of Atypical teratoid/rhabdoid tumors

Yanming Ren[1†], Chuanyuan Tao[1†], Xiliang Wang[2] and Yan Ju[1*] (ID)

## Abstract

**Background:** Rhabdoid tumors (RTs) are aggressive tumors that occur most frequently in children under 2 years old, which often invade kidney (KRTs) and Center Nervous System, named Atypical teratoid/rhabdoid tumors (AT/RTs). RTs often progress fast and lead to a high lethality. RTs have a low incidence, we can hardly accumulate enough samples to elicit the diagnosis. More importantly, histologically, RTs present a host of neural, epithelial, mesenchymal, or ependymal patterns, which makes them rather variable and difficult to diagnose. Molecularly, RTs are diagnosed mainly on the lack of SMARCB1/INI1 protein expression, which, on the one hand, accounts for 75% of RTs, on the other hand, loss of expression of SMARCB1 is not exclusive to RTs. So, there is a need to find more accurate diagnose markers of RTs.

**Methods:** In this study, we analyzed 109 samples including AT/RT, KRT and corresponding normal samples downloaded form NCBI GEO database. First, we identified the differentially expressed lncRNAs and PCGs in AT/RT, KRT and corresponding normal samples. Second, we evaluated the co-expression relationship between lncRNA and PCG, and defined four types of the dysregulated PCG-lncRNA pairs. Third, we compared the differentially expressed genes, the dysregulated PCG-lncRNA pairs and commonly known cancer genes, we get potential diagnostic markers. Then, the potential diagnostic markers were subjected to Receiver operating characteristic (ROC) analysis to assess the diagnostic accuracy. Importantly, differential expression of the marker genes in different tumors was shown to distinguish AT/RT and KRT from other pediatric tumors specifically.

**Results:** We compared the expression profiles between 47 AT/RTs, 31 KRTs, 8 normal brain samples, and 23 normal kidney samples. After applying a stringent set of criteria on the gene expression profiles, we identified 3667 PCGs and 81 lncRNAs differentially expressed in AT/RT, 3809 PCGs and 34 lncRNAs differentially expressed in KRT tissues. Next, we compared the three sets(AT/RT versus control brain samples, KRT versus control kidney samples, and AT/RT versus KRT) of differentially expressed lncRNAs and PCGs, 491 PCGs and 2 lncRNAs appeared in all three sets. We examined the correlation of the expression levels of these genes in the 'three-set overlap' group and identified four types of dysregulated lncRNAs and PCGs. By compared these genes to the well-known cancer driver genes, 19 PCGs were selected as potential candidates of diagnostic markers. Filtered with the number of the corresponding co-expressed lncRNA (namely "degree"), eight PCGs with more than five lncRNAs in the 'three-set overlap' group were selected as candidate diagnostic markers. Among them, RPL5 and RPL10 exhibited high sensitivity and specificity in diagnosis of AT/RT and KRT. However, when these two genes were used to distinguish AT/RT and KRT from other pediatric tumors, only AT/RT can be distinguished from medulloblastoma.

*Correspondence: jvyan@scu.edu.cn
†Yanming Ren and Chuanyuan Tao contribute equally to this paper
[1] Department of Neurosurgery, West China Hospital of Sichuan University, No. 37 Guo Xue Xiang, Chengdu, Sichuan, China
Full list of author information is available at the end of the article

**Conclusions:** Our study mined existing GEO datasets for novel diagnostic markers associated with Rhabdoid tumors, and identified RPL5 and RPL10 as potential diagnostic markers for AT/RT. These two biomarkers may be used as supplementary biomarkers to canonical diagnostic tools such as biopsy and immunohistochemistry.

**Keywords:** Atypical teratoid/rhabdoid tumors, Kidney rhabdoid tumors diagnosis, Bioinformatics, Dysregulation, Biomarker

## Background

Rhabdoid tumors (RTs) are aggressive tumors that occur most frequently in children under 2 years old. RTs often occur in the kidney (KRTs) or the central nervous system (CNS), which are termed Atypical teratoid/rhabdoid tumors (AT/RTs). Extracranial RTs were first recognized as a physiological entity nearly 40 years ago [1]. Later, Haas and colleagues introduced the term rhabdoid in describing KRT, due to the close histological resemblance of the tumor cells to rhabdomyoblasts, although subsequent studies have not confirmed a myogenic origin of these tumor cells [2]. In 1987, AT/RT was recognized as a discrete clinical entity based on pathologic and genetic characteristics [3]. Prior to that, it had been mostly classified as either medulloblastoma, primitive neuroectodermal tumor, or choroid plexus carcinoma. Following this description, the World Health Organization (WHO) began to classify AT/RT as an embryonal grade IV neoplasm in 1993 [4].

Epidemiologic studies of RT have been limited by the fact that this is a rare disease. So far there have been only a handful of epidemiologic reports. In a study conducted in the UK, 106 children under 15 years old were diagnosed with extracranial RT in the UK between in a period of nearly 20 years [5], resulting in an age-standardized annual incidence of 0.6 per 1 million children. In the US, several studies observed that AT/RT accounted for 1–2% in pediatric brain tumors, and for 4.4% of CNS tumors in children aged zero to 5 years [6–9]. Two more recent surveys conducted in China draw consistent results of a prevalence of AT/RT at approximately 5% in pediatric CNS tumors, which is comparable to that in the US study.

Aside from low incidence rate, there are other factors that poses challenges to the diagnosis and treatment of RTs. Histologically, RTs manifest several characteristic features, including eosinophilic cytoplasm, large nucleoli, and filamentous cytoplasmic inclusions. The tumors may present a host of neural, epithelial, mesenchymal, or ependymal patterns, which makes them rather variable and difficult to diagnose [10]. Moreover, RTs often progress fast and lead to a high lethality. In the UK study of extracranial RT, 1-year survival was 31% [5]. The patients usually suffers from metastasis and, to make things worse, the young age of patients limits use of radiotherapy. In an early report of 22 cases of KRTs in children, metastases were found in 82% of cases, either at diagnosis, or developing from 2 weeks to 9 months after diagnosis. Only two patients eventually survived, both with localized disease (stage II) [11]. Therefore, early diagnosis of this formidable disease is of key importance and in urgent demand.

Currently RTs are diagnosed mainly on immunohistochemistry (IHC) results, specifically, the lack of SMARCB1/INI1 protein expression, or less frequently, that of SMARCA4/BRG1 protein expression [4]. Initial genetic studies suggested that approximately 75% of RTs are characterized by biallelic inactivation of the SMARCB1 locus, which indicated a sensitivity of close to 75% [12]. However, loss of expression of SMARCB1 is not exclusive to RTs, but also has been observed in other types of cancers, including chordoma, epithelioid sarcoma, cribriform neuroepithelial tumor, and medullary renal cell carcinoma [13–19]. Together, these lines of evidence suggest that SMARCB1 expression alone is neither sufficiently sensitive nor specific for diagnosing RTs. Moreover, in particular for CNS AT/RTs, another severe limitation in clinical diagnosis is the potential misdiagnosis as medulloblastomas (MBs) or primitive neuroectodermal tumors (PNETs), owing to the close histological resemblance of the rhabdoid cells and neuroepithelial tissue in these tumors [3, 20]. In conclusion, diagnostic markers with improved sensitivity and specificity are needed to complement the current practice, to the end of developing a comprehensive diagnostic strategy with enhanced sensitivity and precision.

In this study, we set out to identify diagnostic markers for RTs by employing a molecular profiling approach. Protein coding genes (PCGs) and long non-coding RNAs (lncRNAs) showing aberrant expression in AT/RT and KRT cases were identified, respectively, and the co-expression between these significantly dysregulated genes was evaluated. Through further comparison of differentially expressed genes, the dysregulated PCG-lncRNA pairs, and commonly known cancer genes, candidate diagnostic markers for AT/RT were identified and subjected to Receiver Operating Characteristic analysis to assess the performance of these candidates. Two PCGs, RPL5 and PRL10, exhibited high sensitivity and specificity not only in diagnosis of AT/RT but also differential diagnosis of AT/RT and KRT, as therefore show considerable promise for AT/RT diagnosis, and warrants further investigation.

## Methods

### Data analysis

The raw data were downloaded from the NCBI GEO database (GSE15641, GSE11482, GSE30946, GSE64019, GSE28026, GSE35493, GSE64019, GSE70421, GSE35493). The limma package was used to deal with the raw data in CEL format, with MAS5 algorithm, to quantify expression level and to identify the difference of gene expression. The biomaRt package was used to convert the probe ID to Ensembl ID. Genes were categorized as "protein coding" and "long non-coding" based on an Ensembl annotation file in the GTF format. Among non-coding genes, rRNAs, tRNAs, miRNAs, snoRNAs and other known classes of RNAs were excluded, and lncRNAs were defined as all non-coding genes longer than 200 nucleotides and not belonging to other RNA categories.

### Pearson's correlation coefficient

Pearson's correlation coefficient (PCC) was calculated by in-house R- scripts and was utilized to evaluate the co-expression relationship between lncRNA and PCG. Co-expressed pairs were defined with a cutoff of $|PCC| \geq 0.7$ and $P < 0.001$.

### Data visualization

Unsupervised hierarchical clustering was done by R software (version 3.3.2, http://www.r-project.org/). The receiver operating characteristic (ROC) and the area under the ROC curves (AUC) values were obtained from the pROC package. Unless otherwise specified, data were analyzed and visualized using R software (version 3.3.2).

### Enrichment analysis

For enrichment analysis to explore their biological effects, PCGs were analyzed using the clusterProfiler package. The GO terms and KEGG pathways with p values or FDR of < 0.05 were considered as significantly enriched function annotations.

### Differential RPL5/10 expression analysis across Affymetrix datasets

We downloaded GSE85217 and GSE2712 from GEO dataset. GSE85217 contains 762 medulloblastoma patients expression data, and GSE2712 contains 18 Wilms' tumors and 14 clear cell sarcoma of the kidney. The former used Affymetrix Human Gene 1.1 ST Array, the latter used Affymetrix Human Genome U133A Array. So in order to make the data comparable, we used the Array Generation based gene Centering (AGC) method to compare the expression value of RPL5/10 between different datasets [21]. The AGC method scaled datasets with a scaling factor that is defined based on the housekeeping genes.

## Results

### Transcriptome expression profiles in AT/RT, KRT and normal samples

We started by comparing the expression profiles between 47 AT/RTs, 31 KRTs, 8 normal brain samples, and 23 normal kidney samples (sample list in Additional file 1: Table S1). Between tumor and normal samples, expression of lncRNAs showed greater level of alteration in AT/RT or KRT (Fig. 1a, b) than that of PCGs (Fig. 1d, e), suggesting a specific expression pattern of lncRNAs in these tumors. However, comparing with KRT, both lncRNAs and PCGs showed weaker changes in expression levels in AT/RT (Fig. 1c, f), suggesting that resemblance in the expression profiles of tumors of RTs and its subtype, AT/RT.

### Differentially expressed lncRNAs and PCGs in AT/RT, KRT and normal samples

After applying a stringent set of criteria on the gene expression profiles, we identified groups of lncRNAs and PCGs differential expressed between tumor and normal tissue samples ($p = 0.00001$ and fold change (FC) = 2 for KRT vs. kidney and AT/RT vs. brain, $p = 0.001$ and fold change = 2 for KRT vs. AT/RT). In total, we identified 3667 PCGs and 81 lncRNAs differentially expressed in AT/RT, with 988 up-regulated and 2679 down-regulated PCGs and 14 up-regulated and 67 down-regulated lncRNAs in the tumor samples (Table 1). Notably, there were more than twice as many down-regulated genes as up-regulated ones. Between KRT and normal samples, 3809 PCGs (1963 up-regulated and 1846 down-regulated) and 34 lncRNAs (14 and 20, respectively) showing aberrant expression in KRT tissues (Table 1). As differentially expressed genes between KRT and AT/RT, 3381 PCGs and 91 lncRNAs showed significantly altered expression levels. Among these genes we identified 2568 up-regulated and 813 down-regulated PCGs along with 59 up-regulated and 32 down-regulated lncRNAs (Table 1). Of note, there were approximately three times as many down-regulated genes as up-regulated ones, suggesting the significance of these genes in differentiating RTs and its subtype AT/RT.

A hierarchical cluster analysis of differentially expressed lncRNAs and PCGs showed that samples derived from AT/RT or KRT were well distinguished from corresponding normal ones based on the expression patterns of these genes (Fig. 2). This clear distinction between tumor and control samples suggests the highly

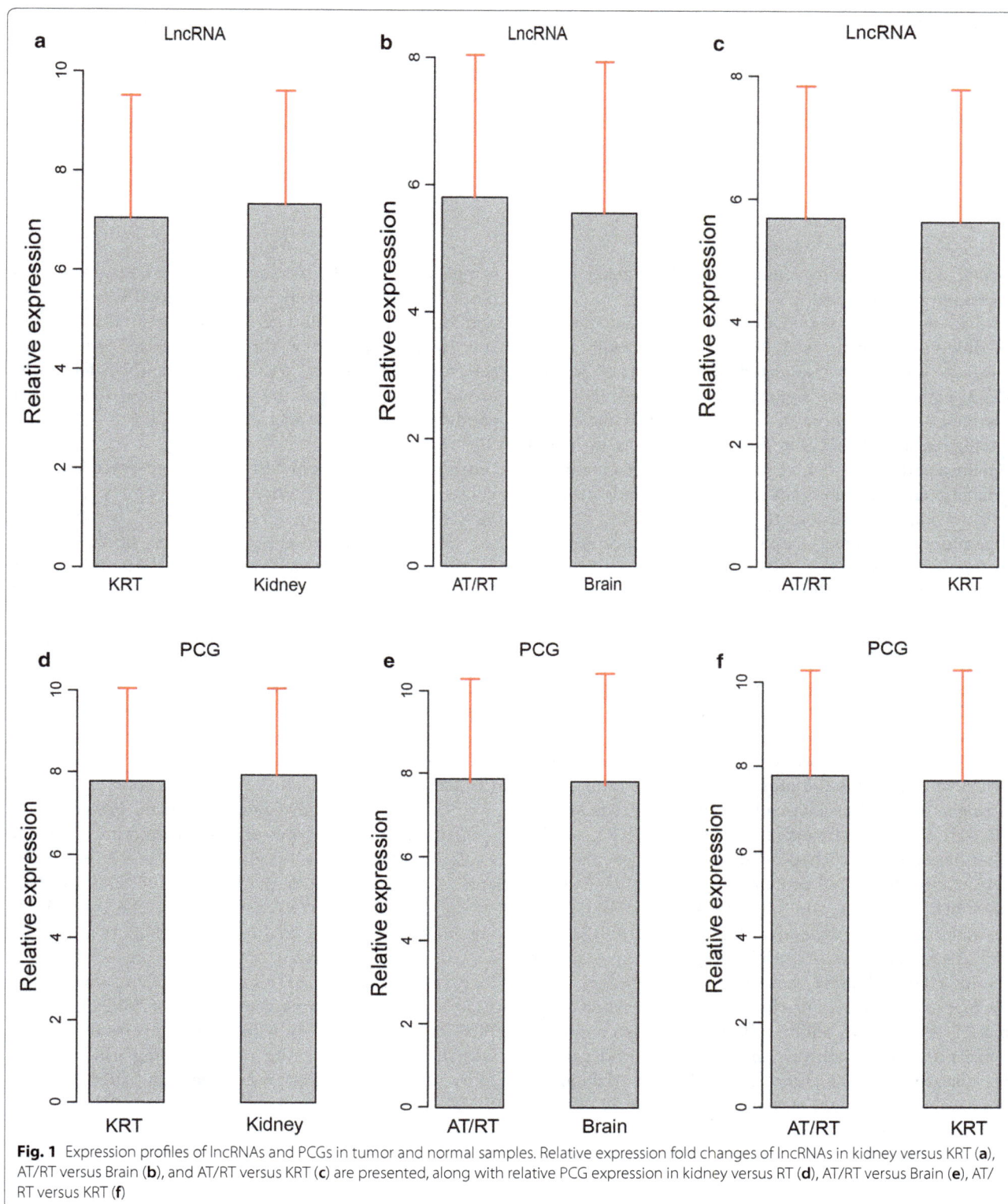

**Fig. 1** Expression profiles of lncRNAs and PCGs in tumor and normal samples. Relative expression fold changes of lncRNAs in kidney versus KRT (**a**), AT/RT versus Brain (**b**), and AT/RT versus KRT (**c**) are presented, along with relative PCG expression in kidney versus RT (**d**), AT/RT versus Brain (**e**), AT/RT versus KRT (**f**)

**Table 1  A summary of differentially expressed lncRNAs and PCGs between AT/RT, KRT and the corresponding normal control samples**

|        | AT/RT vs. Brain | | KRT vs. Kidney | | KRT vs. AT/RT | |
|--------|------|------|------|------|------|------|
|        | Up   | Down | Up   | Down | Up   | Down |
| PCG    | 988  | 2679 | 1963 | 1846 | 2568 | 813  |
| lncRNA | 14   | 67   | 14   | 20   | 59   | 32   |

*AT/RT* atypical teratoid/rhabdoid tumors, *KRT* kidney rhabdoid tumors)

specific nature of the dysregulation of these genes to the corresponding diseases.

Next, we performed pathway enrichment analysis on differentially expressed PCGs to gain insights into pathways potentially implicated in this disease. A total of 72 pathways were significantly enriched (adjusted p value < 0.05). As show in Fig. 3a, many of the differentially expressed PCGs in AR/RT play roles in neural signaling pathways, such as retrograde endocannabinoid signaling (endocannabinoids serve as retrograde messengers at synapses in various regions of the brain [22, 23]), dopaminergic synapse (Dopamine is an important and prototypical slow neurotransmitter in the mammalian brain, where it controls a variety of functions including locomotor activity, motivation and reward, learning and memory, and endocrine regulation [24, 25]), glutamatergic synapse (Glutamate is the major excitatory neurotransmitter in the mammalian central nervous system [26, 27]), "Cholinergic synapse" (Acetylcholine is a neurotransmitter widely distributed in the central nervous system [28, 29]), GABAergic synapse (Gamma aminobutyric acid (GABA) is the most abundant inhibitory neurotransmitter in the mammalian central nervous system [30, 31]). Differentially expression PCGs in KRT, on the other hand, were enriched mainly in processes related to RNA transcription and protein translation, such as RNA transport, ribosome, and spliceosome (Fig. 3b). As for the differentially expressed PCGs between AT/RT and KRT, 19 pathways were enriched significantly (adjusted p value < 0.05). Among these enriched pathways, some overlapped with ones enriched from dysregulated genes in KRT (Fig. 3b). In addition, there were also a considerable number of pathways involved in neurodegenerative diseases, such as Huntington's disease, Alzheimer's disease, and Parkinson's disease (Fig. 3c). As AT/RT and KRT are both subtypes of RT, the overlapping enriched pathways may represent common pathological mechanisms in both subtypes, while the more CNS-specific pathways may be specific to AT/RT.

Next, we compared the three sets of differentially expressed lncRNAs and PCGs, namely those showing significantly different expression levels between AT/RT versus control brain samples, KRT versus control kidney samples, and AT/RT versus KRT. Venn diagrams were plotted for differentially expressed lncRNAs (Fig. 4a) and PCGs (Fig. 4b), and genes that appeared in all three sets (referred to as the 'three-set overlap' group) were selected. A total of 491 PCGs and 2 lncRNAs fell in this group, which served as the pool for further screening of candidate markers for diagnosing AT/RT.

### Dysregulated network of differentially expressed features

Following the identification of differentially expressed lncRNAs and PCGs in AT/RT and KRT, we examined the correlation of the expression levels of these genes in the 'three-set overlap' group. A Pearson's correlation coefficient (PCC) was calculated for the expression levels of each pair of lncRNAs and PCGs across disease states. There were a total of 12,831 PCGs in the microarray profiles (denoted AllPCG in Table 2), among which 491 differentially expressed PCGs (denoted DiffPCG) (Fig. 4b) in all 'three-set overlap' group. Specifically, among these DiffPCGs we focused on the genes reported to be strongly associated with cancer (denoted CancerG). ("cancer genes" were cited from the report of Science [32]; "CancerG" for short, Additional file 2: Figure S1).

We identified four types of dysregulated lncRNAs and PCGs in Table 2. As listed, there were 69236, 18889, and 2773 dysregulated pairs of "AllPCG", "DiffPCG", and "CancerG" in AT/RT, respectively. The overwhelming majority type of the dysregulated pairs was Type I (Table 2) illustrating a massive loss in regulation of lncRNAs to PCGs in AT/RT patients. There were 45175, 13,765, and 1976 dysregulated pairs of "AllPCG", "DiffPCG", and "CancerG" in KRT vs. Kidney, respectively. It was the opposite that the overwhelming majority type of the dysregulated pairs was Type II in "AllPCG", "DiffPCG", and "CancerG", especially in "CancerG" (Table 2). In AT/RT vs. KRT There were 50,862, 7689, and 2011 dysregulated pairs of "AllPCG", "DiffPCG", and "CancerG", respectively, with the majority grouped into Type II (Table 2), showing vast difference of lncRNA dysregulation in AT/RT and KRT. The four types of dysregulated pairs may be one important reason for the aberrance of cancer cells, they may also play important roles in AT/RT or KRT, as well.

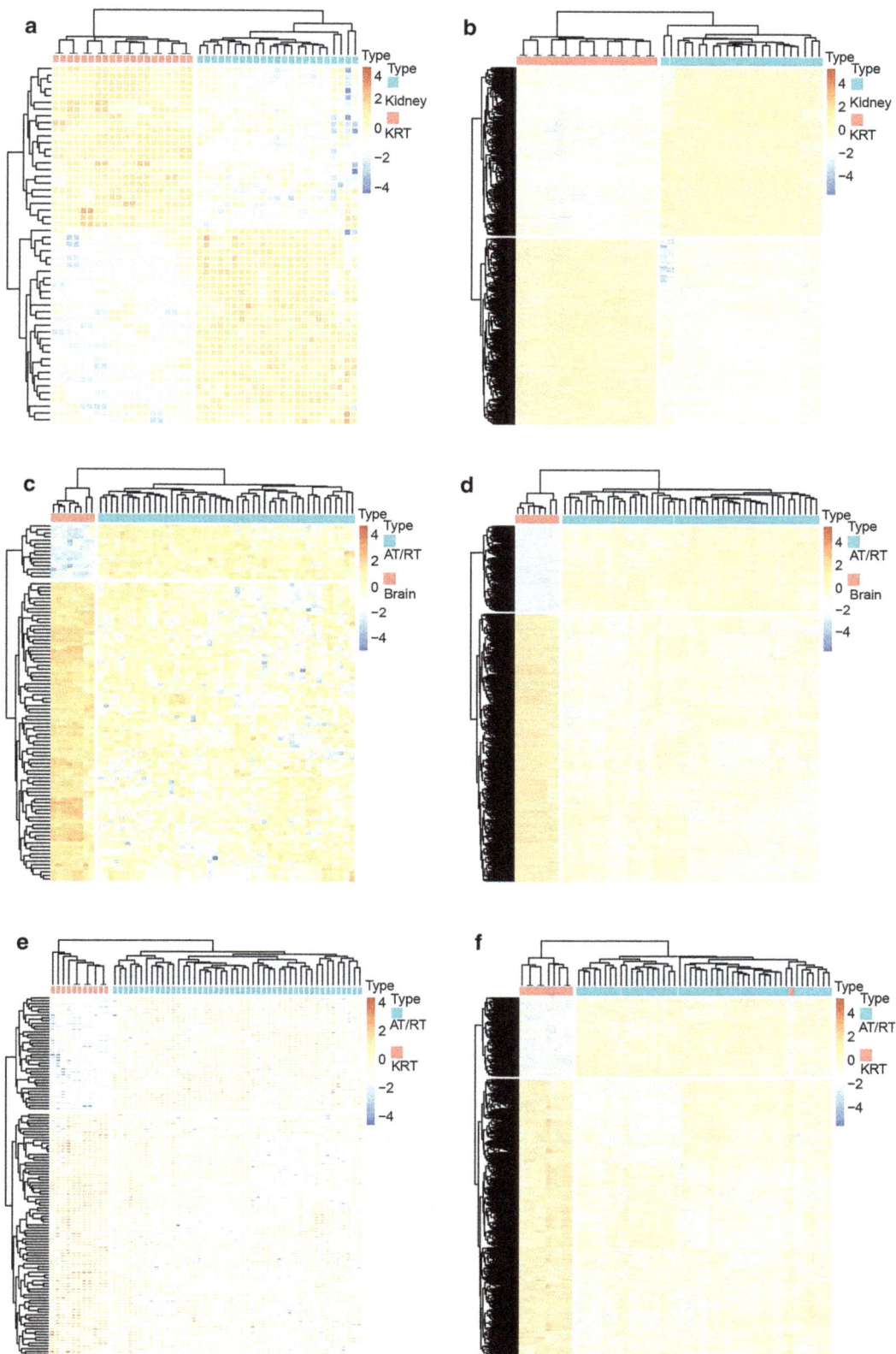

**Fig. 2** Hierarchical clusters of significantly dysregulated lncRNAs and PCGs revealed distinct expression patterns in KRT vs. Kidney (**a**, **b**), AT/RT vs. Brain (**c**, **d**), AT/RT vs. KRT (**e**, **f**)

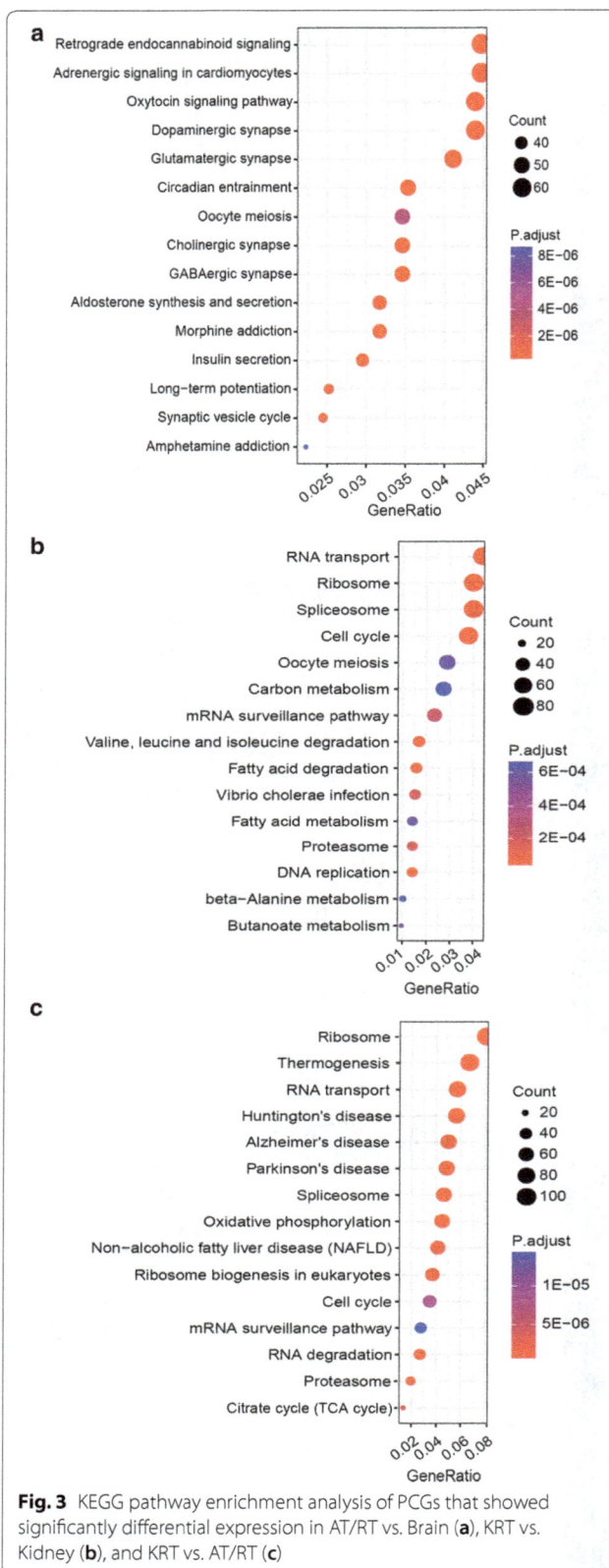

**Fig. 3** KEGG pathway enrichment analysis of PCGs that showed significantly differential expression in AT/RT vs. Brain (**a**), KRT vs. Kidney (**b**), and KRT vs. AT/RT (**c**)

We focused on the "cancer genes" because they have been established to show high relevance in cancer initiation and development. We compared the dysregulated cancer genes in AT/RT vs. Brain, KRT vs. Kidney and AT/RT vs. KRT, there were 268 "cancer genes" dysregulated in all of the 'three-set overlap' group (Fig. 5a). Next, we checked whether those 268 genes were also differentially expressed in the 'three-set overlap' group. After comparing with the 491 DiffPCG (Fig. 4b), 19 PCGs were selected as potential candidates of diagnostic markers (Fig. 5b and Table 3). The dysregulated co-expression pairs were retrieved for these 19 PCGs, and the number of the corresponding co-expressed lncRNA (namely "degree") was showed in Table 4, where a high number is indicative of the complexity of lncRNA regulation to which the corresponding PCG is subjected, and suggests a more central position in the co-expression network. Therefore, eight PCGs with more than five lncRNAs in the 'three-set overlap' group were selected as candidate diagnostic markers, including RPL5, RPL10, NONO, PBRM1, PCM1, PTEN, SF3B1, and ZMYM2. KEGG pathway and Gene Ontology enrichment analysis highlighted ribosome as the main convergence of these aberrantly expressed genes, strongly hinting at a significant role of dysregulation of ribosome-related functions and processes in AT/RT and KRT (Fig. 6).

### Diagnostic values of RPL5 and RPL10 in AT/RT and KRT

To evaluate the performance of the eight candidate markers identified in the last section in diagnosing AT/RT and RT, ROC (Receiver operating characteristic) analysis was performed and the area under curve (AUC) served as the basis for selecting the most sensitive and specific candidates.

Two significantly deregulated cancer-related genes, RPL5 and RPL10, showed outstanding performance in the ROC analysis. As shown in Fig. 7, in KRT versus normal kidney samples, AUC for RPL5 reached 1 (95% CI 1–1), with both sensitivity and specificity level at 1 (Fig. 7a). Also, the AUC of RPL10 reached 0.97 (95% CI 0.924–1), with a sensitivity level of 0.913 and specificity level of 1, respectively (Fig. 7b). Moreover, high levels of diagnostic values were also observed for both genes in AT/RT. AUCs were 0.997 (95% CI 0.99–1) and 0.989 (95% CI 0.969–1) for RPL5 and RPL10, respectively, with sensitivity levels of 0.979 (RPL5) and 0.936 (RPL10), and a specificity level of 1 for both genes (Fig. 7c, d).

More importantly, both genes were powerful indicators for distinguishing AT/RT from KRT. When comparing expression profiles in AT/RT samples with those in KRT samples, AUC for RPL5 was 0.950 (95% CI 0.897–1) with sensitivity and specificity levels of 0.83 and 1, respectively (Fig. 7e). AUC for RPL10 was 0.973 (95% CI 0.933–1)

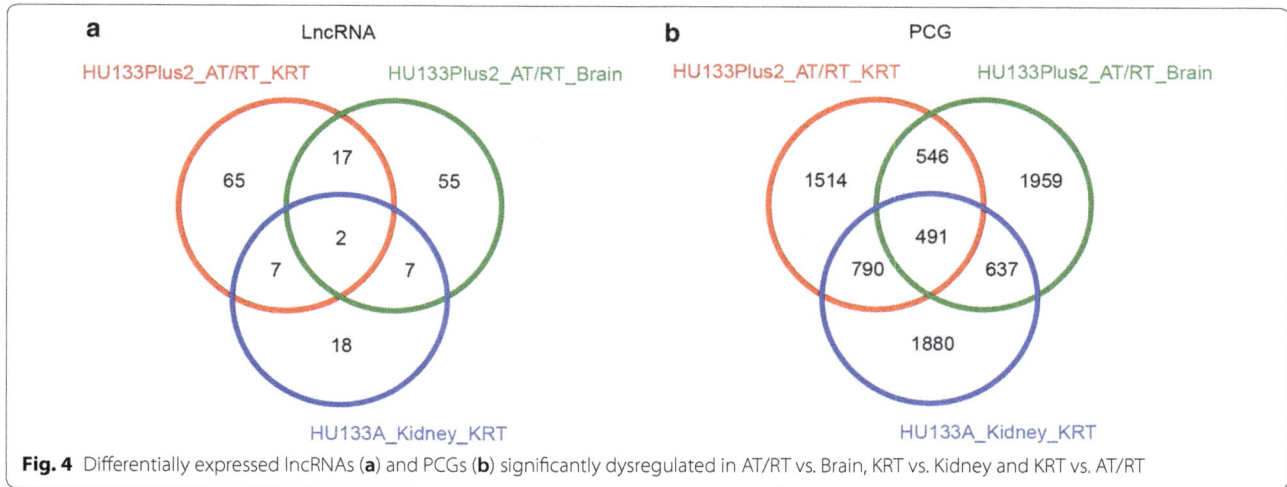

**Fig. 4** Differentially expressed lncRNAs (**a**) and PCGs (**b**) significantly dysregulated in AT/RT vs. Brain, KRT vs. Kidney and KRT vs. AT/RT

**Table 2 Four types of dysregulated pairs of lncRNA-PCG in AT/RT vs. Brain, KRT vs. Kidney and AT/RT vs. KRT**

| AT/RT vs. Brain | | | | | |
|---|---|---|---|---|---|
| Brain | AT/RT | Type | AllPCG | DiffPCG | CancerG |
| Yes | No | I | 66,125 | 18,651 | 2629 |
| No | Yes | II | 3059 | 232 | 138 |
| Positive | Nagetive | III | 16 | 4 | 2 |
| Nagetive | Positive | IV | 36 | 2 | 4 |
| KRT vs. Kidney | | | | | |
| Kidney | KRT | Type | AllPCG | DiffPCG | CancerG |
| Yes | No | I | 16,408 | 6259 | 675 |
| No | Yes | II | 28,350 | 7371 | 1284 |
| Positive | Nagetive | III | 260 | 100 | 12 |
| Nagetive | Positive | IV | 157 | 35 | 5 |
| AT/RT vs. KRT | | | | | |
| AT/RT | KRT | Type | AllPCG | DiffPCG | CancerG |
| Yes | No | I | 5543 | 776 | 263 |
| No | Yes | II | 45,245 | 6908 | 1742 |
| Positive | Nagetive | III | 53 | 2 | 5 |
| Nagetive | Positive | IV | 21 | 3 | 1 |

Co-expressed pair were classified into four types, based on presence and type of regulation of the co-expression in the three sets of comparisons, namely (A) AT/RT vs normal brain samples, (B) KRT vs normal kidney samples, and (C) AT/RT vs KRT samples. Type I: co-expressed pairs that were present in AT/RT (A), KRT (B), and AT/RT (C), and absent in normal brain samples (A), normal kidney samples (B), and KRT(C). Type II: co-expressed pairs that were absent in AT/RT (A), KRT (B), and AT/RT (C), and was present in the corresponding control samples. Type III: co-expression pairs that were positively co-expressed in AT/RT (A), KRT (B), and AT/RT (C) and negatively co-expressed in the corresponding control samples. Type IV: co-expression pairs that were negatively co-expressed in AT/RT (A), KRT (B), and AT/RT (C) and positively co-expressed in the corresponding control samples

and also with high sensitivity (0.957) and specificity (1) (Fig. 7f). In other words, in the samples examined in this analysis, AT/RT and KRT could be accurately diagnosed

based on expression levels of RPL5 and RPL10 (Additional file 3: Figure S2).

**RPL5 and RPL10 can be used to distinguish AT/RT from medulloblastoma**

To evaluate whether RPL5 and RPL10 can be used to distinguish AT/RT and KRT from other tumors, we compared the expression levels of RPL5 and RPL10 in RTs and other types of tumor. Compared with medulloblastoma, RPL5 and RPL10 were signifcantly upregulated in AT/RT, with fold changes of 1.25 and 1.5 (p < 0.001, Fig. 8a, b), respectively. On the other hand, when compared with Wilms' tumor and clear cell sarcoma of the kidney, RPL5 and RPL10 were signifcantly downregulated in KRT (Fig. 8c, d). Together, these results suggest that RPL5 and RPL10 as promising diagnostic markers not only in distinguishing for AT/RT from normal tissues but also in from other types of pediatric tumors.

**Discussion**

Rhabdoid tumors are highly lethal cancers that most frequently observed in young children. Research into the diagnosis and treatment has been hampered by the rare nature of this disease despite its urgency. In a recent study, Chun et al. performed a molecular dissection of Malignant rhabdoid tumors (MRT, mainly KRT) using RNA sequencing [33]. Expression profiles of 40 primary extra-cranial malignant rhabdoid tumors, three human embryonic stem cell lines, and four fetal cerebellum samples were collected and screened for aberrantly expressed genes. Through compare RTs gene expression with genes expressed both in cell lines and fetal cerebellum samples, Author identified 398 up-regulated genes and 615 down-regulated ones. These genes may be used as diagnosis markers of MRT, but this study did not focus on

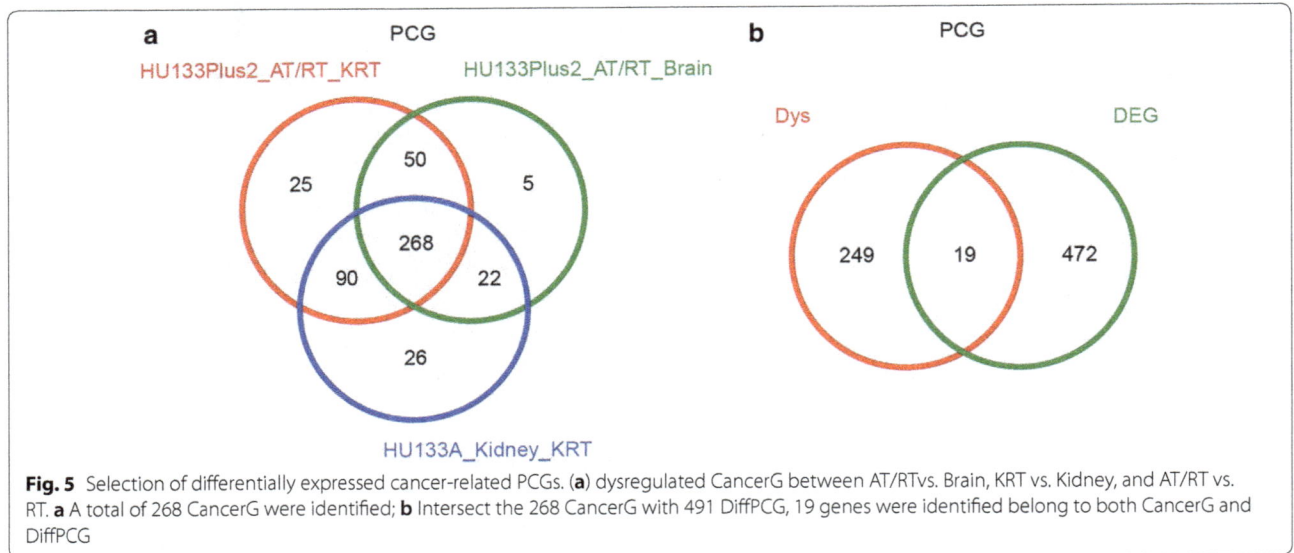

**Fig. 5** Selection of differentially expressed cancer-related PCGs. (**a**) dysregulated CancerG between AT/RTvs. Brain, KRT vs. Kidney, and AT/RT vs. RT. **a** A total of 268 CancerG were identified; **b** Intersect the 268 CancerG with 491 DiffPCG, 19 genes were identified belong to both CancerG and DiffPCG

**Table 3 List of 19 cancer-related PCGs that showed significantly altered expression in AT/RT vs. Brain, KRT vs. Kidney and KRT vs. AT/RT**

| Symbol | Entrezgene |
|--------|-----------|
| ATIC | 471 |
| DDB2 | 1643 |
| FANCA | 2175 |
| GNAS | 2778 |
| NONO | 4841 |
| NPM1 | 4869 |
| PBRM1 | 55,193 |
| PCM1 | 5108 |
| PDE4DIP | 653,513 |
| PTEN | 5728 |
| RPL10 | 6134 |
| RPL22 | 6146 |
| RPL5 | 6125 |
| SF3B1 | 23,451 |
| SMARCE1 | 6605 |
| SRSF3 | 6428 |
| SUZ12 | 23,512 |
| TCF3 | 6929 |
| ZMYM2 | 7750 |

identifying marker candidates for KRT diagnosis. More specifically, similar investigations were conducted in AT/RT over the past few years. Based on patterns in the transcriptional profile, Torchia and colleagues [34] classified AT/RT into three subgroups with distinct genomic profiles, implicated cellular processes, and clinicopathological and survival features. These findings were consistent with those of an independent study [35]. All three

reports, however, focused on the classification and prognosis and AT/RT. Chakravadhanula et al. [36] evaluated the performance of HOTAIR and HOXC as diagnostic markers of AT/RT, however, the authors found that both genes are not sufficient for distinguishing AT/RT from several other forms pediatric brain tumors. In an interesting study, Ho et al. [37] proposed three oncogenes, FGFR2, S100A4 and ERBB2 (HER2/neu), as markers for diagnosing AT/RT, based on the aberrant high expression in tissue samples expressing SMARCB1. Overexpression of these genes may be used as novel markers that complement the current criteria, lack of SMARCB1expression. However, as these results were derived from a limited number of samples, further research is warranted to validate these candidates.

Regulation of PCG expression have been known to occur through a number of mechanisms. Upstream regulators include microRNAs and lncRNAs. In an interesting study into the role of microRNAs in Grupenmacher et al. [38] analyzed the expression profiles of microRNA and PCGs in 13 AT/RT and 10 KRT cases, as well as two human RT cell lines. They found 122 genes significantly differentially expressed between AT/RT and KRT, about 76.22% (93/122) of which down regulated in AT/RT, which was in accordance with our result (Table 1). However, the authors reported a general lack significantly altered expressions in microRNAs between AT/RT and KRT, Therefore, we focused on elucidating the potential of significantly altered lncRNA expression in our investigation, rather than miRNA, as lncRNAs have recently been established as key regulators in cancer. Through identifying differentially expression lncRNAs and constructing lncRNA-PCG co-expression network, 19 PCGs were selected based on co-expression relationship.

**Table 4** The dysregulated co-expression pairs retrieved for the 19 PCGs, and the number of the corresponding co-expressed lncRNA (namely "degree")

| AT/RT vs. KRT | Degree | AT/RT vs. Brain | Degree | KRT vs. Kidney | Degree |
|---|---|---|---|---|---|
| ATIC | 5 | ATIC | 6 | GNAS | 7 |
| FANCA | 7 | GNAS | 13 | NONO | 7 |
| NONO | 7 | NONO | 19 | NPM1 | 10 |
| NPM1 | 11 | PBRM1 | 21 | PBRM1 | 8 |
| PBRM1 | 6 | PCM1 | 6 | PCM1 | 13 |
| PCM1 | 8 | PDE4DIP | 11 | PTEN | 11 |
| PDE4DIP | 9 | PTEN | 15 | RPL10 | 11 |
| PTEN | 13 | RPL10 | 9 | RPL22 | 12 |
| RPL10 | 7 | RPL5 | 6 | RPL5 | 14 |
| RPL5 | 8 | SF3B1 | 26 | SF3B1 | 12 |
| SF3B1 | 13 | SUZ12 | 21 | SRSF3 | 5 |
| SMARCE1 | 5 | ZMYM2 | 26 | TCF3 | 7 |
| SRSF3 | 6 | RPL22 | 4 | ZMYM2 | 12 |
| SUZ12 | 5 | NPM1 | 3 | DDB2 | 3 |
| TCF3 | 8 | DDB2 | 2 | PDE4DIP | 3 |
| ZMYM2 | 13 | SRSF3 | 2 | SMARCE1 | 3 |
| RPL22 | 4 | TCF3 | 2 | SUZ12 | 2 |
| GNAS | 2 | FANCA | 1 | ATIC | 1 |
| DDB2 | 1 | SMARCE1 | 1 | FANCA | 1 |

Further screening, based on numbers of co-expressing lncRNAs, provided a final list of eight candidate markers.

Both *RPL5* and *RPL10* encode members of the 60S subunit of the ribosome [39, 40]. The protein expression of both genes is relative low in the normal brain [41]. RPL5 binds 5S rRNA and forms a stable complex, the 5S ribonucleo protein particle, which is necessary for the 5S rRNA transport, where cytoplasmic 5S rRNA is transported to the nucleolus to be assembled into ribosomes. RPL5 may inhibit tumorigenesis through the activation of downstream tumor suppressors and the down-regulation of oncoprotein expression. A study showed that impaired ribosomes induce a p53-dependent cell cycle arrest [42]. RPL5 has also been reported to play tumor suppressor roles in breast tumors [43].

The functions and significance of RPL10 is largely unknown so far. Existing literature mainly focused on its association with autism and is still in debate [44, 45].

There is one report implicating RPL10 in T cell acute lymphoblastic leukemia (T-ALLs). Exome sequencing analysis identified mutation of RPL5 and RPL10 in 12 of 122 (9.8%) pediatric T-ALLs, with a recurrent mutation of Arg98 in RPL10 [46]. Together, these studies point to a potential role of RPL5 and RPL10 in tumorigenesis, although the relevance of both genes in the KRT and AR/RT has not been elucidated.

In this study, we examined the transcriptome profiles to identify novel prognostic markers for RTs, a rare, lethal, mostly pediatric cancer. After identifying differentially expressed lncRNAs and PCGs, we found intense dysregulation in lncRNA-PCG co-expressed pairs in AT/RT and KRT. Among the key cancer-related PCGs in the co-expression network, RPL5 and RPL10 showed high levels of sensitivity and specificity AT/RT and KRT. After comparison with other common pediatric tumors, RPL5 and RPL10 can also be used to distinguish AT/RT from

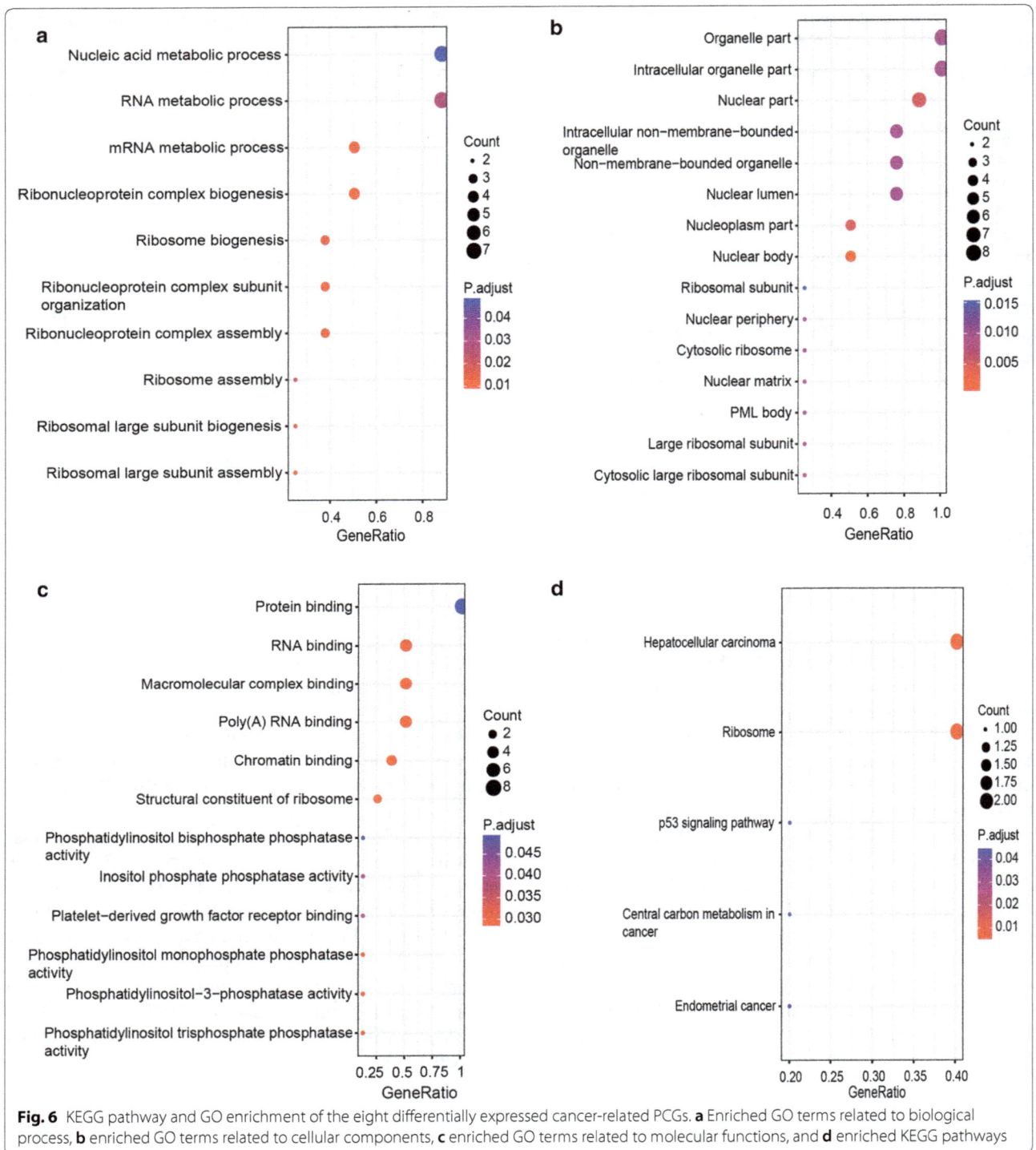

**Fig. 6** KEGG pathway and GO enrichment of the eight differentially expressed cancer-related PCGs. **a** Enriched GO terms related to biological process, **b** enriched GO terms related to cellular components, **c** enriched GO terms related to molecular functions, and **d** enriched KEGG pathways

(See figure on next page.)
**Fig. 7** ROC analysis of assessing the performance of RPL5 and RPL10 as diagnostic markers of AT/RT and KRT. The left column shows ROC analysis of RPL5 in diagnosing **a** KRT, **c** AT/RT, and **e** distinguishing AT/RT from KRT. The right column shows ROC analysis of RPL10 in diagnosing **b** KRT, **d** AT/RT, and **f** distinguishing AT/RT from KRT

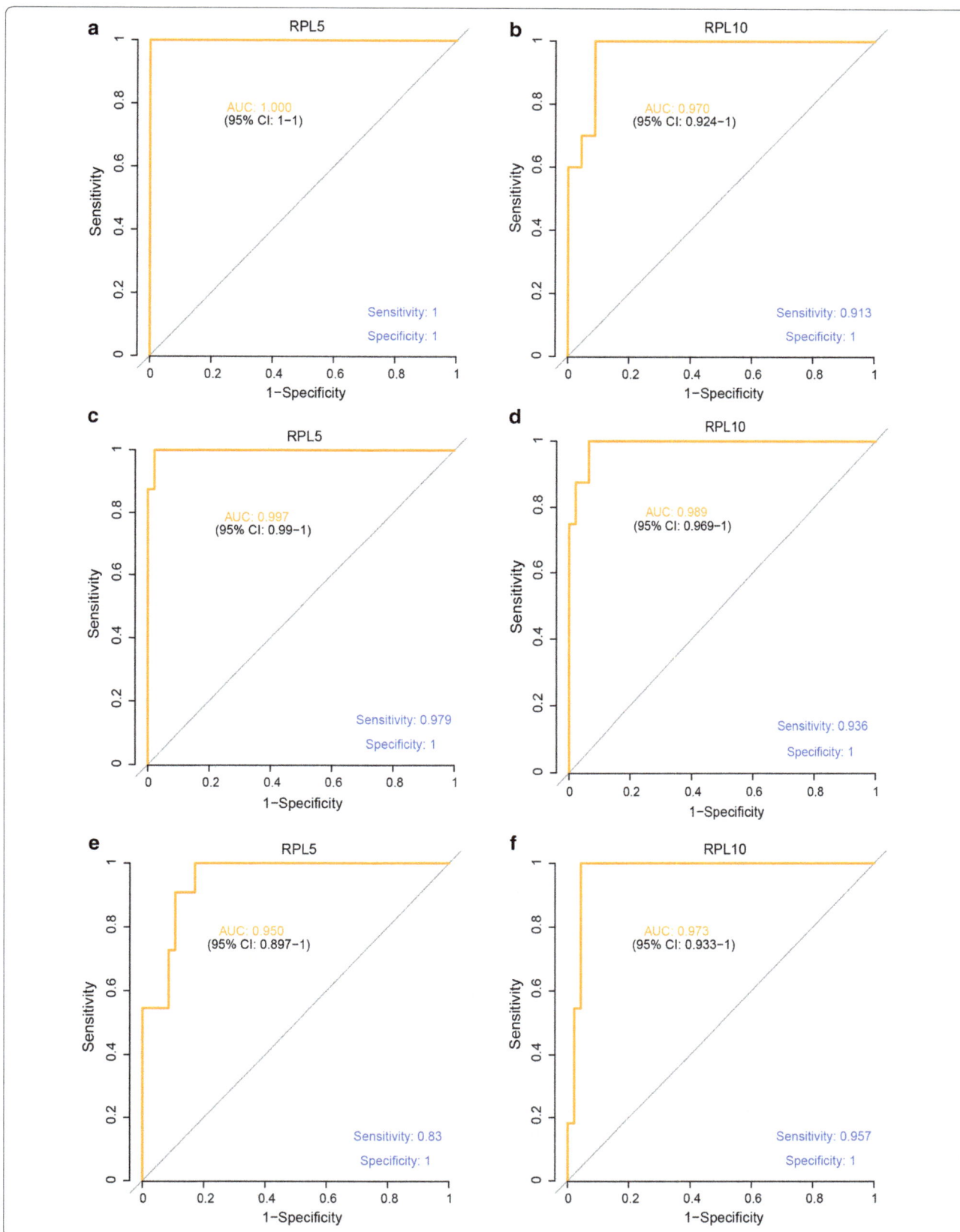

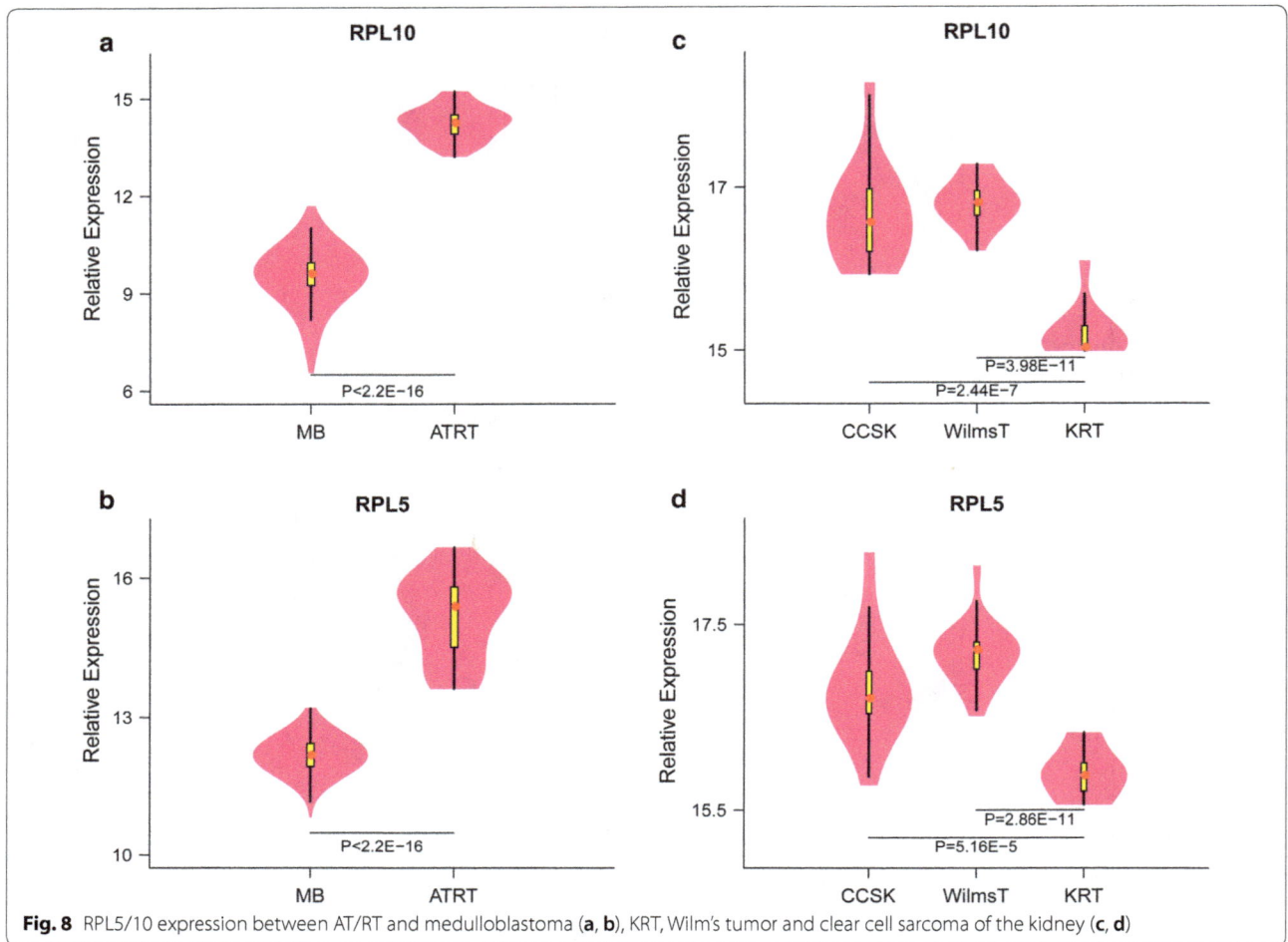

**Fig. 8** RPL5/10 expression between AT/RT and medulloblastoma (**a**, **b**), KRT, Wilm's tumor and clear cell sarcoma of the kidney (**c**, **d**)

medulloblastoma. To our knowledge, this study is the first in associating RPL5 and RPL10 with AT/RT diagnosis. Our results therefore identify two novel promising diagnostic markers for AT/RT, and provide the basis for work to further assess the performance, and to develop a robust diagnosis practice using these markers.

## Conclusions

Our study mined existing GEO datasets for novel diagnostic markers associated with Rhabdoid tumors, and identified RPL5 and RPL10 as potential diagnostic markers for AT/RT. These two biomarkers may be used as supplementary biomarkers to canonical diagnostic tools such as biopsy and immunohistochemistry. Further research is warranted to characterize the roles and significance of RPL5 and RPL10 in AT/RT.

## Additional files

**Additional file 1: Table S1.** Datasets of the 47 AT/RTs, 31 KRTs, 8 normal brain samples and 23 normal kidney samples.

**Additional file 2: Figure S1.** An overview of PCGs used in this study. There were a total of 12831 PCGs in the microarray profiles (denoted All-PCG), among which 491 differentially expressed PCGs AT/RT vs. Brain, KRT vs. Kidney and KRT vs. AT/RT (denoted DiffPCG). DiffPCGs that have been reported to be strongly associated with cancer (denoted CancerG) were highlighted and provide a pool of candidate diagnostic markers.

**Additional file 3: Figure S2.** Relative expression levels of RPL5 (A, B, and C) and RPL10 (D, E, and F) in AT/RT vs. Brain, KRT vs. Kidney and KRT vs. AT/RT.

## Abbreviations

RT: rhabdoid tumors; AT/RT: Atypical teratoid/rhabdoid tumors; KRT: kidney rhabdoid tumors; PCG: protein coding gene; lncRNA: long non-coding RNA; ROC: receiver operating characteristic; MB: medulloblastoma; CCSK: clear cell sarcoma of the kidney.

## Authors' contributions
YR and CT designed the work and contributed equally to the work, XW did the statistical analysis. YJ supervised the work. All authors read and approved the final manuscript.

## Author details
[1] Department of Neurosurgery, West China Hospital of Sichuan University, No. 37 Guo Xue Xiang, Chengdu, Sichuan, China. [2] Beijing Institute of Genomics, Chinese Academy of Sciences, Beijing, China.

## Acknowledgements
We thank all the doctors in our department for their help in patients care so that we can have enough time to conduct this study.

## Competing interests
The authors declare that they have no competing interests.

## Funding
Not applicable.

## References
1. Beckwith JB, Palmer NF. Histopathology and prognosis of Wilms tumors: results from the First National Wilms' Tumor Study. Cancer. 1978;41(5):1937–48.
2. Haas JE, Palmer NF, Weinberg AG, Beckwith JB. Ultrastructure of malignant rhabdoid tumor of the kidney. A distinctive renal tumor of children. Hum Pathol. 1981;12(7):646–57.
3. Rorke LB, Packer RJ, Biegel JA. Central nervous system atypical teratoid/rhabdoid tumors of infancy and childhood: definition of an entity. J Neurosurg. 1996;85(1):56–65.
4. Kleihues P, Louis DN, Scheithauer BW, Rorke LB, Reifenberger G, Burger PC, Cavenee WK. The WHO classification of tumors of the nervous system. J Neuropathol Exp Neurol. 2002;61(3):215–25 (discussion 226–219).
5. Brennan B, Stiller C, Bourdeaut F. Extracranial rhabdoid tumours: what we have learned so far and future directions. Lancet Oncol. 2013;14(8):e329–36.
6. Rickert CH, Paulus W. Epidemiology of central nervous system tumors in childhood and adolescence based on the new WHO classification. Childs Nerv Syst. 2001;17(9):503–11.
7. Wong TT, Ho DM, Chang KP, Yen SH, Guo WY, Chang FC, Liang ML, Pan HC, Chung WY. Primary pediatric brain tumors: statistics of Taipei VGH, Taiwan (1975–2004). Cancer. 2005;104(10):2156–67.
8. Kaderali Z, Lamberti-Pasculli M, Rutka JT. The changing epidemiology of paediatric brain tumours: a review from the Hospital for Sick Children. Childs Nerv Syst. 2009;25(7):787–93.
9. Ostrom QT, Chen Y, M. de Blank P, Ondracek A, Farah P, Gittleman H, Wolinsky Y, Kruchko C, Cohen ML, Brat DJ, et al. The descriptive epidemiology of atypical teratoid/rhabdoid tumors in the United States, 2001-2010. Neuro-oncology. 2014;16(10):1392–9.
10. Parham DM, Weeks DA, Beckwith JB. The clinicopathologic spectrum of putative extrarenal rhabdoid tumors. An analysis of 42 cases studied with immunohistochemistry or electron microscopy. Am J Surg Pathol. 1994;18(10):1010–29.
11. Vujanic GM, Sandstedt B, Harms D, Boccon-Gibod L, Delemarre JF. Rhabdoid tumour of the kidney: a clinicopathological study of 22 patients from the International Society of Paediatric Oncology (SIOP) nephroblastoma file. Histopathology. 1996;28(4):333–40.
12. Biegel JA, Tan L, Zhang F, Wainwright L, Russo P, Rorke LB. Alterations of the hSNF5/INI1 gene in central nervous system atypical teratoid/rhabdoid tumors and renal and extrarenal rhabdoid tumors. Clin Cancer Res. 2002;8(11):3461–7.
13. Le Loarer F, Zhang L, Fletcher CD, Ribeiro A, Singer S, Italiano A, Neuville A, Houlier A, Chibon F, Coindre JM, et al. Consistent SMARCB1 homozygous deletions in epithelioid sarcoma and in a subset of myoepithelial carcinomas can be reliably detected by FISH in archival material. Genes Chromosom Cancer. 2014;53(6):475–86.
14. Sullivan LM, Folpe AL, Pawel BR, Judkins AR, Biegel JA. Epithelioid sarcoma is associated with a high percentage of SMARCB1 deletions. Mod Pathol. 2013;26(3):385–92.
15. Hasselblatt M, Oyen F, Gesk S, Kordes U, Wrede B, Bergmann M, Schmid H, Fruhwald MC, Schneppenheim R, Siebert R, et al. Cribriform neuroepithelial tumor (CRINET): a nonrhabdoid ventricular tumor with INI1 loss and relatively favorable prognosis. J Neuropathol Exp Neurol. 2009;68(12):1249–55.
16. Arnold MA, Stallings-Archer K, Marlin E, Grondin R, Olshefski R, Biegel JA, Pierson CR. Cribriform neuroepithelial tumor arising in the lateral ventricle. Pediatr Dev Pathol. 2013;16(4):301–7.
17. Liu Q, Galli S, Srinivasan R, Linehan WM, Tsokos M, Merino MJ. Renal medullary carcinoma: molecular, immunohistochemistry, and morphologic correlation. Am J Surg Pathol. 2013;37(3):368–74.
18. Calderaro J, Moroch J, Pierron G, Pedeutour F, Grison C, Maille P, Soyeux P, de la Taille A, Couturier J, Vieillefond A, et al. SMARCB1/INI1 inactivation in renal medullary carcinoma. Histopathology. 2012;61(3):428–35.
19. Mobley BC, McKenney JK, Bangs CD, Callahan K, Yeom KW, Schneppenheim R, Hayden MG, Cherry AM, Gokden M, Edwards MS, et al. Loss of SMARCB1/INI1 expression in poorly differentiated chordomas. Acta Neuropathol. 2010;120(6):745–53.
20. Biegel JA. Molecular genetics of atypical teratoid/rhabdoid tumor. Neurosurg Focus. 2006;20(1):E11.
21. Autio R, Kilpinen S, Saarela M, Kallioniemi O, Hautaniemi S, Astola J. Comparison of Affymetrix data normalization methods using 6,926 experiments across five array generations. BMC Bioinformatics. 2009;10(Suppl 1):S24.
22. Basavarajappa BS. Neuropharmacology of the endocannabinoid signaling system-molecular mechanisms, biological actions and synaptic plasticity. Curr Neuropharmacol. 2007;5(2):81–97.
23. Ohno-Shosaku T, Tanimura A, Hashimotodani Y, Kano M. Endocannabinoids and retrograde modulation of synaptic transmission. Neuroscientist. 2012;18(2):119–32.
24. Neve KA, Seamans JK, Trantham-Davidson H. Dopamine receptor signaling. J Recept Signal Transduct Res. 2004;24(3):165–205.
25. Beaulieu JM, Gainetdinov RR. The physiology, signaling, and pharmacology of dopamine receptors. Pharmacol Rev. 2011;63(1):182–217.
26. Ferraguti F, Crepaldi L, Nicoletti F. Metabotropic glutamate 1 receptor: current concepts and perspectives. Pharmacol Rev. 2008;60(4):536–81.
27. Niswender CM, Conn PJ. Metabotropic glutamate receptors: physiology, pharmacology, and disease. Annu Rev Pharmacol Toxicol. 2010;50:295–322.
28. Resende RR, Adhikari A. Cholinergic receptor pathways involved in apoptosis, cell proliferation and neuronal differentiation. Cell Commun Signal. 2009;7:20.
29. Brown DA. Muscarinic acetylcholine receptors (mAChRs) in the nervous system: some functions and mechanisms. J Mol Neurosci. 2010;41(3):340–6.
30. Ben-Ari Y, Khazipov R, Leinekugel X, Caillard O, Gaiarsa JL. GABAA, NMDA and AMPA receptors: a developmentally regulated 'menage a trois'. Trends Neurosci. 1997;20(11):523–9.
31. Farrant M, Kaila K. The cellular, molecular and ionic basis of GABA(A) receptor signalling. Prog Brain Res. 2007;160:59–87.
32. Uhlen M, Fagerberg L, Hallstrom BM, Lindskog C, Oksvold P, Mardinoglu A, Sivertsson A, Kampf C, Sjostedt E, Asplund A, et al. Proteomics. Tissue-based map of the human proteome. Science. 2015;347(6220):1260419.
33. Chun HJ, Lim EL, Heravi-Moussavi A, Saberi S, Mungall KL, Bilenky M, Carles A, Tse K, Shlafman I, Zhu K, et al. Genome-wide profiles of extra-cranial malignant rhabdoid tumors reveal heterogeneity and dysregulated developmental pathways. Cancer Cell. 2016;29(3):394–406.
34. Torchia J, Picard D, Lafay-Cousin L, Hawkins CE, Kim SK, Letourneau L, Ra YS, Ho KC, Chan TS, Sin-Chan P, et al. Molecular subgroups of atypical teratoid rhabdoid tumours in children: an integrated genomic and clinicopathological analysis. Lancet Oncol. 2015;16(5):569–82.
35. Johann PD, Erkek S, Zapatka M, Kerl K, Buchhalter I, Hovestadt V, Jones DT, Sturm D, Hermann C, Segura Wang M, et al. Atypical teratoid/rhabdoid tumors are comprised of three epigenetic subgroups with distinct enhancer landscapes. Cancer Cell. 2016;29(3):379–93.

36. Chakravadhanula M, Ozols VV, Hampton CN, Zhou L, Catchpoole D, Bhardwaj RD. Expression of the HOX genes and HOTAIR in atypical teratoid rhabdoid tumors and other pediatric brain tumors. Cancer Genet. 2014;207(9):425–8.

37. Ho DM, Shih CC, Liang ML, Tsai CY, Hsieh TH, Tsai CH, Lin SC, Chang TY, Chao ME, Wang HW, et al. Integrated genomics has identified a new AT/RT-like yet INI1-positive brain tumor subtype among primary pediatric embryonal tumors. BMC Med Genomics. 2015;8:32.

38. Grupenmacher AT, Halpern AL, Bonaldo Mde F, Huang CC, Hamm CA, de Andrade A, Tomita T, Aredni ST. Study of the gene expression and microRNA expression profiles of malignant rhabdoid tumors originated in the brain (AT/RT) and in the kidney (RTK). Childs Nerv Syst. 2013;29(11):1977–83.

39. Qu LH, Nicoloso M, Michot B, Azum MC, Caizergues-Ferrer M, Renalier MH, Bachellerie JP. U21, a novel small nucleolar RNA with a 13 nt. complementarity to 28S rRNA, is encoded in an intron of ribosomal protein L5 gene in chicken and mammals. Nucleic Acids Res. 1994;22(20):4073–81.

40. Frigerio JM, Dagorn JC, Iovanna JL. Cloning, sequencing and expression of the L5, L21, L27a, L28, S5, S9, S10 and S29 human ribosomal protein mRNAs. Biochem Biophys Acta. 1995;1262(1):64–8.

41. Fagerberg L, Hallstrom BM, Oksvold P, Kampf C, Djureinovic D, Odeberg J, Habuka M, Tahmasebpoor S, Danielsson A, Edlund K, et al. Analysis of the human tissue-specific expression by genome-wide integration of transcriptomics and antibody-based proteomics. Mol Cell Proteomics. 2014;13(2):397–406.

42. Teng T, Mercer CA, Hexley P, Thomas G, Fumagalli S. Loss of tumor suppressor RPL5/RPL11 does not induce cell cycle arrest but impedes proliferation due to reduced ribosome content and translation capacity. Mol Cell Biol. 2013;33(23):4660–71.

43. Fancello L, Kampen KR, Hofman IJ, Verbeeck J, De Keersmaecker K. The ribosomal protein gene RPL5 is a haploinsufficient tumor suppressor in multiple cancer types. Oncotarget. 2017;8(9):14462–78.

44. Chiocchetti A, Pakalapati G, Duketis E, Wiemann S, Poustka A, Poustka F, Klauck SM. Mutation and expression analyses of the ribosomal protein gene RPL10 in an extended German sample of patients with autism spectrum disorder. Am J Med Genet A. 2011;155A(6):1472–5.

45. Gong X, Delorme R, Fauchereau F, Durand CM, Chaste P, Betancur C, Goubran-Botros H, Nygren G, Anckarsater H, Rastam M, et al. An investigation of ribosomal protein L10 gene in autism spectrum disorders. BMC Med Genet. 2009;10:7.

46. De Keersmaecker K, Atak ZK, Li N, Vicente C, Patchett S, Girardi T, Gianfelici V, Geerdens E, Clappier E, Porcu M, et al. Exome sequencing identifies mutation in CNOT3 and ribosomal genes RPL5 and RPL10 in T-cell acute lymphoblastic leukemia. Nat Genet. 2013;45(2):186–90.

# 18

# The miR-199a-3p regulates the radioresistance of esophageal cancer cells via targeting the AK4 gene

Chunbao Zang[1†], Fangfang Zhao[2†], Lei Hua[3] and Youguang Pu[2*]

## Abstract

**Background:** MiRNAs was recognized as vital regulators involved in cancer development. Radioresistance remains a major obstacle for effective treatment of cancers. The mechanisms on the miRNA-mediated radioresistance of cancers are still poorly understood. The main subject of this study is to find new miRNA biomarker that regulates the radioresistance of esophageal cancer (EC).

**Methods:** The cumulative dose of radiation assays were used to screen the EC radioresistant cell lines. Wound-healing and invasion assays were used to characterize the properties of these cell lines. The following survival fraction experiments were performed to test the effects of miR-199a-3p and AK4 in the radioresistance of EC. In addition, we used the luciferase reporter assays to identify the putative underlying mechanism that relates to the miR-199a-3p regulated radio-resistance.

**Results:** We found that the AK4 gene is one of the targets of miR-199a-3p, which promotes the radioresistance of EC cells. The following experiments by force reversal of the miR-199a-3p or AK4 levels confirmed the relationship of miR-199a-3p and AK4 with the radioresistance of EC cells. In addition, the activities of several signaling pathway were drastically altered by the forced changes of the miR-199a-3p level in EC cells.

**Conclusion:** Taken together, we found that miR-199a-3p can be potentially used as a biomarker for the EC radioresistance. Moreover, these results provides new insights into the mechanism on the radioresistance of EC cells, and also might guide the clinical therapy of EC.

**Keywords:** Esophageal cancer, Radioresistance, miR-199a-3p, AK4, TGFβ signaling pathway

## Background

MiRNAs (miRNAs) are small non-coding RNAs that function as post-translational regulators of gene expression [1]. In recent years, increasing studies have been focused on the roles of miRNAs in regulating every biological event in normal cells, as well as in cancer cells [2, 3]. Notably, an individual miRNA can have hundreds of targets, while a single target gene may be regulated by many different miRNAs. Evidently, the dysregulation of miRNAs has been found in cancers, and thus the expression profiling of miRNA levels has already been used as diagnostic and prognostic biomarkers to assess tumor development [4]. Moreover, the previous studies demonstrated the roles of various miRNAs in different types of cancers, such as breast, colon, gastric, lung, and prostate [5–7]. Even more importantly, one type of miRNA might also participate in different cancers. For instance, the accumulating studies showed that the dysregulation of miR-199a is found in various cancers, including hepatocellular carcinoma [8], ovarian cancer [9], renal cell carcinoma [10], osteosarcoma [11] and etc. [12, 13]. All these studies demonstrated the complicated networks on miRNA-regulated cancer biogenesis.

*Correspondence: puyouguang@126.com
†Chunbao Zang and Fangfang Zhao contributed equally to this work
[2] Department of Cancer Epigenetics Program, Anhui Provincial Cancer Hospital, West Branch of the First Affiliated Hospital of USTC, Division of Life Sciences and Medicine, University of Science and Technology of China, Hefei 230001, Anhui, People's Republic of China
Full list of author information is available at the end of the article

Esophageal cancer (EC) is the eighth most commonly occurred cancer worldwide. It has proven to be one of the most difficult malignancies to cure [14, 15]. To date, the chemotherapy or chemoradiotherapy are still the preferred methods for clinical therapy of EC at more advanced stages. However, the chemoresistance and radioresistance are the major obstacles for the effective therapy. Moreover, there is still limited knowledge on the underlying mechanism that governs the chemoresistance and radioresistance of EC. To address this issue, we try to identify new miRNA biomarker that relates to the radioresistance of EC. In our previous studies, we have found that several miRNAs are involved the drug resistance of osteosarcoma by targeting different genes [16–19]. However, whether these miRNAs are involved in the EC radioresistance is still unknown. In this study, using a systematic analysis and profiling methods, we identified that Kyse30-R and Kyse150-R cells are the radioresistant cells of EC. Further investigations in EC cells found that the miR-199a-3p targets AK4, which was reported to be involved in stress, drug resistance, malignant transformation in cancer [20–22]. Taken together, our findings provide a new mechanistic insight into EC radioresistance, which might give us hints for a rational design of the clinical therapy against EC.

## Methods
### Cells and culture

The human esophageal cancer Cells lines Kyse30 and Kyse150 were kindly provided by Professor Zhan (National Laboratory of Molecular Oncology, China, Beijing) [23, 24], Kyse30-R and Kyse150-R were obtained from their parental strains of Kyse30 and Kyse150, respectively. Four cells were cultured and maintained in RPMI medium 1640 (Biological Industries) supplemented with 10% fetal bovine serum (PAN Biotech), 100 U/ml penicillin, and 100 mg/ml streptomycin (WISENT INC) in humidified air at 37 °C with 5% $CO_2$.

### Transient transfection assays

The Homo sapien miR–199a-3p mimic, antagomiR and scrambled negative control (NC) were obtained from Guangzhou Ribobio, China. All the transfection experiments were performed using riboFECT CP transfection kit were supplied by Guangzhou Ribobio, China. Western blot and qRT–PCR assays were performed to confirm the effect of AK4 on the expression of miR–199a-3p. The sequences used in this study are as follows:

si-AK4:
GCCTAATGATGTCCGAGTT
5'-GCCUAAUGAUGUCCGAGUU dTdT-3'
3'-dTdT CGGAUUACUACAGGCUCAA-5'

### Reverse transcription-quantitative polymerase chain reaction (qRT-PCR) assays

Total RNA was extracted from cells using TRIzol reagent (Tiangen) according to the manufacturer's instructions. The reverse-transcription and PCR primers for miR-199a-3p and U6 were purchased from GenePharma. The cDNA library was synthesized using the PrimeScript RT reagent kit (Tiangen). The mRNA expression level of AK4 using TaqMan assay and the miRNA using SYBR Green assay (Biosystems) were quantified in an FTC-3000PCR instrument (Funglyn). Either U6 small nuclear RNA (HmiRQP9001) or β-actin (ShingGene) were used as an internal control. Expression levels were calculated using the relative quantification method ($2^{-\Delta\Delta Ct}$). Each test was repeated in triplicate. The sequences of the primers and probes used for the qRT-PCR analysis are:

hAK4 F: 5'-CACTTCTTGCGGGAGAACATC-3'
hAK4 R: 5'-CCAACTCGGACATCATTAGGC-3'
hAK4 probe: 5'-FAM-CAGCACCGAAGTTGGTGA GATGGC-3'
hACTB F: 5'-GCCCATCTACGAGGGGTATG-3'
hACTB R: 5'-GAGGTAGTCAGTCAGGTCCCG-3'
hACTB probe: 5'CY5-CCCCCATGCCATCCTGCG TC-3'

### Radiation exposure and clonogenic assays

All cells were pretreated by NC, miR-199a-3p mimics, antagomiRs and si-AK4 for 24 h, then were digested and counted according to 0 Gy (500), 2 Gy (1000), 4 Gy (2000), 6 Gy (5000), 8 Gy (8000) cells/well and was inoculated in a 6-well plate in triplicate, the corresponding dose was irradiated after 24 h, using a 6-MV X-ray generated by a linear accelerator (varian trilogy at a dose rate of 2 Gy/min) and the culture was continued for 15 days, then washed and fixed with 10% formaldehyde, and giemsa stained. The number of cloned spheres with > 50 cells was counted, and the number of cells inoculated with 50–200 cloned spheres was selected as the appropriate number of colonies for colony formation experiments. The overall experiment was repeated 3 times and the mean was taken. Calculate the cell clone formation rate (planting efficiency, PE = number of cloned cells/ number of cells inoculated × 100%) and cell survival fraction (SF = each dose of PE/non-irradiated PE × 100%), using the multi-target click model of GraphPad Prism 6 software (GraphPad), The cell dose survival curve was fitted according to the formula $SF = 1 \times (1 - e - D/D0)^N$, and the radiosensitivity parameters (D0, N, Dq and SF2).

### Wound-healing assays

For cell motility assays, cells were grown to near confluence in 24-well plates in full-growth medium and were then incubated overnight in serum-free medium. Cells were scratched with a 10 µl sterile pipette tip and extensively washed with PBS to remove cells debris. Cells were then incubated in medium containing 10% FBS. The wounded areas were photographed and measured after scratching 0, 8, 12, 16, 20, 24, using a CKX41 inverted microscope (Olympus).

### Invasion assays
Invasion assays were conducted in a 24-well plate with 8 µm pore size membranes Matrigel-coated Transwell chambers (Corning). $3 \times 10^4$ cells were seeded into the upper chambers in 200 µl serum-free RPMI-1640, while 600 µl RPMI-1640 supplemented with 10% fetal bovine serum was placed in the lower chamber. After incubation for 36 h at 37 °C and 5% $CO_2$, the invasion potential of the cells that moved to the lower surface invading 8 µm pore size membranes with Matrigel were fixed with 70% ethanol and stained with 0.1% crystal violet for 30 min. The cells were then imaged and counted in five random fields using a CKX41 inverted microscope (Olympus). Each test was repeated in triplicate.

### Cell proliferation assay
The capacity for cellular proliferation was measured by CCK8-based cell proliferation assay. Cells were seeded in 96-well plates at a density of $5 \times 10^3$ cells per well, and cell proliferation assays were performed every 24 h using CCK8. The number of viable cells was measured by their absorbance at 450 nm at the indicated time points.

### Drug resistance profiling
For cell proliferation assay, cells in the logarithmic phase of growth were seeded in triplicate in 96-well plates at a density of $4 \times 10^3$ cells/well and treated with 4-fold serially diluted drugs for 72 h. Then, 10 µl of CCK8 salt (Bimake) was added to the corresponding well, the cells were incubated at 37 °C for an additional 2 h. The optical density was determined with a microplate reader (TECAN) at a wavelength of 450 nm.

### Western blotting assays
Cells protein lysates were separated by 10% SDS-poly acrylamide gel electrophoresis (SDS-PAGE), transferred to 0.45 µm PVDF Transfer Membranes (Immobilon®-P). Next, the PVDF membrane was blocked with 5% non-fat dairy milk in phosphate-buffered saline (PBS) with 0.1% Tween-20. The first antibodies were then detected by second antibodies, which could recognize them conjugated to enzyme horseradish peroxidase. The information of antibodies were as follows: anti-rabbit (San Ying Biotechnology, China), anti-mouse (SanYing Biotechnology, China), anti-GAPDH (San Ying Biotechnology,

China), the rabbit polyclonal antibody of AK4 was bought from Proteintech (AP20571a), the concentration was 45 µg/150 µl. The target bands were visualized by an enhanced chemiluminescence reaction (Pierce), and the relative band intensity was determined by the Gel-Pro Analyzer 4.0 software (Media Cybernetics).

### Luciferase reporter assays
The AK4 wild-type (WT) 3′UTRs, which contain the putative miR-199a-3p binding site, were cloned into the pEZX-MT01-luciferase-report vector (GeneCopoeia™). For the luciferase reporter assay, Kyse30 and Kyse30-R cells were co-transfected with a luciferase reporter vector and negative control, the miR-199a-3p mimic or antago-miR. After 24 h transfection, the cells were assayed for luciferase activity using the Dual-Luciferase Reporter Assay System (Promega) in a Promega GloMax 20/20 luminometer, according to the manufacturer's instructions. The relative firefly luciferase activities of the 3′UTR and pathway reporter vector were analyzed as previously reported [25]. All experiments were repeated in triplicate.

### Signaling pathway analysis
Constructs for the reporters of seventeen signaling pathways were obtained from SABiosciences (USA) and analyzed according to the manufacturer's instructions. The cells were transfected in triplicate with each firefly luciferase reporter construct in combination with the Renilla luciferase-based control construct using transfection reagent, and both the luciferase activities were measured in the cell extracts 48 h after transfection. The luciferase activities (luciferase unit) of the pathway reporter relative to those of the negative control in the transfected cells were calculated as a measurement of the pathway activity.

### Statistical analyses
The data are presented as the mean ± standard deviation. All statistical analyses were conducted by Excel and GraphPad Prism 6. Statistical significance was assessed by a two-tailed unpaired Student's $t$-test, a one-way analysis of variance or Mann–Whitney U test. Results were considered to be statistically significant at $p < 0.05$.

## Results
### Characterization of Kyse30-R and Kyse150-R cells as radioresistant strains of esophageal cancer
To underlie the characteristics of the radioresistance of EC cells, we first aim to screen the radioresistant strains of EC. We thus used the parental strains of Kyse30 and Kyse150 and make them subjected to X-ray radiation at increasing doses. After several rounds of screening against X-ray challenge, we successfully obtained two mutated EC strains that are radioresistant compared to

the parental strains. They can tolerate the X-ray radiation at a dose up to 70 and 82 Gy, respectively, we thus termed them as Kyse30-R and Kyse150-R respectively. During the X-ray challenge, the morphology of the cell lines was obviously changed. Compared to the oval shape of the parental cells, most of the Kyse30-R and Kyse150-R cells were long spindle shaped and protruding outwards to connect with each other. The cell volume was also somewhat enlarged for the radioresistant cell lines (Fig. 1a). The following radiosensitivity detection assays confirmed that Kyse30-R and Kyse150-R are more resistant against radiation (Fig. 1b, c). In addition, we performed the cell proliferation experiment to further characterize these two cell lines. The results showed that the cell proliferation capability of Kyse30-R cells was weaker than that of parental cells, whereas the Kyse150-R cells showed stronger cell proliferation activity than that of parental cells (Fig. 1d, e). Next, we performed the drug-resistance profiling of the two cell lines against the following drugs: CDDP, Dox, ETOP, 5-FU, CBCDA (Fig. 1f, g). In agreement with the radioresistance profiles, these two cell lines are also a little bit more resistant against the above drugs, which indicates that Kyse30-R and Kyse150-R cells are also chemoresistant cells compared to the parental cells.

Generally, the cancer cells are featured with the higher ability of cell migration and invasion. So we detected the migration and invasion ability of resistant cells Kyse30-R and Kyse150-R to see whether they obtained the characteristics of cancer cells. As shown in Fig. 2a, the wound healing assays showed that the cell migration abilities of Kyse30-R and Kyse150-R cells are dramatically increased, as compared to the parental cells. Furthermore, the Kyse150-R cells also showed higher invasion ability compared to the parental cells (Fig. 2b). By contrast, the invasion ability of Kyse30-R cells is lower than that of the parental cells (Fig. 2b). These results demonstrated that the Kyse150-R cells acquired some of the features of the cancer cells, whereas the biological features of Kyse30-R cells is different from the cancer cells. This also indicates that the biogenesis of the cancer cells is rather a complicated process, induced by diverse factors.

### The AK4 is the target of miR-199a-3p

MiRNAs usually down-regulate the target genes to fulfill their functions. To see whether miRNAs participate

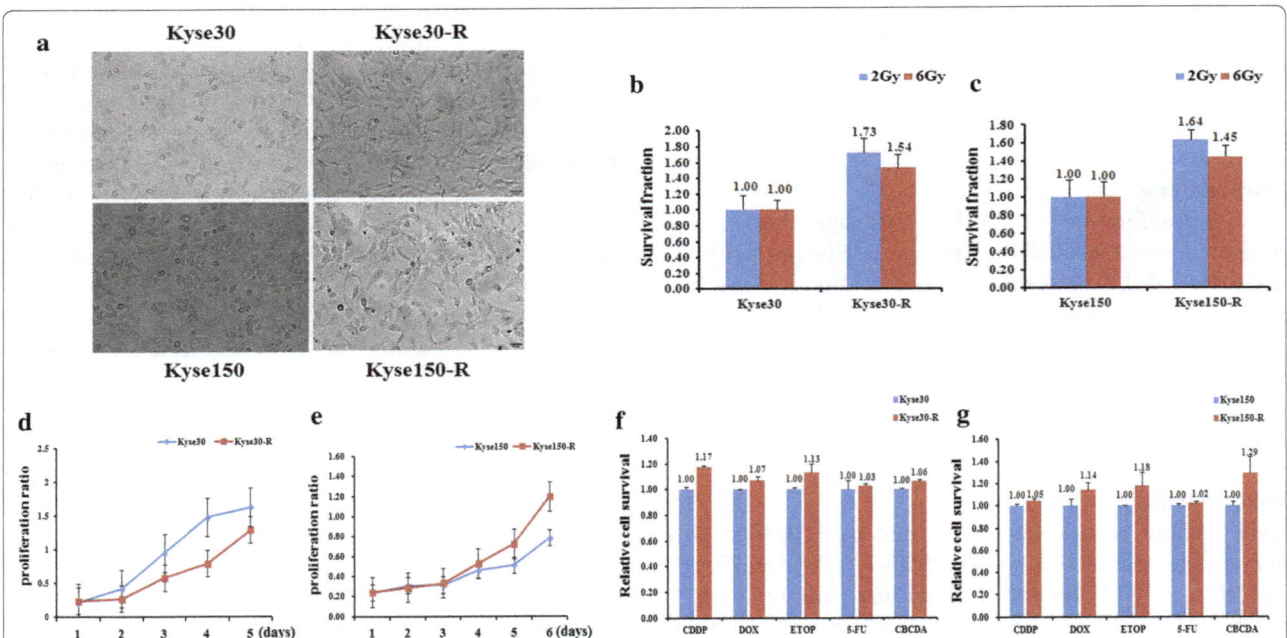

**Fig. 1** Establishment, identification and biological characteristics of radiotherapy resistant strains of esophageal cancer cells. **a** Cell morphology identification. Kyse30-R and Kyse150-R cell lines were established from Kyse30 and Kyse150, respectively. The cumulative dose of radiation of Kyse30-R and Kyse150-R reached to 70 and 82 Gy, respectively. Under the optical microscope, the morphology of the cell line was obviously changed. Most of the cell lines were long spindle shaped and protruding, and the cell space was enlarged and the parental cells were mostly oval and cobblestone, and the cells were closely connected. **b**, **c** Radiosensitivity detection assay showed that the sensitivity of Kyse150-R and Kyse30-R cells was lower than that of parental cells. **d**, **e** Cell proliferation assay showed that the proliferation of Kyse30-R cells was slower than that of parental cells, however, the proliferation activity of Kyse150-R cells was stronger than that of parental cells. **f**, **g** Chemosensitivity and resistance assay showed that Kyse150-R and Kyse30-R cells were drug resistance than that of their parental cells

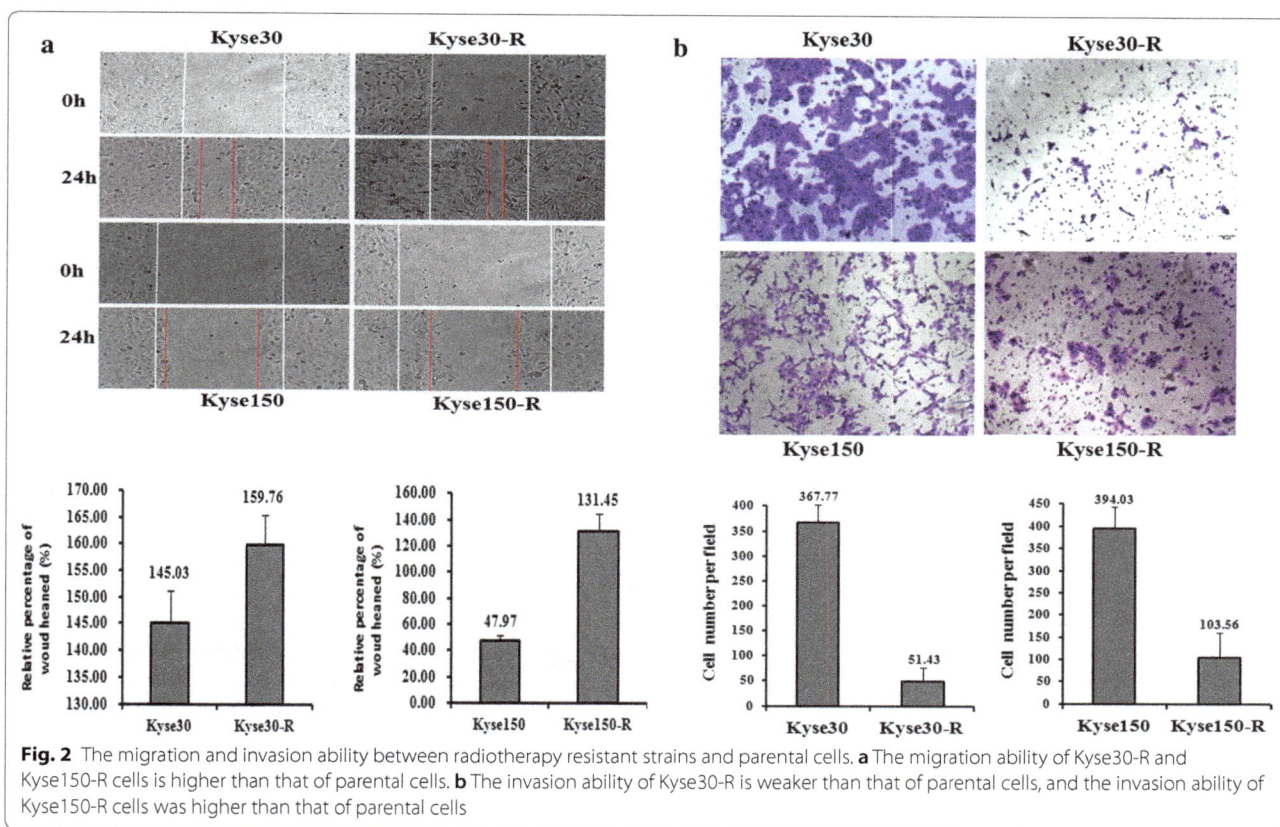

**Fig. 2** The migration and invasion ability between radiotherapy resistant strains and parental cells. **a** The migration ability of Kyse30-R and Kyse150-R cells is higher than that of parental cells. **b** The invasion ability of Kyse30-R is weaker than that of parental cells, and the invasion ability of Kyse150-R cells was higher than that of parental cells

in the process of making the parental cells to be resistant, we select miR-199a-3p as our target for further studies. We first predicted the targets of miR-199a-3p using the following websites: Targetscan and miRDB. Among them, we choose the AK4 gene as our target, which was previously found to be related to cancer drug resistance [26, 27]. We then detected the expression levels of miR-199a-3p and AK4 in the radiosensitive and radioresistant cell lines. The miR-omic and qRT-PCR analyses in Kyse30-R cells versus Kyse30 cells showed that the expression of miR-199a-3p is significantly higher in Kyse30-R cells, resulting in about 16 and 31 folds for the miR-omic and qRT-PCR assays, respectively (Fig. 3a, b). Similarly, the qRT-PCR assay also showed a higher level of Kyse150-R cells compared to the parental cells (Fig. 3a, b). Next we checked the level of AK4 in both the mRNA and protein levels. As shown in Fig. 3c, d, the AK4 mRNA level is reversely correlated with the expression of miR-199a-3p, which means that the AK4 mRNA level is relatively lower in the radioresistant cells (Fig. 3c, d). Consistently, the protein level of AK4 is also down-regulated in Kyse30-R and Kyse150-R cells, with the ratio of about 0.57 and 0.31, respectively (Fig. 3e).

Considering that the AK4 level is negatively correlated with the miR-199a-3p level, we propose that

AK4 might be a direct target of miR-199a-3p. We thus changed the miR-199a-3p level by transfecting miR-199a-3p mimic (3PM) into the Kyse30 and Kyse150 cells or the miR-199a-3p antagomiR (3PA) into the Kyse30-R and Kyse150-R cells. As expected, the transfection of 3PM into the Kyse30 and Kyse150 cells indeed increased the miR-199a-3p level to about 1994 and 900 folds, respectively (Fig. 4a). This conflict indicates that 3PA might cause the dysregulation of other factors that contribute to the up-regulation of miR-199a-3p level in the Kyse150-R cells. Following the changes of the miR-199a-3p, the AK4 level in reversely correlated with the changes of miR-199a-3p, resulting in a much lower AK4 level in Kyse30 and Kyse150 cells whereas a higher AK4 level in Kyse30-R and Kyse150-R cells (Fig. 4b, c). Consistently, the AK4 protein level also showed a similar changing trend to the AK4 mRNA level in these four cell lines (Fig. 4d). Next, to further validate AK4 is indeed the target of miR-199a-3p in EC cells, we constructed a reporter vector pZEX-AK4-UTR WT by the fusion of the 3′-untranslated region (UTR) of the AK4 gene harboring the putative binding site of miR-199a-3p with the *Renilla* luciferase gene (Fig. 4e). The construct was transfected into Kyse30 and Kyse30-R cells to test its

**a**

| gene | cell lines | miR-omic | qRT-PCR |
|------|-----------|----------|---------|
| miR-199a-3p | Kyse30 | 1.00 | 1.00±1.000 |
| | Kyse30-R | 16.36 | 31.10±7.470 |
| | Kyse150 | — | 5.21±1.963 |
| | Kyse150-R | — | 219.94±47.039 |

**c**

| gene | cell lines | miR-omic | qRT-PCR |
|------|-----------|----------|---------|
| AK4 | Kyse30 | 1.00 | 1.00±0.094 |
| | Kyse30-R | 0.61 | 0.29±0.133 |
| | Kyse150 | — | 1.00±0.101 |
| | Kyse150-R | — | 0.10±0.123 |

**b**

**d**

**e**

**Fig. 3** The AK4 level is lower in radiotherapy resistant strains than in parental cells. The relative miR-199a-3p level (fold) in Kyse30-R and Kyse150-R cells versus Kyse30 and Kyse150 cells measured by both miR-omic and qRT-PCR analyses is shown in a table (**a**) and those measured by qRT-PCR are shown in a plot (**b**). The relative level (fold) of the AK4 gene in Kyse30 and Kyse150 cells versus Kyse30-R and Kyse150-R cells are summarized in a table (**c**), with a plot showing the miR-omic and qRT-PCR analyses (**d**) and a figure showing the western blot analysis (**e**). "–" indicates no detection in the omic analysis

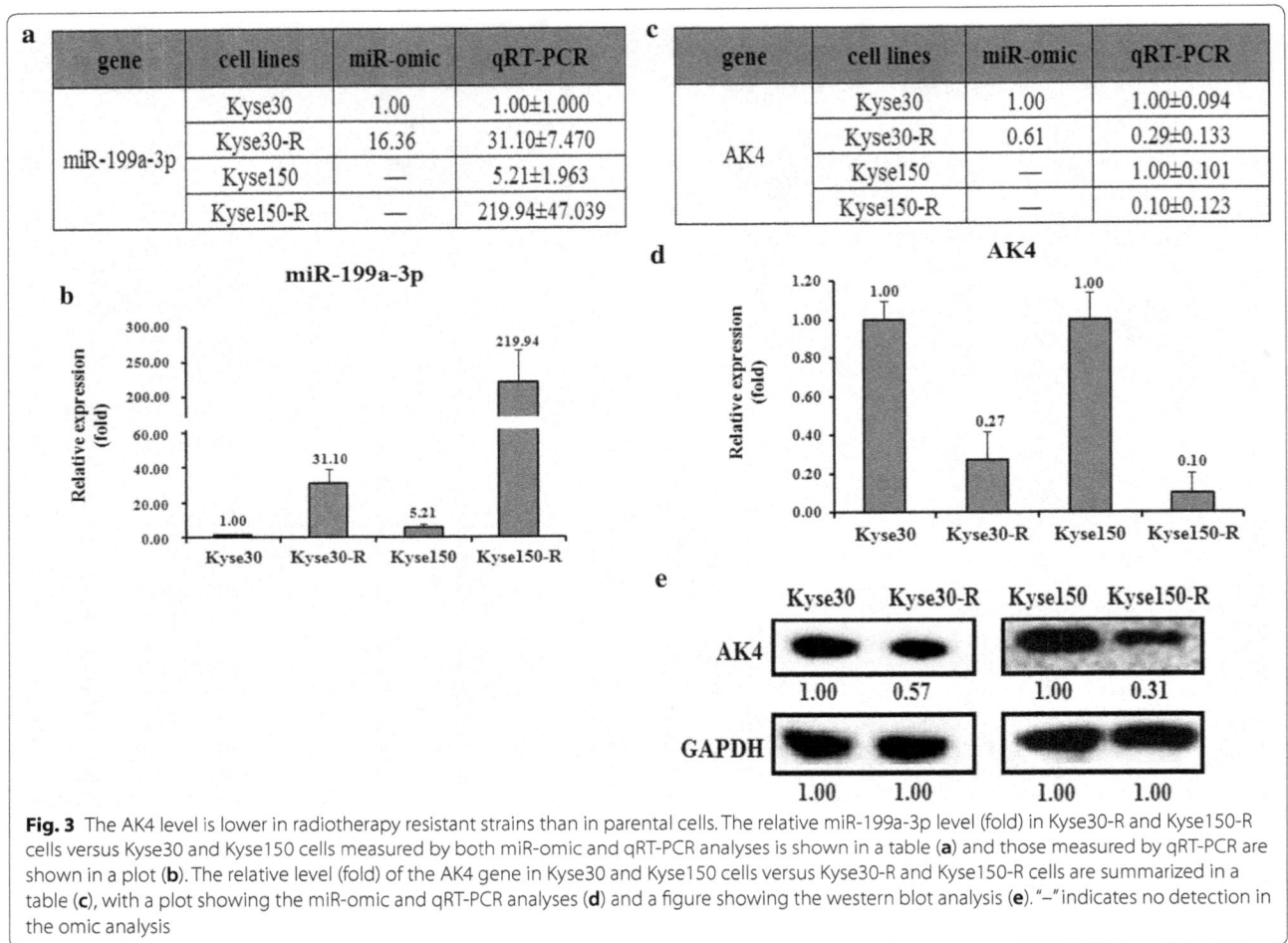

effect. We found that pZEX-AK4-UTR WT led to a significantly higher luciferase activity in Kyse30 cells than that in Kyse30-R cells (Fig. 4f). Furthermore, following the increase of the miR-199a-3p level, the activity of mimic-transfected Kyse30 cells is dramatically decreased whereas a reverse effect was found for the antagomiR-transfected Kyse30-R cells (Fig. 4g, h). All these results suggested that AK4 is indeed a target of miR-199a-3p in EC cells.

**MiR-199a-3p and AK4 expression are related with the radioresistance of EC cells**

We found that AK4 and miR-199a-3p are the differentially expressed targets in EC cells, and miR-199a-3p negatively regulates the expression of AK4. To see whether AK4 and miR-199a-3p are related to the radioresistance of EC cells, we compared the effect on drug-triggered cell death in different EC cell lines. The transfection of miR-199a-3p mimic into Kyse30 or Kyse150 cells increased the

(See figure on next page.)

**Fig. 4** AK4 is a target of miR-199a-3p in esophageal cancer cells. Level of miR-199a-3p (**a**). AK4 mRNA (**b, c**) and protein (**d**) levels in the miR-199a-3p mimic (3PM)-transfected Kyse30 and Kyse150 cells and the miR-199a-3p antagomiR (3PA)-transfected Kyse30-R and Kyse150-R cells versus the negative control (NC) cells, as determined by qRT-PCR or western blot analyses. **e** Sequences in the UTR region of the AK4 gene targeted by miR-199a-3p, with the hatched section showing the combined area and the diagram of the vector. The relative luciferase activities (fold) of the reporter with the wild-type (WT) AK4-UTR or without the UTR (Vec) were determined in the EC cells transfected with the miR-199a-3p mimic (in Kyse30), antagomiR (in Kyse30-R) or Mock (**f–h**) sequences. The Renilla luciferase activity of a co-transfected control plasmid was used as a control for the transfection efficiency. The representative results from three independent experiments are shown. *p value < 0.05, **p value < 0.01 by Student's t-test

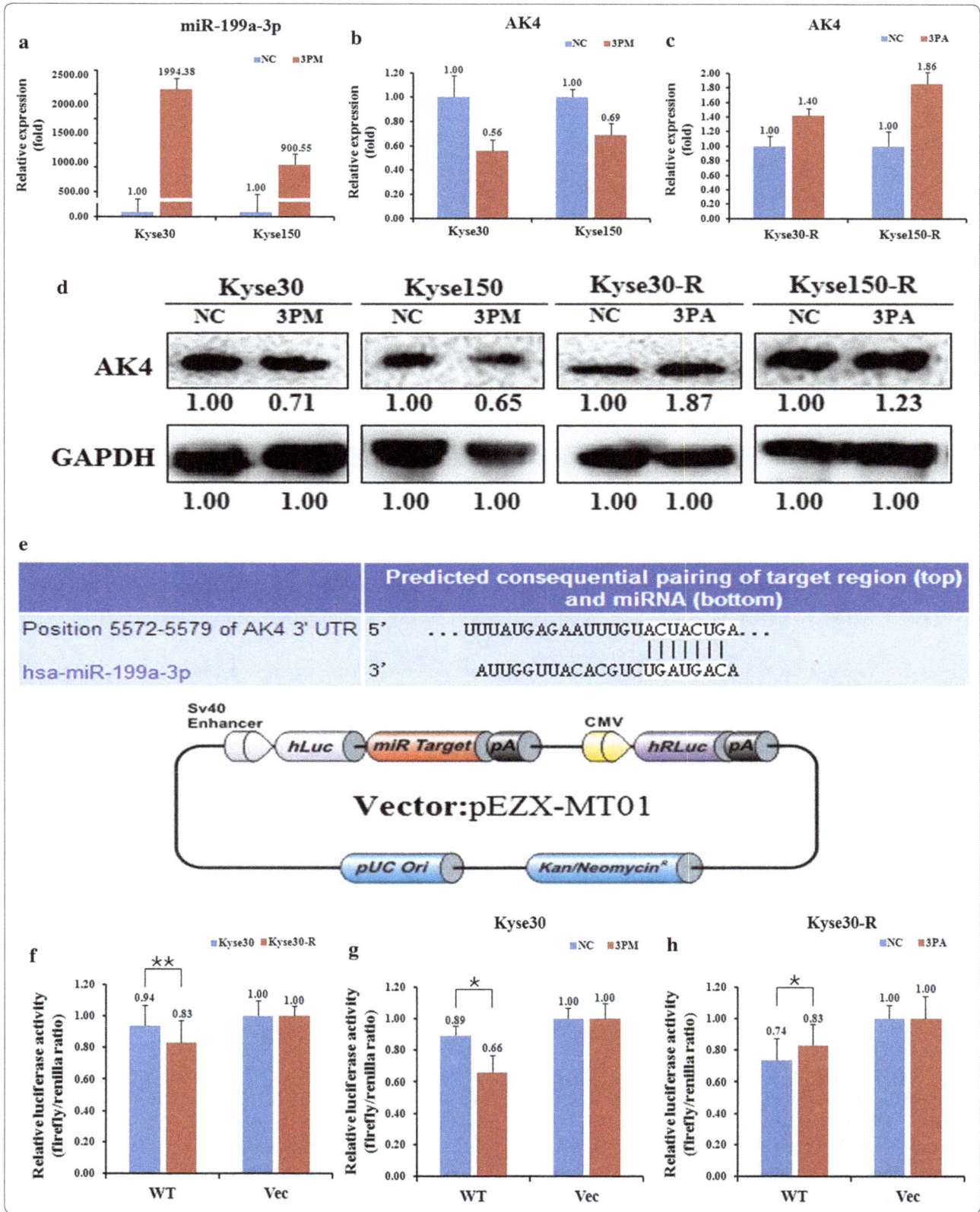

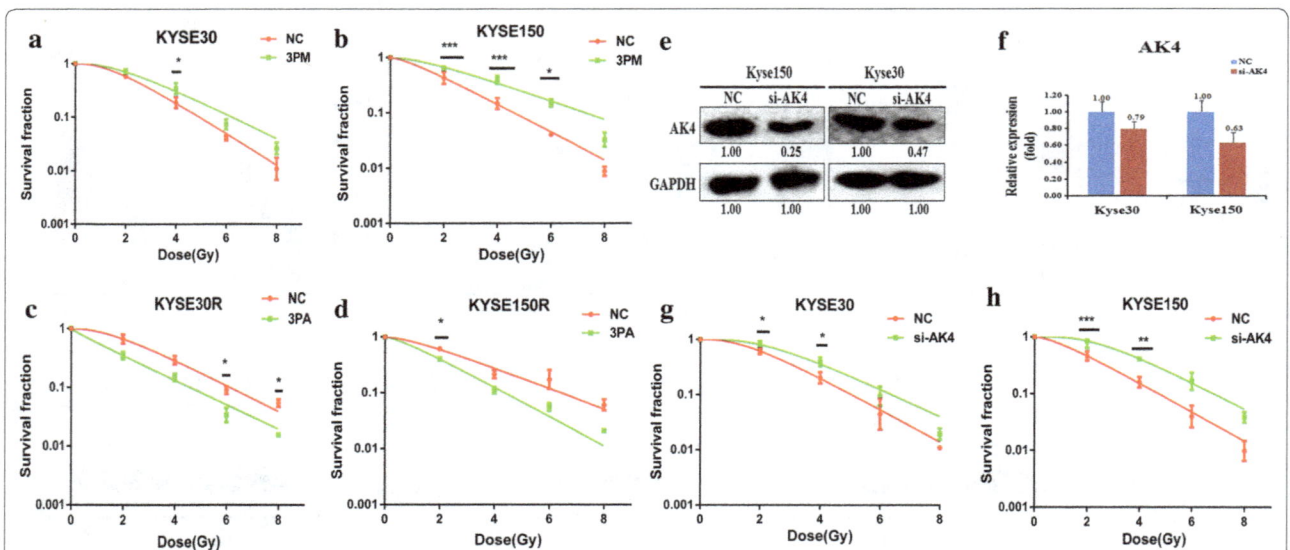

**Fig. 5** Effects of a forced reversal of the miR-199a-3p or AK4 levels on the esophageal cancer cells. The cells were transfected for 24 h, then cells were digested and counted according to 0 Gy (500), 2 Gy (1000), 4 Gy (2000), 6 Gy (5000), 8 Gy (8000) cells/well and was inoculated in a 6-well plate in triplicate, the corresponding dose was irradiated after 24 h, using a 6-MV x-ray generated by a linear accelerator Varian trilogy at a dose rate of 2 Gy/min (varian trilogy at a dose rate of 2 Gy/min). **a**, **b** MiR-199a-3p mimic (3PM)-transfected Kyse30 and Kyse150 increases survival fraction versus the negative control (NC) cells. **c**, **d** MiR-199a-3p antagomiR (3PA)-transfected Kyse30-R and Kyse150-R decreases NC cells survival fraction versus the negative control (NC) cells. AK4 protein level (western blot analysis) and mRNA determined by qRT-PCR in the si-AK4-transfected versus the NC-transfected Kyse30 and Kyse150 cells **e**, **f**. Si-AK4-transfected Kyse30 and Kyse150 cells increases NC cells survival fraction versus the negative control (NC) cells **g**, **h**. The surviving fraction was calculated using the multitarget single-hit model: $Y = 1 - (1 - \exp(-k \ast x))^N$. The data are presented as the mean ± standard deviation of results from 3 independent experiments, and two way anova was used to calculate statistical significance

cell survival rate against radiation (Fig. 5a, b). Reversely, transfection of miR-199a-3p antagomiR into Kyse30-R or Kyse150-R cells somewhat decreased the cell survival rate against radiation (Fig. 5c, d). These results suggest that miR-199a-3p positively correlates with the radioresistance of EC cells. Next we down-regulates the expression of AK4 by transfection of si-AK4 into Kyse30 or Kyse150 cells. Western blot and qRT-PCR analysis showed that the expression of AK4 is significantly down-regulated upon the transfection of si-AK4 (Fig. 5e, f). The resultant radioresistant assays showed that down-regulation of AK4 increased the cell survival capability against radiation, which means that AK4 suppresses the radioresistance of EC cells (Fig. 5g, h).

### MiR-199a-3p regulates the activity of the TGFβ signaling pathway in the context of EC radioresistance

To further elucidate the underlying mechanism of EC radioresistance mediated by miR-199a-3p, we compared the activities of seventeen cancer-related signaling pathways in both Kyse30-R and Kyse150-R versus their parental cells Kyse30 and Kyse150, respectively (Fig. 6a). Notably, all of the tested signaling pathways are up-regulated in the Kyse30 cells, as compared to the resistant cells Kyse30-R. By contrast, most of signaling pathways

are down-regulated in the Kyse150 cells. Only three pathways: TGFβ, MAPK/JNK and IL-6 are up-regulated in the Kyse150 cells, which are in agreement with that of Kyse30 cells. We thus take these three pathways for further studies. We tested the expression level of these three pathways by forced changes in the miR-199a-3p level in both Kyse30 and Kyse150 cells. Upon the transfection of the miR-199a-3p mimic into Kyse30 cells, the activities of TGFβ and MAPK/JNK were down-regulated whereas that of IL-6 was up-regulated accompanied by the elevation of the miR-199a-3p level (Fig. 6b). Similar effect was also found for the TGFβ pathway in the Kyse150 cells upon the transfection of miR-199a-3p mimic. Altogether, only the TGFβ pathway was proposed to be involved in the forced changes of miR-199a-3p level. Generally, the TGFβ pathway was regulated by three transcription factors, SMAD2/3/4, we thus tested the individual levels of SMAD2/3/4 upon the transfection of 3PM in the Kyse30 and Kyse150 cells. The results showed that only SMAD4 is down-regulated in both Kyse30 and Kyse150 cells (Fig. 6c, d). The results demonstrated that the TGFβ signaling pathway might be involved in the miR-199a-3p-regulated EC radioresistance. However, further investigations are needed to further confirm the relationship between AK4 and the TGFβ signaling pathway.

**a**

| Pathway | Transcription Factor | Kyse30/Kyse30-R | Kyse150/Kyse150-R |
|---|---|---|---|
| Wnt | TCF/LEF | 18.54±0.17 | 0.36±0.17 |
| Notch | RBP-Jκ | 1570.90±0.07 | 0.12±0.17 |
| p53/DNA Damage | p53 | 15.17±0.01 | 0.31±0.17 |
| TGFβ | SMAD2/3/4 | 23.37±0.12 | 390.07±1.37 |
| Cell cycle/pRb-E2F | E2F/DP1 | 2.42±0.12 | 0.22±0.02 |
| NFκB | NFκB | 17.28±0.11 | 0.76±0.11 |
| Myc/Max | Myc/Max | 40.67±0.12 | 0.32±0.10 |
| Hypoxia | HIF1A | 51.01±0.07 | 0.28±0.12 |
| MAPK/ERK | Elk-1/SRF | 39.11±0.10 | 0.45±0.09 |
| MAPK/JNK | AP-1 | 9.68±0.10 | 1.74±0.10 |
| ATF2/ATF3/ATF4 | ATF2/ATF3/ATF4 | 130.49±0.09 | 0.01±0.03 |
| cAMP/PKA | CREB | 21.39±0.11 | 0.70±0.04 |
| MEF2 | MEF2 | 30.69±0.04 | 0.74±0.02 |
| Hedgehog | GLI | 21.55±0.16 | 0.75±0.11 |
| PI3K/AKT | FOXO | 20.90±0.10 | 0.75±0.11 |
| IL-6 | STAT3 | 17.32±0.10 | 1.60±0.10 |
| PKC/Ca++ | NFAT | 11.17±0.16 | 2.34±0.10 |
| Negative Control | | 1.00±0.12 | 1.00±0.12 |

**c**

| Transcription Factor | Kyse30 | Kyse150 |
|---|---|---|
| | 3PM/NC | 3PM/NC |
| SMAD2 | 0.66±0.17 | 1.50±0.11 |
| SMAD3 | 2.12±0.20 | 0.04±0.11 |
| SMAD4 | 0.44±0.32 | 0.26±0.24 |

**d**

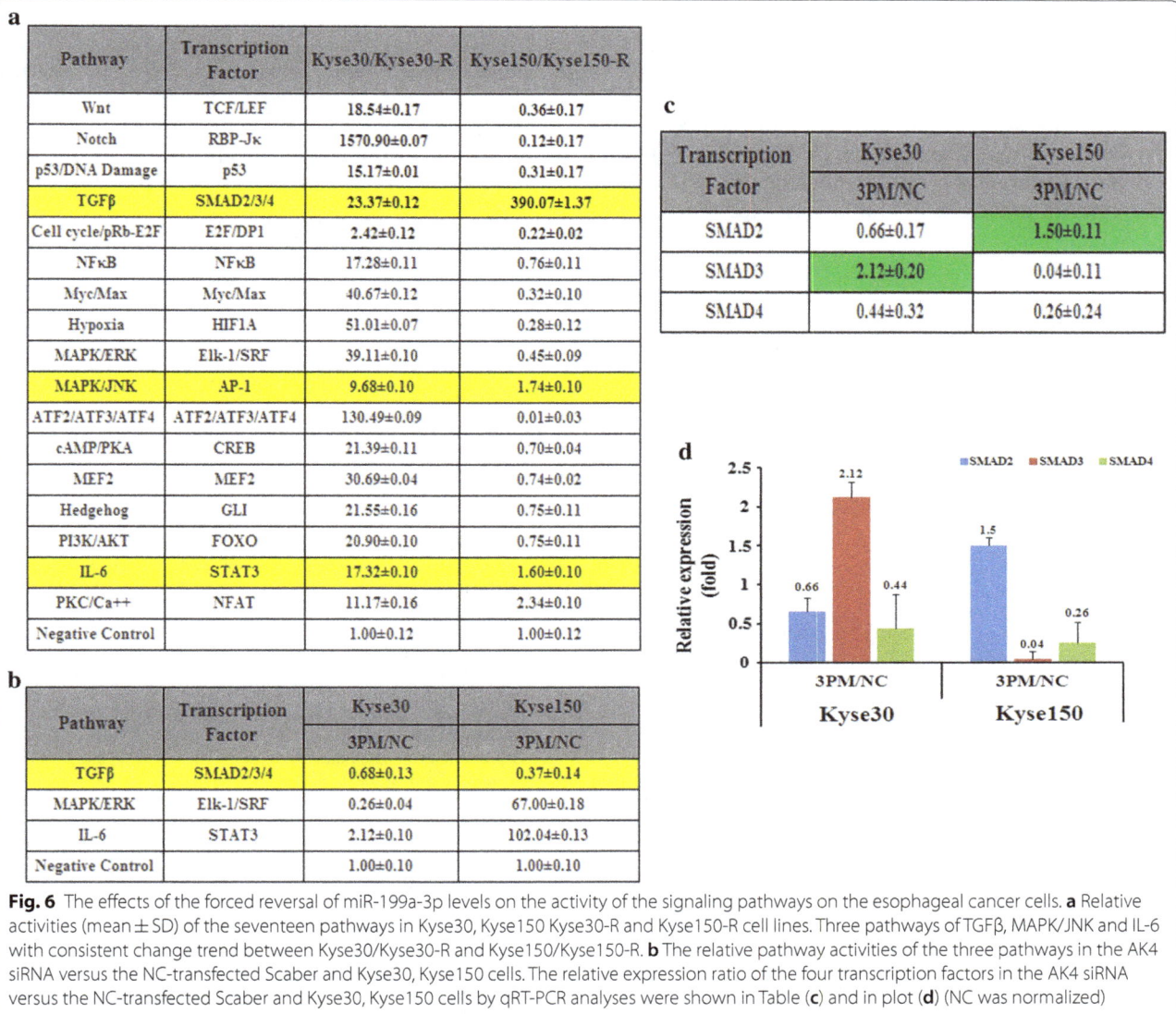

**b**

| Pathway | Transcription Factor | Kyse30 | Kyse150 |
|---|---|---|---|
| | | 3PM/NC | 3PM/NC |
| TGFβ | SMAD2/3/4 | 0.68±0.13 | 0.37±0.14 |
| MAPK/ERK | Elk-1/SRF | 0.26±0.04 | 67.00±0.18 |
| IL-6 | STAT3 | 2.12±0.10 | 102.04±0.13 |
| Negative Control | | 1.00±0.10 | 1.00±0.10 |

**Fig. 6** The effects of the forced reversal of miR-199a-3p levels on the activity of the signaling pathways on the esophageal cancer cells. **a** Relative activities (mean ± SD) of the seventeen pathways in Kyse30, Kyse150 Kyse30-R and Kyse150-R cell lines. Three pathways of TGFβ, MAPK/JNK and IL-6 with consistent change trend between Kyse30/Kyse30-R and Kyse150/Kyse150-R. **b** The relative pathway activities of the three pathways in the AK4 siRNA versus the NC-transfected Scaber and Kyse30, Kyse150 cells. The relative expression ratio of the four transcription factors in the AK4 siRNA versus the NC-transfected Scaber and Kyse30, Kyse150 cells by qRT-PCR analyses were shown in Table (**c**) and in plot (**d**) (NC was normalized)

## Discussion

MiRNAs play vital roles in various biological processes such as proliferation, apoptosis and differentiation, via regulating gene expression at post-modification level [28]. Accumulating evidences have suggested that miR-199a-3p is involved in cancer biology [29, 30]. Moreover, miR-199a showed distinct expression profiles in several types of cancer [31, 32]. For instance, miR-199a-3p is downregulated in hepatocellular carcinoma, resulting in an increased sensitivity to doxorubicin-induced apoptosis [33]. Down-regulation of miR-199a-3p in cisplatin-resistant breast cancer is able to attenuate cisplatin resistance via regulating the mitochondrial transcription factor A [34]. All these studies indicated that miR-199a-3p may be involved

in cancer chemotherapy resistance. In accordance with previous findings, here we showed that miR-199a-3p also involves in EC radioresistance. The results described here increased the knowledge of miR-199a-3p on radioresistance of cancer cells. The multifunctional roles of miR-199a-3p in different types of cancers also indicate miR-199a-3p has a potential to be a biomarker for cancer therapy.

We found that the AK4 gene is a target of miR-199a-3p that positively correlates with the EC radioresistance. AK4 was reported to be involved in the development of cancers, and is used as a potential therapeutic target for anticancer treatment. For example, the AK4 expression level could modulate the anti-cancer drug sensitivity through regulating mitochondrial activity [26]. Of note, a previous study found that AK4 promotes the metastasis of lung cancers by down-regulating the transcription factor ATF3 [21]. In agreement with the previous findings, here we demonstrated that the expression level of AK4 is associated with the EC radioresistance, which might be regulated by miR-199a-3p. However, the fine mechanism for the miR-199a-3p/AK4-mediated EC radioresistance remains to be elucidated.

## Conclusions

In this work, we screened Kyse30-R and Kyse150-R EC radioresistant cells, and find miR-199a-3p/AK4-mediated EC radioresistance, the findings suggest that miR-199a-3p or AK4 may serve as biomarkers for the potential therapeutic treatment of EC.

## Abbreviations

EC: esophageal cancer; miR: microRNA; AK4: adenylate kinase 4; 3PA: miR-199a-3p antagomiR; 3PM: miR-199a-3p mimic; UTR: untranslated region; WT: pEZX-MT01-AK4 UTR wild type; Vec: pEZX-MT01 enhancer control; PBS: phosphate-buffered saline; CDDP: cisplatin; Dox: doxorubicin; Etop: etoposide; 5-FU: 5-fluorouracil; CBCDA: carboplatin.

## Authors' contributions

Conception and design: YGP and CBZ. Acquisition of data (provided animals, provided facilities, etc.): FFZ and LH. Analysis and interpretation of data (e.g., statistical analysis, biostatistics, computational analysis): YGP and FFZ. Writing, review, and/or revision of the manuscript: YGP and CBZ. All authors read and approved the final manuscript.

## Author details

[1] Department of Radiation Oncology, Anhui Provincial Cancer Hospital, West Branch of the First Affiliated Hospital of USTC, Division of Life Sciences and Medicine, University of Science and Technology of China, Hefei 230001, Anhui, People's Republic of China. [2] Department of Cancer Epigenetics Program, Anhui Provincial Cancer Hospital, West Branch of the First Affiliated Hospital of USTC, Division of Life Sciences and Medicine, University of Science and Technology of China, Hefei 230001, Anhui, People's Republic of China. [3] Department of Provincial Clinical College, Anhui Provincial Hospital of Anhui Medical University, Hefei 230031, Anhui, China.

## Acknowledgements

Not applicable.

## Competing interests

The authors declare that they have no competing interests.

## Funding

This work was supported by the Natural Science Foundation of Anhui Province 1608085MH224 and 1608085QH214 Granted to YGP and CBZ, respectively. And the Fundamental Research Funds for the Central Universities Granted to FFZ.

## References

1. Pillai RS, Bhattacharyya SN, Filipowicz W. Repression of protein synthesis by miRNAs: how many mechanisms? Trends Cell Biol. 2007;17(3):118–26.
2. Lu J, Getz G, Miska EA, Alvarez-Saavedra E, Lamb J, Peck D, Sweet-Cordero A, Ebert BL, Mak RH, Ferrando AA, et al. MicroRNA expression profiles classify human cancers. Nature. 2005;435(7043):834–8.
3. Volinia S, Calin GA, Liu CG, Ambs S, Cimmino A, Petrocca F, Visone R, Iorio M, Roldo C, Ferracin M, et al. A microRNA expression signature of human solid tumors defines cancer gene targets. Proc Natl Acad Sci USA. 2006;103(7):2257–61.
4. Cummins JM, Velculescu VE. Implications of micro-RNA profiling for cancer diagnosis. Oncogene. 2006;25(46):6220–7.
5. Michael MZ, O'Connor SM, van Holst Pellekaan NG, Young GP, James RJ. Reduced accumulation of specific microRNAs in colorectal neoplasia. MCR. 2003;1(12):882–91.
6. Iorio MV, Ferracin M, Liu CG, Veronese A, Spizzo R, Sabbioni S, Magri E, Pedriali M, Fabbri M, Campiglio M, et al. MicroRNA gene expression deregulation in human breast cancer. Can Res. 2005;65(16):7065–70.
7. Takamizawa J, Konishi H, Yanagisawa K, Tomida S, Osada H, Endoh H, Harano T, Yatabe Y, Nagino M, Nimura Y, et al. Reduced expression of the let-7 microRNAs in human lung cancers in association with shortened postoperative survival. Can Res. 2004;64(11):3753–6.
8. Duan Q, Wang X, Gong W, Ni L, Chen C, He X, Chen F, Yang L, Wang P, Wang DW. ER stress negatively modulates the expression of the miR-199a/214 cluster to regulates tumor survival and progression in human hepatocellular cancer. PLoS ONE. 2012;7(2):e31518.
9. Wang Z, Ting Z, Li Y, Chen G, Lu Y, Hao X. microRNA-199a is able to reverse cisplatin resistance in human ovarian cancer cells through the inhibition of mammalian target of rapamycin. Oncol Lett. 2013;6(3):789–94.
10. Tsukigi M, Bilim V, Yuuki K, Ugolkov A, Naito S, Nagaoka A, Kato T, Motoyama T, Tomita Y. Re-expression of miR-199a suppresses renal cancer cell proliferation and survival by targeting GSK-3beta. Cancer Lett. 2012;315(2):189–97.
11. Duan Z, Choy E, Harmon D, Liu X, Susa M, Mankin H, Hornicek F. Micro-RNA-199a-3p is downregulated in human osteosarcoma and regulates cell proliferation and migration. Mol Cancer Ther. 2011;10(8):1337–45.
12. Murakami Y, Yasuda T, Saigo K, Urashima T, Toyoda H, Okanoue T, Shimotohno K. Comprehensive analysis of microRNA expression patterns in hepatocellular carcinoma and non-tumorous tissues. Oncogene. 2006;25(17):2537–45.
13. Song G, Zeng H, Li J, Xiao L, He Y, Tang Y, Li Y. miR-199a regulates the tumor suppressor mitogen-activated protein kinase kinase kinase 11 in gastric cancer. Biol Pharm Bull. 2010;33(11):1822–7.
14. Kato H, Fukuchi M, Miyazaki T, Nakajima M, Tanaka N, Inose T, Kimura H, Faried A, Saito K, Sohda M, et al. Surgical treatment for esophageal cancer. Current issues. Dig Surg. 2007;24(2):88–95.
15. Dehdashti F, Siegel BA. Neoplasms of the esophagus and stomach. Semin Nucl Med. 2004;34(3):198–208.
16. Pu Y, Zhao F, Wang H, Cai S. MiR-34a-5p promotes multi-chemoresistance of osteosarcoma through down-regulation of the DLL1 gene. Sci Rep. 2017;7:44218.
17. Pu Y, Zhao F, Li Y, Cui M, Wang H, Meng X, Cai S. The miR-34a-5p promotes the multi-chemoresistance of osteosarcoma via repression of the AGTR1 gene. BMC cancer. 2017;17(1):45.
18. Pu Y, Yi Q, Zhao F, Wang H, Cai W, Cai S. MiR-20a-5p represses multi-drug resistance in osteosarcoma by targeting the KIF26B gene. Cancer Cell Int. 2016;16:64.
19. Pu Y, Zhao F, Wang H, Cai W, Gao J, Li Y, Cai S. MiR-34a-5p promotes the multi-drug resistance of osteosarcoma by targeting the CD117 gene. Oncotarget. 2016;7(19):28420–34.
20. Yamamoto T, Kikkawa R, Yamada H, Horii I. Investigation of proteomic biomarkers in in vivo hepatotoxicity study of rat liver: toxicity differentiation in hepatotoxicants. J Toxicol Sci. 2006;31(1):49–60.
21. Jan YH, Tsai HY, Yang CJ, Huang MS, Yang YF, Lai TC, Lee CH, Jeng YM, Huang CY, Su JL, et al. Adenylate kinase-4 is a marker of poor clinical outcomes that promotes metastasis of lung cancer by downregulating the transcription factor ATF3. Can Res. 2012;72(19):5119–29.
22. Kong F, Binas B, Moon JH, Kang SS, Kim HJ. Differential expression of adenylate kinase 4 in the context of disparate stress response strategies of HEK293 and HepG2 cells. Arch Biochem Biophys. 2013;533(1–2):11–7.

23. Zhao ZT, Zhou W, Liu LY, Lan T, Zhan QM, Song YM. Molecular mechanism and effect of microRNA185 on proliferation, migration and invasion of esophageal squamous cell carcinoma. Zhonghua yi xue za zhi. 2013;93(18):1426–31.

24. Xue LY, Song YM, Tong T, Luo W, Dong LJ, Zou SM, Zheng S, Bi R, Zhan QM, Lu N. Expression of fascin and cytokeratin 14 in esophageal squamous cell carcinoma. Zhonghua yi xue za zhi. 2007;87(35):2494–8.

25. Lv L, Deng H, Li Y, Zhang C, Liu X, Liu Q, Zhang D, Wang L, Pu Y, Zhang H, et al. The DNA methylation-regulated miR-193a-3p dictates the multi-chemoresistance of bladder cancer via repression of SRSF2/PLAU/HIC2 expression. Cell Death Dis. 2014;5:e1402.

26. Fujisawa K, Terai S, Takami T, Yamamoto N, Yamasaki T, Matsumoto T, Yamaguchi K, Owada Y, Nishina H, Noma T, et al. Modulation of anti-cancer drug sensitivity through the regulation of mitochondrial activity by adenylate kinase 4. J Exp Clin Cancer Res. 2016;35:48.

27. Huang D, Wang Y, He Y, Wang G, Wang W, Han X, Sun Y, Lin L, Shan B, Shen G, et al. Paraoxonase 3 is involved in the multi-drug resistance of esophageal cancer. Cancer Cell Int. 2018;18:168.

28. Lynam-Lennon N, Maher SG, Reynolds JV. The roles of microRNA in cancer and apoptosis. Biol Rev Camb Philos Soc. 2009;84(1):55–71.

29. Li SQ, Wang ZH, Mi XG, Liu L, Tan Y. MiR-199a/b-3p suppresses migration and invasion of breast cancer cells by downregulating PAK4/MEK/ERK signaling pathway. IUBMB Life. 2015;67(10):768–77.

30. Hou J, Lin L, Zhou W, Wang Z, Ding G, Dong Q, Qin L, Wu X, Zheng Y, Yang Y, et al. Identification of miRNomes in human liver and hepatocellular carcinoma reveals miR-199a/b-3p as therapeutic target for hepatocellular carcinoma. Cancer Cell. 2011;19(2):232–43.

31. Kong YW, Ferland-McCollough D, Jackson TJ, Bushell M. microRNAs in cancer management. Lancet Oncol. 2012;13(6):e249–58.

32. Ueda T, Volinia S, Okumura H, Shimizu M, Taccioli C, Rossi S, Alder H, Liu CG, Oue N, Yasui W, et al. Relation between microRNA expression and progression and prognosis of gastric cancer: a microRNA expression analysis. Lancet Oncol. 2010;11(2):136–46.

33. Fornari F, Milazzo M, Chieco P, Negrini M, Calin GA, Grazi GL, Pollutri D, Croce CM, Bolondi L, Gramantieri L. MiR-199a-3p regulates mTOR and c-Met to influence the doxorubicin sensitivity of human hepatocarcinoma cells. Can Res. 2010;70(12):5184–93.

34. Fan X, Zhou S, Zheng M, Deng X, Yi Y, Huang T. MiR-199a-3p enhances breast cancer cell sensitivity to cisplatin by downregulating TFAM. Biomed Pharmacother. 2017;88:507–14.

# Permissions

All chapters in this book were first published in CCI, by BioMed Central; hereby published with permission under the Creative Commons Attribution License or equivalent. Every chapter published in this book has been scrutinized by our experts. Their significance has been extensively debated. The topics covered herein carry significant findings which will fuel the growth of the discipline. They may even be implemented as practical applications or may be referred to as a beginning point for another development.

The contributors of this book come from diverse backgrounds, making this book a truly international effort. This book will bring forth new frontiers with its revolutionizing research information and detailed analysis of the nascent developments around the world.

We would like to thank all the contributing authors for lending their expertise to make the book truly unique. They have played a crucial role in the development of this book. Without their invaluable contributions this book wouldn't have been possible. They have made vital efforts to compile up to date information on the varied aspects of this subject to make this book a valuable addition to the collection of many professionals and students.

This book was conceptualized with the vision of imparting up-to-date information and advanced data in this field. To ensure the same, a matchless editorial board was set up. Every individual on the board went through rigorous rounds of assessment to prove their worth. After which they invested a large part of their time researching and compiling the most relevant data for our readers.

The editorial board has been involved in producing this book since its inception. They have spent rigorous hours researching and exploring the diverse topics which have resulted in the successful publishing of this book. They have passed on their knowledge of decades through this book. To expedite this challenging task, the publisher supported the team at every step. A small team of assistant editors was also appointed to further simplify the editing procedure and attain best results for the readers.

Apart from the editorial board, the designing team has also invested a significant amount of their time in understanding the subject and creating the most relevant covers. They scrutinized every image to scout for the most suitable representation of the subject and create an appropriate cover for the book.

The publishing team has been an ardent support to the editorial, designing and production team. Their endless efforts to recruit the best for this project, has resulted in the accomplishment of this book. They are a veteran in the field of academics and their pool of knowledge is as vast as their experience in printing. Their expertise and guidance has proved useful at every step. Their uncompromising quality standards have made this book an exceptional effort. Their encouragement from time to time has been an inspiration for everyone.

The publisher and the editorial board hope that this book will prove to be a valuable piece of knowledge for researchers, students, practitioners and scholars across the globe.

# List of Contributors

**Jing-jing Jing, Ze-yang Wang, Hao Li, Li-ping Sun and Yuan Yuan**
Tumor Etiology and Screening Department of Cancer Institute and General Surgery, The First Hospital of China Medical University, Key Laboratory of Cancer Etiology and Prevention (China Medical University), Liaoning Provincial Education Department, Shenyang, Liaoning, China

**Xu Bin**
Department of Surgery, Zhejiang Rehabilitation Medical Center, Hangzhou 310053, Zhejiang, China

**Yang Hongjian and Zhang Xiping**
Department of Breast Surgery, Zhejiang Cancer Hospital, Banshanqiao, No. 38 Guangji Road, Hangzhou 310022, Zhejiang, China

**Chen Bo and Yang Shifeng**
Department of Pathology, Zhejiang Cancer Hospital, Hangzhou 310022, Zhejiang, China

**Tang Binbin**
Second Outpatient Department of Traditional Chinese Internal Medicine, Tongde Hospital of Zhejiang Province, Hangzhou 310012, Zhejiang, China

**Yong Wang, Yifu He, Gang Wang, Wei Wang, Xinghua Han, Yubei Sun, Lin Lin, Benjie Shan and Yueyin Pan**
Department of Oncology, the First Affiliated Hospital of USTC, Division of Life Sciences and Medicine, University of Science and Technology of China, Hefei 230001, Anhui, People's Republic of China
Department of Oncology, The Affiliated Hospital of Anhui Medical University, Hefei 230001, Anhui, People's Republic of China

**Dabing Huang**
Department of Oncology, the First Affiliated Hospital of USTC, Division of Life Sciences and Medicine, University of Science and Technology of China, Hefei 230001, Anhui, People's Republic of China
Department of Oncology, The Affiliated Hospital of Anhui Medical University, Hefei 230001, Anhui, People's Republic of China

Department of Geriatrics, the First Affiliated Hospital of USTC, Division of Life Sciences and Medicine, University of Science and Technology of China, Hefei 230001, Anhui, People's Republic of China
Anhui Provincial Key Laboratory of Tumor Immunotherapy and Nutrition Therapy, Hefei 230001, Anhui, People's Republic of China
Gerontology Institute of Anhui Province, Hefei 230001, Anhui, People's Republic of China

**Guodong Shen, Min Cheng, Geng Bian, Xiang Fang and Shilian Hu**
Department of Oncology, The Affiliated Hospital of Anhui Medical University, Hefei 230001, Anhui, People's Republic of China
Department of Geriatrics, the First Affiliated Hospital of USTC, Division of Life Sciences and Medicine, University of Science and Technology of China, Hefei 230001, Anhui, People's Republic of China
Anhui Provincial Key Laboratory of Tumor Immunotherapy and Nutrition Therapy, Hefei 230001, Anhui, People's Republic of China
Gerontology Institute of Anhui Province, Hefei 230001, Anhui, People's Republic of China

**Sumitra Shankar, Ahalya Sreekumar, Deepti Prasad, Ani V. Das and M. Radhakrishna Pillai**
Rajiv Gandhi Centre for Biotechnology, Thiruvananthapuram, India

**Rong Hu, Ming-qing Wang, Ling-yu Liu, Juan Zhong, Hai-yan You, Xiao-hui Wu and Lian-bo Wei**
Shenzhen Hospital, Southern Medical University, No. 1333, Xinhu Road, Bao'an District, Shenzhen 518101, Guangdong, China
School of Traditional Chinese Medicine, Southern Medical University, No. 1838, Guangzhou Avenue North, Baiyun District, Guangzhou 510515, Guangdong, China

**Ning Deng**
School of Traditional Chinese Medicine, Southern Medical University, No. 1838, Guangzhou Avenue North, Baiyun District, Guangzhou 510515, Guangdong, China

**Yan-jing Wang and Ming Wang**
Zhujiang Hospital of Southern Medical University, No. 253, Industrial Avenue, Haizhu District, Guangzhou 510280, Guangdong, China

**Lu Lu**
The First Affiliated Hospital, Guangzhou University of Chinese Medicine, No.16 Baiyun Airport Road, Baiyun District, Guangzhou 510405, Guangdong, China

**Wen-bo Niu**
Cancer Research Institute, Southern Medical University, No. 1838, Guangzhou Avenue North, Baiyun District, Guangzhou 510515, Guangdong, China

**Yang-yang Liu**
Zhongshan Huangpu People's Hospital, No. 32, Long'an Street, Huangpu Town, Zhongshan 528429, Guangdong, China

**Yan-Na Jiao, Dong Xue, Shan-Tong Jiang, Shu-Yan Han and Ping-Ping Li**
Key Laboratory of Carcinogenesis and Translational Research (Ministry of Education/Beijing), Department of Integration of Chinese and Western Medicine, Peking University Cancer Hospital & Institute, No. 52 Fucheng Road, Haidian District, Beijing 100142, People's Republic of China

**Li-Na Wu, Xi-Juan Liu and Zhi-Hua Tian**
Key Laboratory of Carcinogenesis and Translational Research (Ministry of Education/ Beijing), Central Laboratory, Peking University Cancer Hospital and Institute, Beijing 100142, People's Republic of China

**Wei Zhang, Han Ge, Yue Song and Yanling Wang**
Jiangsu Key Laboratory of Oral Disease, Nanjing Medical University, 136 Hanzhong Road, Jiangsu 210029, People's Republic of China

**Jin Li, Yaping Wu and Jie Cheng**
Jiangsu Key Laboratory of Oral Disease, Nanjing Medical University, 136 Hanzhong Road, Jiangsu 210029, People's Republic of China
Department of Oral and Maxillofacial Surgery, Affiliated Stomatological Hospital, Nanjing Medical University, 136 Hanzhong Road, Nanjing 210029, People's Republic of China

**Dongmiao Wang, Hua Yuan and Hongbing Jiang**
Department of Oral and Maxillofacial Surgery, Affiliated Stomatological Hospital, Nanjing Medical University, 136 Hanzhong Road, Nanjing 210029, People's Republic of China

**Yujie Feng, Xiao Hu, Lianfang Lu, Wei Zhao, Kai Ma, Chuandong Sun, Chengzhan Zhu and Bingyuan Zhang**
Department of Hepatobiliary and Pancreatic Surgery, The Affiliated Hospital of Qingdao University, No. 16 Jiangsu Road, Qingdao 266003, Shandong, China

**Guangwei Liu**
Department of Outpatient, The Affiliated Hospital of Qingdao University, No. 16 Jiangsu Road, Qingdao 266003, Shandong, China

**Fangzhen Shen**
Department of Oncology, The Affiliated Hospital of Qingdao University, No. 16 Jiangsu Road, Qingdao 266003, Shandong, China

**Xiaojun Zhou, Zhili Shan and Hengying Yang**
Department of General Surgery, The First Affiliated Hospital of Soochow University, Suzhou 215006, China

**Jingjing Xu**
Center for Clinical Laboratory, The First Affiliated Hospital of Soochow University, Suzhou 215006, China

**Wenjing Li**
Department of Clinical Laboratory, Nanjing Medical University Affiliated Suzhou Hospital, Suzhou 215006, China

**Feng Guo**
Department of Oncology, Nanjing Medical University Affiliated Suzhou Hospital, Baita West Road 16, Suzhou 215001, China

**Jie Wang and Zhijun Xi**
Department of Urology, Peking University First Hospital and Institute of Urology, National Research Center for Genitourinary Oncology, No 8, Xishiku Street, Xicheng District, Beijing, China

**Jianzhong Xi and Juan Li**
Department of Biomedical Engineering, College of Engineering, Peking University, No 5, Yiheyuan Road, Haidian District, Beijing, China

**Hanshuo Zhang**
Beijing Genex Health Technology Co Ltd., Beijing, China

**Yuchao Xia and Yuanxue Yi**
Chongqing Institute of Innovation and Entrepreneurship for Precision Medicine, Chongqing, China

**Yong An, Xue-min Chen, Yong Yang, Feng Mo, Yong Jiang, Dong-lin Sun and Hui-hua Cai**
Department of Hepatobiliary Surgery, The First People's Hospital of Changzhou, The Third Affiliated Hospital of Soochow University, 185 Juqian Street, Changzhou 213000, Jiangsu, China

**Zhikui Gao, Han Gao, Lihong Yin and Ran Liu**
Key Laboratory of Environmental Medicine Engineering, Ministry of Education, School of Public Health, Southeast University, Nanjing 210009, China

**Peng Zhang**
Huzhou Center for Disease Control and Prevention, Huzhou 313000, China.

**Ming Xie**
North China Petroleum Bureau General Hospital, Renqiu 062552, China

**Jun Wan, Jie Cui, Kunpeng Wu, Xiaoping Hong, Yulin Zou and Shuang Zhao**
Department of Pharmacy, Third Clinical Medical College, Three Gorges University, Gezhouba Group Central Hospital, Yichang 443002, Hubei, China

**Lei Wang**
Department of Pathogenic Biology, School of Medicine, China Three Gorges University, Yichang 443002, Hubei, China

**Hong Ke**
Department of Oncology, Third Clinical Medical College, Three Gorges University, Gezhouba Group Central Hospital, No. 60 Qiaohu Lake Road, Xiling District, Yichang 443002, Hubei, China

**Xiaoli Hu, Hailing Liu, Miaomiao Ye and Xueqiong Zhu**
Department of Obstetrics and Gynecology, The Second Affiliated Hospital of Wenzhou Medical University, Wenzhou 325000, Zhejiang, China

**Xiaoyan Ding, Wei Sun and Jinglong Chen**
Cancer Center, Beijing Ditan Hospital, Capital Medical University, No 8, Jingshundong Street Chaoyang District, Beijing 100015, China

**Sheng Liu, Sheng Chen, Kaige Ma and Zengwu Shao**
Department of Orthopaedics, Union Hospital, Tongji Medical College, Huazhong University of Science and Technology, Wuhan 430022, China

**Yanming Ren, Chuanyuan Tao and Yan Ju**
Department of Neurosurgery, West China Hospital of Sichuan University, No.37 Guo Xue Xiang, Chengdu, Sichuan, China

**Xiliang Wang**
Beijing Institute of Genomics, Chinese Academy of Sciences, Beijing, China

**Chunbao Zang**
Department of Radiation Oncology, Anhui Provincial Cancer Hospital,West Branch of the First Affiliated Hospital of USTC, Division of Life Sciences and Medicine, University of Science and Technology of China, Hefei 230001, Anhui, People's Republic of China

**Fangfang Zhao and Youguang Pu**
Department of Cancer Epigenetics Program, Anhui Provincial Cancer Hospital, West Branch of the First Affiliated Hospital of USTC, Division of Life Sciences and Medicine, University of Science and Technology of China, Hefei 230001, Anhui, People's Republic of China

**Lei Hua**
Department of Provincial Clinical College, Anhui Provincial Hospital of Anhui Medical University, Hefei 230031, Anhui, China

# Index

www.ingramcontent.com/pod-product-compliance
Lightning Source LLC
Chambersburg PA
CBHW061258190326
41458CB00011B/3706